Nutrition Essentials for Nursing Practice

Eighth Edition

SUSAN G. DUDEK, RD, CDN, BS

Nutrition Instructor, Dietetic Technology Program
Erie Community College
Williamsville, New York

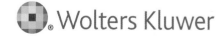

. Wolters Kluwer

Philadelphia · Baltimore · New York · London
Buenos Aires · Hong Kong · Sydney · Tokyo

Acquisitions Editor: Natasha McIntyre
Development Editor: Greg Nicholl
Editorial Coordinator: Lauren Pecarich
Marketing Manager: Katie Schlesinger
Production Project Manager: Marian Bellus
Design Coordinator: Holly McLaughlin
Art Director: Jennifer Clements
Manufacturing Coordinator: Karin Duffield
Prepress Vendor: Absolute Service, Inc.

Eighth Edition

Library of Congress Cataloging-in-Publication Data

Names: Dudek, Susan G., author.
Title: Nutrition essentials for nursing practice / Susan G. Dudek.
Description: Eighth edition. | Philadelphia : Wolters Kluwer, [2018] |
  Includes bibliographical references and index.
Identifiers: LCCN 2017004249 | ISBN 9781496356109
Subjects: | MESH: Diet Therapy | Nutritional Physiological Phenomena |
  Nurses' Instruction
Classification: LCC RM216 | NLM WB 400 | DDC 615.8/54—dc23 LC record
available at https://lccn.loc.gov/2017004249

Dedicated to

My family, for their love, support, and patience: Joe, Kaitlyn, Kara, TJ, and Jared

Charlie, who brings me joy

The memory of my parents, Charles and Annie Maedl, and my son Chris—their impact is infinite

The memory of Jeanne C. Scherer, who planted, nurtured, and championed the idea that I could write a book

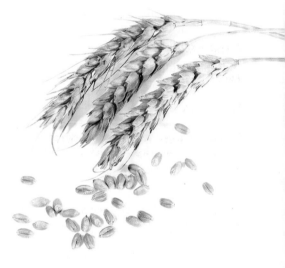

Reviewers

Krista L. Angell, MEd, BSN, RN
Nursing Instructor
Willoughby-Eastlake School of Practical Nursing
Eastlake, Ohio

Rita C. Bergevin, MA, RN-BC, CWCN
Adjunct Lecturer
North Carolina Central University School of Nursing
Durham, North Carolina

Sophia Beydoun, RN, MSN
Madonna University
Livonia, Michigan

Staci Boruff, PhD
Professor of Nursing
Walters State Community College
Morristown, Tennessee

Margaret Bultas, PhD, RN, CNE, CNL, CPNP
Assistant Professor
Saint Louis University
St. Louis, Missouri

Susan Capasso, BA, MS, EdD, CGC
Professor
Vice President of Academic Affairs
Dean of Faculty
St. Vincent's College
Bridgeport, Connecticut

Suzy Cook, MN, RN, CHSE, CNE
Professor
Olympic College
Bremerton, Washington

Vicky King, MS
Faculty
Cochise College
Douglas, Arizona

Loretta Moreno, RN, MSN
Nursing Program Director
Schreiner University
Kerrville, Texas

Lillian A. Rafeldt, RN, MA, CNE
Professor of Nursing
Three Rivers Community College
Norwich, Connecticut

Anita K. Reed, MSN, RN
Assistant Professor
St. Elizabeth School of Nursing
Lafayette, Indiana

Helen Rogers-Koon, MSN, RN
Instructor, Practical Nursing Program
Central Pennsylvania Institute of Science and Technology
Pleasant Gap, Pennsylvania

Elizabeth Rudshteyn, MSN, RN
RN Program Chair
Jersey College
Teterboro, New Jersey

Colleen Tracy Snell, MS, RN
Nursing Instructor
Anoka-Ramsey Community College
Coon Rapids, Minnesota

Julie Stefanski, MEd, RDN, CSSD, LDN, CDE
Owner
Stefanski Nutrition Services
York, Pennsylvania

Boniface Stegman, PhD, MSN, RN
Assistant Professor
Coordinator RN–BSN Completion Program
Maryville University
St. Louis, Missouri

Deborah Leann Vallery, MSN, RN
Assistant Professor
West Kentucky Community and Technical College
Paducah, Kentucky

Victoria Warren-Mears, PhD, RD, FAND
Adjunct Instructor
School of Nursing
University of Portland
Portland, Oregon

Debbie Yarnell, RN, BSN
Program Coordinator/Nursing Instructor
State Fair Community College
Eldon, Missouri

Like air and sleep, nutrition is a basic human need essential for survival. From curing hunger to reducing the risk of chronic disease, nutrition is ever changing in response to technological advances and cultural shifts. Because nutrition at its most basic level is food—for the mind, body, and soul—it is a complex blend of science and art.

Although considered the realm of the dietitian, nutrition is a vital and integral component of nursing care across the life cycle and along the wellness–illness continuum. By virtue of their close contact with patients and families, nurses are often on the front line in facilitating nutrition. Nutrition is woven into all steps of the nursing care process, from assessment and nursing diagnoses to implementation and evaluation. This textbook seeks to give student nurses an essential nutrition foundation to better serve themselves and their patients.

NEW TO THIS EDITION

This eighth edition of *Nutrition Essentials for Nursing Practice* is "new and improved." Content is updated throughout and reflects available evidence-based practice.

- New unfolding cases appear at the beginning of each chapter and are threaded throughout the chapter to give students the opportunity to apply critical thinking skills to nutrition issues.

- New to this edition are Concept Mastery Alerts, which clarify fundamental nursing concepts to improve the reader's understanding of potentially confusing topics, as identified by Misconception Alerts in Lippincott's Adaptive Learning Powered by prepU. Data from thousands of actual students using this program in courses across the United States identified common misconceptions for the authors to clarify in this new feature.

- Chapter 1 shifts from "Nutrition in Nursing" to "Nutrition in Health and Health Care." This chapter explains the role of nutrition in chronic disease prevention, the interdisciplinary nature of nutrition care, and how technology is affecting the future of nutrition.

- The term "diet" has been largely replaced with "eating pattern" to connote lifestyle versus a therapeutic approach.

- Focus moves away from single nutrients toward eating patterns, with the Dietary Approaches to Stop Hypertension (DASH) and Mediterranean-style eating patterns repeatedly cited as examples of healthy patterns.

- The *2015-2020 Dietary Guidelines for Americans* and its companion MyPlate have been updated.

- The topic of antibiotics in the food supply is now included.

- The newly revised "Nutrition Facts" label is featured, which will be implemented for most packaged foods by July 26, 2018.

- Coverage of the significance and treatment of obesity throughout the life cycle has been expanded.

- Proposed changes in how malnutrition is defined are included.

- New guidelines included for the provision of enteral and parenteral nutrition support.

- Increased focus in the "Nutrition for Obesity and Eating Disorders" chapter on obesity prevention and treatment, including lifestyle modification, medication, and bariatric surgery.

- Focus placed on carbohydrate counting versus the Food Lists for diabetes.

ORGANIZATION OF THE TEXT

The 22 chapters are organized into three units. Unit One is devoted to **Principles of Nutrition**. It begins with Chapter 1, "Nutrition in Health and Health Care," which focuses on the increasingly recognized role eating patterns have on health and illness and how nutrition affects the practice of all health-care professionals. Chapters devoted to carbohydrates, protein, lipids, vitamins, and water and minerals provide a foundational understanding of nutrients, their sources, and their physiological functions. The second part of each of these chapters focuses on the role of nutrients in health promotion with emphasis on why and how Americans are urged to shift their eating patterns to reduce the risk of chronic disease. The final chapter in this unit, "Energy Balance," explains how calorie needs are estimated, how body weight is evaluated, and strategies for balancing calorie intake with expenditure.

Unit Two, **Nutrition in Health Promotion**, begins with Chapter 8, "Guidelines for Healthy Eating." This chapter features the Dietary Reference Intakes, the Dietary Guidelines for Americans, and MyPlate. Other chapters in this unit examine consumer issues and cultural and religious influences on food and nutrition. The nutritional needs and issues associated with the life cycle are presented in chapters devoted to pregnant and lactating women, children and adolescents, and older adults.

In Unit Three, the order of the first two chapters has been reversed for better flow. **Nutrition in Clinical Practice** now begins with "Hospital Nutrition: Defining Risk and Feeding Patients." This chapter forms the basis on which the remaining chapters are built. Nutrition therapy is presented for obesity and eating disorders, metabolic and respiratory stress, gastrointestinal disorders, diabetes, cardiovascular disorders, renal disorders, cancer, and HIV/AIDS. Pathophysiology is tightly focused as it pertains to nutrition.

FEATURES

This edition of *Nutrition Essentials for Nursing Practice* incorporates popular features to facilitate learning and engage students.

- **New Unfolding Case Studies** present relevant nutrition information—in real-life scenarios—to provide an opportunity for students to apply theory to practice. Questions regarding the scenarios provide critical thinking opportunities for the student.

- **Check Your Knowledge** presents true/false questions at the beginning of each chapter to assess the students' baseline knowledge. Questions relate to chapter Learning Objectives.

- **Key Terms** are defined in the margin for convenient reference.

- **Quick Bites**—fewer and more condensed to improve layout and readability in the new edition—provide quick nutrition facts, valuable information, and current research.

- **Concept Mastery Alerts** that clarify common misconceptions as identified by Lippincott's Adaptive Learning Powered by prepU.

- **Nursing Process** tables clearly present sample application of nutrition concepts in context of the nursing process.

- **How Do You Respond?** helps students identify potential questions they may encounter in the clinical setting and prepares them to think on their feet.

- The Case Study at the end of each chapter has been renamed **Review Case Study** to distinguish it from the newly added Unfolding Case Studies. The Review Case Studies, along with the **Study Questions**, challenge students to apply what they have learned.

- **Key Concepts** summarize important information from each chapter.

TEACHING AND LEARNING RESOURCES

To facilitate mastery of this textbook's content, a comprehensive teaching and learning package has been developed to assist faculty and students.

Lippincott CoursePoint

Lippincott CoursePoint is a comprehensive, digital, integrated course solution for nursing education. Lippincott CoursePoint is designed for the way students learn, providing content in context, exactly where and when students need it. Lippincott CoursePoint is an integrated learning solution featuring:

- Leading content in context: Content provided in the context of the student learning path engages students and encourages interaction and learning on a deeper level.
  - The interactive ebook features content updates based on the latest evidence-based practices and provides students with anytime, anywhere access on multiple devices.
  - Multimedia resources, including videos, animations, and interactive tutorials, walk students through knowledge application and address multiple learning styles.
  - Full online access to *Stedman's Medical Dictionary for Health Professions and Nursing* ensures students work with the best medical dictionary available.
- Powerful tools to maximize class performance: Course-specific tools, such as adaptive learning powered by *prepU*, provide a personalized learning experience for every student.
- Real-time data to measure students' progress: Student performance data provided in an intuitive display lets instructors quickly spot which students are having difficulty or which concepts the class as a whole is struggling to grasp

Resources for Instructors

Tools to assist you with teaching your course are available upon adoption of this textbook at http://thePoint.lww.com/Dudek8e.

- A **Test Generator** lets you put together exclusive new tests from a bank containing hundreds of questions to help you in assessing your students' understanding of the material. Test questions link to chapter learning objectives.

- **PowerPoint Presentations** provide an easy way for you to integrate the textbook with your students' classroom experience, either via slide shows or handouts. Multiple-choice and true/false questions are integrated into the presentations to promote class participation and allow you to use i-clicker technology.

- An **Image Bank** lets you use the photographs and illustrations from this textbook in your PowerPoint slides or as you see fit in your course.

- **Answers to Case Studies**

- **QSEN Map**

Resources for Students

An exciting set of free resources is available to help students review material and become even more familiar with vital concepts. Students can access all these resources at http://thePoint.lww.com/Dudek8e using the codes printed in the front of their textbooks.

- **Journal Articles** provided for each chapter offer access to current research available in Wolters Kluwer journals.

- **Concepts in Action Animations** bring physiologic and pathophysiologic concepts to life.

- **Interactive Case Studies** provide realistic case examples and offer students the opportunity to apply nutrition essentials to nursing care.

- **Drug Monographs**

I hope this textbook and teaching/learning resource package provide the impetus to embrace nutrition on both a personal and professional level.

Susan G. Dudek, RD, CDN, BS

Acknowledgments

When I wrote the first edition of this book, I never imagined that the privilege would extend through eight editions. I am both humbled and thankful for the opportunity. It amazes me how much our understanding of nutrition evolves from one edition to the next. This project has been professionally rewarding, personally challenging, and rich with opportunities to grow. In large part, the success of this book rests with the dedicated and creative professionals at Wolters Kluwer. Because of their support and talents, I am able to do what I love—write, create, teach, and learn. I especially thank

- **Natasha McIntyre,** Acquisitions Editor, for her vision that helped launch the eighth edition.

- **Greg Nicholl,** Senior Development Editor, who is the best of the best. His energy, dedication, and thoughtful suggestions are responsible for keeping the project on course and on time. I am sincerely grateful for all his effort and support.

- **Holly McLaughlin,** Design Coordinator, and Jennifer Clements, Art Director, the talented behind-the-scene professionals.

- **The reviewers of the seventh edition,** whose insightful comments and suggestions helped shape a new and improved edition.

Contents

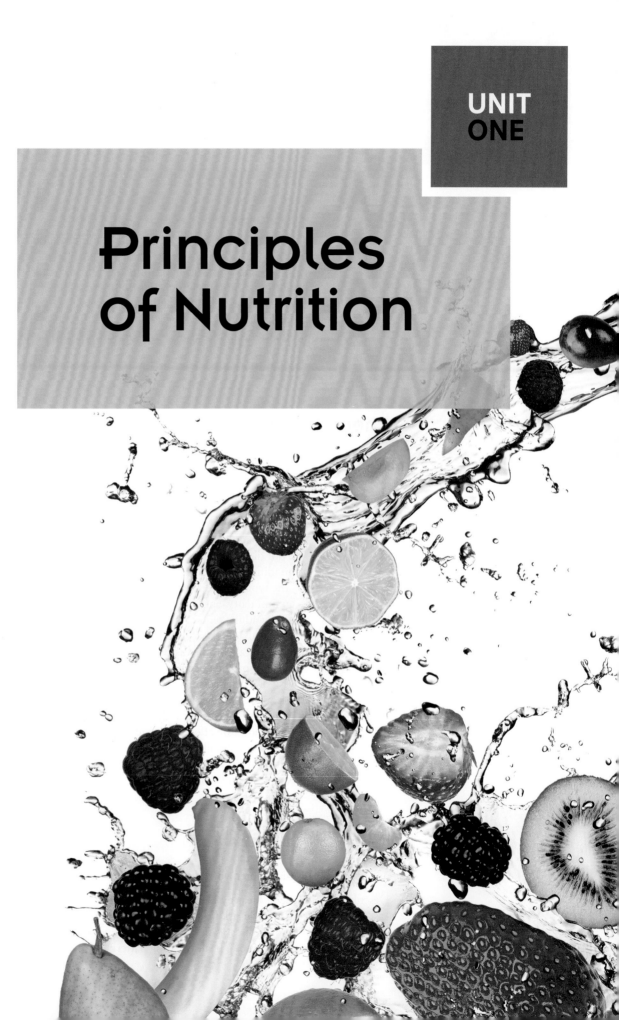

Principles of Nutrition

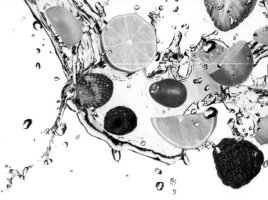

Chapter 1

Nutrition in Health and Health Care

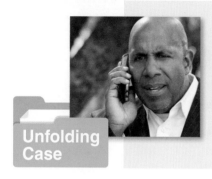

Tyrone Green

Tyrone is a 46-year-old national account executive who spends 4 out of 5 weekdays traveling on business. He was recently diagnosed with prediabetes and hypertension, two of the five diagnostic components of metabolic syndrome that increases the risk of diabetes and cardiovascular disease. He blames his 25-pound weight gain on eating out while traveling. He is taking omega-3 fatty acid supplements because he read they can lower blood pressure.

Check Your Knowledge

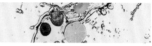

True	False		
☐	☐	1	Chronic diseases, such as cardiovascular disease and type 2 diabetes, are responsible for approximately 25% of deaths worldwide.
☐	☐	2	Chronic health conditions such as hypertension and type 2 diabetes occur only in adults.
☐	☐	3	Poor diet quality, physical inactivity, smoking, and excess body weight are modifiable risk factors that increase the risk of chronic disease.
☐	☐	4	The typical American eating pattern is low in fruits, vegetables, whole grains, dairy, and oils.
☐	☐	5	Older adults tend to have worse eating patterns than young and middle-aged adults.
☐	☐	6	For several chronic diseases, healthier eating and increased physical activity may provide benefits equal to medication, with lower cost and reduced risk of side effects.
☐	☐	7	Genomics will help researchers determine how specific nutrients interact with genes and other body substances to predict the health of an individual.
☐	☐	8	Nutrition care affects the practice of all health-care professionals.
☐	☐	9	Nurses are usually responsible for completing nutrition screening.
☐	☐	10	Most nutrition screenings address body mass index (BMI), appetite, weight change, and severity of disease.

Learning Objectives

Upon completion of this chapter, you will be able to

1 Describe the purpose of Healthy People 2020.
2 List four modifiable lifestyle risk factors for chronic disease.
3 Give examples of chronic diseases that are linked to a poor quality diet.
4 Describe the characteristics of a healthy eating pattern.

5   Give examples of questions that are driving nutrition research.
6   Compare nutrition screening to nutrition assessment.
7   Describe nutrition care responsibilities of the nurse.

When nutrition was a young science, the focus of healthy eating was to consume enough of all essential nutrients to avoid deficiency diseases. Today, nutrient deficiency diseases are generally rare in the United States except among specific population subgroups such as the elderly, alcoholics, fad dieters, and hospitalized patients. In fact, several of the leading causes of death in the United States are associated with dietary excesses—namely, heart disease, cancer, stroke, and diabetes. Many other health problems, such as obesity, hypertension, and hypercholesterolemia, are related, at least in part, to dietary excesses. But nutritional excesses are only part of the story: Americans are not eating enough of the specific foods or food groups that may help protect against chronic disease.

This chapter discusses the relationship between nutrition and human health, the future of nutrition research, and nutrition in health care.

NUTRITION AND HEALTH

Throughout time, all civilizations have linked nutrition with health (Meyer-Abich, 2005). Across the lifespan, good nutrition supports all aspects of health, including healthy pregnancy outcomes; normal growth, development, and aging; healthy body weight; lower risk of disease; and helping to treat acute and chronic disease (DiMaria-Ghalili et al., 2014). Nutrition is intimately entwined with health.

The World Health Organization (WHO, 1948) defines *health* as "a state of complete physical, mental, and social well-being, not merely the absence of disease or infirmity." In practice, health is subjectively and individually defined along a continuum which is influenced by an individual's perception of health. For instance, a recent survey found that although 57% of respondents ranked their health as very good or excellent, 55% of those are overweight or obese (International Food Information Council Foundation, 2015). Likewise, older adults may consider themselves healthy despite having arthritis because they consider it a normal part of aging, not a chronic disease.

Healthy People 2020

Under the jurisdiction of the U.S. Department of Health and Human Services (USDHHS), Healthy People is a program that focuses on improving the health of all Americans and eliminating health disparities. Updated every 10 years after its inception 30 years ago, Healthy People sets public health goals and objectives and monitors the nation's progress toward meeting those objectives.

The newest edition, Healthy People 2020, has approximately 1200 objectives organized into 42 focus areas ranging from cancer and diabetes to substance abuse and immunizations. At the time of its launch in December 2010, 911 objectives were measurable with baseline data and established targets (USDHHS, 2010). The overall objectives under nutrition and weight status are listed in Box 1.1.

Chronic Disease

Preventable chronic disease is a major challenge to global health, responsible for 68% of all worldwide deaths in 2012 (WHO, 2014). In the United States, chronic diseases are responsible for 7 of the top 10 causes of death (Box 1.2) and are the main causes of poor health and disability (Bauer et al., 2014). In 2012, about half of all American adults had one or more chronic health conditions and 1 in 4 adults had two or more chronic health conditions (Table 1.1) (Ward, Schiller, & Goodman, 2014). Children and adolescents also have chronic diseases, such as hypertension and type 2 diabetes. At all ages, chronic disease risk is linked to overweight and obesity (Dietary Guidelines Advisory Committee, 2015).

BOX 1.1 Healthy People 2020: Summary of Nutrition and Weight Status Objectives

Goal: Promote health and reduce chronic disease risk through consumption of healthful diets and achievement and maintenance of healthy body weights.

Healthier Food Access

1. Increase the number of states with nutrition standards for foods and beverages provided to preschool-aged children in child care.
2. Increase the proportion of schools that offer nutritious foods and beverages outside of school meals.
3. Increase the number of states that have state-level policies that incentivize food retail outlets to provide foods that are encouraged by the *Dietary Guidelines for Americans*.
4. (Developmental) Increase the proportion of Americans who have access to a food retail outlet that sells a variety of foods that are encouraged by the *Dietary Guidelines for Americans*.

Health Care and Worksite Settings

1. Increase the proportion of primary care physicians who regularly measure the body mass index of their patients.
2. Increase the proportion of physician office visits that include counseling or education related to nutrition or weight.
3. (Developmental) Increase the proportion of worksites that offer nutrition or weight management classes or counseling.

Weight Status

1. Increase the proportion of adults who are at a healthy weight.
2. Reduce the proportion of adults who are obese.

3. Reduce the proportion of children and adolescents who are considered obese.
4. (Developmental) Prevent inappropriate weight gain in youth and adults.

Food Insecurity

1. Eliminate very low food security among children.
2. Reduce household food insecurity and in doing so reduce hunger.

Food and Nutrient Consumption

1. Increase the contribution of fruits to the diets of the population aged 2 years and older.
2. Increase the variety and contribution of vegetables to the diets of the population aged 2 years and older.
3. Increase the contribution of whole grains to the diets of the population aged 2 years and older.
4. Reduce consumption of calories from solid fats and added sugars in the population aged 2 years and older.
5. Reduce consumption of saturated fat in the population aged 2 years and older.
6. Reduce consumption of sodium in the population aged 2 years and older.
7. Increase consumption of calcium in the population aged 2 years and older.

Iron Deficiency

1. Reduce iron deficiency among young children and females of childbearing age.
2. Reduce iron deficiency among pregnant females.

The mix of food consumed throughout the life cycle can determine whether a chronic disease develops or regresses (Hiza, Casavale, Guenther, & Davis, 2013). Effective and timely nutrition and lifestyle intervention can prevent or minimize morbidity and mortality related to many major chronic diseases such as obesity, cardiovascular disease, diabetes, and certain cancers (Slawson, Fitzgerald, & Morgan, 2013). Other modifiable lifestyle factors that contribute to chronic disease risk are smoking, physical inactivity, obesity, and excessive alcohol intake (Box 1.3).

BOX 1.2 Ten Leading Causes of Death in the United States (Data for 2013)

1. Heart disease
2. Cancer
3. Chronic lower respiratory diseases
4. Accidents (unintentional injuries)
5. Stroke
6. Alzheimer's disease
7. Diabetes
8. Influenza and pneumonia
9. Nephritis, nephrotic syndrome, and nephrosis
10. Suicide

Source: Centers for Disease Control and Prevention. (2016). *Leading causes of death.* Available at http://www.cdc.gov /nchs/fastats/leading-causes-of-death.htm. Accessed on 3/2/16.

Table 1.1	Facts about Nutrition- and Physical Activity–Related Health Conditions in the United States

Health Condition	Facts
Overweight and Obesity	● For more than 25 years, more than half of the adult population has been overweight or obese. ● Obesity is most prevalent in those ages 40 years and older and in African American adults, and is least prevalent in adults with highest incomes. ● Since the early 2000s, abdominal obesity[a] has been present in about half of U.S. adults of all ages. Prevalence is higher with increasing age and varies by sex and race/ethnicity. ● In 2009–2012, 65% of adult females and 73% of adult males were overweight or obese. ● In 2009–2012, nearly one in three youth ages 2 to 19 years were overweight or obese.
Cardiovascular Disease (CVD) and Risk Factors: ● Coronary heart disease ● Stroke ● Hypertension ● High total blood cholesterol	● In 2010, CVD affected about 84 million men and women ages 20 years and older (35% of the population). ● In 2007–2010, about 50% of adults who were normal weight, and nearly three-fourths of those who were overweight or obese, had at least one cardiometabolic risk factor (i.e., high blood pressure, abnormal blood lipids, smoking, or diabetes). ● Rates of hypertension, abnormal blood lipid profiles, and diabetes are higher in adults with abdominal obesity. ● In 2009–2012, almost 56% of adults ages 18 years and older had either prehypertension (27%) or hypertension (29%).[b] ● In 2009–2012, rates of hypertension among adults were highest in African Americans (41%) and in adults ages 65 years and older (69%). ● In 2009–2012, 10% of children ages 8 to 17 years had either borderline hypertension (8%) or hypertension (2%).[c] ● In 2009–2012, 100 million adults ages 20 years or older (53%) had total cholesterol levels ≥200 mg/dL; almost 31 million had levels ≥240 mg/dL. ● In 2011–2012, 8% of children ages 8 to 17 years had total cholesterol levels ≥200 mg/dL.
Diabetes	● In 2012, the prevalence of diabetes (type 1 plus type 2) was 14% for men and 11% for women ages 20 years and older (more than 90% of total diabetes in adults is type 2). ● Among children with type 2 diabetes, about 80% were obese.
Cancer[d] ● Breast cancer ● Colorectal cancer	● Breast cancer is the third leading cause of cancer death in the United States. ● In 2012, an estimated 3 million women had a history of breast cancer. ● Colorectal cancer is the second leading cause of cancer death in the United States. ● In 2012, an estimated 1.2 million adult men and women had a history of colorectal cancer.
Bone Health	● A higher percent of women are affected by osteoporosis (15%) and low bone mass (51%) than men (about 4% and 35%, respectively). ● In 2005–2010, approximately 10 million (10%) adults ages 50 years and older had osteoporosis and 43 million (44%) had low bone mass.

[a]Abdominal obesity, as measured by waist circumference, is defined as a waist circumference of >102 centimeters in men and >88 centimeters in women.
[b]For adults, prehypertension was defined as a systolic blood pressure of 120–139 mm mercury (Hg) or diastolic blood pressure of 80–89 mm Hg among those who were not currently being treated for hypertension. Hypertension was defined as systolic blood pressure (SBP) >140 mm Hg, diastolic blood pressure (DBP) >90 mm Hg, or taking antihypertensive medication.
[c]For children, borderline hypertension was defined as systolic or diastolic blood pressure at the 90th percentile or higher but lower than the 95th percentile or as blood pressure levels of 120/80 mm Hg or higher (but less than the 95th percentile). Hypertension was defined as a systolic or diastolic blood pressure at the 95th percentile or higher.
[d]The types of cancer included here are not a complete list of all diet- and physical activity-related cancers.
Source: U.S. Department of Health and Human Services & U.S. Department of Agriculture. (2015). *2015-2020 Dietary Guidelines for Americans* (8th ed.). Available at http://www.http://health.gov/dietaryguidelines/2015/guidelines/introduction/nutrition-and-health-are-closely-related/#table-i-. Accessed on 3/14/16.

Food: More than Just Nutrients

Food is a complex mix of essential and nonessential components in various ratios and combinations. Essential nutrients, such as most vitamins, minerals, amino acids, fatty acids, and water, must be obtained through food because the body cannot make them. Plants provide fiber and a variety of nonnutrient compounds that have health-enhancing biological activity in the body. These beneficial nonnutrient compounds are known as *phytonutrients*.

Nutrients have long been studied as singular substances and intake recommendations have focused on nutrients more so than food, such as to limit total fat without consideration of the source of fat. Such a narrow focus underestimates the complexity of food and the interactions between its components and ignores the possibility that many constituents of food and eating patterns may act synergistically to impact health (Jacobs & Orlich, 2014). For instance, because populations who consume high amounts of fruits and vegetables were observed to have lower

BOX 1.3   Modifiable Risk Factors for Chronic Disease

Smoking

- Almost 20% of adults smoke cigarettes.
- Is the leading cause of preventable death, contributing to 480,000 deaths annually
- Damages nearly every body organ and causes respiratory disease, heart disease, stroke, cancer, preterm birth, low birth weight, and premature death
- Shortens lifespan by an average of 10 years

Obesity

- Approximately one-third of U.S. adults are obese; it is a leading risk factor for several preventable conditions such as heart disease, type 2 diabetes, stroke, cancer, hypertension, liver disease, kidney disease, and osteoarthritis.
- Obesity contributes to an estimated 200,000 deaths annually.

Excessive Alcohol

- Can lead to fetal damage, liver diseases, hypertension, cardiovascular diseases, and other major health problems
- Contributes to lost workplace productivity, motor vehicle accidents, and property damage

Physical Inactivity

- Responsible for 10% of deaths annually; increases the risk of coronary heart disease, type 2 diabetes, hypertension, obesity, certain cancers, and premature death
- Only 21% of adults meet the U.S. Department of Health and Human Services' recommendation of at least 150 minutes of physical activity weekly.

Source: United Health Foundation. (2015). *The America's Health Rankings Annual Report.* Available at http://www.americashealthrankings.org. Accessed on 3/3/16.

rates of epithelial cancers, researchers speculated that beta-carotene intake was protective. However, a study of large doses of supplemental beta-carotene resulted in an increase in cancer, necessitating a premature halt to the study (Bjelakovic, Nikolova, Gluud, Simonetti, & Gluud, 2007). This is a glaring example of how although certain food patterns may be associated with lower risk of disease, it is not known which components of a food, in what proportion, acting singularly or synergistically with other substances, are protective or detrimental to health. Thus, the health effects of foods may not be simply and accurately reduced to the effects of single nutrients (Jacobs & Orlich, 2014).

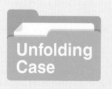

Unfolding Case

Consider Tyrone. Although eating seafood is associated with lowering blood pressure, it is not certain that supplemental omega-3 fatty acids provide the same benefit. Is he willing to try seafood twice a week in place of supplements? What are the potential health benefits Tyrone may reap by adopting a healthy eating pattern and increasing his physical activity?

Healthy Eating

There is a shift away from focusing on nutrients to examining the bigger picture of eating patterns (Mozaffarian & Ludwig, 2010). The Dietary Guidelines Advisory Committee (2015) defines *dietary patterns* as "the quantities, proportions, variety or combinations of different foods and beverages in diets, and the frequency with which they are habitually consumed." Nutritional epidemiology consistently shows that healthy eating patterns reduce the risk of chronic disease (Jacobs & Orlich, 2014). For instance, a prospective cohort study of participants in the Women's Health Initiative Observational Study found that women having better diet quality had 18% to 26% lower all-cause and cardiovascular disease mortality risk and that better diet quality scores were associated with a 20% to 23% lower risk of cancer mortality (George et al., 2014). Likewise, in the Iowa Women's Health Study, the diet quality score was found to be inversely related to mortality: A high quality score was related to lower total mortality rates during the 22 years of follow-up (Mursu, Steffen, Meyer, Duprez, & Jacobs, 2013). Furthermore, healthier eating and increased physical activity have increasingly shown benefits that equal if not surpass those of pharmacologic intervention for several chronic diseases, often with less risk, fewer side effects, and lower costs (Estruch et al., 2013; Sacks et al., 2001; Wing et al., 2013).

Measures of Diet Quality

Healthy Eating Index-2010 (HEI-2010)
a density-based (e.g., amounts per 1000 calories) measure of diet quality based on conformance to the *2010 Dietary Guidelines for Americans*. It is composed of food and nutrient characteristics that have established relationships with health outcomes. The Healthy Eating Index-2015 is currently being updated to align with the *2015-2020 Dietary Guidelines for Americans*. Previous versions were based on previous editions of the *Dietary Guidelines for Americans*.

Mediterranean-Style Diet
not uniformly defined but generally characterized as a pattern high in olive oil, fruits, nuts, vegetables, and cereals; moderate in fish and poultry; low in dairy products, red meat, processed meats, and sweets; and includes wine consumed in moderation with meals.

Dietary Approaches to Stop Hypertension (DASH) Diet
an eating pattern high in fruit, vegetables, low-fat dairy products, whole grains, poultry, fish, and nuts and low in fat, red meat, sweets, and sugar-sweetened beverages.

Although "poor diet quality" is considered to be a major risk factor for several chronic diseases, there is not a universal definition or measure of diet quality. Numerous indices have been developed to assess diet quality according to how closely eating patterns conform to (1) dietary recommendations, such as the *Dietary Guidelines for Americans* (e.g., **Healthy Eating Index-2010 [HEI-2010]**), or (2) healthy eating patterns, such as the **Mediterranean-style diet** and the **Dietary Approaches to Stop Hypertension (DASH) diet**. Many indices have several versions and are distinguished by the words "adapted," "revised," "alternative," or by other descriptions added to the name.

Diet quality indices assign a numeric score based on how closely a person's intake correlates to specified criteria. For components with positive health benefits, such as fruits, vegetables, and whole grains, high intakes receive a high score. Conversely, high intakes of components that should be limited, such as saturated fat, trans fats, and added sugar, are given low scores. All indices emphasize intakes of fruit, vegetables, whole grains, and plants or plant-based proteins. Most of the indices emphasize unsaturated fats over saturated fats, include consideration of sodium, and stress nut consumption. Some include moderate alcohol consumption and a seafood component and give a higher score for low red meat and processed meat intakes. In general, high diet quality scores are a reflection of phytonutrient-rich plant foods; fish and poultry favored over red meat; inclusion of low-fat dairy, coffee, tea, and moderate alcohol consumption; and less-processed foods (Jacobs & Orlich, 2014).

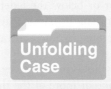

Think of Tyrone. His typical intake while traveling is two sandwiches containing eggs, cheese, and bacon for breakfast; a foot-long assorted deli meat submarine on a white roll with a soft drink and bag of chips for lunch; and a dinner of steak, French fries, and salad. In between meals, he snacks on candy, soft drinks, and granola bars. How would you evaluate Tyrone's diet quality? Which food groups does he need to eat more of? Less of? What potential health benefits may be experience by increasing his physical activity?

Diet Quality in the United States

The typical American eating pattern is low in fruits, vegetables, whole grains, dairy, seafood, and oils; is excessive in calories, saturated fat, added sugars, and sodium; and lacks variety in protein choices (USDHHS & U.S. Department of Agriculture [USDA], 2015). When assessed with the HEI-2010, Americans fall short of nearly every component of diet quality measured (Wilson et al., 2016).

In general, women have been found to have a higher diet quality than men, and older adults have higher diet quality than younger and middle-aged adults as assessed by Healthy Eating Index-2005 (HEI-2005) (Hiza et al., 2013). As adults get older, they generally increase their scores for several variables, including fruit, vegetables, whole grains, calories from solid fats, and added sugars. Adults 75 years and older scored even better than 65- to 74-year-olds for several variables. Possible reasons for the improvement in diet quality with aging include participation in home-delivered and congregate meals, greater health consciousness, and using nutrition therapy to manage or prevent chronic disease. It is also possible that older adults have better eating patterns over their lifetime, contributing to their longevity (Hiza et al., 2013).

Although overall diet quality improved in the United States from 1999 through 2010, diet quality remains poor overall (Wang et al., 2014). Findings show

- Diet quality was lowest in participants who had completed 12 years of education or less and highest in those who had completed college.
- Mexican Americans had the best diet quality, whereas non-Hispanic Blacks had the poorest.

- Adjusting for income and education eliminated the difference between non-Hispanic Whites and non-Hispanic Blacks; however, diet quality among Mexican Americans remained significantly higher, suggesting the differences between non-Hispanic Whites and Mexican Americans may be related to dietary traditions and culture.
- Participants with a lower BMI had more improvement in dietary quality over time. Improvement in the highest BMI group was negligible.
- Socioeconomic status was strongly associated with diet quality, and the difference in diet quality between the highest and lowest socioeconomic status levels widened over time.

Food Insecurity

Household food insecurity describes households whose access to adequate food is limited by a lack of money and other resources (Coleman-Jensen, Rabbit, Gregory, & Singh, 2016). The extent and severity of food insecurity is monitored by the USDA via a nationally representative annual survey. In 2015 (Coleman-Jensen et al., 2016):

- The percentage of food-insecure households was 12.7%, of which 7.7% had low food security and 5.0% had very low food security. This figure represents a decline in food insecurity from 14.0% in the previous year.
- The most commonly reported indicators of food insecurity were being worried food would run out, that food purchased would not last, inability or lack of means to afford balanced meals, reduced size of meals or skipping meals, and eating less than the participant felt he or she should. Among very low food security households, 98% reported being worried that their food would run out before they got money to buy more and 45% reported having lost weight because they did not have enough money for food.
- For households with incomes near or below the federal poverty line, the rates of food insecurity were substantially higher than the national average in households with children headed by single women or single men, women and men living alone, and Black- and Hispanic-headed households.
- Almost 59% of food-insecure households in the survey reported that within the previous month, they had participated in one or more of the three largest federal nutrition assistance programs including Supplemental Nutrition Assistance Program (SNAP, formerly the Food Stamp Program); Special Supplemental Nutrition Program for Women, Infants, and Children (WIC); and National School Lunch Program.

Food Deserts

Food deserts occur predominately in low-income areas where a substantial proportion of the residents experience a lack of access to a supermarket. A food desert is defined as living more than 1 mile from a supermarket in an urban area or more than 10 miles from a supermarket in a rural area. Without ready access to supermarkets, access to fresh fruits, vegetables, and other healthy whole foods is low. Poor access to healthy foods could lead to poor diet quality and increased risk of chronic diseases such as obesity or diabetes.

Since 2011, the federal government has spent almost $500 million to improve access to healthy food in neighborhoods that do not have large supermarkets (Ver Ploeg & Rahkovsky, 2016). State and local governments have also created programs to improve food choices in food deserts. One example is requiring corner stores and drug stores to stock fresh fruits and vegetables and whole grain bread. Although early research showed a correlation between supermarket access and diet quality, more recent studies show the effect of food store access on diet quality may be limited.

Data from USDA's National Household Food Acquisition and Purchase Survey (FoodAPS) revealed that both low-income and higher income households consider store characteristics other than proximity when deciding where to shop (Ver Ploeg & Rahkovsky, 2016). Approximately 90% of households that participate in SNAP or WIC did their primary grocery shopping in a supermarket or supercenter. Likewise, 90% of food-insecure households usually shopped at larger stores. Households often do not shop at the nearest supermarket to obtain groceries regardless of whether the mode of transportation is driving, walking, biking, or public transit (Ver Ploeg & Rahkovsky, 2016).

Economic Research Service researchers used Nielsen Homescan data to understand the relationship between food access and food choices (Ver Ploeg & Rahkovsky, 2016). Households included in the dataset scanned receipts of food purchased for at-home consumption, which provided information on food quantity, price, and place of purchase. Researchers found that in low-income neighborhoods, limited access to a supermarket showed only a modest negative effect on diet quality. Data confirm that diet quality did improve, but only slightly, when consumers with limited shopping options shopped farther from home. When consumers drove to a store farther away, they bought 0.42% more fruit, 0.55% more vegetables, 0.61% more low-fat dairy products, and 0.33% less nondiet beverages. However, a limitation of the Nielsen dataset is that it undersamples minority, poor, and less educated consumers.

SNAP households are more sensitive to price than proximity, which may explain why households bypass the closest store for stores farther away that offer lower prices (Ver Ploeg & Rahkovsky, 2016). The prices of different food groups have a larger effect on what is purchased than does access. In fact, the effects of food access were negligible when price and demographic factors were accounted for. Low income is more strongly associated with buying unhealthy food than is living in an area with limited access to supermarkets (Rahkovsky & Snyder, 2015). Results suggest that improving access to healthy foods by itself will not likely have a major impact on diet quality (Ver Ploeg & Rahkovsky, 2016). The cost of food, income available to spend on food, consumer knowledge about nutrition, and food preferences may be more important factors in food purchase decisions than access.

The Future of Nutrition and Health

Nutrition has the potential to help individuals live healthier, more productive lives and reduce the worldwide strain of chronic disease. As a relatively young science, the importance of nutrition as part of the solution to societal, environmental, and economic challenges facing the world has just begun to be fully recognized (Ohlhorst et al., 2013). Research is needed to expand our knowledge of how nutrition can effectively prevent or treat both infectious and chronic diseases; reduce or end food insecurity; and ensure a safe, sustainable, affordable, and nutritionally adequate food supply for the world's growing population. Some of the questions driving nutrition research are featured in Box 1.4.

New technology and scientific discoveries are deepening our understanding of how nutrients and eating patterns affect health and disease. Technology will enable researchers to expand and update nutrition **databases** to include more food items and substances in food previously not quantified, such as lycopene, resveratrol, and other phytonutrients, which will provide a more accurate and complete picture of food composition. **Bioinformatics** will enable researchers to make connections between intake and health that were not previously possible. Nutritional **genomics** has the potential to redefine the role of nutrition in health and disease risk.

Database
a comprehensive collection of related information organized for convenient access.

Bioinformatics
an interdisciplinary field that uses computer science and information technology to develop and improve techniques to make it easier to acquire, store, organize, retrieve, and use complex biological data.

Genomics
an area of genetics that studies all genes in cells or tissues at the DNA and messenger RNA (mRNA) level.

BOX 1.4 — Some of the Questions Driving Nutrition Research

- How do an individual's genes determine how the body handles specific nutrients?
- What role does a person's microbiota have in an individual's response to diet and food components? What is its role in disease prevention and progression?
- How does food intake affect a person's microbiota?
- How does an individuals' genome affect responses to diet and food?
- How does diet during critical periods of development "program" long-term health and well-being? For instance, how does undernutrition during fetal life increase the risk of diabetes in adulthood?
- How can obesity be prevented? Can obesity be cured?
- How does nutrition influence the initiation of disease and its progression?
- What are the nutritional needs of aging adults?
- What are the biochemical and behavior bases for food choices? How can we most effectively measure, monitor, and evaluate dietary change?
- How can we get people to change their eating behaviors?

Source: Ohlhorst, S., Russell, R., Bier, D., Klurfeld, D., Li, Z., Mein, J., . . . Konopka, E. (2013). Nutrition research to affect food and a health life span. *American Journal of Clinical Nutrition, 98,* 620–625.

Nutrigenetics
the effect of genetic differences on the response to dietary intake and the ultimate impact on disease risk.

Nutrigenomics
the interaction between dietary components and the genome and the resulting changes in proteins and other substances that impact gene expression.

Epigenomics
the impact of diet on changes in gene expression without changing the DNA sequence.

Biomarker
a measurable biological molecule found in blood, other body fluids, or tissues that is a sign of a normal or abnormal process or of a condition or disease.

Nutritional Genomics

Nutritional genomics is an umbrella term that includes **nutrigenetics**, **nutrigenomics**, and nutritional **epigenomics**, all of which pertain to how nutrients and genes interact and are expressed to reveal phenotype outcomes, including disease risk (Camp & Trujillo, 2014).

Genomics has the potential to produce major nutrition breakthroughs in the prevention of chronic disease and obesity and to identify new **biomarkers** that will more accurately assess a person's health and nutritional status. However, most chronic diseases, such as cardiovascular disease, diabetes, and cancer, are multigenetic and multifactorial, and therefore, genetic mutations only partially predict disease risk (Camp & Trujillo, 2014). Other factors, such as family history, laboratory values, and environmental risk factors (e.g., smoking), impact disease risk and nutrition therapy. In the future, nutritional genomics may lead to tailored dietary advice based on genotype in place of current population-wide dietary recommendations. However, the science of nutritional genomics is young, and it is not yet known whether knowledge gained from it will have practical application in the everyday life of consumers (Camp & Trujillo, 2014).

NUTRITION AND HEALTH CARE

Nutrition affects the practice of all health-care professionals. Throughout the life cycle and through all degrees of health and illness, understanding and applying nutrition knowledge and skills enables all members of the health-care team to effectively assess dietary intake and provide appropriate guidance, counseling, and treatment to patients (DiMaria-Ghalili et al., 2014). Patient care is improved when evidence-based nutrition care is synchronized and reinforced by all health professionals, including physicians, physician assistants, nurses, nurse practitioners, pharmacists, dentists, dental hygienists, occupational therapists, physical therapists, speech and language pathologists, exercise physiologists, psychologists, and others. Although the dietitian is the primary nutrition authority, it takes an interprofessional team to provide optimal nutrition care.

Nutrition in Nursing

Nutrition has been an integral component of nursing care since Florence Nightingale noted nutrition as the second most important area for nursing (Nightingale, 1992). Until the profession of dietetics was founded, nurses were responsible for preparing and serving food to the sick. The differentiation between nurses and dietitians continued during the period from 1950 to 1970 (DiMaria-Ghalili et al., 2014). Today, nutrition is 1 of 13 domains in nursing practice. National Council Licensure Examination (NCLEX) exams include a variety of nutrition topics, including assessment and monitoring, nutrition therapy, and enteral and parenteral nutrition.

Nurses have a variety of nutrition care responsibilities (Box 1.5). Nurses provide assessment data through a nursing history and physical exam that the dietitian uses to complete a nutritional assessment. Nurses monitor the patient's intake, weight, and tolerance to food. Nurses often serve as the liaison between the dietitian and physician as well as with other members of the health-care team. As the team member with the greatest contact with the patient and family, nurses serve as a nutrition resource when dietitians are not available, such as during the evening, on weekends, and during discharge instructions. In home care and wellness settings, dietitians may be available only on a consultative basis. Nurses reinforce nutrition counseling provided by the dietitian, provide basic nutrition education, and stress the importance of eating healthy and participating in regular physical activity. An especially important function of nurses is to screen hospitalized patients for **malnutrition** risk.

Malnutrition
literally, bad nutrition. In practice, malnutrition refers specifically to protein–calorie undernutrition.

BOX 1.5 Some Nutrition Care Responsibilities of the Nurse

Create a Culture that Values Nutrition

- Recognize the importance of nurses in the achieving successful patient outcomes
- Include assessment of the patient's intake in team meetings
- Include nutrition into routine care checklists and processes; for instance, a nursing history and physical that includes questions about the number of meals consumed daily; food allergies and intolerances; nutrition concerns of the patient; whether the patient has access to enough food

Recognize At-Risk Patients

- Screen every patient for malnutrition
- Communicate screening results
- Rescreen patients within established time frame

Implement Nutrition Interventions

- Ensure that screening occurs within established time frame
- Ensure that dietitian-prescribed interventions occur in a timely manner
- Facilitate nursing interventions to treat patients who have or are at risk of malnutrition
- Ensure patients receive automated nutrition intervention (e.g., food, oral supplements) if there is a delay between nutrition screening and nutrition assessment
- Maximize food and oral supplement intake
  - Avoid disconnecting enteral or parenteral nutrition for patient repositioning, ambulation, procedures, etc.
  - Advocate discontinuation of intravenous therapy as soon as feasible
  - Be aggressive about diet progressions
  - Replace meals withheld for diagnostic tests
  - Promote congregate dining if appropriate
  - Question diet orders that appear inappropriate
  - Display a positive attitude when serving food or discussing nutrition
  - Help the patient select appropriate foods; offer standby choices for patients who do not like menu selections
  - Gently motivate the patient to eat
  - Encourage patients who feel full quickly to eat the most nutrient dense items first, such as meat and milk over juice, soup or coffee
  - Order snacks and nutritional supplements

- Request assistance with feeding or meal setup
- Get the patient out of bed to eat if possible
- Encourage good oral hygiene
- Screen the patient from offensive sights and remove unpleasant odors from the room
- Down grade the consistency of the diet (e.g., provide a soft diet) if the patient has difficulty chewing swallowing

Monitor

- Observe intake of food and supplements whenever possible
- Document appetite and take action when the client does not eat
- Order supplements if intake is low or needs are high
- Initiate calorie counts
- Request a nutritional consult
- Assess tolerance (i.e., absence of side effects)
- Monitor weight
- Monitor progression of nothing by mouth (NPO) status and restrictive diets
- Monitor the client's grasp of the information and motivation to change

Communicate

- Consult with dietitian about nutrition concerns
- Communicate changes in the patient's condition that may indicate nutrition risk
- Include nutrition discussions into handoff of care and nursing care plans

Educate

- Include nutrition in all discussions with patients and their family members or caregivers
- Reinforce the importance of obtaining adequate nutrition
- Review basic principles of the eating plan and avoid the term "diet"
- Counsel the client about drug–nutrient interactions
- Emphasize things "to do" instead of things "not to do"
- Keep the message simple
- Review written handouts with the client
- Advise the client to avoid foods that are not tolerated

Source: Tappenden, K., Quatrara, B., Parkhurst, M., Malone, A., Fanjiang, G., & Ziegler, T. (2013). Critical role of nutrition in improving quality of care: An interdisciplinary call to action to address adult hospital malnutrition. *Journal of the Academy of Nutrition and Dietetics, 113*, 1219–1237.

Concept Mastery Alert

When nurses prepare discharge plans for obese older adults who will be staying with family members, they should emphasize the positive, not the negative, and encourage their clients to make choices for themselves. Nurses should avoid using terms such as "diet" and keep the message simple, taking care to review any written handouts with clients.

Nutrition Screening

In acute care settings, **nutrition screening** is designed to detect actual or potential malnutrition based on a few selected criteria that are readily available. Note that when a patient is found to *not* have malnutrition, it does not mean the patient is without health risks. For instance, a patient admitted with symptoms of a myocardial infarction may not have malnutrition but still be at high risk for morbidity and mortality related to the admitting diagnosis.

Patients identified as high or moderate risk are referred to a dietitian for further nutrition assessment, diagnosis, and intervention. Patients determined to be at low risk are rescreened within a specified timeframe to identify changes in risk (Field & Hand, 2015).

The Joint Commission, a nonprofit organization that sets health-care standards and accredits health-care facilities that meet those standards, specifies that nutrition screening be conducted within 24 hours after admission to a hospital or other health-care facility. Because the standard applies 24 hours a day, 7 days a week, staff nurses are usually responsible for completing the screen as part of the admission process. Each facility is able to determine the criteria it uses for screening, who completes nutrition screening, and when rescreening is required.

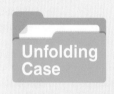

Unfolding Case

Think of Tyrone. He is admitted to the hospital for chest pain. The nurse performs a nutrition screening and determines he is at low nutritional risk because his weight is stable, his appetite is stable, and his BMI is >18.5. Is he at low health risk overall? What criteria will the nurse monitor to identify if a change in his nutritional status occurs?

Various screening tools are available, depending on the setting, such as in community settings, hospitals, and long-term care. To be useful, screening tools should be simple, reliable, valid, and specific. Most clinical screening tools address four basic questions: recent weight loss, recent food intake, current BMI, and disease severity (Rasmussen, Holst, & Kondrup, 2010).

An example of a widely used validated tool for screening older adults is the Mini Nutritional Assessment–Short Form (MNA-SF) (Fig. 1.1). It is the newest version of a nutrition screening tool designed as a stand-alone tool to identify protein–calorie malnutrition in people 65 years and older (Skates & Anthony, 2012). It consists of six questions with a maximum possible score of 14. A score from 12 to 14 indicates normal nutritional status, 8 to 11 indicates at risk for malnutrition, and 7 or less indicates malnutrition. A score less than 12 warrants further assessment by a dietitian.

Nutrition Assessment

Patients found to be at moderate or high risk for malnutrition through screening are referred to a dietitian for a **nutrition assessment** to identify specific risks or diagnose and document malnutrition (Box 1.6). Using the same problem-solving model as the nursing process, dietitians use a nutrition care process to develop an

BOX 1.6   General Characteristics for the Diagnosis of Adult Malnutrition

- Weight loss over time
- Inadequate food and nutrition intake compared to requirements
- Loss of muscle mass
- Loss of fat mass
- Local or generalized fluid accumulation
- Measurably reduced hand grip strength

Source: Malone, A., & Hamilton, C. (2013). The Academy of Nutrition and Dietetics/The American Society for Parenteral and Enteral Nutrition Consensus Malnutrition Characteristics: Application in practice. *Nutrition in Clinical Practice, 28,* 639–650.

individualized nutritional care plan (Fig. 1.2). Assessment data includes medical history and clinical diagnosis, physical exam findings, anthropometric data, laboratory data, food/nutrient intake, and functional assessment. Table 1.2 lists examples of nutrition assessment data used to identify malnutrition. Review of the assessment data leads to a nutrition diagnosis. A plan is formulated and implemented; monitoring, evaluation, and patient and family education follow. Figure 1.3 illustrates the interdisciplinary nature of nutrition care from screening through discharge.

Figure 1.1 ▶

Mini Nutritional Assessment screening tool.

Mini Nutritional Assessment
MNA®

Nestlé
NutritionInstitute

Last name:			First name:		
Sex:	Age:	Weight, kg:	Height, cm:		Date:

Complete the screen by filling in the boxes with the appropriate numbers. Total the numbers for the final screening score.

Screening

A Has food intake declined over the past 3 months due to loss of appetite, digestive problems, chewing or swallowing difficulties?
0 = severe decrease in food intake
1 = moderate decrease in food intake
2 = no decrease in food intake ☐

B Weight loss during the last 3 months
0 = weight loss greater than 3 kg (6.6 lbs)
1 = does not know
2 = weight loss between 1 and 3 kg (2.2 and 6.6 lbs)
3 = no weight loss ☐

C Mobility
0 = bed or chair bound
1 = able to get out of bed / chair but does not go out
2 = goes out ☐

D Has suffered psychological stress or acute disease in the past 3 months?
0 = yes   2 = no ☐

E Neuropsychological problems
0 = severe dementia or depression
1 = mild dementia
2 = no psychological problems ☐

F1 Body Mass Index (BMI) (weight in kg) / (height in m)²
0 = BMI less than 19
1 = BMI 19 to less than 21
2 = BMI 21 to less than 23
3 = BMI 23 or greater ☐

IF BMI IS NOT AVAILABLE, REPLACE QUESTION F1 WITH QUESTION F2.
DO NOT ANSWER QUESTION F2 IF QUESTION F1 IS ALREADY COMPLETED.

F2 Calf circumference (CC) in cm
0 = CC less than 31
3 = CC 31 or greater ☐

Screening score (max. 14 points)

12 - 14 points: Normal nutritional status
8 - 11 points: At risk of malnutrition
0 - 7 points: Malnourished ☐☐

References
1. Vellas B, Villars H, Abellan G, et al. Overview of the MNA® - Its History and Challenges. *J Nutr Health Aging.* 2006;**10**:456-465.
2. Rubenstein LZ, Harker JO, Salva A, Guigoz Y, Vellas B. Screening for Undernutrition in Geriatric Practice: Developing the Short-Form Mini Nutritional Assessment (MNA-SF). *J. Geront.* 2001; **56A**: M366-377
3. Guigoz Y. The Mini-Nutritional Assessment (MNA®) Review of the Literature - What does it tell us? *J Nutr Health Aging.* 2006; **10**:466-487.
4. Kaiser MJ, Bauer JM, Ramsch C, et al. Validation of the Mini Nutritional Assessment Short-Form (MNA®-SF): A practical tool for identification of nutritional status. *J Nutr Health Aging.* 2009; **13**:782-788.
® Société des Produits Nestlé, S.A., Vevey, Switzerland, Trademark Owners © Nestlé, 1994, Revision 2009. N67200 12/99 10M
For more information: www.mna-elderly.com

Figure 1.2 ▶

The nutrition care process.
Like the nursing process, the
nutrition care process is a
problem-solving method used
to evaluate and treat nutrition-
related problems.

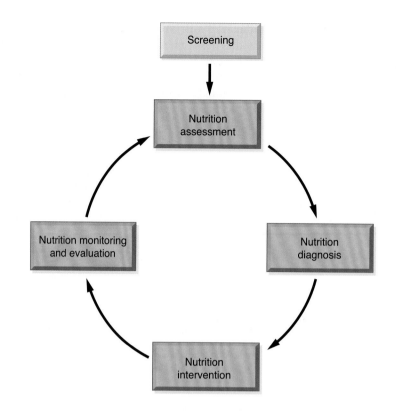

Table 1.2   Nutrition Assessment Data to Identify Malnutrition

Component	Specific Examples
Medical history and clinical diagnosis	The chief complaint and past medical history may suggest clues about nutrition status and nutrient requirements. Medical conditions often associated with malnutrition include AIDS, alcoholism, cancer, cardiovascular disease, celiac disease, chronic kidney disease, diabetes, liver disease, and dementia and other mental illness.
Physical exam	Findings that may diagnose malnutrition include loss of muscle (e.g., quadriceps or deltoids), loss of subcutaneous fat (e.g., triceps/biceps, ribs, lower back), and fluid accumulation (e.g., ankle or sacral edema or ascites).
Anthropometric data	Measured height and weight is obtained to calculate BMI. BMI <18.5 may be used to diagnosis malnutrition. However, obese people may lose substantially more than 10% of their weight and still have a normal or above normal BMI. The percentage of unintentional weight loss over specified time, such as >5% over 3 months or >10% of usual weight regardless of the timeframe (Cederholm et al., 2015).
Laboratory data	Currently, there is no universally agreed upon biochemical indicators to diagnose malnutrition. Although serum albumin has been used to screen or diagnose malnutrition, the major cause of low albumin and other visceral proteins is inflammation, not malnutrition (Cederholm et al., 2015). Inflammation is considered an etiologic factor, not a diagnostic feature, of malnutrition. However, albumin and other visceral proteins are good indicators of disease severity and outcome.
Food/nutrient intake	Information about food and nutrient intake can be obtained through patient or caregiver interview, food records, or observation. It is compared to estimated needs to assess adequacy.
Functional assessment	Hand grip strength is measured via a dynamometer by someone trained in its use.

Sources: White, J., Guenter, P., Jensen, G., Malone, A., & Schofield, M. (2012). Consensus statement of the Academy of Nutrition and Dietetics/American Society for Parenteral and Enteral Nutrition: Characteristics recommended for the identification and documentation of adult malnutrition (undernutrition). *Journal of the Academy of Nutrition and Dietetics, 112,* 730–738; and Cederholm, T., Bosaeus, I., Barazzoni, R., Bauer, J., Van Gossum, A., Klek, S., . . . Singer, P. (2015). Diagnostic criteria for malnutrition—an ESPEN Consensus Statement. *Clinical Nutrition, 34,* 335–340.

Figure 1.3 ▶
The Alliance to Advance
Patient Nutrition Approach
to Interdisciplinary Nutrition
Care.

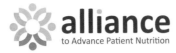 **alliance**
to Advance Patient Nutrition

Approach to Interdisciplinary
Nutrition Care

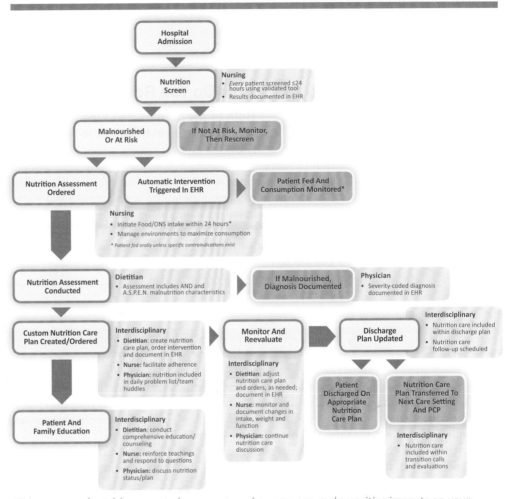

Visit *www.malnutrition.com to learn more on how you can make positive impacts on your patients' outcomes.*

Abbreviations: AND, Academy of Nutrition and Dietetics; A.S.P.E.N., American Society for Parenteral and Enteral Nutrition; EHR, electronic health record; ONS, oral nutrition supplement; PCP, primary care physician. Source: Adapted from Tappenden et al, *JPEN* 2013 37(4):482-497

© 2014 Alliance to Advance Patient Nutrition
88879-002/February 2014 LITHO IN USA
www.malnutrition.com

alliance | AMSN | Academy of Nutrition and Dietetics | shm | Abbott Nutrition

These health organizations are dedicated to the education of effective hospital nutrition practices to help improve patients' medical outcomes and support all clinicians in collaborating on hospital-wide nutrition procedures. The Alliance to Advance Patient Nutrition is made possible with support from Abbott Nutrition.

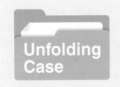 **Unfolding Case**

Recall Tyrone. Although screening did not find him to be at nutritional risk, he and his wife have many questions about how to implement a healthy eating pattern. Do you feel competent to reinforce the written and verbal instructions they've been given? How will you assure the patient that he can improve his eating pattern? What benefits may he realize with improved eating and exercise?

The process of screening and nutrition assessment is an example of the cooperative effort of how nurses and dietitians identify patients with actual or potential malnutrition. Patients who are not found to have malnutrition may also benefit from contact with a dietitian for a number of other reasons, such as patients who need additional nutrition education, have difficulty choosing culturally appropriate foods, or are eating poorly. Nurses, by virtue of their close contact with patients and families, are in an ideal position to identify these patients and make a referral to the dietitian.

How Do You Respond?

Both of my parents had type 2 diabetes so I know I'm doomed. Why should I eat healthier to reduce my risk if it's in the genes?
Although eating healthier cannot guarantee to prevent type 2 diabetes, a healthy eating pattern and physical activity have been found to be effective in preventing or delaying the onset of diabetes among individuals with prediabetes. There are other potential health benefits to adopting a healthy eating pattern and increasing physical activity, such as improvements in weight status, blood pressure, low high-density lipoprotein (HDL) cholesterol, and high triglyceride levels as well as possible reduced risk of certain cancers. There is not a downside to adopting healthier lifestyle behaviors, even though the benefits cannot be guaranteed.

REVIEW CASE STUDY

Mildred is an 80-year-old woman who lives independently in her own home. She was brought to the emergency department due to worsening generalized weakness that resulted in a fall with probable hip fracture. She has a history of lower gastrointestinal (GI) bleeding and presents with anemia. She is alert and oriented. Her BMI is 16.8. Three months ago, she weighed 135 pounds, and she currently weighs 104 pounds. She admits to being hungry but states that she has not had an appetite for several months. Her health has been stable since her last hospital admission for GI bleeding 2 years ago.

- Using Figure 1.1, what is Mildred's nutrition screening score?
- Mildred is admitted and ordered a regular diet. What nutrition interventions would you initiate to help maximize Mildred's intake?
- The nutrition diagnosis is "underweight related to loss of appetite and poor intake as evidenced by BMI of 16.8." What criteria will you monitor that will enable the dietitian to evaluate Mildred's progress?

STUDY QUESTIONS

1 Nurses are in an ideal position to
   a. Screen patients for risk of malnutrition
   b. Order therapeutic diets
   c. Conduct nutrition assessments
   d. Calculate a patient's calorie and protein needs

2 Which of the following criteria would most likely be on a nutrition screen in the hospital?
   a. Prealbumin value
   b. Weight change
   c. Serum potassium value
   d. Cultural food preferences

3 Which of the following statements is accurate regarding characteristics of a healthy eating pattern?
   a. "The only healthy eating pattern is a vegetarian one."
   b. "Healthy eating patterns eliminate foods that are high in saturated fat, added calories, and sodium, such as fried foods, desserts, and snack chips."
   c. "Healthy eating patterns may reduce the risk of several chronic diseases, including cardiovascular disease, type 2 diabetes, and certain cancers."
   d. "Most young and middle-aged adults consume a healthy eating pattern."

4 Your patient has a question about the cardiac diet the dietitian reviewed with him yesterday. What is the nurse's best response?
   a. "Ask your doctor when you go for your follow-up appointment."
   b. "What is the question? If I can't answer it, I will get the dietitian to come back to answer it."
   c. "Just do your best. The handout she gave you is simply a list of guidelines, not rigid instructions."
   d. "If I see the dietitian around, I will tell her you need to see her."

5 Which of the following statements regarding nutrition screening is false?
   a. A nutrition screen is completed only when a patient is suspected of having a nutritional problem.
   b. A nutrition screen must be completed within 24 hours after admission to a hospital or other health-care facility.
   c. The purpose of nutrition screening is to detect actual or potential malnutrition.
   d. Health-care facilities are free to choose their own screening criteria and to determine how quickly a patient must be rescreened.

KEY CONCEPTS

- Initially, the science of nutrition was concerned with preventing and correcting nutrient deficiency diseases. Today, dietary excesses threaten health and Americans are underconsuming certain types of food that are protective against disease.
- Nutrition plays a vital role in all aspects of health, including healthy pregnancies; normal growth, development, and aging; maintenance of healthy body weight; reducing the risk of chronic disease; and managing chronic disease.
- Healthy People 2020 is a comprehensive blueprint for monitoring the nation's progress toward becoming healthier. It states a healthful diet contains a variety of nutrient-dense foods; is limited in saturated fat, trans fat, cholesterol, added sugar, sodium, and alcohol; and has a calorie level that is in balance with calorie need.
- Chronic disease is a global problem. It was responsible for 68% of worldwide deaths in 2012. Seven of the top 10 causes of death in the United States are from chronic disease. Half of American adults have one or more chronic diseases; children and adolescents are also being diagnosed with chronic disease. At all ages, overweight and obesity are linked to an increased risk of chronic disease.
- Modifiable lifestyle risk factors linked to chronic disease include poor quality eating pattern, physical inactivity, smoking, excess body weight, and excessive alcohol intake.
- The impact of a food on health may be greater than the sum of its parts. Both essential and nonessential components of food, working alone or synergistically, in certain proportions and mixtures, may be reasons why eating patterns, more so than individual components, are associated with lower risk of chronic disease.
- A healthy eating pattern is rich in fruits and vegetables; contains whole grains in place of refined grains; includes low-fat milk, coffee, tea, and moderate alcohol; provides adequate dairy and oil and a variety of proteins; and is low in processed foods. No foods are prohibited in a healthy eating pattern.
- Generally older adults have healthier eating patterns than young and middle-aged adults, women eat healthier than

men, Hispanic Americans have the highest diet quality, and eating patterns generally improve with level of education.
- Socioeconomic status is strongly associated with diet quality.
- Food-insecure households have limited access to food due to lack of money or other resources.
- Food deserts occur in low-income areas with limited access to supermarkets. Increasing access to healthy food by itself is not likely to improve diet quality. The price of food, available income, nutrition knowledge, and food preferences may have a greater effect on food choices than access.
- Technology will dramatically improve the science of nutrition. Genomics has the potential to create a major breakthrough in the prevention of obesity and chronic diseases. Bioinformatics will facilitate better management of data to make nutrition and health connections that were previously impossible. Improved biomarkers will enable researchers to more accurately assess nutrient intake and its effect on health. In the future, dietary advice may evolve from population-based recommendations to personalized prescriptions based on genotype.
- All health-care professions are impacted by nutrition. Patient care is improved when all interdisciplinary team members work together to achieve patient nutrition outcomes.
- Nutrition is an integral part of nursing care. Nurses have many nutrition care responsibilities including maximizing patient intake; monitoring intake, weight, and function; providing basic nutrition education; reinforcing nutrition counseling; and completing nutrition screening.
- Nutrition screening is used to identify people with actual or potential malnutrition.
- Patients who are identified to be a low or no nutritional risk are rescreened within a specified period of time to determine whether their nutritional risk status has changed.
- The Joint Commission stipulates that nutrition screening be performed within 24 hours of admission to a health-care facility, but facilities are free to decide what criteria to include on a screen, what findings indicate risk, who is to conduct the screen, and when rescreening occurs. Nutrition screening is usually the responsibility of staff nurses because

they can be completed during a history and physical examination upon admission.
- Screening tools are simple, quick, valid, easy to use, and rely on available data.
- Most nutritional screening address four areas of concern: BMI, weight loss, appetite, and severity of disease.

- Patients who are found to be a moderate to high nutritional risk at screening receive a nutrition assessment by the dietitian that includes the steps of assessment, diagnosis, intervention, and monitoring and evaluation. Dietitians also document the proper code for malnutrition for hospital reimbursement purposes.

Check Your Knowledge Answer Key

1 **FALSE** Chronic diseases were responsible for 68% of worldwide deaths in 2012.

2 **FALSE** Chronic health conditions such as hypertension and type 2 diabetes are affecting children and adolescents. As with adults, lifestyle risk factors such as poor diet, physical inactivity, and excess body weight are likely involved.

3 **TRUE** Poor diet quality, physical inactivity, smoking, and excess body weight are modifiable risk factors that increase the risk of chronic disease.

4 **TRUE** The typical American eating pattern is low in fruits, vegetables, whole grains, dairy, and oils. It also contains excessive calories, saturated fat, added sugars, and sodium.

5 **FALSE** Older adults tend to have better eating patterns than young and middle-aged adults.

6 **TRUE** For several chronic diseases, healthier eating and increased physical activity may provide benefits equal to medication, with lower cost and risk of side effects.

7 **TRUE** Genomics will help researchers determine how specific nutrients interact with genes and other body substances to predict the health of an individual.

8 **TRUE** Nutrition care affects the practice of all health-care professionals. Nutrition is intimately intertwined with all aspects of health and illness across the life cycle.

9 **TRUE** Nurses are usually responsible for completing nutrition screening.

10 **TRUE** Most nutrition screenings address body mass index (BMI), appetite, weight change, and severity of disease.

Websites

2015-2020 Dietary Guidelines for Americans at health.gov/dietaryguidelines/2015/guidelines

Healthy People 2020 at https://www.healthypeople.gov

Healthy Eating Index available at http://www.cnpp.usda.gov/healthyeatingindex

United Health Foundation, a private, not-for-profit foundation dedicated to improving health and health care at www.unitedhealthfoundation.org

A guide to completing the MNA-SF at www.mna-elderly.com/forms/mna_guide_english_sf.pdf

References

Bauer, U., Briss, P., Goodman, R., & Bowman, B. (2014). Prevention of chronic disease in the 21st century: Elimination of the leading preventable causes of premature death and disability in the USA. *Lancet, 384,* 45–52.

Bjelakovic, G., Nikolova, D., Gluud, L., Simonetti, R., & Gluud, C. (2007). Mortality in randomized trials of antioxidant supplements for primary and secondary prevention: Systematic review and meta-analysis. *JAMA, 297,* 842–857.

Camp, K., & Trujillo, E. (2014). Position of the Academy of Nutrition and Dietetics: Nutritional genomics. *Journal of the Academy of Nutrition and Dietetics, 114,* 299–312.

Coleman-Jensen, A., Rabbit, M., Gregory, C., & Singh, A. (2016). *Household food security in the United States in 2015 (ERR-215).* Washington, DC: U.S. Department of Agriculture, Economic Research Service. Available at http://www.ers.usda.gov/media/2137663/err215.pdf. Accessed on 9/26/16.

Dietary Guidelines Advisory Committee. (2015). *Scientific report of the 2015 Dietary Guidelines Advisory Committee.* Available at http://health.gov/dietaryguidelines/2015-scientific-report/. Accessed on 2/22/16.

DiMaria-Ghalili, R., Mirtallo, J., Tobin, B., Hark, L., Van Horn, L., & Palmer, C. (2014). Challenges and opportunities for nutrition education and training in the health care professions: Intraprofessional and interprofessional call to action. *American Journal of Clinical Nutrition, 99,* 1184S–1193S.

Estruch, R., Ros, E., Salas-Salvadó, J., Covas, M., Corella, D., Arós, F., . . . Martínez-Gonzáles, M. (2013). Primary prevention of cardiovascular disease with a Mediterranean diet. *New England Journal of Medicine, 368,* 1279–1290.

Field, L., & Hand, R. (2015). Differentiating malnutrition screening and assessment: A nutrition care process perspective. *Journal of the Academy of Nutrition and Dietetics, 115,* 824–828.

George, S., Ballard-Barbash, R., Manson, J., Reedy, J., Shikany, J., Subar, A., . . . Neuhouser, M. L. (2014). Comparing indices of diet quality with chronic disease mortality risk in postmenopausal women in the Women's Health Initiative Observational Study: Evidence to inform national dietary guidance. *American Journal of Epidemiology, 180,* 616–625.

Hiza, H., Casavale, K., Guenther, P., & Davis, C. (2013). Diet quality of Americans differs by age, sex, race/ethnicity, income, and education level. *Journal of the Academy of Nutrition and Dietetics, 113,* 297–306.

International Food Information Council Foundation. *Food & Health Survey 2015.* Available at http://www.foodinsight.org/sites/default/files/2015%20Food%20And%20Health%20Survey-%20Executive%20Summary%20-%20Final.pdf. Accessed on 3/1/16.

Jacobs, D., & Orlich, M. (2014). Diet pattern and longevity: Do simple rules suffice? A commentary. *American Journal of Clinical Nutrition, 100*(Suppl. 1), 313S–319S.

Meyer-Abich, K. (2005). Human health in nature—towards a holistic philosophy of nutrition. *Public Health Nutrition, 8,* 738–742.

Mozaffarian, D., & Ludwig, D. (2010). Dietary guidelines in the 21st century—a time for food. *JAMA, 304,* 681–682.

Mursu, J., Steffen, L., Meyer, K., Duprez, D., & Jacobs, D. (2013). Diet quality indices and mortality in postmenopausal women: The Iowa Women's Health Study. *American Journal of Clinical Nutrition, 98,* 444–453.

Nightingale, F. (1992). *Notes of nursing: What is it, and what it is not.* Philadelphia, PA: J.B. Lippincott.

Ohlhorst, S., Russell, R., Bier, D., Klurfeld, D., Li, Z., Mein, J., . . . Konopka, E. (2013). Nutrition research to affect food and a healthy life span. *American Journal of Clinical Nutrition, 98,* 620–625.

Rahkovsky, I., & Snyder, S. (2015). *Food choices and store proximity* (EER-195). Washington, DC: U.S. Department of Agriculture, Economic Research Service. Available at http://www.ers.usda.gov/media/1909239/err195.pdf. Accessed on 9/27/16.

Rasmussen, H., Holst, M., & Kondrup, J. (2010). Measuring nutritional risk in hospitals. *Clinical Epidemiology, 2,* 209–216.

Sacks, F., Svetkey, L., Vollmer, W., Appel, L., Bray, G., Harsha, D., . . . Cutler, J. (2001). Effects on blood pressure of reduced dietary sodium and the Dietary Approaches to Stop Hypertension (DASH) diet. *New England Journal of Medicine, 344,* 3–10.

Skates, J., & Anthony, P. (2012). Identifying geriatric malnutrition in nursing practice: The Mini Nutritional Assessment (MNA®)—an evidence-based screening tool. *Journal of Gerontological Nursing, 38,* 18–27.

Slawson, D., Fitzgerald, N., & Morgan, K. (2013). Position of the Academy of Nutrition and Dietetics: The role of nutrition in health promotion and chronic disease prevention. *Journal of Academy of Nutrition and Dietetics, 113,* 972–979.

U.S. Department of Health and Human Services. (2010). *HHS announces the nation's new health promotion and disease prevention agenda.* Available at http://www.healthypeople.gov/2020/about/DefaultPress Release.pdf. Accessed on 10/9/12.

U.S. Department of Health and Human Services & U.S. Department of Agriculture. (2015). *Scientific Report of the 2015 Dietary Guidelines Advisory Committee.* Available at http://health.gov/dietaryguidelines/2015-scientific-report/PDFs/Scientific-Report-of-the-2015-Dietary-Guidelines-Advisory-Committee.pdf. Accessed on 3/6/16.

Ver Ploeg, M., & Rahkovsky, I. (2016). *Recent evidence on the effects of food store access on food choice and diet quality.* Available at http://www.ers.usda.gov/amber-waves/2016-may/recent-evidence-on-the-effects-of-food-store-access-on-food-choice-and-diet-quality.aspx#.V-ptvU3rvIX. Accessed 9/27/16.

Wang, D., Leung, C., Li, Y., Ding, E., Chiuve, S., Hu, F., & Willett, W. (2014). Trends in dietary quality among adults in the United States, 1999 through 2010. *JAMA Internal Medicine, 174,* 1587–1595.

Ward, B. W., Schiller, J. S., & Goodman, R. A. (2014). Multiple chronic conditions among US adults: A 2012 update. *Preventing Chronic Disease, 11,* 130389. doi:10.5888/pcd11.130389

Wilson, M., Reedy, J., & Krebs-Smith, S. (2016). American diet quality: Where it is, where it is heading, and what it could be. *Journal of the Academy of Nutrition and Diet, 116,* 302–310.

Wing, R., Bolin, P., Brancati, F., Bray, G., Clark, J., Coday, M., . . . Yanovski, S. (2013). Cardiovascular effects of intensive lifestyle intervention in type 2 diabetes. *New England Journal of Medicine, 369,* 145–154.

World Health Organization. (2014). *Global Status Report on noncommunicable diseases 2014.* Geneva, Switzerland: Author. Available at http://apps.who.int/iris/bitstream/10665/148114/1/9789241564854_eng.pdf. Accessed on 3/7/16.

World Health Organization Preamble to the Constitution of the World Health Organization as adopted by the International Health Conference, New York, 19-22 June, 1946; signed on 22 July 1946 by the representatives of 61 States (Official Records of the World Health Organization, no. 2, p. 100) and entered into force on 7 April 1948.

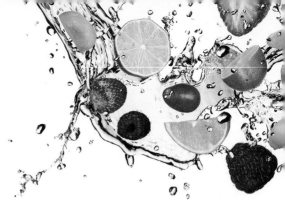

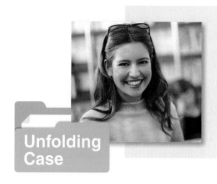

Krista Larson

Krista is 24-year-old graduate student who complains of chronic constipation. In an effort to control her weight, she has used laxatives for years and eliminates as much carbohydrate from her diet as she can. She recently tried to stop using laxatives but is unable to have a bowel movement on her own.

Check Your Knowledge

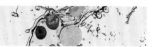

True	False		
☐	☐	1	Starch is made from glucose molecules.
☐	☐	2	Sugar is higher in calories than starch.
☐	☐	3	The sugar in fruit is better for you than the sugar in candy.
☐	☐	4	Most commonly consumed American foods provide adequate fiber to enable people to meet the recommended intake.
☐	☐	5	Enriched wheat bread is nutritionally equivalent to whole wheat bread.
☐	☐	6	Beverages, such as soft drinks, fruit drinks, sports drinks, and sweetened coffee and tea, contribute more added sugars to the typical American diet than any other food or beverage.
☐	☐	7	Bread is just as likely as candy to cause cavities.
☐	☐	8	The Dietary Guidelines recommend Americans limit their intake of added sugars to less than 10% of total calories consumed.
☐	☐	9	The safety of nonnutritive sweeteners is questionable.
☐	☐	10	Sugar causes hyperactivity in kids.

Learning Objectives

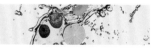

Upon completion of this chapter, you will be able to

1 Classify the type(s) of carbohydrate found in various foods.
2 Describe the functions of carbohydrates.
3 Modify a menu to ensure that the adequate intake for fiber is provided.
4 Calculate the calorie content of a food that contains only carbohydrates.
5 Debate the usefulness of using glycemic load to make food choices.
6 Suggest ways to limit sugar intake.
7 Discuss the benefits and disadvantages of using sugar alternatives.

Sugar and starch come to mind when people hear the word "carbs," but carbohydrates are so much more than just table sugar and bread. Foods containing carbohydrates can be empty calories, nutritional powerhouses, or something in between. Globally, carbohydrates provide the majority of calories in almost all human diets.

This chapter describes what carbohydrates are, where they are found in the diet, and how they are handled in the body. Recommendations regarding intake and the role of carbohydrates in health are presented.

CARBOHYDRATE CLASSIFICATIONS

Carbohydrates (CHO)
a class of energy-yielding nutrients that contain only carbon, hydrogen, and oxygen, hence the common abbreviation of CHO.

Simple Sugars
a classification of carbohydrates that includes monosaccharides and disaccharides; commonly referred to as sugars.

Complex Carbohydrates
a group name for starch, glycogen, and fiber; composed of long chains of glucose molecules.

Monosaccharide
single (mono) molecules of sugar (saccharide); the most common monosaccharides in foods are hexoses that contain six carbon atoms.

Disaccharide
"double sugar" composed of two (di) monosaccharides (e.g., sucrose, maltose, lactose).

Polysaccharides
carbohydrates consisting of many (poly) sugar molecules.

Starch
the storage form of glucose in plants.

Carbohydrates (CHO) are composed of the elements carbon, hydrogen, and oxygen arranged into basic sugar molecules. They are classified as either **simple sugars** or **complex carbohydrates** (Fig. 2.1).

Simple Sugars

Simple sugars contain only one (mono-) or two (di-) sugar (saccharide) molecules; they vary in sweetness and sources (Table 2.1). **Monosaccharides**, such as glucose, fructose, and galactose, are absorbed "as is" without undergoing digestion; **disaccharides**, such as sucrose (table sugar), maltose, and lactose, must be split into their component monosaccharides before they can be absorbed. Glucose, also known as dextrose, is the simple sugar of greatest distinction: It circulates through the blood to provide energy for body cells, it is a component of all disaccharides and is virtually the sole constituent of complex carbohydrates, and it is the sugar to which the body converts all other digestible carbohydrates.

Complex Carbohydrates

Complex carbohydrates, also known as polysaccharides, are composed of hundreds to thousands of glucose molecules linked together. Despite being made of sugar, **polysaccharides** do not taste sweet because their molecules are too large to fit on the tongue's taste bud receptors that sense sweetness. Starch, glycogen, and fiber are types of polysaccharides.

Starch

Through the process of photosynthesis, plants synthesize glucose, which they use for energy. Glucose not used by the plant for immediate energy is stored in the form of **starch** in seeds, roots, or stems. Grains, such as wheat, rice, corn, barley, millet, sorghum, oats, and rye, are the world's major food crops and the foundation of all diets. Other sources of starch include potatoes, legumes, and other starchy vegetables.

Glycogen

Glycogen
storage form of glucose in animals and humans.

Glycogen is the animal (including human) version of starch; it is stored carbohydrate available for energy as needed. Humans have a limited supply of glycogen stored in the liver and muscles. Liver glycogen breaks down and releases glucose into the

Figure 2.1 ▶
Carbohydrate classifications.

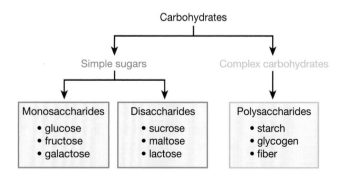

Table 2.1   Simple Sugars

	Relative Sweetness	Sources
Monosaccharides		
Glucose (also known as dextrose)	70	Fruit, vegetables, honey, corn syrup, cornstarch
Fructose (also known as fruit sugar)	170	Fruit, honey, some vegetables
Galactose	60	Does not occur in appreciable amounts in foods; significant only as it combines with glucose to form lactose
Disaccharides		
Sucrose (composed of glucose and fructose)	100	Fruit, vegetables Extracted from sugarcane and sugar beets into white, brown, confectioners, and turbinado sugars
Maltose (composed of two glucose molecules)	50	Not found naturally in foods; added to some foods for flavoring (e.g., malted milk shakes) and to beer for coloring Is an intermediate in starch digestion
Lactose (composed of glucose and galactose)	40	"Milk sugar"; used as an additive in many foods and drugs

Concept Mastery Alert

Typically, two-thirds of the body's glycogen is stored in the muscle, where it is available only for use in the muscle, and the remaining one-third is stored in the liver, where it is available for all body cells.

bloodstream between meals to maintain normal blood glucose levels and provide fuel for tissues. Muscles do not share their supply of glycogen but use it for their own energy needs. There is virtually no dietary source of glycogen because any glycogen stored in animal tissue is quickly converted to lactic acid at the time of slaughter. Miniscule amounts of glycogen are found in shellfish, such as scallops and oysters, which is why they taste slightly sweet compared to other fish.

Fiber

Fiber is a group name for polysaccharides that cannot be digested and absorbed in the human small intestine. Types of fiber include cellulose, pectin, gums, hemicellulose, inulin, oligosaccharides, fructans, lignin, and some resistant starch. Often referred to as "roughage" or "bulk," fiber is found only in plants as a component of plant cell walls or intercellular structure.

Historically, fibers have been categorized as **insoluble** or **soluble** for the purpose of assigning specific functions to each category. For instance, soluble fibers dissolve in water to a gel-like substance. They are credited with slowing gastric emptying time to promote a feeling of fullness, delaying and blunting the rise in postprandial serum glucose, and lowering serum cholesterol. Oatmeal, legumes, lentils, and citrus fruits are sources of soluble fiber. Insoluble fiber absorbs water to make stools larger and softer and speed intestinal transit time. Whole grains, bran, and the skins and seeds of fruits and vegetables provide insoluble fiber. Although sources of fiber may be identified as either soluble (e.g., oats) or insoluble (e.g., wheat bran), almost all sources of fiber provide a blend of both soluble and insoluble fibers.

Unfolding Case

Recall Krista. Her restricted carbohydrate intake provides negligible fiber because fiber occurs naturally only in plant sources of carbohydrates. What other nutrients may be lacking in her eating pattern due to her restricted intake of grains, fruits, vegetables, and legumes? What would you teach Krista about the role of carbohydrates and fiber in health? What does she need to know about increasing her fiber intake?

Insoluble Fiber
nondigestible carbohydrates that absorb but do not dissolve in water.

Soluble Fiber
nondigestible carbohydrates that dissolve to a gummy, viscous texture.

Dietary Fiber
carbohydrates and lignin that are natural and intact components of plants that cannot be digested by human enzymes.

Functional Fiber
as proposed by the Food and Nutrition Board, functional fiber consists of extracted or isolated nondigestible carbohydrates that have beneficial physiologic effects in humans.

Total Fiber
total fiber = dietary fiber + functional fiber.

The National Academy of Sciences recommends that the terms *insoluble* and *soluble* be phased out in favor of ascribing specific physiologic benefits to a particular fiber. **Dietary fiber** refers to the intact and naturally occurring fiber in plants; **functional fiber** refers to fiber that has been isolated or extracted from plants and added to food, such as inulin added to some yogurt. The sum of dietary and functional fiber equals **total fiber**. The rationale for discontinuing soluble and insoluble fiber is that the amounts of soluble and insoluble fibers measured in a mixed diet are dependent on methods of analysis that are not able to exactly replicate human digestion.

It is commonly assumed that fiber does not provide any calories because it is not truly digested by human enzymes and may actually trap macronutrients eaten at the same time and prevent them from being absorbed. Yet most fibers, particularly soluble fibers, are fermented by bacteria in the colon to produce carbon dioxide, methane, hydrogen, and short-chain fatty acids, which serve as a source of energy (calories) for the mucosal lining of the colon. Although the exact energy value available to humans from the blend of fibers in food is unknown, it is estimated that the fermentation of fiber in the average human gut yields between 1.5 and 2.5 cal/g (Institute of Medicine, 2005).

SOURCES OF CARBOHYDRATES

Added Sugars
caloric sugars and syrups added to foods during processing or preparation or consumed separately; do not include sugars naturally present in foods, such as fructose in fruit and lactose in milk.

Sources of carbohydrates include natural sugars in fruit and milk; starch in grains, vegetables, legumes, and nuts; and **added sugars** in foods with empty calories. Servings of most of the commonly consumed grains, fruit, and vegetables contain only 1 to 3 g of dietary fiber. Table 2.2 shows the fiber content of fiber rich foods. Figure 2.2 shows the average carbohydrate and fiber content of each MyPlate food group.

	Fruits Focus on whole fruits	**Vegetables** Vary your veggies	**Grains** Make half your grains whole grains	**Protein** Vary your protein routine		**Dairy** Move to low-fat or fat-free milk or yogurt
				Legumes	Seeds & Nuts	
Carbohydrate g/svg	15	Watery veg: 5 Starchy veg: 15	15	15	4	12
Fiber g/svg	2	2–3	Refined grains 0–1 Whole grains 2+	5–8	2	0
Serving sizes **	1 small fresh fruit 1/2 c canned fruit or unsweetened fruit juice 2 Tbsp dried fruit	1/2 c cooked or 1 c raw non-starchy vegetables 1/2 c most starchy vegetables	1 slice bread 1 oz ready to eat cereal 1/2 c cooked rice, pasta, or cereal	1/2 c cooked	1/2 oz	1 c milk, yogurt, or soy beverage
Exceptions	Fruit juice does not supply fiber	Vegetables with skin (e.g., baked potato) and seeds (e.g., tomato) provide more fiber than skinless, seedless	Added sugars increase CHO content of sweetened cereals High fiber cereals may have 10+ g fiber/svg	No other items in this group naturally contain CHO or fiber		Natural cheese does not provide CHO Sweetened yogurts may have 45 g CHO or more per cup

* No CHO or fiber in the oils category.
** Serving sizes as per the American Diabetes Association/Academy of Nutrition and Dietetics.

Figure 2.2 ▲ **Carbohydrate and fiber content of MyPlate food groups.** *(Sources: U.S. Department of Agriculture, Center for Nutrition Policy and Promotion. [2016]. Available at www.choosemyplate.gov. Accessed on 1/25/16; and American Diabetes Association & Academy of Nutrition and Dietetics. [2014].* Choose your foods: Food lists for weight management. *Alexandria, VA: American Diabetes Association; Chicago, IL: American Dietetic Association.)*

Table 2.2   Fiber Content of Fiber-Rich Foods

Food	Total Fiber (g)
Fruit (1 medium unless otherwise specified)	
Apple with skin	4.0
Banana	3.0
Orange	4.0
Pear	6.0
Strawberries (1 cup)	3.0
Grains (½ cup unless otherwise specified)	
All-Bran cereal	10.0
Brown rice	2.0
Bulgur	4.0
Oats (dry)	4.0
Quinoa	2.5
Whole wheat pasta	3.0
Whole wheat bread (1 slice)	2.0
Legumes (½ cup cooked)	
Black	7.5
Kidney	8.0
Lentils	8.0
Lima	7.0
Navy	9.5
White	9.5
Nuts (1 oz)	
Almonds (24 nuts)	4.0
Cashews (18 nuts)	1.0
Flaxseed	8.0
Pistachios (47 nuts)	3.0
Walnuts (14 halves)	2.0
Vegetables (½ cup cooked)	
Broccoli	2.5
Brussels sprouts	3.0
Savoy cabbage	2.0
Collards	2.5
Mustard greens	2.5
Green peas	7.0
Edamame	3.0

Source: Palmer, S. (2008). The top fiber-rich foods list. *Today's Dietitian, 10*(7), 28. Available at http://www.todaysdietitian.com /newarchives/063008p28.shtml. Accessed on 11/13/16.

Grains

This group is synonymous with "carbs" and consists of grains (e.g., wheat, barley, oats, rye, corn, and rice) and products made with flours from grains (e.g., bread, crackers, pasta, and tortillas).

Grains are classified as "whole" or "refined" (Box 2.1). **Whole grains** consist of the entire kernel of a grain (Fig. 2.3). They may be eaten whole as a complete food (e.g., oatmeal, brown rice, or popcorn) or milled into flour to be used as an ingredient in bread, cereal, pasta, and baked goods. Even when whole grains are ground, cracked, or flaked, they must have the same proportion of the original three parts:

- The bran, or tough outer coating, which provides fiber, antioxidants, B vitamins, iron, zinc, copper, magnesium, and **phytonutrients**
- The endosperm, the largest portion of the kernel, which supplies starch, protein, and small amounts of vitamins and minerals
- The germ (embryo), the smallest portion of the kernel that contains B vitamins, some protein, unsaturated fat, vitamin E, antioxidants, and phytonutrients. Its unsaturated fat content makes whole wheat flour more susceptible to rancidity than refined flour.

Whole Grains
contain the entire grain, or seed, which includes the endosperm, bran, and germ.

Phytonutrients
also known as phytochemicals, are bioactive, nonnutrient plant compounds associated with a reduced risk of chronic diseases.

Refined Grains
consist of only the endosperm (middle part) of the grain and therefore do not contain the bran and germ portions.

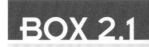

BOX 2.1 Sources of Whole and Refined Grains

Whole Grains	Refined Grains
Whole wheat grain, including varieties of spelt, emmer, farro, einkorn, bulgur, cracked wheat, and wheat berries	Original Cream of Wheat, puffed wheat, refined ready-to-eat wheat cereals
Products made with whole wheat flour, such as 100% whole wheat bread, whole wheat pasta, shredded wheat, Wheaties, whole wheat tortillas, whole wheat crackers	Products made with enriched white or wheat flour as found in white or wheat bread, white pasta, flour tortillas, refined crackers
Whole oats, oatmeal, Cheerios	Oat flour
Brown rice	White rice, Rice Krispies, cream of rice, puffed rice
Corn, popcorn	Cornstarch, grits, hominy, cornflakes
Whole-grain barley, whole rye, teff, triticale, millet, amaranth*, buckwheat*, sorghum*, quinoa*, wild rice*	

*Considered whole grains but are technically not cereals but rather pseudocereals.

Enrichment
adding back certain nutrients (to specific levels) that were lost during processing.

Fortified
adding nutrients that are not naturally present in the food or were present in insignificant amounts.

Bran cereals and wheat germ are not whole grains because they come from only one part of the whole.

"Refined" grains have most of the bran and germ removed. They are rich in starch but lack the fiber, B vitamins, vitamin E, trace minerals, unsaturated fat, and most of the phytonutrients found in whole grains (International Food Information Council, 2014). The process of **enrichment** restores some B vitamins (thiamin, riboflavin, and niacin) and iron to levels found prior to processing. Other substances that are lost, such as other vitamins, other minerals, fiber, and phytonutrients, are not replaced by enrichment. Enriched grains are also required to be **fortified** with folic acid, a mandate designed to reduce the risk of neural tube defects. Examples of refined grains include white flour,

Figure 2.3 ▶
Whole wheat. The components of the whole wheat kernel are the *bran*, the *germ*, and the *endosperm*.

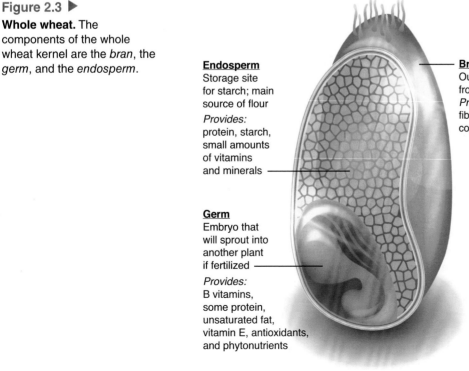

Endosperm
Storage site for starch; main source of flour
Provides:
protein, starch, small amounts of vitamins and minerals

Germ
Embryo that will sprout into another plant if fertilized
Provides:
B vitamins, some protein, unsaturated fat, vitamin E, antioxidants, and phytonutrients

Bran
Outer layer that protects rest of kernel from sunlight, pests, water, and disease
Provides:
fiber, antioxidants, B vitamins, iron, zinc, copper, magnesium, and phytonutrients

Refined grains:
• made only from endosperm
• are enriched with thiamin, riboflavin, niacin, and iron lost through processing
• are fortified with folic acid
• are inferior to whole grains in vitamin B6, protein, pantothenic acid, vitamin E, phytonutrients, antioxidants, fiber

white bread, white rice, flour tortillas, and grits. Whether whole or refined, an ounce-equivalent of grain (e.g., one slice of bread or ½ cup of pasta) is estimated to provide 15 g of carbohydrates. Fiber content can range from 0 to 1 g in refined grains to 10 g or more per serving of high-fiber cereals. Some items in this group, such as sweetened ready-to-eat cereals, muffins, and pancakes, have added sugar.

Vegetables

Starch and some sugars provide the majority of calories in vegetables, but the content varies widely among individual vegetables. Generally, a ½ cup serving of starchy vegetables, such as corn, peas, potatoes, and yams, provides approximately 15 g carbohydrates. In comparison, "watery" vegetables, such as asparagus, broccoli, carrots, and green beans provide 5 g carbohydrate or less per ½ cup serving.

Fruits

Generally, almost all of the calories in fruit come from the natural sugars fructose and glucose. (The exceptions to this are avocado, olives, and coconut, which get the majority of their calories from fat.) According to the American Diabetes Association's Food Lists, a serving of fruit, defined as ½ cup of 100% juice, 1 small fresh fruit, ½ cup of canned or frozen fruit, or 2 tbsp of dried fruit, provides 15 g carbohydrate (American Diabetes Association & Academy of Nutrition and Dietetics, 2014). Because the skin of fruits provides fiber, fresh whole fruits provide more fiber than do fresh peeled fruits, canned fruits, or fruit juices. The effect of processing on fiber content is demonstrated in the examples on the left.

	Fiber (g/serving)
Unpeeled fresh apple (1)	3.0
Peeled fresh apple (1)	1.9
Applesauce (½ cup)	1.5
Apple juice (½ cup)	Negligible

Dairy

Although milk is considered a "protein," more of milk's calories come from carbohydrate than from protein. One cup of milk, regardless of the fat content, provides 12 g of carbohydrate in the form of lactose. Flavored milk and yogurt have added sugars, as do ice cream and frozen yogurt. With the exception of cottage cheese, which has about 6 g of carbohydrate per cup, natural cheese is virtually lactose free because lactose is converted to lactic acid during production. The carbohydrate content, including both natural and added sugars, of various dairy foods is listed in the box on the left.

	Carbohydrate (g)
Milk, 8 oz	12
Chocolate milk, 8 oz	26
Plain yogurt, 8 oz	15
Strawberry yogurt, 8 oz	48.5
Regular vanilla ice cream, ½ cup	15.6
Swiss cheese, 1 oz	1

Added Sugars

Added sugars are sugars and sweeteners used as an ingredient in a food or beverage, such as white sugar, maple syrup, honey, corn syrup, or agave syrup. Sugar has many functional roles in foods including taste, physical properties, antimicrobial purposes, and chemical properties. Sugar adds flavor and interest. Few would question the value brown sugar adds to a bowl of hot oatmeal. Besides its sweet taste, sugar has important functions in baked goods, such as promoting tenderness in cakes. In jams and jellies, sugar inhibits the growth of mold; in candy, it influences texture.

However, added sugars are considered empty calories because they provide calories with few or no nutrients. Sometimes, 100% of the calories in a food are from added sugar, such as in sweetened soft drinks, pancake syrup, and hard candies. In other products, added sugars account for only some of the calories. For instance, in the chocolate milk listed earlier, added sugars provide 14 g (56 empty calories) of the 26 g total carbohydrate content, with the remaining 12 g coming from the natural sugar lactose. Only the calories of the added sugar are considered "empty."

Figure 2.4 ▶

A molecule of sucrose is half glucose and half fructose.

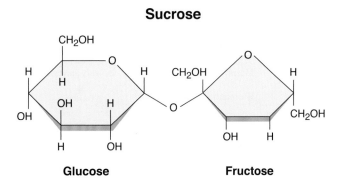

Sucrose

Glucose   Fructose

Figure 2.4 ▶

A molecule of sucrose is half glucose and half fructose.

Quick Bite Carbohydrate and calorie content of selected added sugars

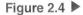

	Carbohydrate (g)	Calories
White sugar, 1 tsp	4.0	16
Jam, 1 tbsp	13.0	52
Gelatin, ½ cup	19.0	76
Pancake syrup, 2 tbsp	25.0	100
Cola drink, 12 oz	40.0	160

An added sugar that generates a lot of controversy is high-fructose corn syrup (HFCS), a commercial sweetener made from enzymatically treated corn syrup. HFCS is composed of glucose and either 42% or 55% fructose, making it similar in composition to sucrose, which is 50% glucose and 50% fructose (Fig. 2.4). HFCS is widely used in food and beverages not only because it provides the same sweetness as white sugar but also because it has other desirable functional properties, such as enhancing spice and fruit flavors. A review of short-term randomized controlled trials, cross-sectional studies, and review articles consistently found little evidence that HFCS differs uniquely from sucrose and other nutritive sweeteners in metabolic effects (e.g., levels of circulating glucose, insulin, postprandial triglycerides), subjective effects (e.g., hunger, satiety, calorie intake at subsequent meals), and adverse effects such as risk of weight gain (Fitch & Keim, 2012).

HOW THE BODY HANDLES CARBOHYDRATES

Digestion and Absorption

Cooked starch begins to undergo digestion in the mouth by the action of salivary amylase, but the overall effect is small because food is not held in the mouth very long (Fig. 2.5). The stomach churns and mixes its contents, but its acid medium halts any residual effect of the swallowed amylase. Fibers delay gastric emptying and thus provide **satiety**.

Most carbohydrate digestion and absorption occurs in the small intestine. Pancreatic amylase, secreted into the intestine by way of the pancreatic duct, reduces polysaccharides to shorter glucose chains and maltose. Disaccharidase enzymes (maltase, sucrase, and lactase) on the surface of the intestinal cells split maltose, sucrose, and lactose, respectively, into monosaccharides. Monosaccharides, whether consumed as monosaccharides or resulting from the digestion of disaccharides or polysaccharides, are absorbed through intestinal mucosa cells and travel to the liver via the portal vein.

Normally, most starches and all sugars are digested within 1 to 4 hours after eating. Small amounts of starch that have not been fully digested pass into the colon and are excreted in the stools. Fibers, which are nondigestible, advance to the large intestine where they attract water, which softens stool and promotes laxation. Some fibers are fermented by **gut microbiota**, which yields water, methane, hydrogen, and short-chain fatty acids. These fatty acids are used by the colon for energy or are absorbed and metabolized by liver cells.

Satiety
the feeling of fullness and satisfaction after eating.

Gut Microbiota
also known as gut flora, is the collective term for the microorganisms that inhabit the gut.

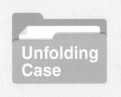

Unfolding Case

Consider Krista. After increasing her fiber and fluid intake, she experiences cramping, distention, and gas and decides to go back to using a laxative daily. Why is Krista experiencing these symptoms? What questions would you ask to help identify the cause?

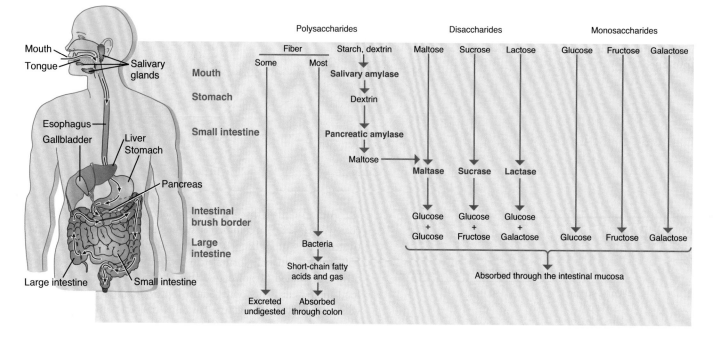

Figure 2.5 ▲ Carbohydrate digestion.

Metabolism

In the liver, fructose and galactose are converted to glucose. The liver releases glucose into the bloodstream, where its level is held fairly constant by the action of hormones. A rise in blood glucose concentration after eating causes the pancreas to secrete insulin, which moves glucose out of the bloodstream and into the cells. Most cells take only as much glucose as they need for immediate energy needs; muscle and liver cells take extra glucose to store as glycogen. The release of insulin lowers blood glucose to normal levels.

Postprandial
following a meal.

In the **postprandial** state, as the body uses the energy from the last meal, the blood glucose concentration begins to drop. Even a slight fall in blood glucose stimulates the pancreas to release glucagon, which causes the liver to release glucose from its supply of glycogen. The result is that blood glucose levels increase to normal.

Glycemic Response

It was commonly believed that sugars produce a greater increase in blood glucose levels, or **glycemic response**, than complex carbohydrates because they are rapidly and completely absorbed. This proved to be too simplistic of an assumption, as illustrated by the lower glycemic index of cola (sugar) compared to that of baked potatoes (complex carbohydrate) (Table 2.3). A food's glycemic response is actually influenced by many variables including the amounts of fat, fiber, and acid in the food; the degree of processing; the method of preparation; the amount eaten; the degree of ripeness (for fruits and vegetables); and whether other foods are eaten at the same time.

On a scale of 0 to 100, glycemic index ranks carbohydrates based on how quickly they raise blood glucose levels after eating. A food's **glycemic index** is determined by comparing the impact on blood glucose after 50 g of a food sample is eaten to the impact of 50 g of pure glucose or white bread. For instance, a baked potato with a glycemic index of 76 elicits 76% of the blood glucose response as an equivalent amount of pure glucose.

Glycemic Response
the effect a food has on the blood glucose concentration; how quickly the glucose level rises, how high it goes, and how long it takes to return to normal.

Glycemic Index
a numeric measure of the glycemic response of 50 g of a food sample; the higher the number, the higher the glycemic response.

Because the amount of carbohydrate contained in a typical portion of food also influences glycemic response, the concept of glycemic load was created to define a food's impact on blood glucose levels more accurately (see Table 2.3). It takes into account both the glycemic index of a food and the amount of carbohydrate in a serving of that food. For example, watermelon has a high glycemic index of 72, but because its carbohydrate content is low (it is mostly water), the glycemic load is only 4.

Table 2.3	Glycemic Index and Glycemic Load of Selected Foods	
Item	Glycemic Index (Glucose = 100)	Glycemic Load/Serving
White spaghetti	58	28
Baked potato	85	26
White bagel	72	25
Cornflakes	92	24
Long-grain white rice	56	24
Snickers bar	68	23
Jelly beans	78	22
Macaroni	45	22
Sweet corn	60	20
Honey	87	18
Boiled sweet potato	59	18
Shredded wheat	83	17
Coca-Cola	56	16
Steamed brown rice	50	16
Pound cake	54	15
Unsweetened clear apple juice	44	13
Banana	46	12
White bread	70	10
Chickpeas	33	10
All-Bran cereal	38	9
Reduced-fat yogurt	26	8
Watermelon	72	4
Orange	40	4
Premium ice cream	37	4
Low-fat ice cream	50	3
Peanuts	17	1

Source: Foster-Powell, K., Holt, S., & Brand-Miller, J. (2002). International table of glycemic index and glycemic load values: 2002. *The American Journal of Clinical Nutrition, 76*, 50–56.

Glycemic Load
a food's glycemic index multiplied by the amount of carbohydrate it contains to determine impact on blood glucose levels.

In a practical sense, **glycemic load** is not a reliable tool for choosing a healthy diet, and claims that a low glycemic index diet promotes significant weight loss or helps control appetite are unfounded. Soft drinks, candy, sugars, and high-fat foods may have a low to moderate glycemic index, but these foods are not nutritious and eating them does not promote weight loss. In addition, a food's actual impact on glucose levels is difficult to predict because of the many factors influencing glycemic load. However, glycemic index may help people with diabetes fine-tune optimal meal planning (see Chapter 19), and athletes can use the glycemic index to choose optimal fuels for before, during, and after exercise.

FUNCTIONS OF CARBOHYDRATES

Glucose metabolism is a dynamic state of balance between burning glucose for energy (*catabolism*) and using glucose to build other compounds (*anabolism*). This process is a continuous response to the supply of glucose from food and the demand for glucose for energy needs.

Glucose for Energy

The primary function of carbohydrates is to provide energy for cells. Glucose is burned more efficiently and more completely than either protein or fat, and it does not leave an end product that the body must excrete. Although muscles use a mixture of fat and glucose for energy, the brain is normally totally dependent on glucose for energy. All digestible carbohydrates—namely, simple sugars and complex carbohydrates—provide 4 cal/g. Depending on the extent to which fibers are fermented in the colon into short-chain fatty acids and metabolized, fibers provide 1.5 to 2.5 cal/g.

Protein Sparing

As a primary source of energy, carbohydrates spare protein and prevent ketosis. Although protein provides 4 cal/g just like carbohydrates, it has other specialized functions that only protein can perform, such as replenishing enzymes, hormones, antibodies, and blood cells. Consuming adequate carbohydrate to meet energy needs has the effect of "sparing protein" from being used for energy, leaving it available to do its special functions. An adequate carbohydrate intake is especially important whenever protein needs are increased such as for wound healing and during pregnancy and lactation.

Preventing Ketosis

Ketone Bodies
intermediate, acidic compounds formed from the incomplete breakdown of fat when adequate glucose is not available.

Fat normally supplies about half of the body's energy requirement. Yet, glucose fragments are needed to efficiently and completely burn fat for energy. Without adequate glucose, fat oxidation prematurely stops at the intermediate step of **ketone body** formation. Although muscles and other tissues can use ketone bodies for energy, they are normally produced only in small quantities. An increased production of ketone bodies and their accumulation in the bloodstream cause nausea, fatigue, loss of appetite, and ketoacidosis. Dehydration and sodium depletion may follow as the body tries to excrete ketones in the urine.

Using Glucose to Make Other Compounds

After energy needs are met, excess glucose can be converted to glycogen, be used to make nonessential amino acids and specific body compounds, or be converted to fat and stored.

Glycogen

The body's backup supply of glucose is liver glycogen. Liver and muscle cells pick up extra glucose molecules during times of plenty and join them together to form glycogen, which can quickly release glucose in times of need. Typically one-third of the body's glycogen reserve is in the liver and can be released into circulation for all body cells to use, and two-thirds is in muscle, which is available only for use by muscles. Unlike fat, glycogen storage is limited and may provide only enough calories for about a half-day of moderate activity.

Nonessential Amino Acids

If an adequate supply of essential amino acids is available, the body can use them and glucose to make nonessential amino acids.

Carbohydrate-Containing Compounds

The body can convert glucose to other essential carbohydrates such as ribose, a component of RNA and DNA, keratin sulfate (in fingernails), and hyaluronic acid (found in the fluid that lubricates the joints and vitreous humor of the eyeball).

Fat

Any glucose remaining at this point—after energy needs are met, glycogen stores are saturated, and other specific compounds are made—is converted by liver cells to triglycerides and stored in the body's fat tissue. The body does this by combining acetate molecules to form fatty acids, which then are combined with glycerol to make triglycerides. Although it sounds easy for excess carbohydrates to be converted to fat, it is not a primary pathway; the body prefers to make body fat from dietary fat, not carbohydrates.

DIETARY REFERENCE INTAKES

Total Carbohydrate

The Recommended Dietary Allowance (RDA) for total carbohydrate (starch, natural sugar, added sugar) is set at 130 g for both adults and children, based on the average *minimum* amount of glucose that is needed to fuel the brain and assuming total calorie intake is adequate (National Research Council, 2005). Yet at this level, total calorie needs are not met unless protein and fat intakes exceed levels considered healthy. A more useful guideline for determining appropriate carbohydrate intake is the Acceptable Macronutrient Distribution Range (AMDR), which recommends carbohydrates provide 45% to 65% of total calories consumed (National Research Council, 2005). As illustrated in Figure 2.6, the carbohydrate content using AMDR standards is significantly higher than the minimum of 130 g/day. The Daily Value for carbohydrate on the new "Nutrition Facts" label (to be fully implemented by July 26, 2018) is set at 275 g, which equates to 55% of total calories in the reference 2000-calorie meal plan.

According to the National Health and Nutrition Examination Survey (NHANES) 2011–2012 data, the mean carbohydrate intake for men 20 years and older was 305 g or 48% of total calories consumed. For women in the same age category, the mean intake of carbohydrate was 228 g or 50% of total calories consumed (U.S. Department of Agriculture & Agricultural Research Service, 2014a, 2014 b).

Fiber

An Adequate Intake (AI) for total fiber is set at 14 g/1000 calories or approximately 25 g/day for women and 38 g/day for men (National Research Council, 2005). Fiber is not an essential nutrient that must be consumed through food in order to prevent a deficiency disease; the recommendation is based on intake levels that have been observed to protect against coronary heart disease based on epidemiologic and clinical data. Mean fiber intake among American men and women 20 years and older is 20.3 g and 16.1 g, respectively (U.S. Department of Agriculture & Agricultural Research Service, 2014a), about half as much fiber as recommended.

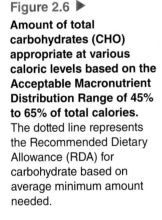

Figure 2.6 ▶

Amount of total carbohydrates (CHO) appropriate at various caloric levels based on the Acceptable Macronutrient Distribution Range of 45% to 65% of total calories. The dotted line represents the Recommended Dietary Allowance (RDA) for carbohydrate based on average minimum amount needed.

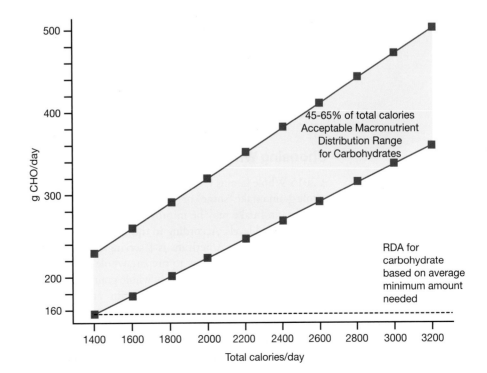

CARBOHYDRATES IN HEALTH PROMOTION

Americans, on average, consume an appropriate percentage of their calories from carbohydrates but are urged to make healthier choices, namely more whole grains and less refined grains and less added sugars. Fiber is identified as a shortfall nutrient in the typical American intake and a public health concern because under consumption is linked to adverse health outcomes—and under consumption of fiber is linked to low intakes of fruits, vegetables, and whole grains (U.S. Department of Health and Human Services [USDHHS] & U.S. Department of Agriculture [USDA], 2015).

Increase Whole Grains

Although more than half of all Americans meet or exceed the recommended intake of total grains, they do not eat enough whole grains. The *2015-2020 Dietary Guidelines for Americans* state that healthy eating patterns include whole grains and to limit refined grains and products made with refined grains, especially those high in saturated fat, added sugars, or sodium. At least half of total grain intake should be from whole grains. Consumers need to understand that the recommendation to eat whole grains is qualified by the advice that whole grains *replace* refined grains, not that they are simply added to usual grain intake.

Although whole grains may be best known for their fiber content, the health benefits are likely due to the "whole package" of healthful components, including essential fatty acids, antioxidants, vitamins, minerals, and phytonutrients (International Food Information Council, 2014). A position of the American Society for Nutrition states that consuming foods rich in cereal fiber or mixtures of whole grains and bran is modestly associated with a lower risk of obesity, type 2 diabetes, and cardiovascular disease (Cho, Lu, Fahey, & Klurfeld, 2013). Potential health benefits are highlighted below.

- Two large prospective cohort studies indicate that higher whole grain intake is associated with lower total and cardiovascular mortality in American men and women, independent of other dietary and lifestyle factors (Wu et al., 2015).
- A study among low-income and African Americans living in the southeast showed that eating a healthy diet that included at least 1.5 servings of whole grains per day is associated with a 14% to 23% lower death rate from all diseases combined as well as from cardiovascular disease, cancer, and other diseases (Yu et al., 2015).
- Observational studies in the United States suggest a strong inverse relationship between whole-grain intake and gastrointestinal cancers, certain hormone-related cancers, and pancreatic cancer (Jonnalagadda et al., 2011).
- Epidemiologic studies suggest populations that have higher intakes of dietary fiber have lower body weights (Dahl & Stewart, 2015).
- The fiber in whole grains is credited with promoting laxation by increasing stool bulk and hastening intestinal transit time.
- The fermentation of fiber to short-chain fatty acids in the large intestine may be protective against systemic inflammation and thereby play an important role in immunity (Meijer, de Vox, & Priebe, 2010).

Choosing Whole Grains

A 2015 Whole Grains Consumer Insights Survey indicates 64% of Americans have increased their whole grain intake "some" or "a lot" since 2010 (Oldways Whole Grains Council, 2015). Although whole grain intake may be improving among some Americans, overall intake still remains below recommended levels. According to the *2015-2020 Dietary Guidelines for Americans*, average whole grain intake among Americans is 1 serving/day or less (USDHHS & USDA, 2015). Cost, taste, and unfamiliarity with how to prepare whole grains are barriers to increasing whole grain intake, as is consumer inability to identify whole grain products. For instance, breads, ready-to-eat cereals, and pastas labeled "made with whole grain" and "100% wheat flour" are not whole grains. Labels that state a product is "100% whole wheat" or "stoneground whole (grain)" indicate whole grains. "Whole wheat" or "whole (grain)" should be the first ingredient on the list or second ingredient after water (Fig. 2.7). Enriched wheat flour indicates the product is not whole grain. Tips for eating more whole grains appear in Box 2.2.

BOX 2.2   Tips for Increasing Whole Grain Intake

Substitute

- Whole wheat bread or rolls for white bread or rolls
- Brown rice for white rice
- Whole wheat pasta or pasta that is part whole wheat, part white flour for white pasta
- Whole wheat pita for white pita
- Whole wheat tortillas for flour tortillas
- Whole wheat English muffins for white English muffins
- Whole grain for refined cereals
- Whole wheat flour or oats for half of the white flour in pancakes, waffles, or muffins
- Whole wheat bread or cracker crumbs for white crumbs as a coating or breading for meat, fish, and poultry
- Whole corn meal for refined corn meal in corn cakes, corn bread, and corn muffins

Add

- Barley, brown rice, or bulgur to soups, stews, bread stuffing, and casseroles
- A handful of oats or whole grain cereal to yogurt

Snack on

- Ready-to-eat whole grain cereal, such as shredded wheat or toasted oat cereal
- Whole grain baked tortilla chips
- Whole grain crackers
- Popcorn

Decrease

- Desserts and sweet snacks made with refined flour, such as cakes, cookies, and pastries, which are also high in added sugars, solid fats, or both and a source of excess calories

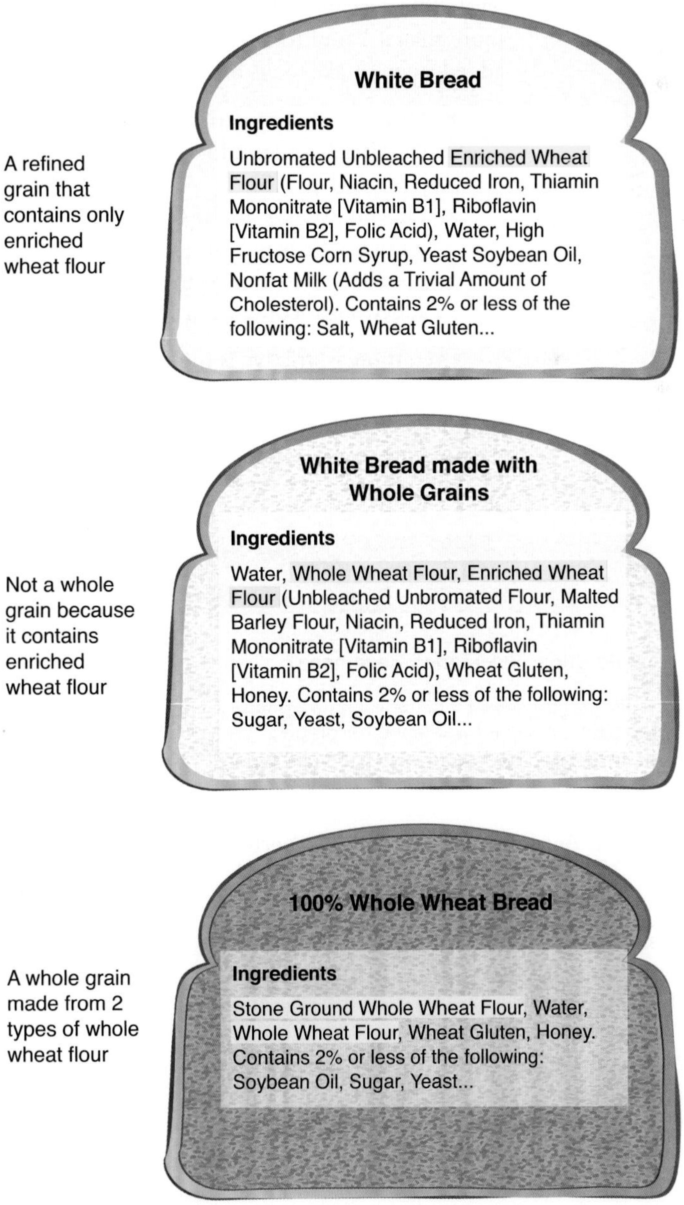

Figure 2.7 ▶

A comparison of ingredient lists to identify whole grains.

A refined grain that contains only enriched wheat flour

White Bread

Ingredients

Unbromated Unbleached Enriched Wheat Flour (Flour, Niacin, Reduced Iron, Thiamin Mononitrate [Vitamin B1], Riboflavin [Vitamin B2], Folic Acid), Water, High Fructose Corn Syrup, Yeast Soybean Oil, Nonfat Milk (Adds a Trivial Amount of Cholesterol). Contains 2% or less of the following: Salt, Wheat Gluten...

Not a whole grain because it contains enriched wheat flour

White Bread made with Whole Grains

Ingredients

Water, Whole Wheat Flour, Enriched Wheat Flour (Unbleached Unbromated Flour, Malted Barley Flour, Niacin, Reduced Iron, Thiamin Mononitrate [Vitamin B1], Riboflavin [Vitamin B2], Folic Acid), Wheat Gluten, Honey. Contains 2% or less of the following: Sugar, Yeast, Soybean Oil...

A whole grain made from 2 types of whole wheat flour

100% Whole Wheat Bread

Ingredients

Stone Ground Whole Wheat Flour, Water, Whole Wheat Flour, Wheat Gluten, Honey. Contains 2% or less of the following: Soybean Oil, Sugar, Yeast...

People who choose whole grains for all of their grain choices are urged to choose some whole grains that are fortified with folic acid because the content of folic acid is naturally lower in whole grains than in enriched refined grains. This is especially true for women who are capable of becoming pregnant because folic acid helps lower the risk of neural tube defects.

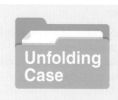

Think of Krista. She has increased her intake of grains, fruits, vegetables, and legumes but admits she doesn't like whole wheat bread or whole grains in any form. What other specific strategies should she try to increase her fiber intake?

Limit Added Sugars

The *2015-2020 Dietary Guidelines for Americans* recommend added sugars be limited to less than 10% of total calories to help ensure an adequate intake of nutrients while keeping calorie intake at an appropriate level, not because research shows sugar causes negative health effects above that level. The average added sugar intake in the United States accounts for almost 270 calories or more than 13% of total calories per day (USDHHS & USDA, 2015). Suggestions for limiting added sugar intake focus on (Box 2.3)

- Limiting or eliminating sugar-sweetened beverages. Beverages (excluding milk and 100% fruit juice) account for the greatest percentage of added sugars in a typical American eating pattern (Fig. 2.8).
- Limiting sweets and desserts. Added sugars and % Daily Value for added sugars are required to be listed on the new Nutrition Facts label for most manufactured foods by July 26, 2018. This change in food labeling regulations will enable consumers to easily identify added sugar content for the first time since packaged foods began using food labels.

Even more restrictive is the American Heart Association's recommendation that most American women limit added sugar intake to a maximum of 100 calories per day (25 g or 6 tsp) and that most American men limit their added sugar intake to 150 calories or less per day (38 g or 9 tsp) (American Heart Association, 2015).

BOX 2.3   Ways to Limit Added Sugars

Cut Back or Eliminate Sugar-Sweetened Beverages

- Choose beverages with no added sugars, such as water or flavored water, in place of sugar sweetened beverages.
- Consume sugar-sweetened beverages less often and reduce the portion size consumed.

Limit Sweetened Grain-Based and Dairy-Based Desserts and Candy

- Limit desserts and snacks made with added sugars, such as candy, cookies, brownies, doughnuts, sweet rolls, pastries, cakes, ice cream, other frozen desserts, and puddings.
- Eat smaller portions less often.

Rely on Natural Sugars in Fruit to Satisfy a "Sweet Tooth"

- Choose fruit instead of sweetened desserts and snacks to reduce the intake of added sugars and boost vitamin, mineral, phytonutrient, and fiber intake.

Read Labels

- "Nutrition Facts" labels (see Chapter 9) list the amount of total sugars; added sugars are required to be listed by July 26, 2018. The Daily Value for added sugars will be 50 g, based on the recommendation that added sugars provide 10% or less of total calories consumed. If total calories consumed are less than 2000, the %Daily Value listed on the food label will underestimate the actual percent of calories from added sugar.

Consider Using Sugar Alternatives Such as Sugar Alcohols or Nonnutritive Sweeteners

- Artificially sweetened low-calorie or calorie-free beverages can reduce calorie and added sugar intake, but their effectiveness as a long-term weight loss strategy is not certain. The high-intensity sweeteners approved for use in the United States are safe for the general population when consumed under intended conditions of use.

Figure 2.8 ▶

Sources of added sugar in the U.S. population ages 2 years and older. *(Source: U.S. Department of Agriculture & U.S. Department of Health and Human Services. [2015]. 2015-2020 Dietary guidelines for Americans [8th ed.]. Available at health.gov /dietaryguidelines/2015. Accessed on 2/1/16.)*

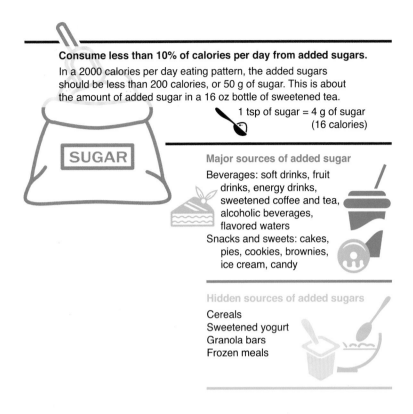

Consume less than 10% of calories per day from added sugars.
In a 2000 calories per day eating pattern, the added sugars should be less than 200 calories, or 50 g of sugar. This is about the amount of added sugar in a 16 oz bottle of sweetened tea.

1 tsp of sugar = 4 g of sugar
(16 calories)

Major sources of added sugar

Beverages: soft drinks, fruit drinks, energy drinks, sweetened coffee and tea, alcoholic beverages, flavored waters
Snacks and sweets: cakes, pies, cookies, brownies, ice cream, candy

Hidden sources of added sugars

Cereals
Sweetened yogurt
Granola bars
Frozen meals

To some extent, sugar is inaccurately blamed for a variety of health problems. The idea that sugar causes hyperactivity in children has been around for decades, even though there is no supporting evidence, even among children who are reported to be sensitive to sugar. Clinical practice guidelines for the treatment of attention deficit-hyperactivity disorder (ADHD) in children state there is a lack of evidence that removing sugar from the diet of a child with ADHD results in fewer symptoms (Ballard, Hall, & Kaufmann, 2010). Similarly, type 2 diabetes is commonly blamed on a high-sugar diet, even though increasing intakes of sugar is not linked to increasing risk of diabetes. Type 2 diabetes is related to excess body weight, not to eating too much sugar.

Although some health problems may be wrongly attributed to sugar, excess added sugar intake may be harmful. Epidemiologic studies suggest that higher intakes of added sugar are linked to cardiovascular disease risk factors and a prospective cohort study recently showed that people who consumed 17% to 21% of their daily calories from added sugar had a 38% higher risk of dying from cardiovascular disease compared to those who consumed 8% of their total calories from added sugar (Yang et al., 2014). In addition, diets high in added sugar are more likely to be inadequate in essential nutrients (if empty calorie foods displace more nutritious ones), excessive in calories (if empty calorie foods are added to the diet), or both.

Polyols
sugar alcohols produced from the fermentation or hydrogenation of monosaccharides or disaccharides; most originate from sucrose or glucose and maltose in starches.

Nonnutritive Sweeteners
synthetically made sweeteners that provide minimal or no carbohydrate and calories; also known as artificial sweeteners.

Sugar Alternatives

One way to reduce sugar intake and not forsake sweetened foods is to consume sugar alternatives, such as **polyols** and **nonnutritive sweeteners**, in place of regular sugar.

Polyols

Polyols, or sugar alcohols, are used as sweeteners but are not true sugars or alcohols; they are derived from hydrogenated sugars and starches (Table 2.4). Although polyols occur naturally in some fruits, vegetables, and fermented foods such as wine and soy sauce, the majority of polyols in the food supply are commercially synthesized. With the exception of xylitol, they are all less sweet than sucrose, so they are often combined with nonnutritive sweeteners in sugarless foods. Sugar alcohols are approved for use in a variety of products, including candies, chewing gum, jams and jellies, baked goods, and frozen confections.

Foods containing polyols and no added sugars can be labeled as sugar free (Fitch & Keim, 2012). Polyols offer some advantages to sugar:

- They are not fermented by mouth bacteria and thus do not cause dental caries. Because they are noncariogenic, they are often used in items held in the mouth, such as chewing gum and breath mints.
- They are considered low-calorie sweeteners because they are incompletely absorbed. Their calorie value ranges from 1.6 to 3.0 cal/g.
- Because they are generally slowly and incompletely absorbed and/or metabolized differently than true sugars, they produce a smaller effect on blood glucose levels and insulin response, making them attractive to people with diabetes.
- Polyols that are not fully absorbed in the small intestine enter the large intestine where they function as a prebiotic; they are fermented into short-chain fatty acids, which foster the growth of colonic bacteria.

The disadvantage of polyols is that because they are incompletely absorbed, they can produce a laxative effect (abdominal gas, discomfort, osmotic diarrhea) when they are fermented in the large intestine. Laxation thresholds are included in Table 2.4.

Table 2.4   Polyols

Polyol	Relative Sweetness (Sucrose = 100)	Calories per Gram	Laxation Threshold (per day)	Sources/Uses
Sorbitol	60	2.6	50 g	Made from corn syrup or glucose Used in sugar-free candies and chewing gums and sugar-free foods such as frozen desserts and baked goods
Mannitol	50	1.6	20 g	Extracted from seaweed or made from mannose Used as dusting powder on chewing gum, in chocolate-flavored coatings for ice cream and candy
Xylitol	100	2.4	50 g	Produced from birch and other hardwood trees Used in chewing gum, hard candies
Maltitol	90	2.1	40–100 g	Made from maltose in corn syrup Used in sugarless hard candies, chewing gum, baked goods, ice cream
Lactitol	40	2.0	20–50 g	Derived from lactose Used in low-calorie, low-fat, and/or low-sugar foods such as ice cream, chocolate candy, baked goods, chewing gum
Isomalt	45–65	2.0	40–50 g	Made from sucrose Used in hard candies, toffee, chewing gum, baked goods, nutritional supplements
Hydrogenated starch hydrolysates	40–90	3.0 or less	40–100 g	Produced from partial breakdown of corn, wheat, or potato starch Used in candy, baked goods
Erythritol	70	0.2	Because it is rapidly absorbed in the small intestine, it is not likely to produce laxative side effects.	Derived from glucose in corn or wheat starch Used as a bulk sweetener in reduced-calorie foods

Sources: Calorie Control Council. (2016). *Facts about polyols*. Available at http://polyol.org/facts-about-polyols/. Accessed on 1/24/16; and Fitch, C., & Keim, K. S. (2012). Position of the Academy of Nutrition and Dietetics: Use of nutritive and non-nutritive sweeteners. *Journal of the Academy of Nutrition and Dietetics, 112,* 739–758.

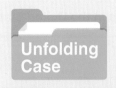

Consider Krista. She wondered if eating several pieces of dietetic chocolate candy sweetened with sugar alcohols every day would help prevent constipation. She was shocked to discover that 5 pieces of sugarless dark chocolate contains almost 200 calories, mostly from fat, and quickly ruled candy out as an option. She asks if she can chew several pieces of sugarless gum every day to improve laxation without consuming calories. How do you respond?

Nonnutritive Sweeteners

Nonnutritive sweeteners are virtually calorie free and are hundreds to thousands of times sweeter than sugar. Sometimes, combinations of nonnutritive sweeteners are used in a food to produce a synergistically sweeter taste, decrease the amount of sweetener needed, and minimize aftertaste. They have different functional properties, which influences how they are used in foods. Because they do not raise blood glucose levels, nonnutritive sweeteners appeal to people with diabetes. The nonnutritive sweeteners approved by the U.S. Food and Drug Administration (FDA) for use in the United States are featured in Table 2.5.

Risks and Benefits of Nonnutritive Sweeteners

At first glance, nonnutritive sweeteners appear to answer Americans' passion for calorie-free sweetness. But are they safe for everyone, including pregnant and lactating women? Do they help people manage their weight? Are they appropriate for people with diabetes?

> **Acceptable Daily Intake (ADI)**
> the estimated amount of a food additive that a person can safely consume every day over a lifetime without risk.

Safety. The FDA is responsible for approving the safety of all food additives, including nonnutritive sweeteners. When consumed at levels within the **Acceptable Daily Intake (ADI)**, all FDA-approved nonnutritive sweeteners are safe for use by the general public, including pregnant and lactating women. Although it is difficult to determine the intake of food additives, including nonnutritive sweeteners, the FDA has determined that estimated daily intake would not exceed ADI limits even among high users (USDHHS& USDA, 2015).

Weight Management. Nonnutritive sweeteners are not a panacea for weight control. In theory, use of nonnutritive sweeteners in place of sugar can save 16 cal/tsp, or 160 calories in a 12-oz can of cola. Eliminating one regularly sweetened soft drink per day for 22 days (160 calories × 22 days = 3520 calories) translates to a 1-pound loss (3500 calories equals 1 pound of body weight) without any other changes in eating or activity. This is because all calories in the regular soft drink have been eliminated. But foods whose calories come from a mixture of sugar, starch, protein, and fat still provide calories after sugar calories are reduced or eliminated. For instance, sugar-free cookies can provide as many or more calories than cookies sweetened with sugar. Many people inaccurately believe that low sugar means low calories and will overeat because they overestimate the calories saved by replacing sugar. Evidence that nonnutritive sweeteners are effective in weight management is limited (Fitch & Keim, 2012).

Appropriateness for Patients with Diabetes Mellitus. Contrary to what was previously believed, regular sugar does not raise blood glucose levels more than complex carbohydrates do; a food's glycemic load is influenced by several factors, not just sugar content. The focus in management of blood glucose levels has shifted from avoiding simple sugars to maintaining a relatively consistent total carbohydrate intake with less emphasis on the source. For that reason, sweets can be included within the context of a nutritious, calorie-appropriate, carbohydrate-controlled diet. However, because most people with type 2 diabetes are overweight, substitution of calorie-free sweets for calorie-containing ones has the potential to improve blood glucose levels by promoting weight management. The full benefit of this is seen when "diet" soft drinks, jellies, syrups, and hard candies replace those containing sugar. The American Diabetes Association 2016 nutrition therapy recommendations urge people with diabetes and those at risk of diabetes avoid sugar-sweetened beverages to control weight and reduce their risk for cardiovascular disease (American Diabetes Association, 2016).

Table 2.5   Nonnutritive Sweeteners Approved for Use in the United States

Sweetener	Times Sweeter than Sucrose	Taste Characteristics	Uses	Comments/ADI
Acesulfame K (Sunette, Sweet One)	200	Bitter aftertaste like saccharin	Tabletop sweeteners, dry beverage mixes, and chewing gum	Often mixed with other sweeteners to synergize the sweetness and minimize the aftertaste Not digested; excreted unchanged in the urine ADI: 15 mg/kg BW/day
Advantame	20,000		Approved as general sweetener and to enhance flavor under certain conditions of use such as baked goods, soft drinks, frozen desserts, and chewing gum	Chemically similar to aspartame but because it is much sweeter, it does not have to contain a warning about phenylalanine for people with PKU ADI: 32.8 mg/kg BW/day
Aspartame (NutraSweet, Equal, Spoonful)	160–220	Similar to sucrose; no aftertaste	Tabletop sweeteners, dry beverage mixes, chewing gum, beverages, confections, fruit spreads, toppings, and fillings	Made from the amino acids aspartic acid and phenylalanine; people with PKU must avoid aspartame Degrades during heating ADI: 50 mg/kg BW/day
Luo han guo (Swingle fruit extract)	100–250	Aftertaste at high levels	Intended as tabletop sweetener, a food ingredient, and a component of other sweetener blends	Approved as GRAS (generally recognized as safe), so it is not officially considered a food additive and is exempt from legal requirement to prove safety ADI: not specified
Neotame (Newtame)	7000–13,000	Clean, sugar-like taste; enhances flavors of other ingredients	Rarely used in foods	Made from aspartic acid and phenylalanine but is not metabolized to phenylalanine so a warning label is not required Has the potential to replace both sugar and HFCS ADI: 0.3 mg/kg BW/day
Saccharin (Sweet Twin, Sweet'N Low)	300	Persistent aftertaste; bitter at high concentrations	Soft drinks, assorted foods, tabletop sweetener	Potential (weak) carcinogen; the FDA has officially withdrawn its proposed ban so warning labels no longer required ADI: 15 mg/kg BW/day
Stevia (Truvia, Pure Via)	200–400	Sweet clean taste in usual amounts; may taste bitter in higher amounts	Intended for use in cereal, energy bars, beverages, and as a tabletop sweetener	Refined stevia products are GRAS; whole leaf or crude extracts are not approved because of concerns about health effects ADI: 4 mg/kg BW
Sucralose (Splenda)	600	Maintain flavor even at high temperatures	Soft drinks, baked goods, chewing gums, and tabletop sweeteners	Poorly absorbed; excreted unchanged in the feces ADI: 5 mg/kg BW

ADI, Acceptable Daily Intake; BW, body weight; FDA, U.S. Food and Drug Administration; HFCS, high-fructose corn syrup; PKU, phenylketonuria.
Sources: Academy of Nutrition and Dietetics. (2012). Position of the Academy of Nutrition and Dietetics: Use of nutritive and non-nutritive sweeteners. *Journal of the Academy of Nutrition and Dietetics, 112,* 739–758; and U.S. Food and Drug Administration. (2015). *Additional information about high-intensity sweeteners permitted for use in food in the United States.* Available at http://www.fda.gov/food/ingredientspackaginglabeling/foodadditivesingredients/ucm397725.htm#Neotame. Accessed on 1/24/16.

Dental Caries

Feeding on sugars and starches, bacteria residing in the mouth produce an acid that erodes tooth enamel. Although whole-grain crackers and orange juice are more nutritious than caramels and soft drinks, their potential damage to teeth is the same. How often carbohydrates are consumed, what they are eaten with, and how long after eating brushing occurs may be more important than whether or not they are "sticky." Anticavity strategies include the following:

- Choose between-meal snacks that are healthy and teeth friendly, such as fresh vegetables, apples, cheese, and popcorn.
- Limit between-meal carbohydrate snacking including drinking soft drinks.

- Avoid high-sugar items that stay in the mouth for a long time, such as hard candy, suckers, and cough drops.
- Brush promptly after eating.
- Chew gum sweetened with sugar alcohols (e.g., sorbitol, mannitol, and xylitol) or with nonnutritive sweeteners after eating. This may reduce the risk of cavities by stimulating production of saliva, which helps to rinse the teeth and neutralize plaque acids. Unlike sucrose and other nutritive sweeteners, sugar alcohols and nonnutritive sweeteners are not fermented by bacteria in the mouth so they do not promote cavities.
- Use fluoridated toothpaste.

How Do You Respond?

Aren't carbohydrates fattening? At 4 cal/g, carbohydrates are no more fattening than protein and are less than half as fattening as fat at 9 cal/g. Whether or not a food is "fattening" has more to do with frequency and total calories provided than whether the calories are in the form of carbohydrates, protein, or fat.

Is whole "white" wheat bread as nutritious as whole wheat? Whole "white" wheat flour is made from albino wheat that is white in color, not the characteristic brown color of whole wheat. Because it is a whole grain, it is nutritionally comparable to whole wheat. Many people not only prefer its lighter color but also its milder flavor.

"Light" or "diet" breads are high in fiber. Can I use them in place of whole-grain breads? "Light breads" usually have processed fiber from peas or other foods substituted for some starch; the result is a lower calorie, higher fiber bread that may help to prevent constipation but lacks the unique "package" of vitamins, minerals, and phytonutrients found in whole grains.

REVIEW CASE STUDY

Amanda is convinced that white flour and white sugar cause her to overeat, resulting in an extra 30 pounds of weight she is carrying around. To control her impulse to overeat, she has decided to eliminate all foods made with white or whole wheat flour and white sugar from her diet. Her total calorie needs are estimated to be 2000 per day. Yesterday, she ate the the foods on the right:

- What foods did she eat yesterday that contained carbohydrates? Estimate how many grams of carbohydrate she ate. How does her intake compare with the amount of total carbohydrate recommended for someone needing 2000 cal/day? How could she increase her carbohydrate intake within the restrictions she has set for herself?
- What sources of fiber did she consume? Estimate how many grams of fiber she ate. How does her fiber intake compare with the AI amount recommended for women? What would you tell her about her fiber intake?
- What would you tell her about her idea to forsake white and whole wheat flour and white sugar to manage her weight? What are the benefits and potential problems with her diet? What suggestions would you make about her intake?

Breakfast: 2 scrambled eggs and 2 sausage links; 1 cup orange juice; lots of black coffee
Snack: 2 oz of cashews and a diet soft drink
Lunch: tossed salad with 1 hard cooked egg, 3 oz of sliced turkey, 2 oz of sliced cheese, 3 tbsp of Italian dressing; 1 can diet soft drink; 1 cup of diet gelatin
Snack: 2 oz of cheese curds and a diet soft drink
Dinner: 6 oz of fried chicken; 1 cup of French fries; ½ cup corn; ½ cup diet pudding with whipped cream; 1 can diet soft drink
Snack: 5 chicken wings with ¼ cup bleu cheese dressing

STUDY QUESTIONS

1 The nurse knows her explanation of glycemic index was effective when the client says which of the following?
   a. "Choosing foods that have a low glycemic index is an effective way to eat healthier."
   b. "Low glycemic index foods promote weight loss because they do not stimulate the release of insulin."
   c. "Glycemic index may help me choose the best foods to eat before, during, and after training."
   d. "Glycemic index is a term to describe the amount of refined sugar in a food."

2 Which of the following recommendations would be most effective for someone wanting to eat more fiber?
   a. Eat legumes more often.
   b. Eat raw vegetables in place of cooked vegetables.
   c. Use potatoes in place of white rice.
   d. Eat fruit for dessert in place of ice cream.

3 A client asks why sugar should be limited in the diet. Which of the following is the nurse's best response?
   a. "A high sugar intake increases the risk of heart disease and diabetes."
   b. "Foods high in sugar generally provide few nutrients other than calories and may make it hard to consume a diet that has enough of all the essential nutrients."
   c. "There is a direct correlation between sugar intake and the risk of obesity."
   d. "Sugar provides more calories per gram than starch, protein, or fat."

4 Compared to refined grains, whole grains have more
   a. Folic acid
   b. Vitamin A
   c. Vitamin C
   d. Phytonutrients

5 The nurse knows her instructions about choosing dairy products that are lactose free have been effective when the client verbalizes she may tolerate
   a. Whole milk
   b. Fat-free milk
   c. Cheddar cheese
   d. Pudding

6 A client who has eaten too many dietetic candies sweetened with sorbitol may experience which of the following?
   a. Diarrhea
   b. Heartburn
   c. Vomiting
   d. Low blood glucose

7 The client wants to eat fewer calories and lose weight by substituting regularly sweetened foods with those that are sweetened with sugar alternatives. Which of the following would be the most effective substitution?
   a. Sugar-free cookies for regular cookies
   b. Sugar-free chocolate candy for regular chocolate candy
   c. Sugar-free soft drinks for regular soft drinks
   d. Sugar-free ice cream for regular ice cream

8 A client is on a low-calorie diet that recommends she test her urine for ketones to tell how well she is adhering to the guidelines of the diet. What does the presence of ketones signify about her intake?
   a. It is too high in protein.
   b. It is too high in fat.
   c. It is too high in carbohydrates.
   d. It is too low in carbohydrates.

KEY CONCEPTS

- Carbohydrates, which are found almost exclusively in plants, provide the major source of energy in almost all human diets.
- The two major groups are simple sugars (monosaccharides and disaccharides) and complex carbohydrates (polysaccharides).
- Monosaccharides and disaccharides are composed of one or two sugar molecules, respectively. They vary in sweetness.
- Polysaccharides—namely, starch, glycogen, and fiber—are made up of many glucose molecules. They do not taste sweet because their molecules are too large to sit on taste buds in the mouth that perceive sweetness.
- Fiber, the nondigestible part of plant cell walls or intracellular structure, is commonly classified as either water soluble or water insoluble. All foods that contain fiber have a mix of different fibers.
- The most popular American foods are not rich sources of fiber. Whole grains, bran cereals, legumes, and unpeeled fruits and vegetables are the best sources of fiber.
- Carbohydrates are found in every MyPlate group except Oils. Starches are most abundant in grains, vegetables, and the plant foods found in the Protein foods group; natural sugars occur in Fruits and in the Dairy group. Added sugars can be found in any food group.
- The majority of carbohydrate digestion occurs in the small intestine, where disaccharides and starches are digested to monosaccharides. Monosaccharides are absorbed through intestinal mucosal cells and transported to the liver through the portal vein. In the liver, fructose and galactose are converted to glucose. The liver releases glucose into the bloodstream.

- Fiber is not digested, but some types can be fermented by gut microbiota in the large intestine to water, gas, and short-chain fatty acids. Fatty acids may be used for energy by gut microbiota or may be absorbed and metabolized in the liver.
- The glycemic response is based on the glycemic index of a food and the carbohydrate content of that food. Because there are so many variables that influence the rise in blood glucose after eating, glycemic response is hard to predict in practice.
- The major function of carbohydrates is to provide energy, which includes sparing protein and preventing ketosis. Glucose can be converted to glycogen, used to make non-essential amino acids, used for specific body compounds, or converted to fat and stored in adipose tissue.
- The RDA for total carbohydrates is set as the minimum amount needed to fuel the brain but not as an amount adequate to satisfy typical energy needs. Most experts recommend that 45% to 65% of total calories come from carbohydrates and that added sugars be limited. Twenty-five and 38 g of fiber is recommended daily for adult women and men, respectively.
- The *2015-2020 Dietary Guidelines for Americans* urge Americans to choose healthy eating patterns that include grains, at least half of which are whole grains, and limit refined grains. Added sugars should be limited to less than 10% of total calories consumed. The amount and % Daily Value for added sugars is being added to the "Nutrition Facts" label. Whole grains offer health benefits

beyond the benefits of fiber. Whole grains may decrease the risk of heart disease, certain cancers, and type 2 diabetes. Whole grains also promote digestive health and weight management.
- Added sugar is sugar added to food during processing or preparation. It is considered a source of empty calories. The higher the intake of empty calories, the greater is the risk of an inadequate nutrient intake, an excessive calorie intake, or both. A high intake of added sugars is also associated with increased risk of cardiovascular disease.
- Polyols are considered to be low-calorie sweeteners because they are incompletely absorbed and, therefore, provide fewer calories per gram than regular sugar does. Because they do not promote dental decay, they are well suited for use in gum and breath mints that stay in the mouth a long time. Most have a laxation effect depending on the dose consumed.
- Nonnutritive sweeteners provide negligible or no calories. Their use as food additives is regulated by the FDA, which sets safety limits known as ADI. The ADI, a level per kilogram of body weight, reflects an amount 100 times less than the maximum level at which no observed adverse effects have occurred in animal studies. Nonnutritive sweeteners have intense sweetening power, ranging from hundreds to thousands of times sweeter than that of sucrose.
- Acids produced from fermentation of sugars and starches in the mouth by bacteria lead to dental decay.

Check Your Knowledge Answer Key

1 **TRUE** Starch, the storage form of carbohydrates in plants, is made from hundreds to thousands of glucose molecules.
2 **FALSE** All digestible carbohydrates—whether sugars or starch—provide 4 cal/g. Insoluble fiber does not provide calories because it is not digested; the mix of fiber in food may provide 1.5 to 2.5 cal/g because some are fermented to short-chain fatty acids.
3 **FALSE** The body cannot distinguish between the sugar in fruit and the sugar in candy. However, the package of nutrients in fruit (vitamins, minerals, fiber, phytonutrients) is better than the package of nutrients in candy (few to no other nutrients with the possible exception of fat).
4 **FALSE** The most commonly consumed American foods provide 1 to 3 g fiber per serving, which is why most Americans typically eat only about one-half the recommended intake of fiber.
5 **FALSE** Although enrichment returns certain B vitamins and iron lost through processing, other vitamins, minerals, phytonutrients, and fiber are not replaced, so whole wheat

bread is nutritionally superior to white or "wheat" bread. Enriched white bread offers the advantage of being fortified with folic acid.
6 **TRUE** Beverages, such as soft drinks, fruit drinks, sports drinks, and sweetened coffee and tea, contribute more added sugar to the average American diet than any other food or beverage.
7 **TRUE** All fermentable carbohydrates, whether sweet or not, promote dental decay by feeding bacteria in the mouth that damage tooth enamel.
8 **TRUE** Americans are urged to limit their intake of added sugars to less than 10% of total calories consumed. In a 2000-calorie diet, this translates to less than 50 g of added sugar.
9 **FALSE** Nonnutritive sweeteners approved for use in the United States are safe in amounts within the ADI. The exception is the use of aspartame by people who have phenylketonuria.
10 **FALSE** Sugar has not been proven to cause hyperactivity in children.

Websites

Learn about grains at www.wholegrainscouncil.org

References

American Diabetes Association. (2016). Standards of medical care in diabetes—2016. *Diabetes Care, 39*(Suppl. 1), 23–35.

American Diabetes Association & Academy of Nutrition and Dietetics. (2014). *Choose your foods: Food lists for weight management.* Alexandria, VA: American Diabetes Association; Chicago IL: Academy of Nutrition and Dietetics.

American Heart Association. (2015). *Added sugars add to your risk of dying from heart disease.* Available at http://www.heart.org/HEARTORG /HealthyLiving/HealthyEating/Nutrition/Added-Sugars-Add-to -Your-Risk-of-Dying-from-Heart-Disease_UCM_460319_Article.jsp# .VqaCqMtwXIU. Accessed on 1/25/16.

Ballard, W., Hall, M., & Kaufmann, L. (2010). Clinical inquiries. Do dietary interventions improve ADHD symptoms in children? *The Journal of Family Practice, 59,* 234–235.

Cho, S., Lu, Z., Fahey, G., Jr., & Klurfeld, D. (2013). Consumption of cereal fiber, mixtures of whole grains and bran, and whole grains and risk reduction in type 2 diabetes, obesity, and cardiovascular disease. *The American Journal of Clinical Nutrition, 98,* 594–619.

Dahl, W., & Stewart, M. (2015). Position of the Academy of Nutrition and Dietetics: Health implications of dietary fiber. *Journal of the Academy of Nutrition and Dietetics, 115,* 1861–1870.

Fitch, C., & Keim, K. (2012). Position of the Academy of Nutrition and Dietetics: Use of nutritive and nonnutritive sweeteners. *Journal of the Academy of Nutrition and Dietetics, 112,* 739–758.

Institute of Medicine. (2005). *Dietary reference intakes for energy, carbohydrates, fiber, fat, fatty acids, cholesterol, protein, and amino acids (macronutrients).* Washington, DC: The National Academies Press.

International Food Information Council. (2014). *Whole grains fact sheet.* Available at http://www.foodinsight.org/Whole_Grains_Fact_Sheet. Accessed on 1/25/16.

Jonnalagadda, S., Harnack, L., Lui, R., McKeown, N., Seal, C., Liu, S., & Fahey, G. C. (2011). Putting the whole grain puzzle together: Health benefits associated with whole grains—summary of American Society for Nutrition 2010 Satellite Symposium. *The Journal of Nutrition, 141,* 1011S–1022S.

Meijer, K., de Vox, P., & Priebe, M. (2010). Butyrate and other short-chain fatty acids as modulators of immunity: What relevance for health? *Current Opinion in Clinical Nutrition and Metabolic Care, 13*(6), 715–721.

National Research Council. (2005). *Dietary reference intakes for energy, carbohydrate, fiber, fat, fatty acids, cholesterol, protein, and amino acids (macronutrients).* Washington, DC: The National Academies Press.

Oldways Whole Grains Council. (2015). Survey: *Two-thirds of Americans make half their grains whole grains.* Available at http://wholegrainscouncil .org/newsroom/blog/2015/08/survey-two-thirds-of-americans-make -half-their-grains-whole. Accessed on 8/22/16.

U.S. Department of Agriculture & Agricultural Research Service. (2014a). *Energy intakes: Percentages of energy from protein, carbohydrate, fat, and alcohol, by gender and age. What We Eat in America. NHANES 2011-2012.* Available at www.ars.usda.gov/nea/bhnrc/fsrg. Accessed on 1/22/16.

U.S. Department of Agriculture & Agricultural Research Service. (2014b). *Nutrient intakes from food and beverages: Mean amounts consumed per individual, by gender and age. What We Eat in America, NHANES 2011-2012.* Available at www.ars.usda.gov/ba/bhnrc/fsrg. Accessed on 1/22/16.

U.S. Department of Health and Human Services & U.S. Department of Agriculture. (2015). *2015-2020 Dietary guidelines for Americans* (8th ed.). Available at www.health.gov/dietaryguidelines/2015. Accessed on 11/7/16.

Wu, H., Flint, A., Qibin, Q., van Dam, R. M., Sampson, L. A., Rimm, E. B., . . . Hu, F. B. (2015). Association between dietary whole grain intake and risk of mortality: Two large prospective studies in US men and women. *JAMA Internal Medicine, 17*(3), 373–384.

Yang, Q., Zhang, Z., Gregg, E., Flanders, W. D., Merritt, R., & Hu, F. B. (2014). Added sugar intake and cardiovascular diseases mortality among US adults. *JAMA Internal Medicine, 174*(4), 516–524.

Yu, D., Sonderman, J., Buchowski, M., McLaughlin, J. K., Shu, X. O., Steinwandel, M., . . . Zheng, W. (2015). Healthy eating and risks of total and cause-specific death among low-income populations of African-Americans and other adults in the southeastern United States: A prospective cohort study. *PLoS Medicine, 12*(5), e1001830.

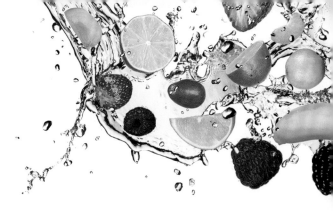

Chapter 3   Protein

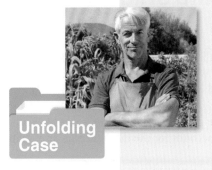

Unfolding Case

Robert Santos

Three years ago, Robert, a 50-year-old farmer, learned he has alpha-gal allergy, an allergy caused by a lone star tick bite that causes a delayed anaphylactic reaction after eating meat. He must avoid beef, pork, lamb, rabbit, venison, and buffalo meat. Prior to the tick bite, his usual weight was 185 pounds (84 kg), which was within healthy range for his height. However, after years of restricting the variety of protein foods he eats, he is now underweight and continues to lose weight. He does not like seafood and is tired of eating poultry.

Check Your Knowledge

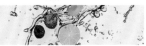

True	False		
☐	☐	**1**	Most Americans eat more than their Recommended Dietary Allowance (RDA) for protein.
☐	☐	**2**	Protein is the nutrient most likely to be deficient in a purely vegetarian diet.
☐	☐	**3**	The body stores extra amino acids in muscle tissue.
☐	☐	**4**	The quality of soy protein is comparable to or greater than that of animal proteins.
☐	☐	**5**	A high protein intake over time leads to kidney damage.
☐	☐	**6**	A protein classified as "high quality" has the majority of calories provided by protein with few fat or carbohydrate calories.
☐	☐	**7**	Protein is found in all MyPlate groups.
☐	☐	**8**	Healthy adults are in a state of positive nitrogen balance.
☐	☐	**9**	Vegetarian diets are not adequate during pregnancy.
☐	☐	**10**	In the United States, protein–energy malnutrition (PEM) occurs most often in hospitalized patients, especially older patients.

Learning Objectives

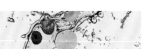

Upon completion of this chapter, you will be able to

1 Discuss the functions of protein.
2 Compare complete and incomplete proteins.
3 Explain protein "sparing."
4 Calculate an individual's protein requirement.
5 Estimate the amount of protein in a sample meal plan.
6 Give examples of conditions that increase a person's protein requirement.
7 Select appropriate sources of nutrients that are most likely to be deficient in a vegetarian diet.
8 Describe nitrogen balance and how it is determined.

In Greek, *protein* means "to take first place," and truly life could not exist without protein. Protein is a component of every living cell: plant, animal, and microorganism. In the adult, protein accounts for 20% of total weight. Dietary protein seems relatively immune to the controversy over optimal intake that surrounds both carbohydrates and fat.

This chapter discusses the composition of protein, its functions, and how it is handled in the body. Sources, Dietary Reference Intakes, and the role of protein in health promotion are presented.

PROTEIN COMPOSITION AND STRUCTURE

Amino Acids

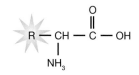

Figure 3.1 ▲
Generic amino acid structure.

Amino acids are the basic building blocks of all proteins and the end products of protein digestion. All amino acids have a carbon atom core with four bonding sites, one of which holds a hydrogen atom, one an amino group (NH_2), and one an acid group (COOH) (Fig. 3.1). Attached to the fourth bonding site is a side group (R group), which contains the atoms that give each amino acid its own distinct identity. Some side groups contain sulfur, some are acidic, and some are basic. The differences in these side groups account for the differences in size, shape, and electrical charge among amino acids.

There are 20 common amino acids that make up proteins, 9 of which are classified as essential or indispensable because the body cannot make them so they must be supplied through the diet (Box 3.1). The remaining 11 amino acids are classified as nonessential or dispensable because cells can make them as needed through the process of transamination. Some dispensable amino acids may become indispensable when metabolic need is great and endogenous synthesis is not adequate. Note that the terms essential and nonessential refer to whether or not they must be supplied by the diet, not to their relative importance: All 20 amino acids must be available for the body to make proteins.

Protein Structure

Amino acids are joined end to end with a peptide bond. The types and amounts of amino acids and the unique sequence in which they are joined determine a protein's primary structure. A dipeptide is a molecule of two joined amino acids. Many amino acids bonded together form a polypeptide. Most proteins are several dozen to several hundred amino acids in length: Just as the 26 letters of the alphabet can be used to form an infinite number of words, so can amino acids be joined in different amounts, proportions, and sequences to form a great variety of proteins.

Proteins also vary in shape and may be straight, folded, coiled along one dimension, or a three-dimensional shape such as a sphere or globe. Larger proteins are created when two or more three-dimensional polypeptides combine. A protein's shape determines its function.

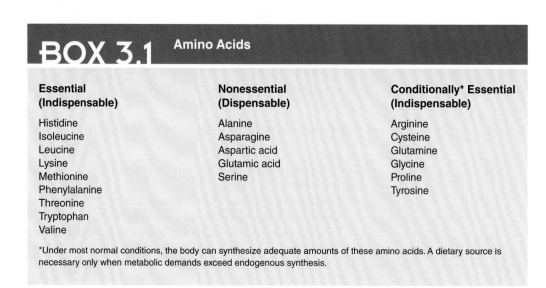

BOX 3.1   Amino Acids

Essential (Indispensable)	Nonessential (Dispensable)	Conditionally* Essential (Indispensable)
Histidine	Alanine	Arginine
Isoleucine	Asparagine	Cysteine
Leucine	Aspartic acid	Glutamine
Lysine	Glutamic acid	Glycine
Methionine	Serine	Proline
Phenylalanine		Tyrosine
Threonine		
Tryptophan		
Valine		

*Under most normal conditions, the body can synthesize adequate amounts of these amino acids. A dietary source is necessary only when metabolic demands exceed endogenous synthesis.

FUNCTIONS OF PROTEIN

Protein is the major structural and functional component of every living cell. Except for bile and urine, every tissue and fluid in the body contains some protein. In fact, the body may contain as many as 10,000 to 50,000 different proteins that vary in size, shape, and function. Amino acids or proteins are components of or involved in the following:

Body structure and framework. More than 40% of protein in the body is found in skeletal muscle, and approximately 15% is found in each the skin and the blood. Proteins also form tendons, membranes, organs, and bones.

Enzymes. Enzymes are proteins that facilitate specific chemical reactions in the body without undergoing change themselves. Some enzymes (e.g., digestive enzymes) break down larger molecules into smaller ones; others (e.g., enzymes involved in protein synthesis in which amino acids are combined) combine molecules to form larger compounds.

Other body secretions and fluids. Neurotransmitters (e.g., serotonin, acetylcholine), antibodies, and peptide hormones (e.g., insulin, thyroxine, epinephrine) are made from amino acids, as are breast milk, mucus, sperm, and histamine.

Fluid balance. Proteins help to regulate fluid balance because they attract water, which creates osmotic pressure. Circulating proteins, such as albumin, maintain the proper balance of fluid among the **intravascular**, **intracellular**, and **interstitial** compartments of the body. A symptom of a low albumin level is **edema**.

Acid–base balance. Because amino acids contain both an acid (COOH) and a base (NH_2), they can act as either acids or bases depending on the pH of the surrounding fluid. The ability to buffer or neutralize excess acids and bases enables proteins to maintain normal blood pH, which protects body proteins from being **denatured**.

Transport molecules. **Globular** proteins transport other substances through the blood. For instance, lipoproteins transport fats, cholesterol, and fat-soluble vitamins; hemoglobin transports oxygen; and albumin transports free fatty acids and many drugs.

Other compounds. Amino acids are components of numerous body compounds such as opsin, the light-sensitive visual pigment in the eye, and thrombin, a protein necessary for normal blood clotting.

Some amino acids have specific functions within the body. For instance, tryptophan is a precursor of the vitamin niacin and is also a component of serotonin. Tyrosine is the precursor of melanin, the pigment that colors hair and skin and is incorporated into thyroid hormone.

Fueling the body. Like carbohydrates, protein provides 4 cal/g. Although it is not the body's preferred fuel, protein is a source of energy when it is consumed in excess or when calorie intake from carbohydrates and fat is inadequate.

Intravascular
within blood vessels.

Intracellular
within cells.

Interstitial
between cells.

Edema
the swelling of body tissues secondary to the accumulation of excessive fluid.

Denatured
an irreversible process in which the structure of a protein is disrupted, leading to partial or complete loss of function.

Globular
spherical.

HOW THE BODY HANDLES PROTEIN

Digestion and Absorption

Chemical digestion of protein begins in the stomach, where hydrochloric acid denatures protein to make the peptide bonds more available to the actions of enzymes (Fig. 3.2). Hydrochloric acid also converts pepsinogen to the active enzyme pepsin, which begins the process of breaking down proteins into smaller polypeptides and some amino acids.

The majority of protein digestion occurs in the small intestine, where pancreatic proteases reduce polypeptides to shorter chains, tripeptides, dipeptides, and amino acids. The enzymes trypsin and chymotrypsin act to break peptide bonds between specific amino acids. Carboxypeptidase breaks off amino acids from the acid (carboxyl) end of polypeptides and dipeptides. Enzymes located on the surface of the cells that line the small intestine complete the digestion: Aminopeptidase splits amino acids from the amino ends of short peptides, and dipeptidase reduces dipeptides to amino acids. **Protein digestibility** is 90% to 99% for animal proteins, over 90% for soy and legumes, and 70% to 90% for other plant proteins.

Protein Digestibility
how well a protein is digested to make amino acids available for protein synthesis.

Figure 3.2 ▶
Protein digestion.

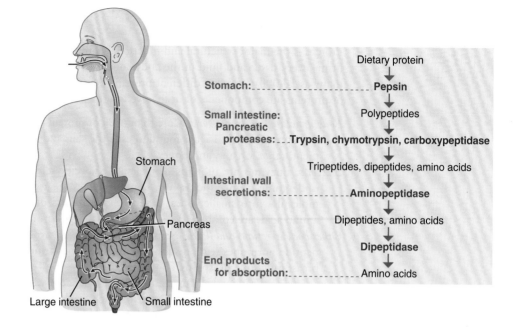

Figure 3.2 ▶
Protein digestion.

Dietary protein
↓
Stomach: .... **Pepsin**
↓
Polypeptides
Small intestine:
Pancreatic
proteases: .... **Trypsin, chymotrypsin, carboxypeptidase**
↓
Tripeptides, dipeptides, amino acids
↓
Intestinal wall
secretions: .... **Aminopeptidase**
↓
Dipeptides, amino acids
↓
Dipeptidase
End products ↓
for absorption: .... Amino acids

Stomach
Pancreas
Large intestine   Small intestine

Amino acids, and sometimes a few dipeptides or larger peptides, are absorbed through the mucosa of the small intestine by active transport with the aid of vitamin B_6. Intestinal cells release amino acids into the bloodstream for transport to the liver via the portal vein.

Metabolism

The liver acts as a clearinghouse for the amino acids it receives: it uses the amino acids it needs, releases those needed elsewhere, and handles the extra. For instance, the liver

- Retains amino acids to make liver cells, nonessential amino acids, and plasma proteins such as heparin, prothrombin, and albumin
- Regulates the release of amino acids into the bloodstream and removes excess amino acids from the circulation
- Synthesizes specific enzymes to degrade excess amino acids
- Removes the nitrogen from amino acids so that they can be burned for energy
- Converts certain amino acids to glucose, if necessary
- Forms urea from the nitrogenous wastes when protein and calories are consumed in excess of need
- Converts protein to fatty acids that form triglycerides for storage in adipose tissue

Protein Synthesis

Protein synthesis (anabolism) is a complicated but efficient process that quickly assembles amino acids provided through food or released from the breakdown of existing body proteins into proteins the body needs, such as those needed for growth and development or lost through normal wear and tear. The body prioritizes muscle protein synthesis; cells in the liver, heart, and diaphragm are replenished even during short-term periods of catabolism.

In the 1990s, researchers discovered that the essential amino acid leucine has the ability to stimulate muscle protein synthesis. It appears that the amount of protein in a meal necessary to promote protein synthesis may be dependent on its leucine content (Layman et al., 2015). In adults, an intake of 25 to 30 g protein per meal with 2.2 g or more of leucine may be optimal for muscle protein synthesis. A rich source of leucine is whey, a protein in milk.

Part of what makes every individual unique is the minute differences in body proteins, which are caused by variations in the sequencing of amino acids determined by genetics. Genetic codes created at conception hold the instructions for making all of the body's proteins. Cell function and life itself depend on the precise replication of these codes. Some important concepts related to protein synthesis are protein turnover, metabolic pool, and nitrogen balance.

Protein Turnover

Protein turnover is a continuous process that occurs within each cell as proteins are broken down from normal wear and tear and replenished. Body proteins vary in their rate of turnover. For example, red blood cells are replaced every 60 to 90 days, gastrointestinal cells are replaced every 2 to 3 days, and enzymes used in the digestion of food are continuously replenished.

Metabolic Pool

Although protein is not truly stored in the body as are glucose and fat, a supply of each amino acid exists in a metabolic pool of free amino acids within cells and circulating in blood. This pool consists of recycled amino acids from body proteins that have broken down and also amino acids from food. Because the pool accepts and donates amino acids as they become available or are needed, it is in a constant state of flux.

Nitrogen Balance

Nitrogen balance reflects the state of balance between protein breakdown (catabolism) and protein synthesis (anabolism). It is determined by comparing nitrogen intake with nitrogen excretion over a specific period of time, usually 24 hours. To calculate nitrogen intake, protein intake is measured (in grams) over a 24-hour period and divided by 6.25 because protein is 16% nitrogen. The result represents total nitrogen intake for that 24-hour period. Nitrogen excretion is computed by analyzing a 24-hour urine sample for the amount (grams) of urinary urea nitrogen it contains and adding a coefficient of 4 to this number to account for the estimated daily nitrogen loss in feces, hair, nails, and skin. Comparing grams of nitrogen excretion to grams of nitrogen intake will reveal the state of nitrogen balance, as illustrated in Box 3.2.

A neutral nitrogen balance, or state of equilibrium, exists when nitrogen intake equals nitrogen excretion, indicating protein synthesis is occurring at the same rate as protein breakdown. Healthy adults are in neutral nitrogen balance. When protein synthesis exceeds protein breakdown, as is the case during growth, pregnancy, or recovery from injury, nitrogen balance is positive. A negative nitrogen balance indicates that protein catabolism is occurring at a faster rate than protein synthesis, which occurs during starvation or the catabolic phase after injury.

Protein Catabolism for Energy

Using protein for energy is a physiologic and economic waste because amino acids used for energy are not available to be used for protein synthesis, a function unique to amino acids. Normally, the body uses very little protein for energy as long as intake and storage of carbohydrate and fat are adequate. If insufficient carbohydrate and fat are available for energy use (e.g., when calorie intake is inadequate), dietary and body proteins are sacrificed to provide amino acids that can be burned for energy. Over time, loss of lean body tissue occurs and, if severe, can lead to decreased muscle

---

BOX 3.2 Calculating Nitrogen Balance

Mary is a 25-year-old woman who was admitted to the hospital with multiple fractures and traumatic injuries from a car accident. A nutritional intake study indicated a 24-hour protein intake of 64 g. A 24-hour urinary urea nitrogen (UUN) collection result was 19.8 g.

1. Determine nitrogen intake by dividing protein intake by 6.25:

$$64 \text{ g} \div 6.25 = 10.24 \text{ g of nitrogen}$$

2. Determine total nitrogen output by adding a coefficient of 4 to the UUN:

$$19.8 + 4 \text{ g} = 23.8 \text{ g of nitrogen}$$

3. Calculate nitrogen balance by subtracting nitrogen output from nitrogen intake:

$$10.24 - 23.8 \text{ g} = -13.56 \text{ g in 24 hours}$$

4. Interpret the results.

A negative number indicates that protein breakdown is exceeding protein synthesis. Mary is in a catabolic state.

strength, altered immune function, altered organ function, and ultimately death. To "spare" protein—both dietary and body—from being burned for calories, an adequate supply of energy from carbohydrate and fat is needed.

SOURCES OF PROTEIN

The protein group consists of meat, poultry, seafood, eggs, legumes, and nuts and seeds. As a group, protein provides a variety of other nutrients, such as iron, riboflavin, niacin, vitamin B_6, vitamin B_{12}, choline, potassium, zinc, copper, vitamin D, vitamin E, and fiber (Phillips et al., 2015). Not all items within the group provide the same array of nutrients. For instance, red meat is the best source of heme iron, poultry provides niacin, vitamin D is found in seafood, legumes provide fiber, and nuts and seeds provide vitamin E. Protein is also found in dairy, grains, and vegetables (Fig. 3.3).

The protein content of individual foods within the protein group varies with what is defined as an "ounce-equivalent." For instance, for meat, poultry, and seafood, 1 ounce equals an ounce-equivalent. For nuts and seeds, an ounce-equivalent is actually ½ ounce because they are higher in calories than lean meats, poultry, and seafood. At ½ oz as an "ounce-equivalent," nuts and seeds provide approximately ½ or less the amount of protein as an ounce of animal protein (Berner, Becker, Wise, & Doi, 2013). Table 3.1 shows the MyPlate recommendations for the protein group at various calorie levels.

Protein Quality

Dietary proteins differ in quality based on their content of essential amino acids. For most Americans, protein quality is not important because the amounts of protein and calories consumed over the course of a day are more than adequate. But when protein needs are increased or protein intake is marginal, quality becomes a crucial concern.

Terms that refer to protein quality are complete and incomplete. Complete proteins provide all nine essential amino acids in adequate amounts and proportions needed by the body for protein synthesis. These high-quality proteins include all animal sources of protein plus soy and quinoa. Sources of complete protein include the following:

- Meat, poultry, seafood, eggs
- Milk, yogurt, cheese
- Soybeans, soybean products, quinoa

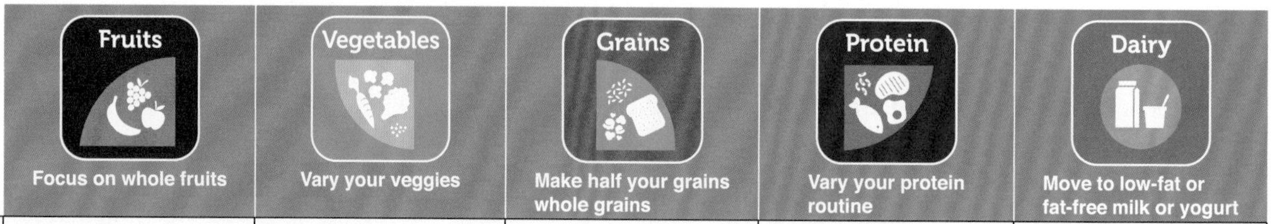

	Fruits Focus on whole fruits	**Vegetables** Vary your veggies	**Grains** Make half your grains whole grains	**Protein** Vary your protein routine	**Dairy** Move to low-fat or fat-free milk or yogurt
Protein g/svg	0	2	3	1 oz lean meat, poultry, or seafood — 7; 1 egg — 7; 1 Tbsp peanut butter — 3½; ½ c cooked beans or peas — 7; ½ oz nuts or seeds — 2½–3½	8
Serving sizes **	1 med piece of fruit; ½ c canned fruit or fruit juice	½ c cooked or raw; 1 c leafy salad greens	1 slice bread; 1 oz ready to eat cereal; ½ c cooked rice, pasta, or cereal	As specified above	1 c milk, yogurt, or soy beverage

* No protein in the oils category.
** Serving sizes as per the American Diabetes Association/Academy of Nutrition and Dietetics.

Figure 3.3 ▲ Protein content of MyPlate. *(Source: U.S. Department of Agriculture, Center for Nutrition Policy and Promotion. [2016]. Available at www.choosemyplate.gov. Accessed 2/7/16.)*

Table 3.1	**The Number of Protein Group Equivalents Recommended at Various Calorie Levels in Healthy U.S.-Style Eating Patterns**	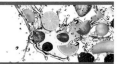

Total Daily Calories	Recommended Number of Ounce-Equivalents
1000	2
1200	3
1400	4
1600–1800	5
2000	5.5
2200	6
2400–2600	6.5
2800–3200	7

Source: U.S. Department of Health and Human Services & U.S. Department of Agriculture. (2015). *2015-2020 Dietary guidelines for Americans* (8th ed.). Available at https://health.gov/dietaryguidelines/2015/guidelines/appendix-3/. Accessed on 2/7/16.

Incomplete proteins also provide all the essential amino acids, but one or more are present in insufficient quantities to support protein synthesis. These amino acids are considered "limiting" in that they limit the process of protein synthesis. All plant proteins, with the exception of soy and quinoa, are incomplete proteins, as is gelatin. Sources of incomplete protein include the following:

- Grains and products made with grains
- Legumes and lentils
- Nuts and seeds
- Vegetables
- Gelatin

Different sources of incomplete proteins differ in their limiting amino acids. For instance, grains are typically low in lysine and isoleucine, and legumes are low in methionine and cysteine. Two incomplete proteins that have different limiting amino acids are known as complementary proteins because together they form the equivalent of a complete protein. Likewise, a complete protein combined with any incomplete protein is complementary. Examples of food that contain complementary proteins appear in Box 3.3. It is not necessary to eat complementary proteins at the same meal; what is important is eating a variety of proteins over the course of a day and consuming adequate calories.

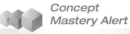

Concept Mastery Alert

Two kinds of beans (such as black beans and kidney beans) do not create a complete, or complementary, protein because they have the same incomplete proteins. Consuming one of those kinds of beans with a different incomplete or complete protein (such as rice or a toasted cheese sandwich) would create a complete protein.

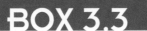

BOX 3.3 Sources of Foods with Complementary Proteins

Two Incomplete Proteins

Black beans and rice
Bean tacos
Pea soup with toast
Lentils and rice curry
Falafel (ground chickpea patties) sandwich
Peanut butter sandwich
Pasta e fagioli (white beans and pasta soup)
Hummus with crackers
Tofu lasagna

A Complete Protein Combined with an Incomplete Protein

Bread pudding
Rice pudding
Corn pudding
Cereal and milk
Macaroni and cheese
French toast
Cheese sandwich
Vegetable quiche
Cheese enchilada

DIETARY REFERENCE INTAKES

The Recommended Dietary Allowance (RDA) for protein for healthy adults age 19 years and older is 0.8 g/kg, derived from the absolute minimum requirement needed to maintain nitrogen balance plus an additional factor to account for individual variations and the mixed quality of proteins typically consumed (National Research Council, 2005). This figure also assumes calorie intake is adequate. For the reference adult male who weighs 154 pounds, this translates to 56 g protein/day; the reference female weighing 127 pounds needs 46 g/day. The RDA for protein is higher for people younger than 19 years (in gram per kilogram body weight) and for pregnant or lactating women to support growth and development (Table 3.2).

According to the National Health and Nutrition Examination Survey (NHANES) 2011–2012 data, the mean intake for adult men and women aged 20 years and older is 98 g and 68 g, respectively, an amount well above the RDA (U.S. Department of Agriculture, Agricultural Research Service, 2014b). American adults typically consume >60% of daily protein intake at the evening meal and 15 g of protein or less at breakfast (Layman et al., 2015).

Controversy exists over the RDA for protein and whether it is optimal for health. Layman et al. (2015) suggest a daily protein intake of approximately 1 to 1.2 g/kg in adults is beneficial for various metabolic functions. Other research shows modestly higher intakes of high quality protein (1.0–1.5 g/kg/day) evenly consumed throughout the day may be necessary to help maintain muscle mass in older adults (Paddon-Jones et al., 2015). The consensus position paper from the PROT-AGE Study Group recommends >1.0 g/kg for adults and emphasized the need to focus on meal quantity and timing of protein as important factors in adult health (Bauer et al., 2013).

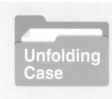

Unfolding Case

Think of Robert. What is his RDA for protein at a healthy weight of 84 kg? His protein calorie intakes are inadequate, as determined by food records and weight loss. He agrees to try in-between meal snacks. What snacks would you specifically suggest?

The Acceptable Macronutrient Distribution Range (AMDR) for protein for adults is 10% to 35% of total calories (National Research Council, 2005). As illustrated in Figure 3.4, the AMDR is a wide range, with the upper end far greater than both the RDA and median protein intake by American adults cited earlier. From a practical standpoint, grams of protein per day is a more valid standard of adequacy than tracking the percentage of total calories from protein. That is because the RDA for protein is based on enough to fulfill specific protein functions, whereas the AMDR is a range that allows for protein to be used for energy. For men aged 20 years and older, protein provides 16% of total calories consumed, whereas among women of the same age group, protein provides 15% of total calories (U.S. Department of Agriculture, Agricultural Research

Table 3.2	Recommended Dietary Allowance for Protein by Age and Life Stage	
By Age		**g protein/kg body weight**
For males and females		
7–12 months		1.2
1–3 years		1.05
4–13 years		0.95
14–18 years		0.85
≥19 years		0.8
By life stage		
Pregnancy		1.1
Lactation		1.3

Figure 3.4 ▶

Amount of total protein appropriate at various calorie levels based on the Acceptable Macronutrient Distribution Range of 10% to 35% of total calories.

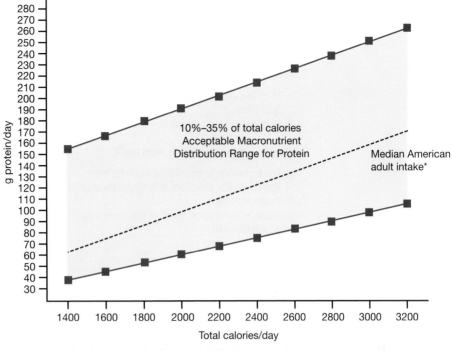

*Median American adult intake of 15% of total calories

Service, 2014a). Although the upper limit of the AMDR for protein is 35% of total calories, a "high-protein" diet is commonly defined as consuming 20% or more of calories from protein (Westerterp-Plantenga, Lemmens, & Westerterp, 2012).

Quick Bite

To calculate a healthy adult's RDA for protein

1. Divide weight in pounds by 2.2 to determine weight in kilograms.
2. Multiply by 0.8 g/kg.
3. Result is total grams of protein per day.

When the Recommended Dietary Allowance Doesn't Apply

The RDA is intended for healthy people only and assumes total calorie intake is adequate. Health impairments that require tissue repair increase a person's protein requirement (Box 3.4). When calorie intake is inadequate, protein may be used for energy instead of its specialized function. For instance, evidence supports the idea that people on calorie-restricted weight loss diets should consume a higher protein intake. Instead of the RDA of 0.8 g/kg, a protein intake of 1.2 to 1.6 g/kg may be optimal for weight loss (Leidy et al., 2015). Meta-analysis of several controlled studies showed higher loss of fat and weight and greater preservation of lean mass with a high-protein low-calorie intake compared to a low-protein low-calorie intake. A higher protein intake also enhances energy expenditure because dietary protein has a higher thermic effect than either carbohydrates or fat, meaning that the body burns more calories to digest, absorb, metabolize, and store protein than it does carbohydrates or fat. Another positive attribute of protein is that it is high in satiety, delaying the return of hunger, which may help people better adhere to a low calorie intake. People on high-protein weight loss plans also had improvements in cardiometabolic risk factors, such as the triglyceride levels, blood pressure, and waist circumference. To achieve these protein-related benefits, it may be necessary to consume at least 25- to 30-g protein at each meal.

Conversely, protein restriction is appropriate for people with severe liver disease (because the liver metabolizes amino acids) and for those who are unable to adequately excrete nitrogenous wastes from protein metabolism due to impaired renal function.

Protein Deficiency

Macronutrients
nutrients required by the body in large amounts (gram quantities); namely, carbohydrate, protein, and fat.

Kwashiorkor
a type of PEM resulting from a deficiency of protein or infections.

Marasmus
a type of PEM resulting from severe deficiency or impaired absorption of calories, protein, vitamins, and minerals.

Protein–energy malnutrition (PEM) is a calorie deficit due to a deficiency of all **macronutrients**. **Kwashiorkor** and **marasmus** are generally viewed as two distinctly

BOX 3.4   Conditions that Increase the Need for Protein

When Calorie Intake Is Inadequate Resulting in Protein Being Used for Energy

- Very-low-calorie weight loss diets
- Starvation
- Protein–energy malnutrition

When the Body Needs to Heal Itself

- Hypermetabolic conditions such as burns, sepsis, major infection, and major trauma
- Postsurgically
- Acute inflammation such as inflammatory bowel disease
- Skin breakdown
- Multiple fractures
- Hepatitis

When Excessive Protein Losses Need Replacement

- Long-term peritoneal or hemodialysis dialysis
- Protein-losing renal diseases
- Malabsorption syndromes such as protein-losing enteropathy and short bowel syndrome

When Periods of Normal Tissue Growth Occur

- Pregnancy
- Lactation
- Infancy through adolescence

different forms of PEM (Table 3.3). Although there is controversy as to whether kwashiorkor and marasmus simply represent the same disease at different stages, Di Giovanni et al. (2016) found that children with kwashiorkor have different metabolic alterations and are prone to more severe metabolic disorders than children with marasmus.

Although PEM can affect people of any country or age, it is most prevalent in developing countries and in children under the age of 5 years. Approximately 50% of the 10 million annual deaths in developing countries occur from malnutrition in children aged 5 years or younger (Scheinfeld, 2015). In the United States, PEM is predominately seen in hospitals with as many as half of all patients exhibiting some degree of malnutrition. The elderly are particularly at risk with

Table 3.3   Comparison Between Kwashiorkor and Marasmus

	Kwashiorkor	Marasmus
Intake	Fair to normal calorie intake; inadequate protein intake	Inadequate calorie and protein intake
Cause	Acute critical illness or infections that cause loss of appetite while increasing nutrient requirements and losses. Stressors in children in developing countries may be measles or gastroenteritis and often occurs during weaning; in American adults, trauma or sepsis.	Severe prolonged starvation may occur in children from chronic or recurring infections with marginal food intake; in adults from developed countries, may occur secondary to chronic illness.
Onset	Rapid, acute; may develop in a matter of weeks	Slow, chronic; may take months or years to develop
Edema	Characterized by bilateral pitting edema that begins in the lower legs and feet and progresses to generalized edema	Absent
Appearance	May look plump due to fluid retention	"Skin and bones" due to severe muscle loss with virtually no body fat
Weight loss	Children present with poor weight gain or weight loss; adults lose weight	Severe
Other clinical symptoms that may be present	Skin lesions; shedding skin Hair loss, loss of hair color, easy pluckability Enlarged fatty liver Loss of appetite Apathy and lethargy	Dry, thin skin that easily wrinkles Hair is sparse; easy pluckability No fatty liver Hypothermia Infection

estimates of up to 85% of institutionalized elderly undernourished (Scheinfeld, 2015). Other groups at risk include people with certain chronic diseases, such as cancer, AIDS, chronic pulmonary disease, cirrhosis, and those on long-term hemodialysis. Additionally, homeless people, fad dieters, adults who are addicted to drugs or alcohol, and people with eating disorders are at risk. Protein deficiency affects all body organs and many body systems. An impaired immune system increases the risk of infection. Infection in the intestinal tract impairs nutrient digestion and absorption. Anemia occurs from a decreased production of hemoglobin, and diminished levels of serum albumin leads to edema. Wound healing is impaired, and in elderly patients, risk of hip fractures and pressure ulcers increase. With acute or chronic severe PEM, cardiac output decreases, blood pressure falls, and respiratory rate decreases. Liver, kidney, or heart failure may occur.

In both children and adults, nutrition therapy begins with correcting fluid and electrolyte imbalances to help raise blood pressure and increase heart rate. Infections are treated (Scheinfeld, 2015). After the first 24 to 48 hours, protein and calories are provided in small amounts that are gradually increased as tolerated. Severely malnourished people, especially those with edema, may recover better when protein intake is limited to 10% of total calories. Actual protein and calorie needs may be double that of normal.

Protein Excess

There are no proven risks from eating an excess of protein. Data are conflicting as to whether high-protein eating patterns increase the risk of osteoporosis or renal stones. Although a UL has not been established, this does not mean there is no potential for adverse effects from a high protein intake from food or supplements (National Research Council, 2005). Data are limited on adverse effects of high levels of amino acid intakes from supplements, so caution is advised in taking any single amino acid in amounts significantly higher than what is found in food (National Research Council, 2005).

PROTEIN IN HEALTH PROMOTION

The *2015-2020 Dietary Guidelines for Americans* urge people to consume a healthy eating pattern that includes a variety of protein foods, including seafood, lean meats and poultry, eggs, legumes (beans and peas), nuts, seeds, and soy products (U.S. Department of Health and Human Services [USDHHS] & U.S. Department of Agriculture [USDA], 2015). Although Americans, on average, consume an appropriate percentage of their calories from protein, average intakes of seafood are low for all age-sex groups and intakes of meats, poultry, and eggs are high for teenage boys and adult men. Legumes, a vegetable subgroup that provides significant protein, is also underconsumed. The *Guidelines* urge a shift in protein selections, such as to

- Eat seafood twice a week in place of other meats or poultry. In a 2000-calorie eating pattern, at least 8 oz of seafood per week is recommended. Eating seafood, especially salmon, trout, or herring, in place of other animal proteins lowers saturated fat intake and increases unsaturated fat intake, particularly of the omega-3 fatty acids eicosapentaenoic acid (EPA) and docosahexaenoic acid (DHA), which help lower the risk of cardiac deaths in people with or without cardiovascular disease (USDHHS & USDA, 2015).
- Use legumes, quinoa, or soy products occasionally as a main dish instead of meat, such as black bean burritos, soy veggie burgers, hummus on pita bread, quinoa chili, or split pea soup. Eating plant proteins lowers saturated fat intake and increases fiber intake.
- Choose lean meats and lean poultry (Box 3.5).
- Consume processed meats and processed poultry only if they fit within an individual's sodium, saturated fat, and total calories intake goals. Strong evidence from prospective cohort and randomized controlled trials shows that eating patterns that include lower intakes of meats, processed meats, and processed poultry are associated with a decreased risk of cardiovascular disease in adults (USDHHS & USDA, 2015).

BOX 3.5   Sources of Lean Animal Protein

- The leanest beef cuts are round steaks and roasts (eye of round, top round, bottom round, round tip) top loin, and top sirloin.
- Lean pork choices include pork loin, tenderloin, center loin, and ham.
- Choose ground beef that is at least 90% lean.
- Buy skinless poultry; chicken breasts and turkey cutlets are the leanest choices of poultry.
- Choose lean turkey, roast beef, ham, or low-fat luncheon meats instead of luncheon or deli meats with more fat, such as bologna or salami.

Source: Tips to help you make wise choices from the protein foods group. (2015). Available at https://www.choosemyplate.gov/protein-foods-tips. Accessed on 8/22/16.

Many leading health organizations, including the American Institute for Cancer Research (World Cancer Research Fund & American Institute for Cancer Research, 2016) and the American Cancer Society (Kushi et al., 2012), recommend a plant-based diet, which means replacing some or most animal sources of protein with vegetable sources, such as soy, legumes, nuts, and seeds. The American Institute for Cancer Research also advises consumers to limit consumption of red meats, such as beef, pork, and lamb, and to avoid processed meat, such as ham, bacon, salami, hot dogs, and sausages, based on evidence that red meat increases the risk of colorectal cancer (World Cancer Research Fund & American Institute for Cancer Research, 2016). The health benefits of a plant-based diet may come from eating less of certain substances (such as saturated fat), eating more of others (such as fiber, antioxidants, and phytonutrients), or a combination of the two.

Vegetarian Diets

Vegetarianism is a general term assigned to plant-based eating patterns with restrictions ranging from total elimination of all animal products to simply excluding one or more types of animal proteins. Once a rarity, plant-based eating patterns are becoming mainstream for a variety of reasons including moral, religious, environmental, and health. In the United States, the prevalence of vegetarianism, defined as "never" eating meat, fish, or poultry, is reported to be approximately 4% (Vegetarian Resource Group, 2015). The *2015-2020 Dietary Guidelines for Americans* includes healthy vegetarian-style eating patterns as one of three eating patterns that reflect the Guidelines (USDHHS & USDA, 2015). Categories of vegetarian eating patterns are the following:

- Vegan, which excludes all animal products including eggs, dairy products, and sometimes honey
- Raw vegan: a strictly uncooked food eating pattern based on fruit, nuts, seeds, and vegetables
- Lacto-ovo vegetarian, excludes flesh foods but includes dairy products and eggs
- Lacto-vegetarian, excludes flesh foods and eggs but includes dairy products
- Ovo-vegetarian, excludes flesh foods and dairy products but includes eggs
- Pesco-vegetarian, excludes all animal products except fish
- Macrobiotic diet: a strict whole-foods, plant-based eating pattern that includes no flesh foods except fish and seafood and includes mostly brown rice and whole grains supplemented with locally grown vegetables and tofu, tempeh, miso, beans, nuts, seeds, certain fruits, and sea vegetables such as seaweed, nori, and agar
- Semi-vegetarian or flexitarian: a plant-based pattern that includes occasional intake (perhaps up to twice a week) of meat, fish, poultry, or dairy products

Unfolding Case

Recall Robert. Is it appropriate to recommend vegetarian resources that feature nonmeat recipes and meal patterns to him even though he is not a vegetarian?

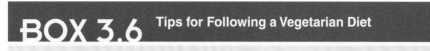

BOX 3.6 Tips for Following a Vegetarian Diet

- *Eat a variety of foods that provide protein including whole grains, vegetables, legumes, nuts, seeds, and, if desired, dairy products and eggs.* Consider meatless versions of familiar favorites, such as vegetable pizza, vegetable lasagna, vegetable stir-fry, vegetable lo mein, and vegetable kabobs.
- *Experiment with meat substitutes made from vegetables.* For variety, try soy sausage patties or links, veggie burgers, quinoa chili, or scrambled tofu.
- *Include legumes.* Try vegetarian chili, three bean salad, navy bean soup, hummus, bean burritos, or black bean burgers.
- *Include nuts.* Snack on unsalted nuts or add to salads or main dishes.
- *Eat enough calories.* Adequate calories are necessary to avoid using amino acids for energy, which could lead to a shortage of amino acids for protein synthesis.
- *Consume a rich source of vitamin C at every meal.* Eating a good source of vitamin C at every meal helps to maximize iron absorption from plants. Try orange and citrus fruits, tomatoes, kiwi, red and green peppers, broccoli, Brussels sprouts, cantaloupe, and strawberries.
- *Include foods that supply omega-3 fats,* such as flaxseeds, chia seeds, walnuts, and canola and soybean oils.
- *Don't go overboard on high-fat cheese as a meat substitute.* Full-fat cheese has more saturated fat and calories than many meats.
- *Experiment with ethnic cuisines.* Many Asian, Middle Eastern, and Indian restaurants offer a variety of meatless dishes.
- *Choose vitamin B_{12}–fortified foods or take a vitamin B_{12} supplement daily.* See Table 3.4 for sources of other nutrients of concern.
- *Supplement nutrients that are lacking from food.*

Within each defined category of vegetarianism, individuals differ as to how strictly they adhere to their eating pattern. For instance, some vegans do not eat refried beans that contain lard because lard is an animal product, but other vegans do not avoid animal products so conscientiously. Properly planned vegetarian and vegan eating patterns are healthful and are nutritionally adequate during all phases of the life cycle, including pregnancy, lactation, infancy, childhood, and adolescence (Craig & Mangels, 2009). Vegetarian eating patterns can provide health benefits in the prevention and treatment of certain health conditions, including ischemic heart disease, type 2 diabetes, hypertension, certain cancers, and obesity, and are associated with increased longevity (Leitzmann, 2014). Compared to meat eaters, vegetarians eat less total fat, saturated fat, and cholesterol and more fiber (Ha & de Souza, 2015) as well as more micronutrients and phytonutrients. Although the cardiometabolic benefits of vegetarian diets are widely attributed to the absence of red meat, reciprocal increases in the intake of healthy foods, such as legumes, vegetables, fruit, and grains, are also significant (Ha & de Souza, 2015).

However, vegetarian eating patterns are not automatically healthier than nonvegetarian patterns. Poorly planned vegetarian eating patterns may lack certain essential nutrients, which endangers health. They can also be excessive in fat and cholesterol if whole milk, whole-milk cheeses, eggs, and high-fat desserts are used extensively. Whether a vegetarian eating pattern is healthy or detrimental to health depends on the actual food choices made over time. Tips for vegetarians appear in Box 3.6.

Nutrients of Concern

The concerns that vegetarian eating patterns are deficient in total protein or provide poor overall protein quality are unfounded. Most vegetarian eating patterns, even vegan ones, meet or exceed the RDA for protein; if calorie needs are met, eating a variety of plant proteins ensures that the supply of essential amino acids are adequate. It is not necessary to combine complementary proteins at every meal as long as a variety of proteins are consumed daily. Box 3.7 illustrates how a vegan menu can exceed the RDA for the average adult.

Iron, zinc, calcium, vitamin D, omega-3 fatty acids, and iodine are nutrients of concern not because they cannot be obtained in sufficient quantities from plants but because they may not be adequately consumed, depending on an individual's food choices. Vitamin B_{12} is of concern because it does not occur naturally in plants. Table 3.4 lists vegetarian sources of these nutrients of concern.

BOX 3.7   Protein Content of a Sample Vegan Menu

Food item	g protein
Breakfast	
1 cup oatmeal	6
With 2 tbsp walnuts	1
1 cup soymilk	6
Banana	
Lunch	
Black bean burger	10
On whole wheat bun	6
Condiments as desired	
Side salad with dressing	2
Fresh orange	
Dinner	
4 oz tofu	12
Stir fried with 1½ cup vegetables	6
Served over 1 cup brown rice	4
Fresh watermelon	
Snack	
1 cup Greek yogurt	20
With 2 tbsp almonds	2
Total gram protein/day	75 g

RDA for "reference" male is 56 g/day and for reference female, 46 g/day.

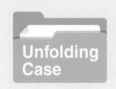

Unfolding Case

Think of Robert. Because he does not eat red meat, his intake of heme iron is low. What other nutrients may he consume in inadequate amounts? Would he benefit from a multivitamin with minerals?

Protein for Muscle Building

High-protein diets and protein supplements are popular among athletes based on the rationale that muscle is protein tissue thus eating more protein makes more muscle. Although protein recommendations for athletes are higher than for nonathletes, building muscle is not simply a matter of increasing protein intake. To increase muscle mass, both resistance training and an adequate overall intake are necessary.

Resistance training, also called weight or strength training, is exercise that causes muscle to contract against an external force for the purpose of increasing strength, tone, mass, or endurance. Resistance training causes microscopic tears in muscle tissue (catabolism), which the body quickly repairs to regenerate and strengthen muscle (anabolism). Although an adequate protein is important, so is an adequate intake of overall calories—energy to fuel the activity as well as repair the tissue. Recommendations for protein intake typically range from 1.2 to 2.0 g protein/kg/day (Thomas, Erdman, & Burke, 2016). This amount of protein can generally be met through food alone, without the need for protein or amino acid supplements. Bodybuilders may need 1.8 to 2.7 g/kg or more of protein daily, especially lean athletes who are restricting their calorie intake to lose body fat (Helms, Aragon, & Fitschen, 2014). The type of protein consumed and timing of intake affects muscle anabolism. Only essential amino acids in food stimulate protein synthesis, and leucine in particular appears to have the most impact on muscle protein synthesis (Pasiakos et al., 2011). High-quality proteins—namely, eggs, dairy, lean meat, seafood, quinoa, and soy—provide all essential amino acids in balanced proportions. Dairy proteins seem to be superior to other proteins in stimulating muscle protein synthesis mostly because of the leucine content and

Table 3.4 Sources of Nutrients of Concern in Vegan Eating Patterns

Nutrient	Vegetarian Sources	Comments
Iron	Iron-fortified bread and cereals Baked potato with skin Kidney beans, black-eyed peas, and lentils Cooked soybeans Tofu Veggie "meats" Dried apricots, prunes, and raisins Cooking in a cast iron pan, especially with acidic foods such as tomatoes	Because of the lower bioavailability of iron from plants, it is recommended that vegetarians consume good sources of iron such as iron-fortified breads and cereals, legumes, lentils, and raisins, with a source of vitamin C.
Zinc	Whole grains Legumes Zinc-fortified cereals Soybean products Pumpkin seeds Nuts	Recommended zinc intake is 50% higher in vegetarians than nonvegetarians because zinc from plants is not absorbed as well as zinc from meats.
Calcium	Bok choy Broccoli Chinese/napa cabbage Collard greens Kale Calcium-fortified orange juice Calcium-set tofu Calcium-fortified soy milk, breakfast cereals Legumes Spinach	Beet greens and Swiss chard are also high in calcium, but their oxalate content interferes with calcium absorption. Calcium supplements are recommended for people who do not meet their calcium requirement through food.
Vitamin D	Sunlight Fortified milk Fortified ready-to-eat cereals Fortified soy milk Fortified nondairy milk products	Supplements may be necessary depending on the quality of sunlight exposure and adequacy of food choices.
Omega-3 fatty acids	Fortified foods, such as breakfast cereals, soy milk, and yogurt Sources of alpha-linolenic acid are the following: Ground flaxseed and flaxseed oil Chia seeds Walnuts and walnut oil Canola oil Soybean oil	Diets that exclude fish and sea vegetables do not contain a direct source of the omega-3 fatty acids DHA and EPA. The body can convert small amounts of alpha-linolenic acid into one of the omega-3 fatty acids (DHA). Adequate DHA and EPA is especially important during pregnancy, infancy, and in the elderly.
Vitamin B_{12}	Fortified soy milk, breakfast cereals, and veggie burgers	Seaweed, algae, spirulina, tempeh, miso, beer, and other fermented foods contain a form of vitamin B_{12} that the body cannot use. Supplemental vitamin B_{12} through food or pills is recommended for all people over the age of 50 years regardless of the type of diet they consume because absorption decreases with age. Vitamin B_{12} deficiency during pregnancy and lactation may lead to severe developmental problems in the fetus and infant.

digestion and absorption of its amino acids (Pennings et al., 2011). Eating a high-quality protein within 2 hours after exercise promotes muscle repair and growth, whether the protein is eaten alone or with carbohydrates (Caspero, 2014). An even distribution of protein intake at each meal may optimize muscle protein synthesis (Layman et al., 2015).

Protein Powders and Amino Acid Supplements

Protein powders appeal to athletes by claiming to build muscle, promote recovery, and strengthen muscle. They may be made from whey, casein, soy, beef, or plants (e.g., peas, hemp, and brown rice). Unlike whole foods, they are not balanced sources of nutrition. As a supplement, they can easily provide excessive protein, which is not automatically converted to muscle but rather metabolized in the liver so it can be used for energy or stored as fat. Protein consumed in excess of need challenges the kidneys to excrete unused nitrogen.

Amino acid supplements often provide only one or few particular amino acids unlike the natural array of amino acids found in food. An imbalance of amino acids is not beneficial: An excess of one amino acid can interfere with the absorption of other amino acids, causing them to become the limiting amino acid for protein synthesis. Second, an abnormally high serum concentration of an amino acid raises the possibility of toxicity. Amino acid supplements are not recommended.

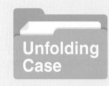

Unfolding Case

Consider Robert. He wants to know if whey protein powder or amino acid supplements would be appropriate for him. How would you respond?

How Do You Respond?

Is ground turkey a low-fat alternative to ground beef? Not necessarily. Ground turkey may contain skin, dark meat, and fat along with the breast, making it a higher fat product than 95% lean ground beef. Ground turkey breast and ground chicken breast are made only from white meat and are lower in fat (approximately 3 g/3 oz cooked) than all varieties of ground beef (5.5–15 g fat/3 oz cooked).

Does "vegetarian" on the label mean the product is also low fat? No, vegetarian is not synonymous with low fat, particularly for items such as vegetarian hot dogs, soy cheese, soy yogurt, and refried beans. Advise clients to read the "Nutrition Facts" label to determine if a vegetarian item is a good nutritional buy.

REVIEW CASE STUDY

For ethical reasons, Emily does not eat meat, eggs, or milk, although she is not so strict as to avoid baked goods that may contain milk or eggs. Over the last 6 months, she has gained 15 pounds, although she actually expected to lose weight. She needs 2000 cal/day according to MyPlate. A typical daily intake for her is shown on the right:

- What kind of vegetarian is Emily? What sources of protein is she consuming? Is she consuming enough protein? How does her daily intake compare to MyPlate recommendations for a 2000-calorie diet? What suggestions would you make to her to improve the quality of her diet?
- Is Emily at risk of any nutrient deficiencies? If so, what would you recommend she do to ensure nutritional adequacy?
- What would you tell Emily about her weight gain? What foods would you recommend she eat less of if she wants to lose weight? What could she substitute for those foods?

Breakfast:	A smoothie made with soy milk, tofu, and fresh fruit; a glazed doughnut
Snack:	Potato chips and soda
Lunch:	A peanut butter sandwich; soy yogurt; oatmeal cookies; soda
Snack:	A candy bar
Dinner:	Stir-fried vegetables over rice; bread with margarine; a glass of soy milk; apple pie
Snack:	Buttered popcorn

STUDY QUESTIONS

1 What is the RDA for protein for a healthy adult who weighs 165 pounds?
   a. 60 g
   b. 75 g
   c. 100 g
   d. 165 g

2 The client asks what foods are rich in protein and are less expensive than meat. Which of the following foods would the nurse recommend she eat more of?
   a. Breads and cereals
   b. Legumes
   c. Fruit and vegetables
   d. Fish and shellfish

3 Which of the following sources of protein is lowest in fat?
   a. Eggs
   b. Ground chicken
   c. 80% lean ground beef
   d. Turkey breast without skin

4 Which statement indicates the client understands vegetarian diets?
   a. "Vegetarians need to eat more calories than nonvegetarians in order to spare protein."
   b. "Vegetarian diets are always healthier than nonvegetarian diets."
   c. "Vegetarians usually do not consume enough protein."
   d. "Vegetarians may need to take supplements of iron, vitamin B_{12}, and calcium."

5 A client who is in a positive nitrogen balance is most likely to be
   a. A healthy adult
   b. Starving
   c. Pregnant
   d. Losing weight

6 An adult in the hospital has been diagnosed with marasmus. Which of the following would you expect?
   a. The client has experienced severe weight loss.
   b. The client denies hunger.
   c. The client has edema and a swollen abdomen.
   d. The onset of the deficiency was rapid.

7 The nurse knows that instructions have been effective when the client verbalizes that a source of complete, high-quality protein is found in
   a. Peanut butter
   b. Black-eyed peas
   c. Cottage cheese
   d. Corn

8 A client says that she doesn't eat much meat. After teaching the client about serving sizes, the nurse determines that the teaching has been effective when the client states that an ounce of meat provides approximately the same amount of protein as which of the following?
   a. 8 oz of milk
   b. 8 oz of nuts
   c. 2 oz of cheese
   d. 2 eggs

KEY CONCEPTS

- Protein is a component of every living cell. Protein in the body provides structure and framework. Amino acids are also components of enzymes, hormones, neurotransmitters, and antibodies. Proteins play a role in fluid balance and acid–base balance and are used to transport substances through the blood. Protein provides 4 cal/g of energy.
- Amino acids, which are composed of carbon, hydrogen, oxygen, and nitrogen atoms, are the building blocks of protein. Of the 20 common amino acids, 9 are considered essential because the body cannot make them. The remaining 11 amino acids are no less important but are considered nonessential because they can be made by the body if nitrogen is available. Some of these are considered conditionally essential under certain circumstances.
- Amino acids are joined in different amounts, proportions, and sequences to form the thousands of different proteins in the body.
- The small intestine is the principal site of protein digestion; amino acids and some dipeptides are absorbed through the portal bloodstream.
- In the body, amino acids are used to make proteins, nonessential amino acids, and other nitrogen-containing compounds. Some amino acids can be converted to glucose. Amino acids consumed in excess of need are burned for energy or converted to fat and stored.
- Healthy adults are in nitrogen balance, which means that protein synthesis is occurring at the same rate as protein breakdown. Nitrogen balance is determined by comparing the amount of nitrogen consumed with the amount of nitrogen excreted in urine, feces, hair, nails, and skin.
- Except for the Fruits and Oils, all MyPlate groups provide protein in varying amounts.
- The quality of proteins varies. Complete proteins provide adequate amounts and proportions of all essential amino

acids needed for protein synthesis. Animal proteins, quinoa, and soy protein are complete proteins. Incomplete proteins lack adequate amounts of one or more essential amino acids. Except for soy and quinoa, all plants are sources of incomplete proteins. Gelatin is also an incomplete protein.

- The RDA for protein for healthy adults is 0.8 g/kg of body weight; other age and lifecycle categories have higher protein needs to support growth and development. The AMDR for protein among adults is 10% to 35% of total calories. Most Americans consume more than the RDA for protein and approximately 15% of their total calories from protein.

- Pure vegans eat no animal products. Most American vegetarians are lacto-vegetarians or lacto-ovo vegetarians, whose diets include milk products or milk products and eggs, respectively.

- Most vegetarian diets meet or exceed the RDA for protein. Specific nutrients may be underconsumed depending on actual food choices. Pure vegans who do not have reliable sources of vitamin B_{12} and vitamin D need supplements.

- To gain muscle mass, resistance exercise is necessary. The increase in protein that is needed can be easily met by an increase in calorie intake. Nutritionally, adequate calories are the most important factor for increasing muscle mass.

Check Your Knowledge Answer Key

1 **TRUE** Most Americans consume more than their RDA for protein.

2 **FALSE** Over the course of a day, if the food consumed is varied and contains sufficient calories, most vegetarian diets meet or exceed the RDA for protein.

3 **FALSE** Unlike glucose and fat, the body is not able to store excess amino acids for later use.

4 **TRUE** Soy protein is complete. It is a high biologic value protein and is comparable in quality to animal protein.

5 **FALSE** There are no proven risks to having a high dietary protein intake.

6 **FALSE** The quality of a protein is determined by the balance of essential amino acids provided.

7 **FALSE** Fruits generally provide negligible protein, and oils are protein free.

8 **FALSE** Healthy adults are in neutral nitrogen balance: Protein synthesis is occurring at the same rate as protein breakdown.

9 **FALSE** Properly planned vegetarian diets are nutritionally adequate during all phases of pregnancy and lactation.

10 **TRUE** In the United States, PEM occurs most often in hospitalized patients, especially older patients. Others at risk include people with chronic diseases such as AIDS, cancer, and chronic obstructive pulmonary disease (COPD).

Student Resources on *the*Point®
For additional learning materials, activate the code in the front of this book at
http://thePoint.lww.com/activate

Websites

Food and Nutrition Information Center, U.S. Department of Agriculture at http://fnic.nal.usda.gov/

Soyfoods Association of North America at www.soyfoods.org

The Vegan Society at www.vegansociety.com

Vegan Health at www.veganhealth.org

Vegetarian Nutrition Dietetic Practice Group's consumer website at www.vegetariannutrition.net

Vegetarian Resource Group at www.vrg.org

The Vegetarian Society of the United Kingdom at www.vegsoc.org /health/

VegWeb at www.vegweb.com

References

Bauer, J., Biolo, G., Cederholm, T., Cesari, M., Cruz-Jentoft, A. J., Morley, J. E., . . . Boirie, Y. (2013). Evidence-based recommendations for optimal dietary protein intake in older people: A position paper from the PROT-AGE Study Group. *Journal of the American Medical Directors Association, 14,* 542–559.

Berner, L., Becker, G., Wise, M., & Doi, J. (2013). Characterization of dietary protein among older adults in the United States: Amount, animal sources, and meal patterns. *Journal of the Academy of Nutrition and Dietetics, 113,* 809–815.

Caspero, A. (2014). *Protein and the athlete—how much do you need?* Available at www.eatright.org/resource/fitness/sports-and-performance-fueling -your-workout/protein-and-the-athlete. Accessed on 1/30/16.

Craig, W., & Mangels, A. (2009). Position of the American Dietetic Association: Vegetarian diets. *Journal of the American Dietetic Association, 109*, 1266–1282.

Di Giovanni, V., Bourdon, C., Wang, D. X., Seshadri, S., Senga, E., Versloot, V. J., . . . Bandsma, R. H. J. (2016). Metabolomic changes in serum of children with different clinical diagnoses of malnutrition. *Journal of Nutrition.* Advance online publication. doi:10.3945/jn.116.239145

Ha, V., & de Souza, R. (2015). "Fleshing out" the benefits of adopting a vegetarian diet. *Journal of the American Heart Association, 4*, e002654. doi:10.1161/JAHA.115.002654

Helms, E., Aragon, A., & Fitschen, P. (2014). Evidence-based recommendations for natural bodybuilding contest preparation: Nutrition and supplementation. *Journal of the International Society of Sports Nutrition, 11*, 20. doi:10.1186/1550-2783-11-20

Kushi, L., Doyle, C., McCullough, M., Rock, C. L., Demark-Wahnefried, W., Bandera, E. V., . . . Gansler, T. (2012). American Cancer Society Guidelines on nutrition and physical activity for cancer prevention: Reducing the risk of cancer with healthy food choices and physical activity. *CA: A Cancer Journal for Clinicians, 62*, 30–67.

Layman, D., Anthony, T., Rasmussen, B., Adams, S. H., Lynch, C. J., Brinkworth, G. D., & Davis, T. A. (2015). Defining meal requirements for protein to optimize metabolic roles of amino acids. *The American Journal of Clinical Nutrition, 101*(Suppl.), 1330S–1338S.

Leidy, H., Clifton, P., Astrup, A., Wycherley, T. P., Westerterp-Plantenga, M. S., Luscombe-Marsh, N. D., . . . Mattes, R. D. (2015). The role of protein in weight loss and maintenance. *The American Journal of Clinical Nutrition, 101*(Suppl.), 1320S–1329S.

Leitzmann, C. (2014). Vegetarian nutrition: Past, present, future. *The American Journal of Clinical Nutrition, 100*(Suppl. 1), 496S–502S.

National Research Council. (2005). *Dietary reference intakes for energy, carbohydrate, fiber, fat, fatty acids, cholesterol, protein, and amino acids (macronutrients).* Washington, DC: The National Academies Press.

Paddon-Jones, D., Campbell, W., Jacques, P., Kritchevsky, S., Moore, L. L., Rodriguez, N. R., . . . van Loon, L. J. (2015). Protein and healthy aging. *The American Journal of Clinical Nutrition, 101*(Suppl.), 1339S–1345S.

Pasiakos, S., McClung, H., McClung, J., Margolis, L. M., Andersen, N. E., Cloutier, G. J., . . . Young, A. J. (2011). Leucine-enriched essential amino acid supplementation during moderate steady state exercise enhances postexercise muscle protein synthesis. *The American Journal of Clinical Nutrition, 94*, 809–818.

Pennings, B., Boirie, Y., Senden, J., Gijsen, A., Kuipers, H., & van Loon, L. J. (2011). Whey protein stimulates postprandial muscle protein accretion more effectively than do casein and casein hydrolysate in older men. *The American Journal of Clinical Nutrition, 93*, 997–1005.

Phillips, S., Fulgoni, V., III, Heaney, R., Nicklas, T. A., Slavin, J. L., & Weaver, C. M. (2015). Commonly consumed protein foods contribute to nutrient intake, diet quality, and nutrient adequacy. *The American Journal of Clinical Nutrition, 101*(Suppl), 1346S–1352S.

Scheinfeld, N. (2015). Protein-energy malnutrition. Available at http://emedicine.medscape.com/article/1104623-overview. Accessed on 2/1/16.

Thomas, D., Erdman, K., & Burke, L. M. (2016). Position of the Academy of Nutrition and Dietetics, Dietitians of Canada, and the American College of Sports Medicine: Nutrition and athletic performance. *Journal of the Academy of Nutrition and Dietetics, 116*, 501–528.

U.S. Department of Agriculture, Agricultural Research Service. (2014a). *Energy intakes: Percentages of energy from protein, carbohydrate, fat, and alcohol, by gender and age. What We Eat in America, NHANES 2022-2012.* Available at www.ars.usda.gov/nea/bhnrc/fsrg. Accessed on 1/22/16.

U.S. Department of Agriculture, Agricultural Research Service. (2014b). *Nutrient intakes from food and beverages: Mean amounts consumed per individual, by gender and age. What We Eat in America, NHANES 2011-2012.* Available at www.ars.usda.gov/ba/bhnrc/fsrg. Accessed on 1/22/16.

U.S. Department of Health and Human Services & U.S. Department of Agriculture. (2015). *2015-2020 Dietary guidelines for Americans* (8th ed.). Available at www.health.gov/dietaryguidelines/2015. Accessed on 1/7/16.

Vegetarian Resource Group. (2015). *How often do Americans eat vegetarian meals? And how many adults in the US are vegetarian?* Available at http://www.vrg.org/blog/2015/05/29/how-often-do-americans-eat-vegetarian-meals-and-how-many-adults-in-the-u-s-are-vegetarian-2/. Accessed on 8/33/16.

Westerterp-Plantenga, M., Lemmens, S., & Westerterp, K. (2012). Dietary protein—its role in satiety, energetics, weight loss and health. *The British Journal of Nutrition, 108*(Suppl. 2), S105–S112.

World Cancer Research Fund & American Institute for Cancer Research. (2016). *Recommendations for cancer prevention.* Available at http://www.aicr.org/reduce-your-cancer-risk/recommendations-for-cancer-prevention/. Accessed on 3/21/16.

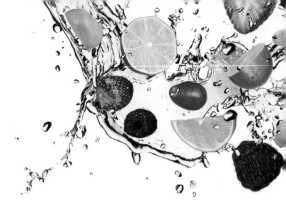

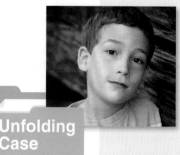

Unfolding Case

Dylan Masters

Dylan is a 7-year-old boy who has up to 20 seizures a day due to epilepsy. Because antiseizure medications have failed to control his seizures, he is a candidate for a ketogenic diet. Although there are several different levels of the diet, it is characterized as a high-fat, adequate-protein, very low carbohydrate diet. Dylan's classic ketogenic diet will provide 1200 calories, 120 g of fat, 18 g of protein, and 12 g of carbohydrate. The family has undergone extensive counseling and has agreed to try the diet for at least 12 weeks; they understand the risks and that all foods must be carefully prepared and weighed on a gram scale. Dylan will be under close medical and nutritional supervision and will start the diet in the hospital where he will be closely monitored by a neurologist and registered dietitian. Lab work will be used to identify metabolic abnormalities and evaluate serum nutrient levels.

Check Your Knowledge

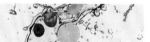

True	False		
☐	☐	1	Fat provides more than double the amount of calories as an equivalent amount of carbohydrate or protein.
☐	☐	2	All fats are bad fats.
☐	☐	3	The body makes two to three times more cholesterol than the typical American consumes.
☐	☐	4	The risk of consuming mercury from fish outweighs any potential benefits for the general population.
☐	☐	5	Tub margarine is healthier than butter.
☐	☐	6	All sources of fat are a blend of saturated and unsaturated fatty acids.
☐	☐	7	All oils are predominately unsaturated fats.
☐	☐	8	Menu items described as being "cooked in vegetable oil" are trans fat free.
☐	☐	9	A dietary intake of "fish oils" is essential.
☐	☐	10	The *2015-2020 Dietary Guidelines for Americans* does not include a recommendation to limit cholesterol intake.

Learning Objectives

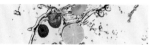

Upon completion of this chapter, you will be able to

1 Compare saturated, monounsaturated, and polyunsaturated fatty acids.
2 Propose ways to limit saturated fat present in a sample eating pattern.

3 Explain the functions of fat in the body.
4 Discuss the digestion and absorption of fat.
5 Give examples of foods that provide omega-3 fatty acids.
6 Discuss strategies for decreasing saturated fat intake and increasing oil intake within the context of a healthy eating pattern.
7 Explain why there is no Recommended Dietary Allowance for total fat, trans fat, and saturated fat.

"Avoid too much fat" appeared in the first edition of the *Dietary Guidelines for Americans* published in 1980 (http://health.gov/dietaryguidelines/1980thin.pdf). Since then, decades of study have shown that the relationship between fat and health is far more complex than that statement implies. The evolving understanding of individual fatty acids and fatty acid groups is emerging as a key factor in health (Vannice & Rasmussen, 2014). Some fatty acids have a positive impact on health (e.g., omega-3 fatty acids) and should be eaten in moderation; other fatty acids have a negative impact on health (e.g., trans fats) and should be limited. Eating less of some fatty acid groups and more of others is a recommendation among many American and international health and government agencies. There are three classes of **lipids**, which are referred to as fat throughout the rest of this chapter and book: triglycerides (fats and oils), which account for 98% of the fat in food; phospholipids (e.g., lecithin); and sterols (e.g., cholesterol). This chapter describes the classes of fats, their dietary sources, and how they are handled in the body. The functions of fat are presented, as are recommendations regarding intake.

Lipids
a group of water-insoluble, energy-yielding organic compounds composed of carbon, hydrogen, and oxygen atoms.

TRIGLYCERIDES

Chemically, **triglycerides** are made of the same elements as carbohydrates, namely, carbon, hydrogen, and oxygen. Because there are proportionately more carbon and hydrogen atoms to oxygen atoms, triglycerides yield more calories per gram than carbohydrates. Structurally, triglycerides are composed of a three-carbon atom glycerol backbone with three fatty acids attached (Fig. 4.1). An individual triglyceride molecule may contain one, two, or three different types of fatty acids.

Triglycerides
a class of lipids composed of a glycerol molecule as its backbone with three fatty acids attached.

Fatty Acids

Fatty acids are basically chains of carbon atoms with hydrogen atoms attached (Fig. 4.2). At one end of the chain is a methyl group (CH_3), and at the other end is an acid group (COOH). Fatty acids are commonly abbreviated by a C followed by the number of carbon atoms, a colon, and the number of double bonds. For example, stearic acid, an 18-carbon length fatty acid with no double bonds, is abbreviated as C18:0. The most common fatty acids and their sources are listed in Table 4.1.

Fatty acids attach to **glycerol** molecules in various ratios and combinations to form a variety of triglycerides within a single food fat. The types and proportions of fatty acids present influence the sensory and functional properties of the food fat. For instance, butter tastes and acts differently from corn oil, which tastes and acts differently from lard. Fatty acids vary in the length of their carbon chain and in the degree of unsaturation. These variables account for the differences in physiologic function and impact on disease risk seen between individual fatty acids (Vannice & Rasmussen, 2014).

Fatty Acids
organic compounds composed of a chain of carbon atoms to which hydrogen atoms are attached. An acid group (COOH) is attached at one end, and a methyl group (CH_3) at the other end.

Glycerol
a three-carbon atom chain that serves as the backbone of triglycerides.

Carbon Chain Length

Almost all naturally occurring fatty acids have an even number of carbon atoms in their chain, generally between 4 and 24. Long-chain fatty acids (containing more than 12 carbon atoms) predominate in meats, fish, and vegetable oils and are the most common length fatty acid in the diet. Smaller amounts of medium-chain (8–12 carbon atoms) and short-chain (up to 6 carbon atoms) fatty acids are found primarily in dairy products. The body absorbs short- and medium-chain fatty acids differently than long-chain fatty acids.

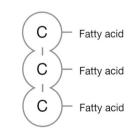

Figure 4.1 ▲
Generic triglyceride molecule.

Figure 4.2 ▶
Fatty acid configurations.

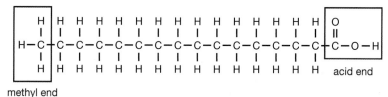

methyl end

Palmitic acid: 16 carbon saturated fatty acid

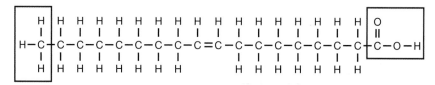

Oleic acid: 18 carbon *n*-9, monounsaturated fatty acid

Degree of Saturation

Saturated Fatty Acids
fatty acids in which all the carbon atoms are bonded to as many hydrogen atoms as they can hold so no double bonds exist between carbon atoms.

Unsaturated Fatty Acids
fatty acids that are not completely saturated with hydrogen atoms, so one or more double bonds form between the carbon atoms.

Monounsaturated Fatty Acids
fatty acids that have only one double bond between two carbon atoms.

Polyunsaturated Fatty Acids
fatty acids that have two or more double bonds between carbon atoms.

As dictated by nature, each carbon atom in a fatty acid chain must have four bonds connecting it to other atoms. When all the carbon atoms in a fatty acid have four single bonds each, the fatty acid is saturated with hydrogen atoms. The majority of naturally occurring **saturated fatty acids** are straight-line molecules that can pack tightly together; thus, they are solid at room temperature.

An **"unsaturated" fatty acid** does not have all the hydrogen atoms it can potentially hold; therefore, one (**monounsaturated**) or more (**polyunsaturated**) double bonds form between carbon atoms in the chain. Because of the double bond, unsaturated fatty acids are physically kinked and unable to pack together tightly; they are liquid at room temperature and are referred to as "oils."

All food fats contain a mixture of saturated, monounsaturated, and polyunsaturated fatty acids. When applied to sources of fat in food, "unsaturated" and "saturated" are not absolute terms used to describe the only types of fatty acids present; rather, they are relative descriptions that indicate which kinds of fatty acids are present in the largest proportion. For instance, butter is classified as a saturated fat; however, 34% of

Table 4.1   The Most Common Fatty Acids in Food

	Common Abbreviation	Chemical Abbreviation	Common Food Sources
Saturated fatty acids	SFA		
Lauric acid	Medium-chain triglyceride (MCT)	C12:0	Palm kernel oil, coconut oil
Myristic acid		C14:0	Beef tallow, cocoa butter
Palmitic acid		C16:0	Main SFA that naturally occurs in animal fats (meat, poultry, eggs, dairy products) and vegetable oils
Stearic acid		C18:0	Meat, fully hydrogenated vegetable oils
Monounsaturated fatty acid	MUFA		
Oleic acid		C18:1	Meats; canola and olive oil; most nuts, avocado
Polyunsaturated fatty acids	PUFA		
n-3			
Alpha-linolenic acid	ALA	C18:3	Walnuts; ground flaxseed and flaxseed oil, soybean oil, canola oil, chia and hemp seeds
Eicosapentaenoic acid	EPA	C20:5	Fatty fish, such as salmon, herring, mackerel, tuna
Docosahexaenoic acid	DHA	C22:6	Fatty fish; marine algae–fortified foods, such as juice
n-6			
Linoleic acid	LA	C18:2	Soybean and corn oils; also in safflower, cottonseed, and sunflower oils; shortening
Arachidonic acid	ARA	C20:4	Meat, poultry, eggs

its fatty acids are unsaturated. Similarly, olive oil is known as a monounsaturated fat because 77% of its fatty acids are monounsaturated, not because all of them are.

Saturated Fats

Fats with a high percentage of saturated fatty acids are referred to as solid fats because they are solid at room temperature. Saturated fatty acids occur to the greatest extent in animal fats—the fat in meats, egg yolks, and whole-milk dairy products (the fat in milk does not appear as a solid due to the process of homogenization). The only vegetable oils that are saturated are palm oil, palm kernel oil, and coconut oil.

As a category, saturated fat is commonly known as a "bad" fat based on early studies that showed a correlation between dietary saturated fat and coronary heart disease (Kato, Tillotson, Nichaman, Rhoads, & Hamilton, 1973). More recent studies have shown a positive, inverse, or no association between dietary saturated fat and cardiovascular disease (CVD) morbidity and/or mortality (Siri-Tarino, Sun, Hu, & Krauss, 2010). In reality, individual saturated fatty acids do not all have the same impact on **low-density lipoprotein (LDL) cholesterol**. The saturated fatty acids lauric, myristic, and palmitic acids increase LDL cholesterol (Nicolosi, 1997), whereas the saturated fatty acid stearic acid has a neutral impact on LDL cholesterol (Grande, Anderson, & Keys, 1970). However, stearic acid is found in foods that also provide the saturated fatty acids that raise LDL cholesterol. Thus, it is recommended that the intake of foods high in saturated fat be limited even though not all saturated fatty acids may be considered "bad."

> **Low-Density Lipoprotein (LDL) Cholesterol**
> the major class of atherogenic lipoproteins that carry cholesterol from the liver to the tissues.

Unsaturated Fatty Acids

Categories of unsaturated fatty acids are polyunsaturated (PUFA) and monounsaturated (MUFA), commonly known as "good fats." Strong consistent evidence shows that replacing saturated fat with unsaturated fat, especially PUFA, is associated with a decrease in LDL cholesterol and lowers the risk of cardiovascular events and death (U.S. Department of Health and Human Services [US-DHHS] & U.S. Department of Agriculture [USDA], 2015). There is some evidence that MUFA also lower CVD risk, but it is not as strong. MUFAs are the predominate fat in olives, olive oil, canola oil, avocado, peanut oil, and most other nuts. Meat fat contains moderate amounts of monounsaturated fats, providing approximately 50% of MUFAs in a typical American eating pattern (National Research Council, 2005). PUFAs are less ubiquitous than monounsaturated fats. They are the predominate fat in corn, soybean, safflower, and cottonseed oils and also in fish.

Unsaturated fatty acids can be classified according to the location of their double bonds along the carbon chain. The most common method of identifying the bond is to count the number of carbon atoms from the methyl (CH_3) end, as denoted by the term "n" or "omega." A PUFA with its first double-bond three carbons from the methyl end is an **omega-3** or **n-3** fatty acid. Likewise, an **omega-6** or **n-6** PUFA has its first double-bond 6 carbons from the methyl end. Omega-9 or n-9 fatty acids are monounsaturated fats.

> **Omega-3 (n-3) Fatty Acid**
> an unsaturated fatty acid whose endmost double bond occurs three carbon atoms from the methyl end of its carbon chain.
>
> **Omega-6 (n-6) Fatty Acid**
> an unsaturated fatty acid whose endmost double bond occurs six carbon atoms from the methyl end of its carbon chain.
>
> **Essential Fatty Acids**
> fatty acids that cannot be synthesized in the body and thus must be consumed through food.

The location of the first double bond is significant because it determines the essentiality of a fatty acid. The body is unable to synthesize fatty acids with double bonds closer than n-9, so one n-6 fatty acid (linoleic acid) and one n-3 fatty acid (alpha-linolenic acid) are **essential fatty acids** and must be consumed through food. MUFAs are n-9 fatty acids and are not essential because they can be synthesized in the body.

Linoleic Acid. Linoleic acid, the essential n-6 PUFA, is the most highly consumed PUFA in Western diets. The richest sources are soybean, corn, and safflower oils; poultry, nuts, and seeds are also sources. The body can make other n-6 fatty acids, such as arachidonic acid, from linoleic acid. However, if a deficiency of linoleic acid develops, arachidonic acid becomes "conditionally essential" because the body is unable to synthesize it without a supply of linoleic acid.

Alpha-Linolenic Acid. Alpha-linolenic acid, the essential n-3 fatty acid, is the most prominent n-3 fatty acid in most Western diets. It is found in walnuts, flaxseed, chia and hemp seeds, and canola and soybean oils.

To a very limited extent, humans can convert alpha-linolenic acid to the *n*-3 fatty acids eicosapentaenoic acid (EPA) and docosahexaenoic acid (DHA). These two *n*-3 fatty acids are commonly referred to as "**fish oils**" because they are primarily found in fatty fish, especially salmon, anchovy, sardines, tuna, herring, and mackerel. Food products fortified with EPA and/or DHA are available, such as soy milks, cooking oils, margarine-like spreads, breakfast cereals, baked goods, infant formulas, and baby food and juices.

Omega-3 fatty acids are probably best known for their heart health benefits, which are attributed to their anti-inflammatory, anticlotting, and anti-arrhythmic effects. Other potential benefits include improvements in symptoms related to hypertension, depression, joint pain, and other rheumatoid issues (International Food Information Council Foundation [IFICF], 2014).

> **Fish Oils**
> a common term for the long-chain, poly-unsaturated omega-3 fatty acids EPA and DHA found in the fat of fish, primarily in cold-water fish.

Stability of Fats

> **Rancidity**
> the chemical change that occurs when fats are oxidized, which causes an offensive taste and smell and the loss of fat-soluble vitamins A and E.
>
> **Hydrogenation**
> a process of adding hydrogen atoms to unsaturated vegetable oils (usually corn, soybean, cottonseed, safflower, or canola oil), which reduces the number of double bonds; the number of saturated and mono-unsaturated bonds increases as the number of polyunsaturated bonds decreases.
>
> **Cis Fats**
> unsaturated fatty acids whose hydrogen atoms occur on the same side of the double bond.
>
> **Trans Fats**
> unsaturated fatty acids that have at least one double bond whose hydrogen atoms are on the opposite sides of the double bond; "trans" means across in Latin.

Although all fats can become oxidized when exposed to light and oxygen over time, the greater the number of double bonds, the greater is the susceptibility to **rancidity**. Therefore, polyunsaturated fats are most susceptible to rancidity, saturated fats are least susceptible, and monounsaturated fats are somewhere in between.

To help extend the shelf life of foods, manufacturers may add antioxidants, such as butylated hydroxyanisole (BHA) and butylated hydroxytoluene (BHT), to polyunsaturated fat–rich foods and oils. Another commercial method to make oils more stable is hydrogenation.

Hydrogenation

Hydrogenation is a process that adds hydrogen atoms to polyunsaturated oils to saturate some of the double bonds so that the resulting product is less susceptible to rancidity and has improved function. Hydrogenation varies in degrees from "light" to "partial" according to the desired outcome. Lightly hydrogenated oils are more stable than polyunsaturated oils because they have fewer double bonds but are still in liquid form. Partial hydrogenation results in a more solid (more saturated) product, such as stick margarine and shortening, yet still maintains some unsaturated (double) bonds. Fully hydrogenated products are virtually completely saturated.

Initially, hydrogenated fats appeared to be superior to both saturated and unsaturated fats, albeit for different reasons. Compared to the saturated fats in butter and lard, hydrogenated fats seemed more heart healthy because they still provide some unsaturated fatty acids. And compared to liquid oils, products made with partially hydrogenated fats have a longer shelf life and improved functionality. Hydrogenated fats make pie crusts flakier, French fries crispier, and frosting creamier. Seemingly a have-your-cake-and-eat-it-too type of product, partially hydrogenated fats permeated the food supply and quickly became a dietary staple in the 1970s.

However, the process of hydrogenation changes the placement of the hydrogen atoms around the remaining double bonds from the natural **cis** position to the rare trans position (Fig. 4.3). Lightly or partially hydrogenated margarines, shortenings, and oils as well as processed foods made with those products, such as fried foods (doughnuts, French fries, potato chips), baked goods (cakes, cookies, pie crusts), and frozen pizza became the major source of artificial trans fats in the food supply. Because fully hydrogenated fats are completely saturated, they are trans fat free. Only small amounts of **trans fats** occur naturally in some animal foods, such as beef, lamb, and dairy products.

Trans Fats

Over time, mounting evidence revealed that trans fats increase LDL cholesterol and reduce high-density lipoprotein (HDL) cholesterol, the lipoprotein that is protective against CVD. Even at low intake levels, trans fat intake is associated with abnormal lipid levels, inflammation, and increased cardiovascular mortality; growing evidence also suggests an increased risk of diabetes, cancer, and stroke (Kiage et al., 2013). Changes in food manufacturing have reduced the prevalence of trans fats in foods. By limiting processed foods and fast foods that are made with light or partially hydrogenated oils, consumers should be able to ideally lower their trans fat intake to <1% of total calories (Vannice & Rasmussen, 2014). Currently, manufactured and natural trans fats account for 3.7% of total calories consumed.

Figure 4.3 ▶
Cis and trans fatty acid configuration.

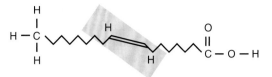

Trans-position: H on opposite sides of double bond

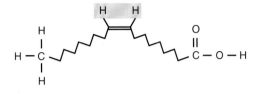

Cis-position: H on same side of double bond

Trans fatty acid content is listed on the "Nutrition Facts" label. However, because amounts less than 0.5 g per serving can be rounded down to zero, the label can claim to have "zero trans fats" even if partially hydrogenated oils or shortenings appear on the ingredient list. And although 0.5 g trans fat per serving may sound insignificant, it can add up. For instance, most people will eat 3 cups of microwave popcorn at a time, which is actually three servings according to the label. At slightly under 0.5 g trans fat per serving, the total trans fat intake comes to almost 1.5 g. Only when the label says "no trans fats" is it actually free of trans fat.

Based on extensive research and public input, the U.S. Food and Drug Administration (FDA) released a final determination in June 2015 that states partially hydrogenated oils are no longer **Generally Recognized as Safe (GRAS)** (FDA, 2016). A 3-year compliance period gives food manufacturers time to reformulate products without partially hydrogenated oils and/or petition the FDA to permit specific uses of partially hydrogenated oils. In the meantime, consumers are urged to read ingredient labels and choose products that do not contain partially hydrogenated oils. Because trans fatty acids occur naturally in meat and dairy products, they will not be eliminated from the food supply.

Generally Recognized as Safe (GRAS) compounds exempt from the definition of "food additive" because they are generally recognized as safe based on "a reasonable certainty of no harm from a product under the intended conditions of use."

FUNCTIONS OF FAT IN THE BODY

The primary function of fat is to fuel the body. At rest, fat provides about 60% of the body's calorie needs. All fat, whether saturated or unsaturated, cis or trans, provides 9 cal/g, more than double the amount of calories as an equivalent amount of either carbohydrate or protein. Although fat is an important energy source, it cannot meet all of the body's energy needs because certain cells, such as brain cells and cells of the central nervous system, normally rely solely on glucose for energy.

Fat has other important functions in the body. Fat deposits insulate and cushion internal organs to protect them from mechanical injury. Fat under the skin helps to regulate body temperature by serving as a layer of insulation against the cold. And dietary fat facilitates the absorption of the fat-soluble vitamins A, D, E, and K when consumed at the same meal.

Specific types of fatty acids have particular functions in the body. For instance,

- Saturated fatty acids provide structure to cell membranes and facilitate normal function of proteins.
- MUFAs are components of lipid membranes, especially nervous tissue myelin.
- Both essential fatty acids play a role in maintaining healthy skin and promoting normal growth in children.
- Omega-6 PUFAs are involved in the synthesis of fatty acids, are components of cell membranes, and play a role in cell signaling pathways.

- Arachidonic acid and EPA are precursors of eicosanoids (e.g., prostaglandins, thromboxanes, and leukotrienes), a group of hormone-like substances that help regulate blood pressure, blood clotting, and other body functions. Observational and randomized controlled trial evidence suggest that fish or fish oil intake may reduce inflammation, improve endothelial function, and normalize variations in heart rate and, at high doses, inhibit platelet aggregation (Mozaffarian, Appel, & Van Horn, 2011).
- EPA and DHA may play a role in preventing and treating heart disease through their anti-inflammatory, antiarrhythmic, and anticlotting effects (IFICF, 2014). They are essential for normal growth and development. DHA is a structural component of red blood cell membranes and is abundant in retinal tissue, neuron cells, the liver, and testes.

Phospholipids

Phospholipids
a group of compound lipids that is similar to triglycerides in that they contain a glycerol molecule and two fatty acids. In place of the third fatty acid, phospholipids have a phosphate group and a molecule of choline or another nitrogen-containing compound.

Emulsifier
a stabilizing compound that helps to keep both parts of an emulsion (oil and water mixture) from separating.

Like triglycerides, **phospholipids** have a glycerol backbone with fatty acids attached. What makes them different from triglycerides is that a phosphate group replaces one of the fatty acids. Although phospholipids occur naturally in almost all foods, they make up a very small percentage of total fat intake.

Phospholipids are both fat soluble (because of the fatty acids) and water soluble (because of the phosphate group), a unique feature that enables them to act as **emulsifiers**. This role is played out in the body as they emulsify fats to keep them suspended in blood and other body fluids. As a component of all cell membranes, phospholipids not only provide structure but also help to transport fat-soluble substances across cell membranes. Phospholipids are also precursors of prostaglandins.

Lecithin is the best-known phospholipid. Claims that it lowers blood cholesterol; improves memory; controls weight; and cures arthritis, hypertension, and gallbladder problems are unfounded. Studies show no benefit from taking supplements because lecithin is digested in the gastrointestinal tract into its component parts and is not absorbed intact to perform super functions. Lecithin is not even an essential nutrient because it is synthesized in the body. Many people who take lecithin supplements do not realize that they provide 9 cal/g, just like all other fats.

Cholesterol

Sterols
one of three main classes of lipids that include cholesterol, bile acids, sex hormones, the adrenocortical hormones, and vitamin D.

Cholesterol is a **sterol**, a waxy substance whose carbon, hydrogen, and oxygen molecules are arranged in a ring. Cholesterol occurs in the tissues of all animals. It is found in all cell membranes and in myelin. Brain and nerve cells are especially rich in cholesterol. The body synthesizes bile acids, steroid hormones, and vitamin D from cholesterol. Although cholesterol is made from acetyl-coenzyme A (acetyl-CoA), the body cannot break down cholesterol into CoA molecules to yield energy, so cholesterol does not provide calories.

Cholesterol is found exclusively in animals, with organ meats and egg yolks the richest sources. The cholesterol in food is just cholesterol; descriptions of "good" and "bad" cholesterol refer to the lipoprotein packages that move cholesterol through the blood (see Chapter 20). You cannot eat more "good" cholesterol, but you can make lifestyle changes, such as quitting smoking, exercising, and losing weight if overweight, that increase the amount of "good" cholesterol in the blood.

Because all body cells are capable of making enough cholesterol to meet their needs, cholesterol is not an essential nutrient. In fact, daily endogenous cholesterol synthesis is approximately two to three times more than average cholesterol intake. When dietary cholesterol decreases, endogenous cholesterol production increases to maintain an adequate supply. The body makes cholesterol from acetyl-CoA, which can originate from carbohydrates, protein, fat, or alcohol. Thus, eating an excess of calories, regardless of the source, can increase cholesterol synthesis.

HOW THE BODY HANDLES FAT

Digestion

A minimal amount of chemical digestion of fat occurs in the mouth and stomach through the action of lingual lipase and gastric lipases, respectively (Fig. 4.4).

Figure 4.4 ▶
Fat digestion.

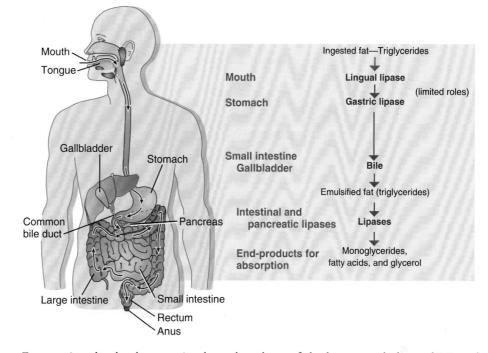

Fat entering the duodenum stimulates the release of the hormone cholecystokinin, which in turn stimulates the gallbladder to release bile. Bile, an emulsifier produced in the liver from bile salts, cholesterol, phospholipids, bilirubin, and electrolytes, prepares fat for digestion by suspending the hydrophobic molecules in the watery intestinal fluid. Emulsified fat particles have enlarged surface areas on which digestive enzymes can work.

Most fat digestion occurs in the small intestine. Pancreatic lipase, the most important and powerful lipase, splits off one fatty acid at a time from the triglyceride molecule, working from the outside in until two free fatty acids and a **monoglyceride** remain. Usually, the process stops at this point, but sometimes, digestion continues and the monoglyceride splits into a free fatty acid and a glyceride molecule. The end products of digestion—mostly monoglycerides with free fatty acids and little glycerol—are absorbed into intestinal cells. It is normal for a small amount of fat (4–5 g) to escape digestion and be excreted in the feces.

> **Monoglyceride**
> a glyceride molecule with only one fatty acid attached.

The digestion of phospholipids is similar, with the end products being two free fatty acids and a phospholipid fragment. Cholesterol does not undergo digestion; it is absorbed as is.

Absorption

About 95% of consumed fat is absorbed, mostly in the duodenum and jejunum. Small fat particles, such as short- and medium-chain fatty acids and glycerol, are absorbed directly through the mucosal cells into capillaries. They bind with albumin and are transported to the liver via the portal vein.

The absorption of larger fat particles—namely, monoglycerides and long-chain fatty acids—is more complex. Although they are insoluble in water, monoglycerides and long-chain fatty acids dissolve into **micelles**, which deliver fat to the intestinal cells. Once inside the intestinal cells, the monoglycerides and long-chain fatty acids combine to form triglycerides. The reformed triglycerides, along with phospholipids and cholesterol, become encased in protein to form **chylomicrons**. Chylomicrons distribute dietary lipids throughout the body.

> **Micelles**
> fat particles encircled by bile salts to facilitate their diffusion into intestinal cells.
>
> **Chylomicrons**
> lipoproteins that transport absorbed lipids from intestinal cells through the lymph and eventually into the bloodstream.

Their job done, most of the released bile salts are reabsorbed in the terminal ileum, transported back to the liver, and recycled (enterohepatic circulation). Some bile salts become bound to fiber in the intestine and are excreted in the feces.

Fat Catabolism

Whether from the most recent meal or from storage, triglycerides that are needed for energy are split into glycerol and fatty acids by lipoprotein lipase and are released into the bloodstream to be picked up by cells.

The catabolism of fatty acids increases when carbohydrate intake is inadequate (e.g., while on a very-low-calorie or low carbohydrate diet) or unavailable (e.g., in the case of uncontrolled diabetes). Without adequate glucose, the breakdown of fatty acids is incomplete, and ketones are formed. Eventually, ketosis and acidosis may result.

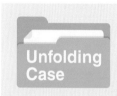

Recall Dylan. It is well known that starvation causes a decrease in seizure activity, although the mechanism of action is not known. Starvation causes acidosis, ketosis, dehydration, and hypoglycemia. The ketogenic diet provides calories and carbohydrate at levels that mimic a starved state where the primary fuel is fat. After fully implementing the diet, Dylan's blood work confirms a low pH related to ketoacids. What does that finding indicate in terms of dietary compliance?

Because fatty acids break down into two-carbon molecules, not three-carbon molecules, they cannot be reassembled to make glucose. Only the glycerol component of triglycerides can be used to make glucose, making fat an inefficient choice of fuel for glucose-dependent brain cells, nerve cells, and red blood cells. Fortunately, most body cells can use fatty acids for energy.

Fat Anabolism

Most newly absorbed fatty acids recombine with glycerol to form triglycerides that end up stored in adipose tissue. Fat stored in adipose cells represents the body's largest and most efficient energy reserve; most other body cells are able to store only minute amounts of fat. Unlike glycogen, which can be stored only in limited amounts and is accompanied by water, adipose cells have a virtually limitless capacity to store fat and carry very little additional weight as intracellular water. Although normal glycogen reserves may last for half a day of normal activity, fat reserves can last up to 2 months in people of normal weight. Each pound of body fat provides 3500 calories.

FAT IN FOODS

Fat has many vital functions in food and serves to improve overall palatability. For instance, it

- Imparts its own flavor, from the mild taste of canola oil and corn oil to the distinctive tastes of peanut oil and olive oil
- Transfers heat to rapidly cook food, as in the case of frying
- Absorbs flavors and aromas of ingredients to improve overall taste
- Adds juiciness to meats
- Creates a creamy and smooth "mouth feel" in items such as ice cream, desserts, and cream soups
- Adds texture or body to many foods, such as flakiness, tenderness, elasticity, and viscosity (e.g., milk is watery and cheese is rubbery when fat is removed)
- Imparts tenderness and moisture in baked goods, such as cookies, pies, and cakes, and delays staling
- Is insoluble in water and thus provides a unique flavor and texture to foods such as salad dressings

The fat content in MyPlate varies greatly among groups and between selections within each group (Fig. 4.5). Vegetables and grains naturally provide little or no fat; however, some items within each group have added fat, such as fried or creamed vegetables and granola cereals and biscuits. With the exception of avocado, coconut, and olives, fruits are naturally fat free. Items in the dairy group range from fat free to full fat. The fat content of the protein group and oils is discussed in the following sections.

	Fruits Focus on whole fruits	Vegetables Vary your veggies	Grains Make half your grains whole grains	Protein Vary your protein routine	Dairy Move to low-fat or fat-free milk or yogurt
Fat g/svg or oz (as specified)**	0 Exceptions: coconut, olives, avocados	0 Exceptions: vegetables prepared with added fat, such as fried onion rings or creamed spinach	Most items: 0–1 Items with 5 g fat/svg ⅓ c bread stuffing 1 biscuit 6 butter-type crackers Items with 10 g fat/svg 3 c buttered popcorn 13 regular potato or tortilla chips	Lean: 2 g/oz Lean beef, 90% lean ground beef Egg whites Catfish, cod, tilapia Lean pork Poultry without skin Medium-fat: 5 g/oz 85% or lower lean ground beef Egg Fried fish (any) Poultry with skin High-fat: 8 g/oz Pork bacon (2 slices) American, cheddar, swiss cheese Beef and/or pork hotdog Pork sausage	Fat-free & low fat: 0–3 g/svg 1 c fat-free or low fat milk ⅔ c fat-free or low fat plain or artificially sweetened yogurt Reduced fat: 5 g/svg 1 c reduced fat milk ⅔ c plain yogurt Whole milk & yogurt: 8g/svg 1 c whole milk 8 oz plain yogurt

* Oils category: 5 g fat per 1 tsp oil, 1 Tbsp low-fat margarine, 2 Tbsp reduced-fat salad dressing
** Serving sizes as per the American Diabetes Association/Academy of Nutrition and Dietetics.

Figure 4.5 ▲ Fat content of MyPlate. *(Source: USDA, Center for Nutrition Policy and Promotion. [2016]. Available at www.choosemyplate.gov. Accessed 2/26/16.)*

Protein Group

The amount of fat in items from the protein group varies from virtually fat free to 8 g/oz or more (see Fig. 4.5). Details worth noting are as follows:

- The 1-oz size cited in MyPlate is simply a reference, not a serving size or a portion size. Typically, a *serving size* (the amount recommended for a meal) is 3 or 4 oz, and a *portion size* (the amount actually eaten at one time) may be much larger. For instance, the portion size of meat in a fast-food triple cheeseburger is approximately 9 oz.
- Fat added during cooking, such as frying or basting with fat, increases the overall fat content and counts as choices from the Oils group. Cooking methods that usually do not require added fat are baking, roasting, broiling, grilling, poaching, and boiling.
- Untrimmed meats are higher in fat than lean-only portions.
- "Red meats"—namely, beef, pork, and lamb—are higher in saturated fat than the "white meats" of poultry and seafood.
- White poultry meat is lower in fat than dark meat; removing poultry skin removes significant fat.
- Fat content varies among different cuts of meat. The leanest beef cuts are round steaks and roasts (eye of round, top round, bottom round, round tip), top loin, and top sirloin. Lean pork choices include pork rib or loin chop or roast and lean ham. The leanest cuts of veal and lamb are loin and leg.
- Beef grades can be used as a guide to fat content because grades are based largely on the amount of **marbling**. Beef graded "prime," sold mostly to restaurants, is the most heavily marbled grade and thus the fattiest. In retail stores, within any cut, "choice" has more marbling and higher fat content than "select."
- Shellfish are very low in fat but have cholesterol.
- Most wild game is very lean. The fat content in bison, venison, elk, ostrich, pheasant (without skin), rabbit, and squirrel ranges from 2 to 5 g per 3-oz serving.
- Processed meats, such as sausage and hot dogs, may provide more fat calories than protein calories.

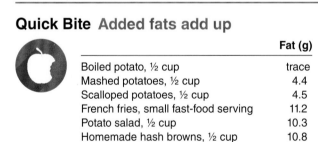

Quick Bite Added fats add up

	Fat (g)
Boiled potato, ½ cup	trace
Mashed potatoes, ½ cup	4.4
Scalloped potatoes, ½ cup	4.5
French fries, small fast-food serving	11.2
Potato salad, ½ cup	10.3
Homemade hash browns, ½ cup	10.8

Marbling
fat deposited in the muscle of meat.

- Nuts have many healthy attributes; they contain plant protein, fiber, vitamin E, selenium, magnesium, zinc, phosphorus, and potassium in a low–saturated fat, cholesterol-free package. Their high fat content of 13 to 20 g/oz comes mostly from monounsaturated fats and polyunsaturated fats. Walnuts are a rich source of alpha-linolenic acid.
- Egg yolks have approximately 186 mg of cholesterol. The cholesterol content of typical cuts of beef, pork, lamb, and poultry is generally around 70 mg/3 oz. Veal averages slightly more at about 90 mg/3 oz. The exceptions are organ meats, which are very high in cholesterol. Egg whites, legumes, and nuts are cholesterol free.

Oils

Oils are not a food group but are part of a healthy eating pattern. Allowances are small, about 6 tsp/day for a 2000-calorie eating plan. Oils include vegetable oils such as soybean, canola, corn, and olive. Most Americans consume the majority of their oils through processed foods such as salad dressing, mayonnaise, prepared vegetables (e.g., French fries), and snack chips (e.g., potato chips). Oils are also in nuts and seeds. Coconut, palm, and palm kernel oils are high in saturated fatty acids and are considered solid fats, not oils.

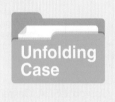

Unfolding Case

Think of Dylan. A typical ketogenic meal consists mostly of fats (e.g., 5 tbsp heavy whipping cream) with approximately an ounce of protein (e.g., chicken) and a small amount of carbohydrate (e.g., less than ½ cup green beans). What serving suggestions would you make to help make the high fat diet more palatable?

DIETARY REFERENCE INTAKES

Total Fat

Because there is insufficient data to define a level of total fat intake at which risk of deficiency or prevention of chronic disease occurs, there is not an Adequate Intake (AI) or Recommended Dietary Allowance (RDA) for total fat (National Research Council, 2005). An Acceptable Macronutrient Distribution Range (AMDR) for total fat intake is estimated to be 20% to 35% of total calories for adults (Fig. 4.6). Generally as total fat intake increases, the amount of saturated

Figure 4.6 ▶

Amount of total fat appropriate at various calorie levels based on AMDR of 20% to 35% of total calories.

AMDR 20%–35% total cal

g fat/day

Total cal/day

fat increases; therefore, limiting total fat intake to 35% of total calories may help limit saturated fat intake.

According to National Health and Nutrition Examination Survey (NHANES) 2011–2012 data, the average intake of total fat for both men and women aged 20 years and older is 33% of total calories (USDA, Agricultural Research Service [ARS], 2014). This translates to a mean intake of 96.2 g/day for men and 69.90 g/day for women.

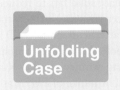

Unfolding Case

Consider Dylan. His eating pattern is for 1200 calories with 18 g of protein, 12 g of carbohydrate, and 120 g of fat. What are the percentages of calories from protein, carbohydrate, and fat? How do these percentages compare to the AMDR for each of these macronutrients? What nutrients are deficient in the diet due to the severe restriction on carbohydrates?

Specific Types of Fat

Fats that the body can synthesize—namely, saturated fatty acids, MUFAs, and cholesterol—do not need to be consumed through food. Trans fats provide no known health benefits, and so they are not essential. Neither an AI nor RDA exists for any of these fats. The essential fatty acids that the body cannot synthesize, namely, alpha-linolenic acid (*n*-3) and linoleic acid (*n*-6), have Daily Reference Intakes (DRIs). Box 4.1 summarizes the DRI for specific types of fatty acids.

Essential Fatty Acid Deficiency

Although the body cannot make essential fatty acids, it does store them, making deficiencies extremely rare in people eating a variety of food. Those at risk for deficiency include infants and children with low-fat intakes (their need for essential fatty acids is proportionately higher than that of adults), clients with anorexia nervosa, and people receiving lipid-free parenteral nutrition for long periods. People with fat malabsorption syndromes are also at risk. Symptoms of essential fatty acid deficiency include growth failure, reproductive failure, scaly dermatitis, and kidney and liver disorders.

BOX 4.1 Dietary Reference Intakes for Adults for Total Fat and Specific Types of Fat

Total Fat

- AMDR 20%–35% of total calories
- No RDA, AI, or UL

Saturated Fatty Acids (SFAs) and Trans Fat

- No RDA or AI because a dietary source is not required
- No UL because any incremental increase in intake increases the risk of coronary heart disease

Monounsaturated Fatty Acids (MUFAs)

- No RDA or AI because a dietary source is not required
- Evidence is insufficient to set a UL

Alpha-Linolenic Acid (*n*-3 Fatty Acid)

- AMDR 0.6%–1.2% of total calories
- AI: 1.1 g/day for women; 1.6 g/day for men
- Evidence insufficient to set a UL

Linoleic Acid (*n*-6 Fatty Acid)

- AMDR 5%–10% of total calories
- AI: 11–12 g/day for women; 14–17 g/day for men
- Evidence insufficient to set a UL

Acceptable Macronutrient Distribution Range (AMDR): an intake range as a percentage of total calories for energy nutrients. Adequate Intake (AI): an intake level thought to meet or exceed the requirement of almost all members of a life stage and gender group; AI is set when there are insufficient data to define an RDA. Recommended Dietary Allowance (RDA): the average daily dietary intake level sufficient to meet the nutrient requirements of 97%–98% of healthy people in a particular life stage and gender group. Tolerable Upper Intake Level (UL): the highest average daily intake level of a nutrient likely to pose no danger to most individuals in the group.

FAT IN HEALTH PROMOTION

In general, health is "promoted" when total fat and the types of fat consumed are in appropriate amounts based on calorie needs. A healthful fat intake means

- A moderate total fat intake of 20% to 35% of total calories, consistent with the AMDR
- Trans fat intake is as low as possible.
- Saturated fats intake is limited to less than 10% of total cal/day.
- Sources of PUFA and MUFA replace solid fats to reduce the risk of CVD. The European Prospective Investigation of Cancer (EPIC)-Norfolk study reported a positive association with blood levels of saturated fatty acids and CHD risk and an inverse relationship with PUFA (Khaw, Friesen, Riboli, Luben, & Wareham, 2012). Similarly, data from a prospective cohort study among women in the Nurses' Health Study showed that, independent of CHD risk factors, as intake of PUFA as a proportion of fat increased, the risk of sudden cardiac death decreased (Chiuve et al., 2012).
- Adequate amounts of omega-3 fatty acids are consumed through seafood.

Saturated and trans fat, cholesterol, and seafood intake are discussed in the following sections.

Limit Saturated Fat and Trans Fat

A key recommendation in the *2015-2020 Dietary Guidelines for Americans* is to limit saturated fats and trans fats; that recommendation is further quantified to limiting saturated fat intake to less than 10% of total calories. To achieve these goals, Americans are urged to choose a healthy eating pattern that includes the following:

- Fat-free or low-fat dairy, including milk, yogurt, cheese, and/or fortified soy beverages
- A variety of protein foods, including fatty fish and other seafood, lean meats and poultry, eggs, legumes, nuts and seeds, and soy products
- Oils, such as olive, canola, and safflower, in place of solid fats, such as butter, stick margarine, shortenings, and products made with palm and coconut oils
- Limited fried foods and foods made with partially hydrogenated oils to keep synthetic trans fat intake as low as possible
- A variety of fruits, vegetables, and whole grains—groups that provide calories, fiber, and essential nutrients in a virtually fat-free package. Avocado and olives, which are both actually fruits, provide unsaturated fat and can be part of a healthy eating pattern.

According to data from NHANES 2011–2012, saturated fat represents 11% of the total calories an average American adult consumes (USDA, ARS, 2014). The biggest source of saturated fat in the typical American eating pattern is mixed dishes, such as pizza, burgers, sandwiches, and tacos (Fig. 4.7). The most effective way to limit saturated fat and solid fats is to eat less animal fats and processed foods containing hydrogenated and partially hydrogenated oils. Strategies for lowering solid fat and increasing oils appear in Box 4.2.

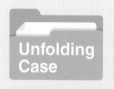

Recall Dylan. The most common adverse side effect of the ketogenic diet is constipation related to the very low carbohydrate intake. Children are closely monitored for other potential side effects, such as kidney stones, hyperlipidemias, dyslipidemias, hypoglycemia, pancreatitis, and cardiomyopathy. How do the potential risks of the diet compare to the risk of uncontrolled seizures, severe adverse side effects from medication, or the possible option of brain surgery?

Eat More Seafood—Especially Fatty Fish

Seafood is known for the *n*-3 fatty acids it provides; yet, it contains an array of other nutrients including protein, selenium, iodine, and vitamin D. Strong evidence indicates that eating

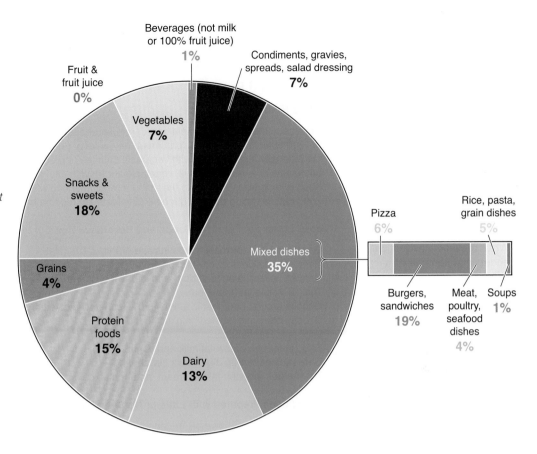

Figure 4.7 ▶

Food category sources of saturated fats in the United States. *(Sources: U.S. Department of Health and Human Services & U.S. Department of Agriculture. 2015-2020 Dietary guidelines for Americans [8th ed.]. Available at http://health .gov.dietaryguidelines/2015. Accessed on 2/26/16; and What We Eat in America [WWEIA] Food Category Analyses for the 2015 Dietary Guidelines Advisory Committee; NHANES 2009-2010.)*

patterns that include seafood are associated with a lower risk of CVD; moderate evidence shows a reduced risk of obesity (USDHHS & USDA, 2015). It is not completely known whether health benefits are solely due to fish oil intake or if other nutrients contribute to its benefits (Gribble et al., 2016).

The *2015-2020 Dietary Guidelines for Americans* recommends 8 oz of seafood per week from a variety of seafood sources. This weekly amount of seafood averages to approximately 250 mg/day of EPA and DHA combined. Likewise, the American Heart Association recommends eating fish, especially fatty fish such as salmon, anchovy, shad, sardines, tuna, herring, and mackerel, at least twice a week for a total of about 7 oz per week (American Heart Association, 2015), and the American Diabetes Association recommends eating fatty fish to prevent or treat CVD (American Diabetes Association, 2016). The term "fatty" here is relative. Atlantic mackerel is a "high-fat" fish that provides approximately 13 g of fat/3 oz; a high-fat meat such as beef brisket that may provide 21 g fat for the same size portion.

Although 80% of American adults eat seafood, an estimated 80% to 90% does not meet the recommended intake amounts (Jahns et al., 2014). In fact, average intakes of seafood are low for all age/gender groups (USDHHS & USDA, 2015). According to NHANES data for 2011–2012, mean intake of both EPA and DHA in men 20 years and older is 100 mg/day and 70 mg/day for women 20 years and older (USDA, ARS, 2014). Barriers to increasing intake include cost and not knowing how to cook seafood.

A potential risk from eating fish is exposure to **methylmercury**, which is found in varying amounts in almost all fish. Most fish have minute amounts that are not harmful to humans; large predatory fish with long lifespans have more. Relatively recent evidence suggests that the effects of mercury may be neutralized by selenium, which is also present in seafood in varying amounts (Gribble et al., 2016). Still, to minimize potential risk from methylmercury, it is recommended that people choose seafood that is high in EPA and DHA and lower in methylmercury, such as salmon, anchovies, herring, shad, sardines, Pacific oysters, and Atlantic and Pacific mackerel. People who eat more than the recommended 8 oz of seafood per week are encouraged to choose a mix of seafood that are relatively low in methylmercury.

Methylmercury
mercury, a neurotoxin, is a heavy metal that occurs naturally in the environment and is released into the air through industrial pollution. It changes to methylmercury when it falls from the air into the water. As a fat-soluble element, it accumulates in the fat tissue of large predatory fish. Pregnant and lactating women and children younger than age 8 years are vulnerable to the toxic effects of mercury because it can damage the developing brain and spinal cord.

BOX 4.2   Strategies for Reducing Solid Fats and Increasing Oils

Reduce Solid Fats

Eat Less Meat

- Replace some of the fatty meat and/or regular cheese in mixed dishes with increased amounts of vegetables, whole grains, lean meat, or low-fat or nonfat cheese.
- Occasionally replace meat with vegetable sources of protein, such as bean burritos, black beans and rice, meatless chili, vegetable stir fry with tofu, and lentil soup.
- Keep portion sizes of meat to the amount recommended with your appropriate calorie level. In a 2000-calorie eating pattern, 5½ oz-equivalents are recommended per day.

Choose Lower Fat Forms of Foods and Beverages that Contain Solid Fats

- Bake, broil, grill, or roast meats instead of frying. Drain fat.
- Remove the skin from chicken before eating.
- Choose "select" grades of beef, which have less marbling than "choice" grades.
- Trim all visible fat from meat.
- Choose ground beef that is at least 90% lean as indicated on the label.
- Choose beef cuts labeled "loin" or "round."
- Limit processed meats.
- Choose fat-free or low-fat milk and yogurt.
- Choose cheese with 3 g or less per serving.
- Try sherbet, reduced-fat ice cream, and nonfat ice cream.

Choose Foods Prepared with Little or No Solid Fats

- Use nonstick spray, olive oil, or canola oil in place of margarine or butter to sauté foods and "butter" pans.
- Use imitation butter spray to season vegetables and hot air popcorn.
- When you eat foods with solid fats, limit portion sizes. Foods high in solid fat include cakes, cookies, desserts, pizza, cheese, fatty meats, and ice cream.

Reduce Trans Fat Intake

- Use soft margarine (liquid or tub) in place of butter or stick margarine. Look for margarine that is "trans fat free," contains no more than 2 g saturated fat per tablespoon, and has liquid vegetable oil as the first ingredient.
- Look for processed foods made with unhydrogenated oil rather than partially hydrogenated oil or saturated fat.
- Avoid fried fast foods that are made with hydrogenated shortenings and oils.

Replace Fatty Foods with Fruit and Vegetables

- Eat fruit for dessert.
- Snack on raw vegetables or fresh fruit instead of snack chips.
- Double up on your usual portion of vegetables.

Increase Oils

- Use oils—especially soybean, canola, corn, or olive—instead of butter or shortening for cooking and baking.
- Eat 8 oz of fatty fish per week, such as salmon, sardines, herring, trout, and mackerel.
- If you eat more than 8 oz of fish per week, choose a variety of seafood.
- Eat nuts and nut butters that are rich in monounsaturated fats: walnuts, almonds, hazelnuts, pecans, pistachios, and pine nuts. Walnuts also contain alpha-linolenic acid. Cashews and macadamia nuts are higher in saturated fats.
- Sprinkle ground flaxseed, chia seeds, or hemp seed (1–2 tbsp/day) over cereal or yogurt. Use ground flaxseed as a fat substitute in many recipes: 3 tbsp of ground flaxseed can replace 1 tbsp of fat or oil.
- Read the "Nutrition Facts" label to identify oils with the highest unsaturated fat content.

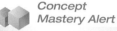

Concept Mastery Alert

When providing instruction about what constitutes a "good" fat, nurses should emphasize flaxseed, walnuts, and tuna. Whereas whole wheat is a healthy choice for sandwiches, processed meats should be limited in the diet.

Because fish provides vital nutrients for developing fetuses and infants, especially *n*-3 fatty acids, pregnant and lactating women are urged to eat 8 to 12 oz of seafood per week (FDA & Environmental Protection Agency [EPA], 2014). They are further advised to avoid certain fish high in mercury, namely, shark, swordfish, king mackerel, and tilefish, and to limit white albacore tuna to 6 oz per week. Likewise, state and local advisories should be adhered to for locally caught fish. Table 4.2 lists the amount of *n*-3 fatty acids and mercury in various types of seafood.

Table 4.2 — Estimated EPA and DHA and Mercury Content in 4 oz of Selected Seafood Varieties

Common Seafood Varieties	EPA+DHA[a] (mg/4 oz)[b]	Mercury[c] (μg/4 oz)[d]
Salmon[e]: Atlantic,[f] Chinook,[f] Coho[f]	1200–2400	2
Anchovies,[e,f] Herring,[e,f] and Shad[e]	2300–2400	5–10
Mackerel: Atlantic and Pacific (not King)	1350–2100	8–13
Tuna: Bluefin[e,f] and Albacore[e]	1700	54–58
Sardines[e]: Atlantic[f] and Pacific[f]	1100–1600	2
Trout: Freshwater	1000–1100	11
Tuna: White (Albacore) canned	1000	40
Salmon[e]: Pink[f] and Sockeye[f]	700–900	2
Pollock[e]: Atlantic[f] and Walleye[f]	600	6
Crab[g]: Blue,[e] King,[e,f] Snow,[e] Queen,[f] and Dungeness[f]	200–550	9
Tuna: Skipjack and Yellowfin	150–350	31–49
Flounder,[e,f] Plaice,[e] and Sole[e,f] (Flatfish)	350	7
Tuna: Light canned	150–300	13
Catfish	100–250	7
Cod[e]: Atlantic[f] and Pacific[f]	200	14
Scallops[e,g]: Bay[f] and Sea[f]	200	8
Lobster[g,h]: Northern[e,f] American[e]	200	47
Tilapia	150	2
Shrimp[g]	100	0
Seafood varieties that should not be consumed by women who are pregnant or breastfeeding[i]		
Shark	1250	151
Tilefish[f]: Gulf of Mexico[e,j]	1000	219
Swordfish	1000	147
Mackerel: King	450	110

[a]A total of 1750 mg of eicosapentaenoic acid (EPA) and docosahexaenoic acid (DHA) per week represents an average of 250 mg/day, which is the goal amount to achieve at the recommended 8 oz of seafood per week for the general public.
[b]EPA and DHA values are for the cooked, edible portion rounded to the nearest 50 mg. Ranges are provided when values are comparable. Values are estimates.
[c]A total of 39 μg of mercury per week would reach the EPA reference dose limit (0.1 μg/kg/day) for a woman who is pregnant or breastfeeding and who weighs 124 pounds (56 kg).
[d]Mercury was measured as total mercury and/or methylmercury. Mercury values of zero were below the level of detection. Values for mercury adjusted to reflect 4-oz weight after cooking, assuming 25% moisture loss. Canned varieties not adjusted; mercury values gathered from cooked forms. Values are rounded to the nearest whole number. Ranges are provided when values are comparable. Values are estimates.
[e]Seafood variety is included in mercury value(s) reported.
[f]Seafood variety is included in EPA+DHA value(s) reported.
[g]Cooked by moist heat.
[h]Spiny lobster has approximately 550 mg of EPA+DHA and 14 μg mercury per 4 oz.
[i]Women who are pregnant or breastfeeding should also limit white (albacore) tuna to 6 oz/week.
[j]Values are for tilefish from the Gulf of Mexico; does not include Atlantic tilefish, which have approximately 22 μg of mercury per 4 oz.
Source: U.S. Food and Drug Administration. (2014). *Fish: What pregnant women and parents should know*. Available at http://www.fda.gov/Food/FoodborneIllness Contaminants/Metals/ucm393070.htm. Accessed on 11/15/16.

How Do You Respond?

Is coconut oil healthy? An attractive attribute of coconut oil is that almost half of its fatty acids are medium-chain triglycerides (MCTs), which the body readily oxidizes instead of storing them as fat in the body. In fact, MCT have been shown to be better at decreasing body fat and improving weight loss when compared to olive oil (St-Onge & Bosarge, 2008). It is no surprise that coconut oil is being touted as a healthy fat. However, because 44% of the fatty acids in coconut oil are saturated and known to raise serum cholesterol levels, the intake of coconut products is not currently recommended (Vannice & Rasmussen, 2014).

What is flaxseed? Flaxseed is derived from the flax plant, the same plant used to make linen. It is a nutritional powerhouse, providing essential fatty acids, fiber, and lignans. Specifically, 57% of its fat is from alpha-linolenic acid, the essential *n*-3 fatty acid that is only found in plants. The fiber in flaxseed is predominately soluble, which helps to lower cholesterol levels and improves glucose levels in people with diabetes. Flaxseed contains 100 to 800 times more lignans than other grains; lignans, a group of plant estrogens, may help to reduce the risk of breast and prostate cancers. Although flaxseed oil and flaxseed oil pills provide the benefits of alpha-linolenic acid, they lack the fiber found in the whole grain, and the lignan content is variable. However, humans are unable to digest the tough outer coating, so flaxseeds must be eaten ground, not whole. Because they are high in polyunsaturated fat, they are prone to rancidity. Ground flaxseed should be refrigerated and used within a few weeks.

REVIEW CASE STUDY

Michael is a 40-year-old man who lost about 25 pounds 10 years ago by reducing his fat intake. He has slowly regained the weight and now wants to go back to a low-fat diet to manage his weight. He gives you a sample of his usual intake on the right:

- What foods and beverages did Michael eat that contain fat? What sources of saturated fat did he eat? What sources of unsaturated fat? What sources of *n*-3 fats? What sources of cholesterol? What specific suggestions would you make for him to eat less fat and/or improve the type of fat he eats?
- What would you tell Michael about cutting fat intake to lose weight? What would you suggest he do to "eat healthier"?

Breakfast: 3 cups of coffee with sugar and nondairy creamer
On the way to work: A bagel with low-fat cream cheese and jelly
Snack before lunch: Low-fat coffee cake; more coffee with sugar and nondairy creamer
Lunch: Usually a burger, large order of French fries, and a diet soda from the fast-food restaurant near his office
Snack before dinner: A glass of wine with cheese and crackers
Dinner: Meat, potato, and vegetable; often double portions of meat; a salad with Italian dressing; bread and butter; Sherbet for dessert
Snack: A bowl of cornflakes with 2% milk and sugar

STUDY QUESTIONS

1 The client asks if the cholesterol in shrimp is the "good" or "bad" type. Which of the following would be the nurse's best response?
   a. "All cholesterol is bad cholesterol."
   b. "Bad and good refer to how cholesterol is packaged for transport through the blood. The cholesterol in food is unpackaged and neither bad nor good."
   c. "Good cholesterol is found in plants; bad cholesterol is found in animal sources."
   d. "Shrimp has good cholesterol because it is low in saturated fat; foods high in cholesterol and saturated fat are a bad source of cholesterol."

2 When developing a teaching plan for a client who needs to limit saturated fat, which of the following foods would the nurse suggest the client limit?
   a. Seafood and poultry
   b. Nuts and seeds
   c. Olive oil and canola oil
   d. Red meat and full-fat dairy products

3 What is the primary function of fat?
   a. To facilitate protein metabolism
   b. To provide energy
   c. To promote the absorption of fat-soluble vitamins
   d. To facilitate carbohydrate metabolism

4 The nurse knows that instructions have been effective when the client verbalizes that the sources of synthetic trans fats are
a. Red meat and full-fat dairy products
b. Commercial baked goods and stick margarine
c. Pretzels and nuts
d. Butter and lard

5 A client asks why lowering saturated fat intake is necessary for lowering serum cholesterol levels. Which of the following is the nurse's best response?
a. "Saturated fats raise the 'bad' cholesterol levels more than any other dietary fat."
b. "Sources of saturated fat also provide monounsaturated fat, and both should be limited to control blood cholesterol levels."
c. "Saturated fat is high in calories, and excess calories from any source increase the risk of high blood cholesterol levels."
d. "Saturated fats make blood more likely to clot, increasing the risk of heart attack."

6 What should the nurse tell a client who likes fish but refuses to eat it because of fear of mercury poisoning?
a. "You are justified to be concerned. To be safe, use fish oil supplements instead."
b. "You can eat as much fish as you want because most fish are not contaminated with even small amounts of mercury."
c. "The benefits of eating 8 oz/week of a variety of fish outweigh any potential risks from mercury."
d. "As a compromise, eat 4 oz of fish per week instead of 8 oz."

7 Which statement indicates the client understands about choosing low-fat foods from MyPlate?
a. "All items within a food group have approximately the same amount of fat."
b. "You don't have to consciously select low-fat items because the empty calorie allowance will account for higher fat choices."
c. "It is best to eliminate as much fat from the diet as possible."
d. "Within each food group, the foods lowest in fat should be chosen most often."

8 Which of the following are the best sources of omega-3 fatty acids?
a. Salmon and trout
b. Flaxseed and walnuts
c. Olive and canola oils
d. Cod fish and haddock

KEY CONCEPTS

- Ninety-eight percent of lipids consumed in the diet are triglycerides, which are composed of one glyceride molecule and three fatty acids. Phospholipids and sterols are the other two types of dietary lipids.
- Saturation refers to each carbon atom in the fatty acid chain having four single bonds. In saturated fats, each carbon is "saturated" with as much hydrogen as it can hold. Unsaturated fats have one (monounsaturated) or more than one (polyunsaturated) double bond between carbon atoms.
- All fats in foods contain a mixture of saturated, monounsaturated, and polyunsaturated fats. When used to describe food fats, these terms are relative descriptions of the type of fatty acid present in the largest amount.
- Generally, saturated fats are "bad" because they raise total and LDL cholesterol, although not all individual saturated fatty acids have a detrimental impact serum cholesterol. Unsaturated fats are "good" because they lower total and LDL cholesterol when consumed in place of saturated fats.
- Trans fatty acids are produced through the process of hydrogenation. They are chemically unsaturated fats; however, like saturated fat, they raise total and LDL cholesterol.
- Linoleic acid (n-6) and alpha-linolenic acid (n-3) are essential fatty acids because they cannot be made by the body. They are important constituents of cell membranes, are involved in eicosanoid synthesis, and function to maintain healthy skin and promote normal growth.

- The major function of fat is to provide energy; 1 g of fat supplies 9 calories of energy. Fat also provides insulation, protects internal organs from mechanical damage, and promotes absorption of the fat-soluble vitamins.
- Fish oils lower the risk of heart disease by their anti-inflammatory, anticlotting, and anti-arrhythmia effects. Although they may also be beneficial in preventing other health problems, the evidence is currently inconclusive or lacking.
- The best sources of n-3 fatty acids are fatty cold-water fish such as salmon, trout, herring, sardines, and mackerel. Walnuts, soybeans, flaxseed, and canola oil are plant sources of the n-3 fatty acid alpha-linolenic acid, but alpha-linolenic acid may not have the same cardioprotective benefits as fish oils.
- Phospholipids are structural components of cell membranes that facilitate the transport of fat-soluble substances across cell membranes. They are widespread but appear in small amounts in the diet.
- Cholesterol, a sterol, is a constituent of all cell membranes and is used to make bile acids, steroid hormones, and vitamin D. Cholesterol is found in all foods of animal origin except egg whites. Most Americans eat about half as much cholesterol as the body makes each day.
- Fat digestion occurs mostly in the small intestine. Short- and medium-chain fatty acids and glycerol are absorbed through mucosal cells into capillaries leading to the portal vein. Larger fat molecules—namely, cholesterol, phospholipids, and reformed triglycerides made from monoglycerides and

long-chain fatty acids—are absorbed in chylomicrons and transported through the lymph system.

- Grains and vegetables are naturally fat free or low in fat, although certain preparation methods can add fat. Only three fruits provide fat: coconut, avocado, and olives. The dairy and protein groups provide fat, with the type and quantity of fat varying among items within each group. Oils are not a food group but are part of a healthy eating pattern.
- The AMDR for total fat is set at 20% to 35% of total calories. The intake of saturated fat and trans fat should be as low as possible within the context of a nutritionally

adequate diet. The *2015-2020 Dietary Guidelines for Americans* do not include a recommendation to limit cholesterol intake. Deficiencies of essential fatty acids are nonexistent in healthy people.

- To achieve a more optimal fat intake, a plant-based diet rich in fruit, vegetables, whole grains, legumes, and nuts is recommended with adequate amounts of fat-free dairy products and lean meats. Fats, such as in margarine and salad dressings, should be trans fat free, and these products should preferably be made with canola or olive oil. A total of 8 oz or more of seafood per week is suggested.

Check Your Knowledge Answer Key

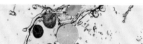

1 **TRUE** All fats, whether saturated or unsaturated, provide 9 cal/g compared to 4 cal/g from carbohydrates and protein.

2 **FALSE** "Good" fats—namely, polyunsaturated and monounsaturated fats—may help to lower LDL cholesterol when used in place of saturated fat. Omega-3 fish oils are also "good": They lower triglyceride levels; decrease platelet aggregation; and may decrease inflammation in rheumatoid arthritis, Crohn disease, and ulcerative colitis.

3 **TRUE** Endogenous cholesterol synthesis is generally two to three times higher than the average cholesterol intake in the United States.

4 **FALSE** The benefits of eating seafood outweigh the potential risks related to the mercury content of fish. Still, eating fish that are lower in mercury is recommended. A high selenium content in the fish may also mitigate the potential risk from mercury.

5 **TRUE** Tub margarine is healthier than butter because it is lower in saturated fat, which is why it has a softer texture than butter, which is hard because saturated fatty acids are physically able to pack together tightly. Unsaturated fatty

acids are physically kinked due to the double bonds and stay liquid at room temperature.

6 **TRUE** All food fats are a blend of saturated fatty acids, PUFAs, and MUFAs. The description of a fat as "saturated" means that there are more saturated fatty acids than PUFAs or MUFAs in that source, not that saturated fatty acids are the only fatty acids present.

7 **FALSE** Although they are oils, palm, palm kernel, and coconut are predominately saturated and are considered solid fats, not oils.

8 **FALSE** Vegetable oils are still vegetable oils, even when they are lightly or partially hydrogenated; therefore, the term "vegetable oil" is not synonymous with trans fat free.

9 **FALSE** Fish oils are not essential in the diet because the body can convert alpha-linolenic acid to EPA and DHA, although only in limited quantities. Essential nutrients cannot be made by the body and so must be supplied through food.

10 **TRUE** Citing lack of evidence of the detrimental role of dietary cholesterol on serum cholesterol levels, the *2015-2020 Dietary Guidelines for Americans* does not include a recommendation on limiting cholesterol intake.

Student Resources on thePoint®
For additional learning materials, activate the code in the front of this book at http://thePoint.lww.com/activate

Websites

American Heart Association at www.heart.org

American Oil Chemists' Society at www.aocs.org

Calorie Control Council's glossary of fat replacers at www.caloriecontrol.org/articles-and-video/feature-articles/glossary-of-fat-replacers

Institute of Shortening and Edible Oils at www.iseo.org

International Food Information Council at www.foodinsight.org/

National Heart, Lung, and Blood Institute at www.nhlbi.nih.gov

References

American Diabetes Association. (2016). Standards of medical care in diabetes—2016. *Diabetes Care, 39*(Suppl. 1), 23–35.

American Heart Association. (2015). *Fish and omega-3 fatty acids.* Available at http://www.heart.org/HEARTORG/HealthyLiving/HealthyEating/HealthyDietGoals/Fish-and-Omega-3-Fatty-Acids_UCM_303248_Article.jsp#.Vrepmsv2bIU. Accessed on 2/7/16.

Chiuve, S., Rimm, E., Sandhu, R., Bernstein, A. M., Rexrode, K. M., Manson, J. E., . . . Albert, C. M. (2012). Dietary fat quality and risk of sudden cardiac death in women. *The American Journal of Clinical Nutrition, 96,* 498–507.

Grande, F., Anderson, J., & Keys, A. (1970). Comparison of effects of palmitic and stearic acids in the diet on serum cholesterol in man. *The American Journal of Clinical Nutrition, 23,* 1184–1193.

Gribble, M., Karimi, R., Feingold, B., Nyland, J., O'Hara, T., Gladyshev, M., & Chen, C. Y. (2016). Mercury, selenium and fish oils in marine food webs and implications for human health. *Journal of the Marine Biological Association of the United Kingdom, 96,* 43–59.

International Food Information Council Foundation. (2014). *Functional foods fact sheet: Omega-3 fatty acids.* Available at http://www.foodinsight.org/Functional_Foods_Fact_Sheet_Omega_3_Fatty_Acids. Accessed on 2/6/16.

Jahns, L., Raatz, S., Johnson, L., Kranz, S., Silverstein, J. T., & Picklo, M. J. (2014). Intake of seafood in the US varies by age, income, and education level but not by race-ethnicity. *Nutrients, 6,* 6060–6075. doi:10.3390/nu6126060

Kato, H., Tillotson, J., Nichaman, M., Rhoads, G., & Hamilton, H. B. (1973). Epidemiologic studies of coronary heart disease and stroke in Japanese men living in Japan, Hawaii and California. *American Journal of Epidemiology, 97,* 372–385.

Khaw, K., Friesen, M., Riboli, E., Luben, R., & Wareham, N. (2012). Plasma phospholipid fatty acid concentration and incident coronary heart disease in men and women: The EPIC-Norfolk prospective study. *PLoS Medicine, 9,* e1001255.

Kiage, J., Merrill, P., Robinson, C., Cao, Y., Malik, T. A., Hundley, B. C., . . . Kabagambe, E. K. (2013). Intake of trans fat and all-cause mortality in the Reasons for Geographical and Racial Differences in Stroke (REGARDS) cohort. *The American Journal of Clinical Nutrition, 97,* 1121–1128.

Mozaffarian, D., Appel, L., & Van Horn, L. (2011). Components of a cardioprotective diet. New insights. *Circulation, 123,* 2870–2891.

National Research Council. (2005). *Dietary reference intakes for energy, carbohydrate, fiber, fat, fatty acids, cholesterol, protein, and amino acids (macronutrients).* Washington, DC: The National Academies Press.

Nicolosi, R. (1997). Dietary fat saturation effects on low-density-lipoprotein concentration and metabolism in various animal models. *The American Journal of Clinical Nutrition, 65*(5, Suppl.), 1617S–1627S.

Siri-Tarino, P., Sun, Q., Hu, F., & Krauss, R. (2010). Meta-analysis of prospective cohort studies evaluating the association of saturated fat with cardiovascular disease. *The American Journal of Clinical Nutrition, 91,* 535–546.

St-Onge, M., & Bosarge, A. (2008). Weight-loss diet that includes consumption of medium-chain triacylglycerol oil leads to a greater rate of weight and fat mass loss than does olive oil. *The American Journal of Clinical Nutrition, 87,* 621–626.

U.S. Department of Agriculture, Agricultural Research Service. (2014). *Nutrient intakes from food: Mean amounts consumed per individual, by gender and age. What We Eat in America, NHANES 2011–2012.* Available at www.ars.usda.gov/ba/bhnrc/fsrg. Accessed on 1/22/16.

U.S. Department of Health and Human Services & U.S. Department of Agriculture. (2015). *2015-2020 Dietary guidelines for Americans* (8th ed.). Available at www.health.gov/dietaryguidelines/2015. Accessed on 2/24/11.

U.S. Food & Drug Administration. (2016). *Final determination regarding partially hydrogenated oils (removing trans fat).* Available at http://www.fda.gov/Food/IngredientsPackagingLabeling/FoodAdditivesIngredients/ucm449162.htm. Accessed on 8/23/16.

U.S. Food and Drug Administration & Environmental Protection Agency. (2014). *Fish: What pregnant women and parents should know.* Available at www.fda.gov/food/foodborneillnesscontaminants/metals/ucm393070.htm. Accessed 2/11/16.

Vannice, G., & Rasmussen, H. (2014). Position of the Academy of Nutrition and Dietetics: dietary fatty acids for healthy adults. *Journal of the Academy of Nutrition and Dietetics, 114,* 136–153.

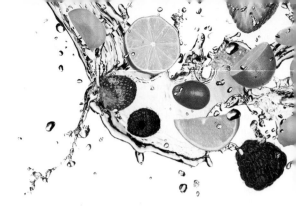

Chapter 5

Vitamins

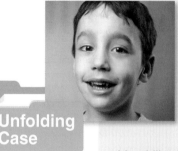

Marcus Skinner

Marcus is a 4-year-old boy with autism spectrum disorder who has communication impairments and social difficulties and exhibits repetitive behavior. His treatment includes medical nutrition therapy, speech-language therapy, occupational therapy, and physical therapy. Marcus does not eat a well-balanced eating pattern for several reasons: a feature of his compulsive behavior is that he only accepts a limited variety of foods, he is unable to eat when overstimulated at mealtime, and he has poor fine motor coordination that impairs his ability to feed himself. He is on a gluten-free/casein-free diet because these peptides are believed to cause a variety of effects in the neurotransmitter systems of the brain. Eliminating all foods containing gluten (foods containing wheat, barley, and rye) and casein (the major protein in milk and other dairy products and used as an additive in other foods such as soy products) may improve behaviors in some children with autism, although there is insufficient evidence of benefit.

Check Your Knowledge

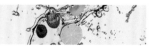

True	False		
☐	☐	1	Daily use of a multivitamin reduces the risk of cardiovascular disease and cancer.
☐	☐	2	Vitamins provide energy.
☐	☐	3	Because underconsumption is linked to adverse health outcomes, Americans' low intake of vitamin D is a public health concern.
☐	☐	4	Vitamins are susceptible to destruction.
☐	☐	5	With vitamin supplements, the higher the price, the better the quality.
☐	☐	6	"Natural" vitamins are superior to "synthetic" ones.
☐	☐	7	Under optimal conditions, vitamin D is not an essential nutrient because the body can make all it needs from sunlight on the skin.
☐	☐	8	Natural folate in foods is better absorbed than synthetic folic acid added to foods.
☐	☐	9	U.S. Pharmacopeia (USP) on a label of vitamin supplements means that the product is safe.
☐	☐	10	All vitamins need to be consumed on a daily basis.

Learning Objectives

Upon completion of this chapter, you will be able to

1 Compare and contrast fat- and water-soluble vitamins.
2 Describe general functions and uses of vitamins.

3 Judge when vitamin supplements may be necessary.
4 Give examples of food sources for individual vitamins.
5 Discuss how Americans can shift their food choices to improve their intake of shortfall vitamins.
6 Identify characteristics to look for when choosing a vitamin supplement.

In 1913, thiamin was discovered as the first vitamin, the "vital amine" necessary to prevent the deficiency disease beriberi. Today, 13 vitamins have been identified as important for human nutrition; vitamin deficiency diseases are generally rare in the United States, and vitamin research focuses on whether consuming various vitamins above the minimum basic requirement can reduce the risk of heart disease, cancer, vision disorders, cognitive decline in the elderly, and other chronic diseases.

This chapter describes vitamins and their uses. Generalizations about fat- and water-soluble vitamins are presented. Unique features of each vitamin are covered individually, and criteria for selecting a vitamin supplement are discussed.

UNDERSTANDING VITAMINS

Vitamins are organic compounds made of carbon, hydrogen, oxygen, and, sometimes, nitrogen or other elements. They differ in their chemistry, biochemistry, function, and availability in foods. Vitamins facilitate biochemical reactions within cells to help regulate body processes such as growth and metabolism. They are essential to life. Unlike the organic compounds covered previously in this unit (carbohydrates, protein, and fat), vitamins

Micronutrients
nutrients that are needed in very small amounts.

- Are individual molecules, not long chains of molecules linked together
- Do not provide energy but are needed for the metabolism of energy
- Are needed in microgram or milligram quantities, not gram quantities, and so are called **micronutrients**

Chemical Substances

Vitamins are extremely complex chemical substances that differ widely in their structures. Because vitamins are defined chemically, the body cannot distinguish between natural vitamins extracted from food and synthetic vitamins produced in a laboratory. However, the absorption rates of natural and synthetic vitamins sometimes differ because of different chemical forms of the same vitamin (e.g., synthetic folic acid is better absorbed than natural folate in foods) or because the synthetic vitamins are "free," not "bound" to other components in food (e.g., synthetic vitamin B_{12} is not bound to small peptides as natural vitamin B_{12} is).

Susceptible to Destruction

As organic substances, vitamins in food are susceptible to destruction and subsequent loss of function. Individual vitamins differ in their vulnerability to heat, light, **oxidation**, acid, and alkalis. For instance,

Oxidation
a chemical reaction in which a substance combines with oxygen; the loss of electrons in an atom.

- Thiamin is heat sensitive and is easily destroyed by high temperatures and long cooking times.
- Riboflavin is resistant to heat, acid, and oxidation but is quickly destroyed by light. That is why riboflavin-rich milk is sold in opaque, not transparent, containers.
- From 50% to 90% of folate in foods may be lost during preparation, processing, and storage.
- Vitamin C is destroyed by heat, air, and alkalis.

Multiple Forms

Many vitamins exist in more than one active form. Different forms perform different functions in the body. For instance, vitamin A exists as retinol (important for reproduction), retinal (needed for vision), and retinoic acid (acts as a hormone to regulate growth). Some vitamins have **provitamins**, an inactive form found in food that the body converts to the active form. Beta-carotene is a provitamin of vitamin A. Dietary Reference Intakes take into account the biologic activity of vitamins as they exist in different forms.

Provitamins
precursors of vitamins.

Essentiality

Vitamins are essential in the diet because, with a few exceptions, the body cannot make them. The body can make vitamin A, vitamin D, and niacin if the appropriate precursors are available. Microorganisms in the gastrointestinal (GI) tract synthesize vitamin K and vitamin B_{12} but not in amounts sufficient to meet the body's needs.

Coenzymes

Enzymes
proteins produced by cells that catalyze chemical reactions within the body without undergoing change themselves.

Coenzymes
organic molecules that activate an enzyme.

Many **enzymes** cannot function without a **coenzyme**, and many coenzymes are vitamins. All B vitamins work as coenzymes to facilitate thousands of chemical conversions. For instance, thiamin, riboflavin, niacin, and biotin participate in enzymatic reactions that extract energy from glucose, amino acids, and fat. Folacin facilitates both amino acid metabolism and nucleic acid synthesis; without adequate folacin, protein synthesis and cell division are impaired. An adequate and continuous supply of B vitamins in every cell is vital for normal metabolism.

Antioxidants

Free Radicals
highly unstable, highly reactive molecular fragments with one or more unpaired electrons.

Free radicals are produced continuously in cells as they burn oxygen during normal metabolism. Ultraviolet radiation, air pollution, ozone, the metabolism of food, and smoking can also generate free radicals in the body. The problem with free radicals is that they oxidize body cells and DNA in their quest to become stable by gaining an electron. These structurally and functionally damaged oxidized cells are believed to contribute to aging and various health problems such as cancer, heart disease, and cataracts. Polyunsaturated fatty acids (PUFAs) in cell membranes are particularly vulnerable to damage by free radicals.

Antioxidants
substances that donate electrons to free radicals to prevent oxidation.

Antioxidants protect body cells from being oxidized (destroyed) by free radicals by undergoing oxidation themselves, which renders free radicals harmless. Vitamins and other substances in fruits, vegetables, and other plant-based food provide dozens, if not hundreds, of antioxidants (Box 5.1). Vitamins that function as major antioxidants are vitamin C, vitamin E, and the provitamin beta-carotene. Each has a slightly different role, so one cannot completely substitute for another. For instance, water-soluble vitamin C works within cells to disable free radicals, and fat-soluble vitamin E functions within fat tissue. Whether high doses of individual antioxidants offer the same health benefits as the package of substances found in food sources is an area of ongoing research.

BOX 5.1   Rich Sources of Antioxidants

- Beverages: coffee, green and black tea, red wine
- Fruits: bilberries, black currants, wild strawberries, blackberries, goji berries, cranberries, dried apples, dried plums, dried apricots, prunes, kiwi, strawberries
- Vegetables: green leafy vegetables, pepper, red and green chili, spinach, carrots, tomato, onion, garlic
- Spices and herbs: cloves, peppermint, allspice, cinnamon, oregano, thyme, sage, rosemary
- Other: dark chocolate, walnuts and pecans with pellicle, sesame oil, canola oil

Food Additives
substances added intentionally or unintentionally to food that affect its character.

Enrich
to add nutrients back that were lost during processing; for example, white flour is enriched with B vitamins lost when the bran and germ layers are removed.

Fortified
to fortify is to add nutrients to a food that were either not originally present or were present in insignificant amounts; for instance, many brands of orange juice are fortified with vitamin D.

Megadoses
amounts at least 10 times greater than the Recommended Dietary Allowance (RDA).

Food Additives

Some vitamins are used as **food additives** in certain foods to boost their nutritional content; examples include vitamin C–**enriched** fruit drinks, vitamin D–**fortified** milk, and enriched flour and breads. Other foods have certain vitamins added to them to help preserve quality. For instance, vitamin C is added to frozen fish to help prevent rancidity and to luncheon meats to stabilize the red color. Vitamin E helps retard rancidity in vegetable oils, and beta-carotene adds color to margarine.

Medications

In **megadoses**, vitamins function like drugs, not nutrients. Large doses of niacin are used to lower cholesterol, low-density lipoprotein (LDL) cholesterol, and triglycerides in people with hyperlipidemia who do not respond to diet and exercise. Tretinoin (retinoic acid, a form of vitamin A) is used as a topical treatment for acne vulgaris and orally for acute promyelocytic leukemia. Gram quantities of vitamin C promote healing in patients with impaired bone and wound healing.

VITAMIN CLASSIFICATIONS BASED ON SOLUBILITY

Vitamins are classified according to their solubility. Vitamins A, D, E, and K are fat soluble. Vitamin C and the B vitamins (thiamin, riboflavin, niacin, folate, B_6, B_{12}, biotin, and pantothenic acid) are water soluble. Solubility determines vitamin absorption, transportation, storage, and excretion.

Fat-Soluble Vitamins

Group characteristics of fat-soluble vitamins are summarized in Table 5.1. Table 5.2 highlights recommended intakes, sources, functions, deficiency symptoms, and toxicity symptoms of each fat-soluble vitamin. The complete table of Dietary Reference Intakes for vitamins appears in Appendix B. Additional features of individual fat-soluble vitamins follow.

Table 5.1   Group Characteristics of Fat-Soluble and Water-Soluble Vitamins

Characteristic	Fat-Soluble Vitamins	Water-Soluble Vitamins
Sources	The fat and oil portion of foods	The watery portion of foods
Absorption	With fat encased in chylomicrons that enter the lymphatic system before circulating in the bloodstream	Directly into the bloodstream
Transportation through the blood	Attach to protein carriers because fat is not soluble in watery blood	Move freely through the watery environment of blood and within cells
When consumed in excess of need	Are stored—primarily in the liver and adipose tissue	Are excreted in the urine, although some tissues may hold limited amounts of certain vitamins
Safety of consuming high intakes through supplements	Can be toxic; this applies primarily to vitamins A and D; large doses of vitamins E and K are considered relatively nontoxic	Are generally considered nontoxic, although side effects can occur from consuming very large doses of vitamin B_6 over a prolonged period
Frequency of intake	Generally do not have to be consumed daily because the body can retrieve them from storage as needed	Must be consumed daily because there is no reserve in storage

Table 5.2   Summary of Fat-Soluble Vitamins

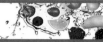

Vitamin and Sources	Functions	Deficiency/Toxicity Signs and Symptoms
Vitamin A **Adult RDA:** **Men: 900 μg** **Women: 700 μg** • Retinol: beef, liver, milk, butter, cheese, cream, egg yolk, fortified milk, margarine, and ready-to-eat cereals • Beta-carotene: "greens" (turnip, dandelion, beet, collard, mustard), spinach, kale, broccoli, carrots, peaches, pumpkin, red peppers, sweet potatoes, winter squash, mango, apricots, cantaloupe	The formation of visual purple, which enables the eye to adapt to dim light Normal growth and development of bones and teeth The formation and maintenance of mucosal epithelium to maintain healthy functioning of skin and membranes, hair, gums, and various glands Important role in immune function	**Deficiency** Slow recovery of vision after flashes of bright light at night is the first ocular symptom; can progress to xerophthalmia and blindness Bone growth ceases; bone shape changes; enamel-forming cells in the teeth malfunction; teeth crack and tend to decay Skin becomes dry, scaly, rough, and cracked; keratinization or hyperkeratosis develops; mucous membrane cells flatten and harden: eyes become dry (xerosis); irreversible drying and hardening of the cornea can result in blindness Decreased saliva secretion → difficulty chewing, swallowing → anorexia Decreased mucous secretion of the stomach and intestines → impaired digestion and absorption → diarrhea, increased excretion of nutrients Impaired immune system functioning → increased susceptibility to respiratory, urinary tract, and vaginal infections increases **Toxicity** Headaches, vomiting, double vision, hair loss, bone abnormalities, liver damage, which may be reversible or fatal Can cause birth defects during pregnancy

Vitamin D
Adult RDA:
Up to age 70 years: 600 IU/day
≥71 years: 800 IU/day
Sunlight on the skin
• Cod liver oil, oysters, mackerel, most fish, egg yolks, beef liver; fortified milk, ready-to-eat cereals, orange juice and margarine
	Maintains serum calcium concentrations by
	Stimulating GI absorption
	Stimulating the release of calcium from the bones
	Stimulating calcium absorption from the kidneys
	Appears to play a role in immune system functioning and inflammation
		Deficiency
		Rickets (in infants and children)
		  Retarded bone growth
		  Bone malformations (bowed legs)
		  Enlargement of ends of long bones (knock-knees)
		  Deformities of the ribs (bowed, with beads or knobs)
		  Delayed closing of the fontanel → rapid enlargement of the head
		  Decreased serum calcium and/or phosphorus
		  Malformed teeth; decayed teeth
		  Protrusion of the abdomen related to relaxation of the abdominal muscles
		  Increased secretion of parathyroid hormone
		Osteomalacia (in adults)
		  Softening of the bones → deformities, pain, and easy fracture
		  Decreased serum calcium and/or phosphorus, increased alkaline phosphatase
		  Involuntary muscle twitching and spasms
		Toxicity
		Kidney stones, irreversible kidney damage, muscle and bone weakness, excessive bleeding, loss of appetite, headache, excessive thirst, calcification of soft tissues (blood vessels, kidneys, heart, lungs), death

Vitamin E **Adult RDA: 15 mg** • Vegetable oils, margarine, salad dressing, other foods made with vegetable oil, nuts, seeds, wheat germ, dark green vegetables, whole grains, fortified cereals	Acts as an antioxidant to protect vitamin A and polyunsaturated fatty acids from being destroyed Protects cell membranes	**Deficiency** Increased red blood cell hemolysis In infants, anemia, edema, and skin lesions **Toxicity** Relatively nontoxic High doses enhance action of anticoagulant medications
Vitamin K **Adult AI:** **Men: 120 μg** **Women: 90 μg** Bacterial synthesis • Brussels sprouts, broccoli, cauliflower, Swiss chard, spinach, loose leaf lettuce, carrots, green beans, asparagus, eggs	Synthesis of blood clotting proteins and a bone protein that regulates blood calcium	**Deficiency** Hemorrhaging **Toxicity** No symptoms have been observed from excessive intake of vitamin K.

Vitamin A

Preformed Vitamin A
the active form of vitamin A.

Carotenoids
a group name of retinol precursors found in plants.

In its preformed state, vitamin A exists as an alcohol (retinol), aldehyde (retinaldehyde), or acid (retinoic acid). **Preformed vitamin A** is found only in animal sources such as liver, whole milk, and fish. Low-fat milk, skim milk, margarine, and ready-to-eat cereals are fortified with vitamin A.

The term vitamin A also includes provitamin A **carotenoids**, natural plant pigments found in deep yellow and orange fruits and vegetables and most dark green leafy vegetables. Although there are over 600 different carotenoids, only a few are considered precursors of retinol. Beta-carotene, lutein, and lycopene are among the most commonly known carotenoids. Carotenoids account for about one-quarter to one-third of the usual intake of vitamin A.

Vitamin A is best known for its roles in normal vision, reproduction, growth, and immune system functioning. It is a relatively poor antioxidant. In contrast, beta-carotene is a major antioxidant in the body, prompting researchers to study whether it can prevent heart disease and cancer. A landmark trial designed to test whether beta-carotene supplements could decrease cancer incidence in people at high risk was prematurely halted when results showed a surprising increase in lung cancer incidence and deaths in smokers and male asbestos workers (Omenn et al., 1996; The Alpha-Tocopherol, Beta-Carotene Cancer Prevention Study Group, 1994). The U.S. Preventive Services Task Force recommends against beta-carotene supplements for the prevention of cardiovascular disease or cancer (Moyer, 2014).

The body can store up to a year supply of vitamin A, 90% of which is in the liver. Because deficiency symptoms do not develop until body stores are exhausted, it may take 1 to 2 years for them to appear. Although severe vitamin A deficiency is rare in the United States, a large percentage of adults may have suboptimal liver stores of vitamin A even though they are not clinically deficient. Worldwide, vitamin A deficiency is a major health problem; an estimated 250,000 to 500,000 vitamin A–deficient children become blind every year. Half of them die within a year of losing their sight from common infections such as diarrheal disease and measles (World Health Organization, 2012).

Only preformed vitamin A, the form found in animal foods, fortified foods, and supplements, is toxic in high doses. The risk of toxicity is much greater when supplements of vitamin A are consumed. Extremely high doses (at least 30,000 μg/day) consumed over months or years may cause central nervous system (CNS) changes, bone and skin changes, and liver abnormalities that range from reversible to fatal. At high doses during pregnancy, such as three to four times the recommended intake, vitamin A is teratogenic. Supplementation is not recommended during the first trimester of pregnancy unless there is specific evidence of vitamin A deficiency.

Beta-carotene is nontoxic because the body makes vitamin A from it only as needed and the conversion is not rapid enough to cause hypervitaminosis A. Instead, carotene is stored primarily in adipose tissue and may accumulate under the skin to the extent that it causes the skin color to turn yellowish orange, a harmless condition known as hypercarotenemia. The Tolerable Upper Intake Level (UL) for vitamin A does not apply to vitamin A derived from carotenoids.

Vitamin D

Essential Nutrient
a nutrient that must be supplied by the diet because it is not synthesized in the body. Essentiality does not refer to importance but to the need for a dietary source.

Vitamin D is unique in that the body has the potential to make all it needs if exposure to sunlight is optimal and liver and kidney functions are normal. Because vitamin D can be endogenously synthesized, it is not an **essential nutrient** in the diet.

Vitamin D exists in two forms: vitamin D_3 or cholecalciferol and vitamin D_2 or ergocalciferol. Vitamin D_3 is synthesized in the skin when exposed to ultraviolet light. Both forms accumulate in the liver where they are converted to 25-hydroxyvitamin D [25(OH)D], which then enters the circulation. The kidneys convert [25(OH)D] to the biologically active form of vitamin D, $1,25(OH)_2D$. This conversion is tightly regulated by parathyroid hormone in response to serum calcium and phosphorus levels.

Because vitamin D is synthesized in one part of the body (skin) and stimulates functional activity elsewhere (e.g., GI tract, bones, kidneys), it is actually a prohormone. The most widely known function of vitamin D is to maintain normal blood concentrations of calcium and phosphorus by

- Stimulating calcium and phosphorus absorption from the GI tract
- Mobilizing calcium and phosphorus from the bone as needed to maintain normal serum levels
- Stimulating the kidneys to retain calcium and phosphorus

Rickets
vitamin D deficiency disease in children, most prominently characterized by bowed legs.

Osteomalacia
adult rickets characterized by inadequate bone mineralization due to the lack of vitamin D.

Overt deficiency of vitamin D causes poor calcium absorption, leading to a calcium deficit in the blood that the body corrects by releasing calcium from bone. In children, the result is **rickets**, a condition characterized by abnormal bone shape and structure. Fortification of milk was instituted as an effective and inexpensive way to boost vitamin D intake. In adults, vitamin D deficiency can result in **osteomalacia**, a softening of the bones. Loss of bone mineral density coincides with osteoporosis and increased risk of falls and fractures (Pludowski et al., 2013).

The inverse relationship between sunlight exposure and increased incidence of several chronic diseases such as cancer, autoimmune diseases, diabetes, and cardiovascular disease led researchers to speculate that vitamin D has functions beyond its role in bone health. The discovery that most tissues and cells have vitamin D receptors (e.g., in the skin, pancreas, colon, kidney, parathyroid and pituitary glands, ovaries, and lymphocytes) suggests vitamin D has many diverse roles. Vitamin D may be involved in (Eich & Kline, 2016)

- Regulating cell growth and differentiation
- Inducing apoptosis
- Modulating T and B cells, cell-mediated immunity and cytokines
- Decreasing proinflammatory immune cells
- Stimulating insulin production.

Low levels of vitamin D have been implicated in autoimmune diseases such as multiple sclerosis (Pender, 2012), hypertension (Witham, Nadir, & Struthers, 2009), cardiovascular diseases (Khaw, Luben, & Wareham, 2014; Muscogiuri et al., 2012), metabolic syndrome (Fung et al., 2012), type 2 diabetes (Lim et al., 2013), several types of cancer (Bolland, Grey, Gamble, & Reid, 2011; Grant, 2011), cognitive decline (Breitling et al., 2012), and depression (Bertone-Johnson et al., 2011). A large cohort study shows vitamin D deficiency is strongly associated with mortality from all causes, including cardiovascular diseases, cancer, and respiratory diseases (Schöttker et al., 2013). There is also evidence that vitamin D plays a role in reducing the risk of respiratory tract infection (Bergman et al., 2012) and sepsis (Watkins, Yamshchikov, Lemonovich, & Salata, 2011).

In 2010, the Institute of Medicine (IOM) established the RDA for vitamin D at 600 **IU**/day for children and adults through age 70 years and 800 IU/day for adults age 71 years and older

IU
to convert micrograms of vitamin D to IU, multiply micrograms by 40.

(Ross et al., 2011). These levels are based on the assumption of minimal or no sun exposure. The basis for determining the RDA for vitamin D is its cause-and-effect relationship with bone health only; the IOM maintains that evidence linking vitamin D with extraskeletal outcomes, including cancer, cardiovascular disease, diabetes, and autoimmune disorders, is inconsistent, inconclusive, and insufficient to use in determining vitamin D requirements (IOM, 2011).

Many researchers criticize the RDA for being too conservative. The Endocrine Society agrees that more studies are needed on vitamin D's extraskeletal roles before those roles are factored into dietary recommendations. However, the Endocrine Society recommends adults consume 1500 to 2000 IU/day to prevent deficiency [25(OH)D <20 ng/mL] or vitamin D insufficiency [25(OH)D levels of 21 to 29 ng/mL] (Holick et al., 2011).

The current UL for vitamin D is set at 4000 IU/day for ages 9 years and older. Factors considered in determining the UL included hypercalcemia, hypercalciuria, vascular and soft tissue calcification, and emerging evidence of a U-shaped relationship for all-cause mortality, cardiovascular disease, certain cancers, falls, and fractures (Ross et al., 2011). Because the body destroys excess vitamin D produced from overexposure to the sun, there has never been a reported case of vitamin D toxicity from too much sun (Food and Nutrition Board, IOM, 1997).

Quick Bite Vitamin D content of selected items

	IUs of Vitamin D
1 tbsp cod liver oil	1360
3 oz swordfish	566
3 oz sockeye salmon	447
3 oz canned tuna in water, drained	154
1 cup fortified orange juice	137
1 cup nonfat, reduced fat, and whole milk fortified with vitamin D	115–124
1 tbsp fortified margarine	60
1 large egg yolk	41

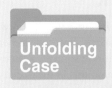

Recall Marcus. His gluten-free/casein-free diet restricts many types of grain and milk products and some children following this diet have developed amino acid deficiencies, which is essentially a form of protein malnutrition. Marcus has difficulty chewing meat, which further limits his intake of protein. What foods can provide protein within the context of his dietary restrictions? Should Marcus take amino acid supplements? Which vitamins may he be underconsuming given his restricted intake of grains, milk, and meats? Will vitamin supplements compensate for the lack of variety in his intake?

Vitamin E

Vitamin E is a group name that describes a group of at least eight structurally related, naturally occurring compounds. Alpha-tocopherol is considered the most biologically active form of vitamin E, although other forms also have important roles in maintaining health. As a group, vitamin E functions as the primary fat-soluble antioxidant in the body, protecting PUFAs and other lipid molecules, such as LDL cholesterol, from oxidative damage. By doing so, it helps to maintain the integrity of PUFA-rich cell membranes, protects red blood cells against hemolysis, and protects vitamin A from oxidation. Vitamin E also has several important functions independent of its antioxidant activity, such as inhibiting cell division, enhancing immune system functioning, regulating gene expression, inhibiting platelet aggregation, and promoting blood vessel dilation.

The need for vitamin E increases as the intake of PUFA increases. Fortunately, vitamin E and PUFA share many of the same food sources, particularly nuts, seeds, fortified cereals, vegetable oils and products made from oil such as margarine, salad dressings, and other prepared foods. However, not all oils are rich in alpha-tocopherol, the active form of vitamin E. Soybean oil, the most commonly used oil in food processing, ranks low in alpha-tocopherol content.

Interest in the role of vitamin E in health stems from its antioxidant and anti-inflammatory activity as well as its role in immune system functioning and blood clotting. One hypothesis is that the antioxidant activity of vitamin E could reduce the risk of cancer by protecting cells from damage caused by unchecked free radicals. Unfortunately, most randomized trials find that vitamin E is not beneficial with regard to total or site-specific cancers (Wang et al., 2014). In addition, a study in the posttrial follow-up to the Selenium and Vitamin E Cancer Prevention Trial (SELECT) found that vitamin E supplementation significantly increased the risk of prostate cancer in healthy men (Klein et al., 2011). The U.S. Preventive Services Task Force position states that supplements of vitamin E do not reduce the risk for cancer or cardiovascular disease and recommends they not be taken (Moyer, 2014).

One promising area of research it the role in age-related macular degeneration (ARMD). The Age-Related Eye Disease Study (AREDS), a large randomized clinical trial, and its follow-up study Age-Related Eye Disease Study 2 (AREDS2), showed that a daily supplement containing vitamin E decreased the risk of ARMD by 25% in people at high risk of developing advanced ARMD (Age-Related Eye Disease Study Research Group, 2001; The Age-Related Eye Disease Study 2 Research Group, 2013). However, it is not clear that vitamin E supplements, taken alone or in combination with other antioxidants, reduces the risk of developing ARMD in people who are not at high risk for the disorder.

Vitamin E deficiency is rare and more likely to occur secondary to fat malabsorption syndromes, such as cystic fibrosis and short bowel syndrome, than from an inadequate intake. Premature infants who have not benefited from the transfer of vitamin E from mother to fetus in the last weeks of pregnancy are at risk for red blood cell hemolysis. The breaking of their red blood cell membranes is caused by oxidation; vitamin E corrects red blood cell hemolysis by preventing oxidation. Prolonged vitamin E deficiency symptoms include peripheral neuropathy, ataxia, and impaired vision and speech.

Large amounts of vitamin E are relatively nontoxic but can interfere with vitamin K action (blood clotting) by decreasing platelet aggregation. Large doses may also potentiate the effects of blood-thinning drugs, increasing the risk of hemorrhage. The UL is 66 times higher than the RDA.

Quick Bite Oils containing active form of vitamin E (in descending order)

Wheat germ oil
Walnut oil
Sunflower oil
Cottonseed oil
Safflower oil
Palm oil
Canola oil
Sesame oil
Peanut oil
Olive oil
Corn oil
Soybean oil

Vitamin K

Vitamin K occurs naturally in two forms. Phylloquinone is found in plants—spinach, broccoli, iceberg lettuce, and soybean and canola oils are common sources. Menaquinones, the animal form, is found in modest amounts in meat, dairy products, and eggs and is the form of vitamin K synthesized in the intestinal tract by microbiota. It is not known how much vitamin K produced by microbiota are absorbed.

Vitamin K is a coenzyme essential for the synthesis of prothrombin and at least 6 of the other 13 proteins needed for normal blood clotting. Without adequate vitamin K, life is threatened: Even a small wound can cause someone deficient in vitamin K to bleed to death. Vitamin K also activates at least three proteins involved in building and maintaining bone.

Newborns are prone to vitamin K deficiency for a few reasons: Vitamin K transport across the placenta is low, the vitamin K content of breast milk is low, and because newborns have sterile GI tracts that cannot synthesize vitamin K. To prevent hemorrhagic disease, a single intramuscular dose of vitamin K is given prophylactically at birth.

Clinically significant vitamin K deficiency is defined as vitamin K–responsive hypoprothrombinemia and is characterized by an increase in prothrombin time. Vitamin K deficiency does not occur from inadequate intake but may occur secondary to malabsorption syndromes or to the use of certain medications that interfere with vitamin K metabolism or synthesis, such as anticoagulants and antibiotics. Anticoagulants, such as warfarin (Coumadin), interfere with hepatic synthesis of vitamin K–dependent clotting factors. People who take warfarin do not need to avoid vitamin K, but they should try to maintain a consistent intake so that the effect on coagulation time is as constant and as predictable as possible. Antibiotics kill the intestinal bacteria that synthesize vitamin K.

Due to the lack of data to estimate an average requirement, an Adequate Intake (AI), not an RDA, has been set. A UL has not been set because no adverse effects are associated with vitamin K intake from food or supplements.

Water-Soluble Vitamins

Group characteristics of water-soluble vitamins are summarized in Table 5.1. Table 5.3 highlights sources, functions, deficiency symptoms, and toxicity symptoms of each water-soluble vitamin. The complete table of Dietary Reference Intakes for vitamins appears in Appendix B. Additional features of individual water-soluble vitamins are summarized in the following sections.

Thiamin

Thiamin (vitamin B_1) is a coenzyme in the metabolism of carbohydrates and branched-chain amino acids. In addition to its role in energy metabolism, thiamin is important in nervous system functioning.

In the United States and other developed countries, the use of enriched breads and cereals has virtually eliminated the thiamin deficiency disease known as beriberi. Today, thiamin deficiency is usually seen only in alcoholics with limited food consumption because chronic alcohol abuse impairs thiamin intake, absorption, and metabolism. Edema occurs in wet beriberi; muscle wasting is prominent in dry beriberi. Cardiac and renal complications can be fatal.

No adverse effects have been noted from high intakes of thiamin from food or supplements, so a UL has not been set.

Riboflavin

Homocysteine
an amino acid correlated with increased risk of heart disease.

Methionine
an essential amino acid.

Riboflavin (vitamin B_2) is an integral component of the coenzymes flavin adenine dinucleotide (FAD) and flavin mononucleotide (FMN) that function to release energy from nutrients in all body cells. Flavin coenzymes are also involved in the formation of some vitamins and their coenzymes and in the conversion of **homocysteine** to **methionine**. Riboflavin is unique among water-soluble vitamins in that milk and dairy products contribute the most riboflavin to the diet.

Table 5.3   Summary of Water-Soluble Vitamins

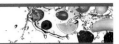

Vitamin and Sources	Functions	Deficiency/Toxicity Signs and Symptoms

Thiamin (vitamin B$_1$)
Adult RDA
Men: 1.2 mg
Women: 1.1 mg
● Whole-grain and enriched breads and cereals, liver, nuts, wheat germ, pork, dried peas and beans
	Coenzyme in energy metabolism
	Promotes normal appetite and nervous system functioning
		Deficiency
		Beriberi
		  Mental confusion, decrease in short-term memory
		  Fatigue, apathy
		  Peripheral paralysis
		  Muscle weakness and wasting
		  Painful calf muscles
		  Anorexia, weight loss
		  Edema
		  Enlarged heart
		  Sudden death from heart failure
		Toxicity
		No toxicity symptoms reported

Riboflavin (vitamin B$_2$) **Adult RDA** **Men: 1.3 mg** **Women: 1.1 mg** ● Milk and other dairy products; whole-grain and enriched breads and cereals; liver, eggs, meat, spinach	Coenzyme in energy metabolism Aids in the conversion of tryptophan into niacin	**Deficiency** Dermatitis Cheilosis Glossitis Photophobia Reddening of the cornea **Toxicity** No toxicity symptoms reported

Niacin (vitamin B$_3$)
Adult RDA
Men: 16 mg
Women: 14 mg
All protein foods, whole-grain and enriched breads and cereals
	Coenzyme in energy metabolism
	Promotes normal nervous system functioning
		Deficiency
		Pellagra: 4 Ds
		  Dermatitis (bilateral and symmetrical) and glossitis
		  Diarrhea
		  Dementia, irritability, mental confusion → psychosis
		  Death, if untreated
		Toxicity (from supplements/drugs)
		Flushing, liver damage, gastric ulcers, low blood pressure, diarrhea, nausea, vomiting

Vitamin B$_6$ **Adult RDA** **Men: 1.3–1.7 mg** **Women: 1.3–1.5 mg** ● Meats, fish, poultry, fruits, green leafy vegetables, whole grains, nuts, dried peas and beans	Coenzyme in amino acid and fatty acid metabolism Helps convert tryptophan to niacin Helps produce insulin, hemoglobin, myelin sheaths, and antibodies	**Deficiency** Dermatitis, cheilosis, glossitis, abnormal brain wave pattern, convulsions, and anemia **Toxicity** Depression, fatigue, irritability, headaches; sensory neuropathy characteristic
Folate **Adult RDA: 400 μg** ● Liver, okra, spinach, asparagus, dried peas and beans, seeds, orange juice; breads, cereals, and other grains are fortified with folic acid	Coenzyme in DNA synthesis; therefore, vital for new cell synthesis and the transmission of inherited characteristics	**Deficiency** Glossitis, diarrhea, macrocytic anemia, depression, mental confusion, fainting, fatigue **Toxicity** Too much can mask vitamin B$_{12}$ deficiency
Vitamin B$_{12}$ **Adult RDA: 2.4 μg** Animal products: meat, fish, poultry, shellfish, milk, dairy products, eggs ● Some fortified foods	Coenzyme in the synthesis of new cells Activates folate Maintains nerve cells Helps metabolize some fatty acids and amino acids	**Deficiency** GI changes: glossitis, anorexia, indigestion, recurring diarrhea or constipation, and weight loss Macrocytic anemia: pallor, dyspnea, weakness, fatigue, and palpitations Neurologic changes: paresthesia of the hands and feet, decreased sense of position, poor muscle coordination, poor memory, irritability, depression, paranoia, delirium, and hallucinations **Toxicity** No toxicity symptoms reported
Pantothenic Acid **Adult AI: 5 mg** Widespread in foods ● Meat, poultry, fish, whole-grain cereals, and dried peas and beans are among best sources.	Part of coenzyme A used in energy metabolism	**Deficiency** Rare; general failure of all body systems **Toxicity** No toxicity symptoms reported, although large doses may cause diarrhea.

(continued)

Table 5.3   Summary of Water-Soluble Vitamins (continued)

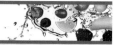

Vitamin and Sources	Functions	Deficiency/Toxicity Signs and Symptoms
Biotin **Adult AI: 30 μg** Widespread in foods Eggs, liver, milk, and dark green vegetables are among best choices. Synthesized by GI flora	Coenzyme in energy metabolism, fatty acid synthesis, amino acid metabolism, and glycogen formation	**Deficiency** Rare; anorexia, fatigue, depression, dry skin, heart abnormalities **Toxicity** No toxicity symptoms reported

Vitamin C
Adult RDA
Men: 90 mg
Women: 75 mg
● Citrus fruits and juices, red and green peppers, broccoli, cauliflower, Brussels sprouts, cantaloupe, kiwifruit, mustard greens, strawberries, tomatoes
	Collagen synthesis
	Antioxidant
	Promotes iron absorption
	Involved in the metabolism of certain amino acids
	Thyroxin synthesis
	Immune system functioning
		Deficiency
		Bleeding gums, pinpoint hemorrhages under the skin
		Scurvy, characterized by
		    Hemorrhaging
		    Muscle degeneration
		    Skin changes
		    Delayed wound healing: reopening of old wounds
		    Softening of the bones → malformations, pain, easy fractures
		    Soft, loose teeth
		    Anemia
		    Increased susceptibility to infection
		    Hysteria and depression
		Toxicity
		Diarrhea, mild GI upset

Biochemical signs of an inadequate riboflavin status can appear after only a few days of a poor intake. The elderly and adolescents are at greatest risk for riboflavin deficiency. Riboflavin deficiency interferes with iron handling and contributes to anemia when iron intake is low. Other deficiency symptoms include sore throat, cheilosis, stomatitis, glossitis, and dermatitis, many of which may be related to the effect riboflavin deficiency has on the metabolism of folate and vitamin B_6. Certain diseases, such as cancer, heart disease, and diabetes, precipitate or exacerbate riboflavin deficiency.

Niacin

Niacin (vitamin B_3) exists as nicotinic acid and nicotinamide. The body converts nicotinic acid to nicotinamide, which is the major form of niacin in the blood. All protein foods provide niacin, as do whole-grain and enriched breads and fortified ready-to-eat cereals.

Niacin Equivalents (NEs)
the amount of niacin available to the body including that made from tryptophan.

A unique feature of niacin is that the body can make it from the amino acid tryptophan: Approximately 60 mg of tryptophan is used to synthesize 1 mg of niacin. Because of this additional source of niacin, niacin requirements are stated in **niacin equivalents (NEs)**. Median intake in the United States generously exceeds the RDA.

Niacin is part of the coenzymes nicotinamide adenine dinucleotide (NAD) and nicotinamide adenine dinucleotide phosphate (NADP), which are involved in energy transfer reactions in the metabolism of glucose, fat, and alcohol in all body cells. Reduced NADP is used in the synthesis of fatty acids, cholesterol, and steroid hormones.

Pellagra, the disorder caused by severe niacin deficiency, is rare in the United States and usually is seen only in alcoholics. However, pellagra is widespread in areas that rely on corn as a staple, such as parts of Africa and Asia, because corn is low in niacin and tryptophan. Before grain products were enriched with niacin in the early 20th century, pellagra was also common in the Southern United States.

Niacin deficiency may be treated with niacin, tryptophan, or both. Because a deficiency of niacin rarely occurs alone, treatment is most effective when other B-complex vitamins are also given, especially thiamin and riboflavin.

Large doses of niacin in the form of nicotinic acid (1 to 6 g/day) are used therapeutically to lower total cholesterol and LDL cholesterol and raise high-density lipoprotein (HDL) cholesterol.

Flushing is a common side effect caused by vasodilation. Large doses, which may cause liver damage and gout, should be used only with a doctor's supervision. The UL of 35 mg of NE does not apply for clinical applications using niacin as a drug.

Vitamin B$_6$

Vitamin B$_6$ and pyridoxine are group names for six related compounds that include pyridoxine, pyridoxal, and pyridoxamine. All forms can be converted to the active form, pyridoxal phosphate, which is involved in nearly 100 enzymatic reactions, mostly involving protein metabolism.

Vitamin B$_6$ plays a role in the synthesis, catabolism, and transport of amino acids and in the conversion of tryptophan to niacin. It is involved in the formation of heme for hemoglobin and in the synthesis of myelin sheaths and neurotransmitters. It facilitates the transfer of carbon groups for DNA synthesis. Vitamin B$_6$ helps to regulate blood glucose levels by assisting in the release of stored glucose from glycogen and is important in the maintenance of cellular immunity. Unlike other B vitamins, vitamin B$_6$ is stored extensively in muscle tissue.

Low concentrations of vitamin B$_6$, folic acid, and vitamin B$_{12}$ are associated with an increase in blood homocysteine levels, a nonessential amino acid linked to an increased risk of stroke (Lonn et al., 2006), coronary heart disease (Humphrey, Fu, Rogers, Freeman, & Helfand, 2008), cognitive decline (Elias et al., 2005), and vascular disease (McCully, 2007). However, most large clinical trials fail to show that supplemental B vitamins reduce the risk of cardiovascular events, even though they lower homocysteine levels (National Institutes of Health [NIH], Office of Dietary Supplements [ODS], 2013a). For example, findings from three major studies, the Heart Outcomes Prevention Evaluation-2 (HOPE-2) trial (Lonn et al., 2006), Norwegian Vitamin (NORVIT) trial (Bønaa et al., 2006), and Vitamin Intervention for Stroke Prevention (VISP) trial (Toole et al., 2004), showed that the combination of vitamin B$_6$, vitamin B$_{12}$, and folic acid lowers homocysteine levels in people with advanced vascular disease but has little effect on recurrent heart attack or stroke. The American Heart Association (AHA) has not defined hyperhomocysteinemia a major risk factor for cardiovascular disease nor does it recommend widespread use of folic acid and B vitamin supplements to reduce the risk of heart disease and stroke (AHA, 2012).

The role of vitamin B$_6$ in the incidence of colorectal cancer is being studied. Results from the Women's Health Initiative show vitamin B$_6$ intake from food and supplements is associated with a decreased risk of colorectal cancer (Zschäbitz et al., 2013). Likewise, a meta-analysis of cohort studies shows an inverse relationship between vitamin B$_6$ intake and colorectal cancer (Liu et al., 2015).

In 2013, the U.S. Food and Drug Administration (FDA) approved vitamin B$_6$ in and doxylamine succinate (an antihistamine) in a delayed-release combination pill for the treatment of nausea and vomiting in pregnancy based on data from a randomized, placebo-controlled clinical trial that shows it is safe (not a teratogen) and effective as an antiemetic for mild to moderate nausea and vomiting during pregnancy (Nuangchamnong & Niebyl, 2014). Vitamin B$_6$ may also help reduce physical symptoms of premenstrual syndrome (Hasani, Kazemi, Afshar, Kazemi, & Tavakoli, 2015). High intakes of vitamin B$_6$ from food do not pose any danger. Long-term use of high-dose supplements (1000 to 4000 mg/day) is associated with neuropathy that is reversible with discontinuation (IOM, 1998).

Deficiencies of vitamin B$_6$ are uncommon but are usually accompanied by deficiencies of other B vitamins, such a folic acid and vitamin B$_{12}$. People at risk of vitamin B$_6$ deficiency include those with impaired renal function, autoimmune diseases, and malabsorption autoimmune disorders such as celiac disease, ulcerative colitis, and Crohn disease. Vitamin B$_6$ deficiency also occurs in people with alcohol dependency (because the metabolism of alcohol promotes the destruction and excretion of vitamin B$_6$) and those on certain drug therapies such as isoniazid, the antituberculosis drug that acts as a vitamin B$_6$ antagonist.

Folate

Folate is the generic term for this B vitamin that includes both synthetic folic acid found in vitamin supplements and fortified foods and naturally occurring folate in foods such as green leafy vegetables, legumes, seeds, liver, and orange juice. **Dietary folate equivalents (DFEs)**, used in establishing folate requirement, are based on the assumption that natural food folate is approximately only half as available to the body as synthetic folic acid. A more recent study showed that bioavailability of food folate may be as high as 80% of synthetic folic acid (Winkels, Brouwer, Siebelink, Katan, & Verhoef, 2007).

Dietary Folate Equivalents (DFEs)
DFE = microgram of food folate + (1.7 × micrograms synthetic folic acid).

As part of the coenzymes tetrahydrofolate (THF) and dihydrofolate (DHF), folate's major function is in the synthesis of DNA. With the aid of vitamin B_{12}, folate is vital for synthesis of new cells and transmission of inherited characteristics. Folate is also involved in homocysteine metabolism.

Because folate is recycled through the intestinal tract (much like the enterohepatic circulation of bile), a healthy GI tract is essential to maintain folate balance. When GI integrity is impaired, as in malabsorption syndromes, failure to reabsorb folate quickly leads to folate deficiency. GI cells are particularly susceptible to folate deficiency because they are rapidly dividing cells that depend on folate for new cell synthesis. Without the formation of new cells, GI function declines and widespread malabsorption of nutrients occurs.

Folate deficiency impairs DNA synthesis and cell division and results in macrocytic anemia and other clinical symptoms. It is prevalent in all parts of the world. In developing countries, folate deficiency commonly is caused by parasitic infections that alter GI integrity. In the United States, alcoholics are at highest risk of folate deficiency because of alcohol's toxic effect on the GI tract. Groups at risk because of poor intake include the elderly, fad dieters, and people of low socioeconomic status. Because new tissue growth increases folate requirements, infants, adolescents, and pregnant women may have difficulty consuming adequate amounts.

Studies show that an adequate intake of folate before conception and during the first trimester of pregnancy reduces the risk of neural tube defects (e.g., spina bifida) in infants (Medical Research Council Vitamin Study Research Group, 1991). This discovery prompted the U.S. Public Health Service to recommend that all women of childbearing age who are capable of becoming pregnant consume 400 μg of synthetic folic acid from fortified food and/or supplements in addition to folate from a varied diet. Mandatory folic acid fortification of enriched bread and grain products began on January 1, 1998.

As mentioned in the section on vitamin B_6, studies using supplements of folic acid alone or in combination with other B vitamins show they effectively lower homocysteine levels but fail to lower the risk of strokes or coronary events (Armitage et al., 2010). The UL for folic acid is 1000 μg/day from fortified food or supplements, exclusive of food folate. After folic acid fortification became mandatory, safety concerns were raised that high intakes of folic acid may increase the risk of certain types of cancer. Several studies show no association between folic acid supplements and cancer incidence (Armitage et al., 2010; Hu, Juan, & Sahyoun, 2016), whereas others show inconsistent results (Heine-Bröing et al., 2015).

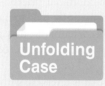

Unfolding Case

Recall Marcus. Because he has a restricted diet and accepts only a limited variety of foods, he may be under- or overconsuming certain nutrients. His parents give him a multivitamin with minerals, plus additional supplements of vitamin D, vitamin C, and calcium. Should Marcus's parents keep a food diary so that his total vitamin intake from food and supplements can be estimated? Which nutrients consumed in excess may cause health problems?

Vitamin B_{12}

Vitamin B_{12} (cobalamin) has several interesting features. First, vitamin B_{12} has an interdependent relationship with folate: Each vitamin must have the other to be activated. Because it activates folate, vitamin B_{12} is involved in DNA synthesis and maturation of red blood cells. Like folate, vitamin B_{12} functions as a coenzyme in homocysteine metabolism. Unlike folate, vitamin B_{12} has important roles in maintaining the myelin sheath around nerves. For this reason, large doses of folic acid can alleviate the anemia caused by vitamin B_{12} deficiency (a function of both vitamins), but folic acid cannot halt the progressive neurologic impairments that only vitamin B_{12} can treat. Nervous system damage may be irreversible without early treatment with vitamin B_{12}.

Vitamin B_{12} also holds the distinction of being the only water-soluble vitamin that does not occur naturally in plants. Fermented soy products and algae may be enriched with vitamin B_{12}, but it is in an inactive, unavailable form. Some ready-to-eat cereals are fortified with vitamin B_{12}. All animal foods contain vitamin B_{12}.

Another unique feature of vitamin B_{12} is that it requires an intrinsic factor, a glycoprotein secreted in the stomach, to be absorbed from the terminal ileum. But before it can bind to the intrinsic factor, vitamin B_{12} must first be separated from the small peptides to which it is bound in food sources. Separation is accomplished by pepsin and gastric acid. Conversely, synthetic vitamin B_{12} found in enriched foods and supplements does not require this separation step because it is in free form.

Vitamin B_{12} deficiency symptoms may take 5 to 10 years or longer to develop because the liver can store relatively large amounts of B_{12} and the body recycles B_{12} by reabsorbing it. Vitamin B_{12} deficiency can be caused by

- Dietary deficiencies, especially in vegans who consume no animal products. Although once thought to be rare, vitamin B_{12} deficiency is relatively common among people adhering to any type of vegetarian pattern including lacto-ovo vegetarians (Pawlak, Parrott, Raj, Cullum-Dugan, & Lucus, 2013). A dietary deficiency is preventable with regular consumption of oral supplements or vitamin B_{12} fortified foods.
- Pernicious anemia, an autoimmune gastritis in which destruction of parietal cells leads to achlorhydria and failure to produce intrinsic factor. Even when intake is adequate, severe vitamin B_{12} malabsorption results in vitamin B_{12} deficiency. Lifelong parenteral injections of vitamin B_{12} are necessary to treat pernicious anemia; sublingual preparations, oral sprays, nasal gels, and transdermal patches are available, but data on the absorption and efficacy of these methods are lacking (Stabler, 2013).
- Conditions that impair the integrity of the stomach (e.g., total or partial gastrectomy, gastric bypass or other bariatric surgery) or bowel (e.g., ileal resection, inflammatory bowel disease). These conditions can cause severe deficiency related to vitamin B_{12} malabsorption.
- Protein-bound vitamin B_{12} malabsorption, a milder form of atrophic gastritis in which low gastric acid secretion impairs the freeing of protein-bound vitamin B_{12} in foods. It is frequently attributed to aging and affects up to 20% of older adults (Lewerin, Jacobsson, Lindstedt, & Nilsson-Ehle, 2008). It may also occur secondary to the use of medications that suppress gastric acid secretion. This mild form of malabsorption can be treated with large doses of oral supplements. As a preventive measure, the National Academy of Sciences IOM recommends that people older than age 50 years obtain most of their requirement from fortified foods or supplements (Food and Nutrition Board, IOM, 1998).

Other B Vitamins

Pantothenic acid is part of coenzyme A (CoA), the coenzyme involved in the formation of acetyl-CoA and in the TCA (tricarboxylic acid) cycle. Pantothenic acid participates in more than 100 different metabolic reactions. It is widespread in the diet. The best sources of pantothenic acid are meat, fish, poultry, whole-grain cereals, and dried peas and beans.

As a coenzyme, biotin is involved in the TCA cycle, gluconeogenesis, fatty acid synthesis, and chemical reactions that add or remove carbon dioxide from other compounds. Biotin is widely distributed in nature, and significant amounts are synthesized by GI flora, but it is not known how much is available for absorption. It is assumed that the average American diet provides adequate amounts of both pantothenic acid and biotin.

Choline is an essential nutrient commonly categorized with the B vitamins. It plays important roles in the synthesis of the neurotransmitter acetylcholine and lethicin and was assigned an AI value in 1998. Since then, studies have shown potential deleterious effects of choline deficiencies (Hollenbeck, 2010). Milk, liver, eggs, and peanuts provide choline.

Non–B Vitamins

Other substances, such as inositol and carnitine, are sometimes inaccurately referred to as B vitamins because they are coenzymes. Research is needed to determine whether these substances are essential in the diet.

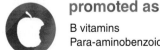

Quick Bite Substances often falsely promoted as

B vitamins
Para-aminobenzoic acid (PABA)
Bioflavonoids
Vitamin P
Hesperidin
Ubiquinone
Vitamin B_{15}
Vitamin B_{17}

Vitamin C

Vitamin C (ascorbic acid), most notably found in citrus fruits and juices, may be the most famous vitamin. Its long history dates back more than 250 years when it was determined that something in citrus fruits prevents scurvy, a disease that killed as many as two-thirds of sailors on long journeys. Years later, British sailors acquired the nickname "Limeys" because of Great Britain's policy to prevent scurvy by providing limes to all navy men. It wasn't until 1932 that the antiscurvy agent was identified as vitamin C. Since then, vitamin C has been touted as a cure for a variety of ills, including cancer, colds, and infertility.

Vitamin C prevents scurvy by promoting the formation of collagen, the most abundant protein in fibrous tissues, such as connective tissue, cartilage, bone matrix, tooth dentin, skin, and tendon. Without adequate vitamin C, the integrity of collagen is compromised; muscles degenerate, weakened bones break, wounds fail to heal, teeth are lost, and infection occurs. Hemorrhaging begins as pinpoints under the skin and progresses to massive internal bleeding and death. Even though scurvy is deadly, it can be cured within a matter of days with moderate doses of vitamin C.

Vitamin C is a water-soluble antioxidant that protects vitamin A, vitamin E, PUFA, and iron from destruction. It is involved in many metabolic reactions including the promotion of iron absorption, the formation of some neurotransmitters, the synthesis of thyroxine, the metabolism of some amino acids, and normal immune system functioning.

Cigarette smokers are advised to increase their intake by 35 mg/day because smoking increases oxidative stress and metabolic turnover of vitamin C (Food and Nutrition Board, IOM, 2000). The need for vitamin C also increases in response to other stresses such as fever, chronic illness, infection, and wound healing as well as from chronic use of certain medications such as aspirin, barbiturates, and oral contraceptives. There is no evidence that mental stress increases the need for vitamin C.

As an antioxidant, vitamin C is being studied for its ability to prevent heart disease, certain cancers, and ARMD. Although most case controlled studies show an inverse relationship between vitamin C intake and cancers of the lung, breast, colon, stomach, oral cavity, and esophagus, evidence is inconsistent as to whether vitamin C affects cancer risk (NIH, ODS, 2013b). Likewise, most intervention trials do not provide convincing evidence that vitamin C supplements reduce the risk of cardiovascular disease. Vitamin C and other antioxidants may help slow the progression of ARMD in people at high risk (Age-Related Eye Disease Study Research Group, 2001; The Age-Related Eye Disease Study 2 Research Group, 2013).

There is no clear and convincing evidence that large doses of vitamin C prevent colds in the general population. However in five trials, vitamin C decreased the risk of colds in people under physical stress (e.g., marathon runners or soldiers in subarctic environments) by 50% (Hemilä & Chalker, 2013). Efficacy is difficult to measure because it may be influenced by how much, how often, and how long supplements are used and by which outcome it is measured, such as frequency of colds, length of cold, and severity of symptoms.

Phytonutrients
bioactive, nonnutrient plant compounds associated with a reduced risk of chronic diseases.

Phytonutrients

Phytonutrients, also known as phytochemicals, are literally plant ("phyto" in Greek) chemicals. They are a broad and diverse class of nonnutritive compounds that function like the immune system of plants to protect them against viruses, bacteria, and fungi. In foods phytochemicals impart color, taste, aroma, and other characteristics When eaten in the "package" of fruit, vegetables, whole grains, or nuts, these chemicals work together with nutrients and fiber to promote health, for example, by acting as antioxidants, detoxifying enzymes, stimulating the immune system, and regulating hormones or by inactivating bacteria and viruses. Thousands of phytochemicals have been identified; often, their actions in the body are complementary and overlapping. Phytonutrients are hypothesized to be a large part of the reason why eating patterns high in fruits, vegetables, whole grains, legumes, tea, and wine are associated with lower risk of chronic disease, such as heart disease, cancer, and diabetes.

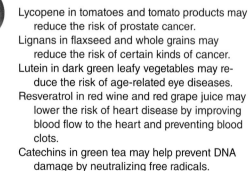

Quick Bite Examples of phytonutrients and their connection to health

Lycopene in tomatoes and tomato products may reduce the risk of prostate cancer.

Lignans in flaxseed and whole grains may reduce the risk of certain kinds of cancer.

Lutein in dark green leafy vegetables may reduce the risk of age-related eye diseases.

Resveratrol in red wine and red grape juice may lower the risk of heart disease by improving blood flow to the heart and preventing blood clots.

Catechins in green tea may help prevent DNA damage by neutralizing free radicals.

Phytonutrients are an emerging area of nutrition research. At this time, researchers simply do not know all the components in plants, how they function, which ones are beneficial, which ones are potentially harmful, and the ideal combination and concentration of these chemicals to be able to create a pill to substitute for a varied diet rich in plants. More than likely, it is the total package and balance of nutrients and nonnutritive substances that make fruits and vegetables so healthy. Until science catches up to nature, the best advice is to eat a diet rich in a variety of plants.

VITAMINS IN HEALTH PROMOTION

A premise of the *2015-2020 Dietary Guidelines for Americans* is that nutrient needs should be met primarily from food, not supplements. Although key vitamins are found in all MyPlate food groups, items within each group vary in the amount and kind of vitamins they provide (Fig. 5.1). Eating a variety of nutrient-dense items within each group is advocated to help ensure nutritional adequacy.

The Dietary Guidelines has identified several shortfall vitamins that Americans under consume namely vitamin A, vitamin D, vitamin E, and vitamin C (U.S. Department of Health and Human Services [USDHHS] & U.S. Department of Agriculture [USDA], 2015). Figure 5.2 illustrates mean intake of these nutrients expressed as a percentage of the RDA for each vitamin. Notice for men and women, vitamin C exceed 100% of the RDA. Still, the intake of these shortfall vitamins is a concern because the majority of the U.S. population has low intakes of key food groups that provide these vitamins, specifically vegetables, fruits, whole grains, and dairy.

Although vitamin E is mentioned as a vitamin that is underconsumed, average intake among Americans may be underestimated because of (1) underreporting of total fat intake, (2) difficulty in estimating the amount of fat used in the food preparation (e.g., frying), and (3) vague ingredient lists that state "may contain one or more of the following oils" because vegetable oils differ in their vitamin E content. It is noteworthy that deficiency symptoms have never been reported in healthy people eating a low–vitamin E diet.

Specific healthy eating pattern recommendations put forth in the Dietary Guidelines that will help to maximize vitamin intake are to

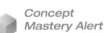

Concept Mastery Alert

Folate is found in fruits, vegetables, and protein foods and is beneficial to everyone, especially pregnant clients. Folic acid is found in fortified grains.

- Shift toward eating more vegetables from all subgroups (dark green, red and orange, legumes, starchy, and other) and more fruit, especially whole fruit. Table 5.4 lists amounts of fruits and vegetables recommended at various calorie levels of the Healthy U.S. Style Eating Pattern. Box 5.2 provides tips for boosting vegetable and fruit intake.
- Shift to more whole grains in place of refined grains.
- Increase intake of fat-free or low fat dairy products, especially those fortified with vitamin D.
- Consume a greater variety of nutrient-dense items within the protein group, such as more seafood (e.g., provides vitamin D) and nuts and seeds (e.g., provide vitamin E).
- Replace solid fats with oils, which will improve vitamin E intake.

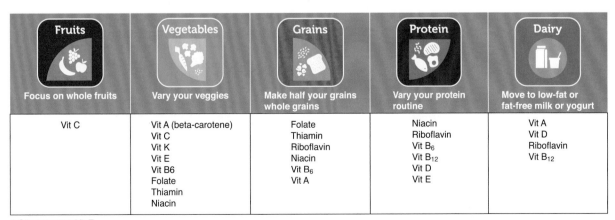

Fruits	Vegetables	Grains	Protein	Dairy
Focus on whole fruits	Vary your veggies	Make half your grains whole grains	Vary your protein routine	Move to low-fat or fat-free milk or yogurt
Vit C	Vit A (beta-carotene)	Folate	Niacin	Vit A
	Vit C	Thiamin	Riboflavin	Vit D
	Vit K	Riboflavin	Vit B_6	Riboflavin
	Vit E	Niacin	Vit B_{12}	Vit B_{12}
	Vit B6	Vit B_6	Vit D	
	Folate	Vit A	Vit E	
	Thiamin			
	Niacin			

* Oils category: Vit E

Figure 5.1 ▲ **Vitamins in MyPlate food groups.** *(Source: U.S. Department of Agriculture, Center for Nutrition Policy and Promotion. [2016]. Available at www.choosemyplate.gov. Accessed 2/13/16.)*

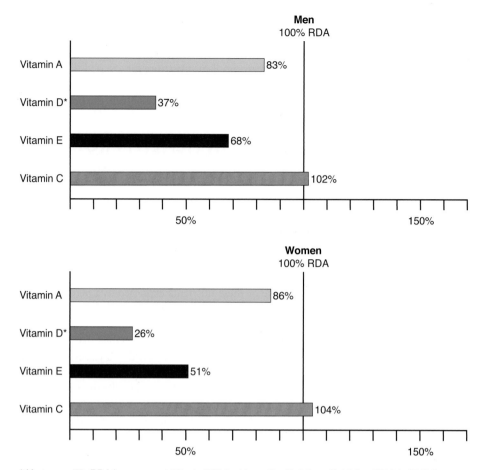

* Up to age 70; RDA increases at 71 y to 800 iu. Mean % of intake with higher RDA is 28% for men, 20% for women.

Figure 5.2 ▲ Mean intake of shortfall vitamins as a percentage of the Recommended Dietary Allowance in adult men and women. *(Source: U.S. Department of Agriculture [USDA], Agricultural Research Service [ARS]. [2014].* Nutrient intakes from food: Mean amounts consumed per individual by gender and age. What We Eat in America, NHANES 2011-2012. *Available at www.ars.usda.gov/ba/bhnrc/fsrg. Accessed 1/22/16.)*

Table 5.4	Amounts of Fruits and Vegetables Recommended at Various Calorie Levels in Healthy U.S. Style Eating Pattern	
Total Calorie Intake	**Amount of Fruit Recommended per Day (in cups)**	**Amount of Vegetables Recommended per Day (in cups)**
1600	1.5	2
1800	1.5	2.5
2000	2	2.5
2200–2400	2	3
2600	2	3.5
2800	2.5	3.5
3000–3200	2.5	4

Source: U.S. Department of Health and Human Services & U.S. Department of Agriculture. (2015). *2015-2020 Dietary Guidelines for Americans* (8th ed.). Available at http://health.gov/dietaryguidelines/2015/guidelines/ Accessed on 2/12/16.

BOX 5.2	Tips for Boosting Fruit and Vegetable Intake

- Eat at least five servings of fruits and vegetables every day. More is even better. Five servings of fruits and vegetables per day may provide more than 200 mg of vitamin C, far more than the RDA of 75 mg for adult women and 90 mg for adult men.
- Concentrate on variety and color. Aim for at least one green, one orange, one red, one citrus, and one legume serving every day.
- Make an effort to preserve the vitamin content of vegetables: Store them in the refrigerator (except for onions, tomatoes, winter squash, and potatoes), prepare them with minimal peeling, and cook for as short a time as possible in as little water as necessary. Microwaving is a better option than boiling.
- Start at least one meal each day with a fresh salad.
- Eat raw vegetables or fresh fruits for snacks.
- Add vegetables to other foods, such as zucchini to spaghetti sauce, grated carrots to meat loaf, and spinach to lasagna.
- Fill half the dinner plate with vegetables or vegetables and fruit.
- Buy a new fruit or vegetable when you go grocery shopping.
- Eat occasional meatless entrees such as pasta primavera, vegetable stir fry, or black beans and rice.
- Order a vegetable when you eat out.
- Choose 100% fruit juice at breakfast and during the day instead of drinks, cocktails, "-ades" (e.g., lemonade), and/or carbonated beverages.
- Eat fruit for dessert.
- Make fruits and vegetables more visible. Leave a bowl of fruit on the center of your table. Keep fresh vegetables on the top shelf of the refrigerator in plain view.

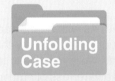

Unfolding Case

Consider Marcus. One of his food obsessions is a fortified gluten-free cereal. It is fortified with 100% of the Daily Value (DV) for many vitamins—but those DVs are based on adult requirements, not recommendations for children. Because he eats a few servings of this cereal daily, he is getting much larger amounts of certain vitamins and minerals than is required. Would you encourage Marcus's parents to find a nonfortified gluten-free cereal? Would you recommend they discontinue his vitamin and mineral supplements?

Of the shortfall vitamins identified, vitamin D is the only one classified as a nutrient of public health concern because under consumption is linked to adverse health outcomes.

Vitamin D

For most children and adults, sun exposure provides 90% of vitamin D, an inconsistent source that is difficult to quantify (Holick, 2007). Although it is possible for the body to make all the vitamin D it needs, a dietary source is considered necessary because few people meet those conditions. Winter, living in northern latitudes, dark skin pigmentation, air pollution, clothing, use of sunscreen, and older age are associated with low vitamin D synthesis. For instance, during the winter months in northern latitudes, the angle of the sun is such that most ultraviolet B rays are absorbed by the earth's ozone layer, preventing most or all endogenous synthesis of previtamin D. Elderly persons are particularly at risk for vitamin D deficiency because of various risk factors, including inadequate intake, limited sun exposure, reduced skin thickness, impaired GI absorption, and impaired activation by the liver and kidneys. Some experts suggest 5 to 30 minutes of sun exposure between 10 AM and 3 PM at least twice a week to the face, arms, legs, or back without sunscreen (NIH, ODS, 2014). Sun exposure may be more effective at raising vitamin D levels than oral vitamin D (Eich & Kline, 2016).

Vitamin D occurs naturally in few foods, such as oily fish, cod liver oil, egg yolks, and beef liver. Most dietary vitamin D is from fortified milk; other fortified foods include orange juice, yogurt, margarine, and ready to eat cereals. Despite the increase in the variety of vitamin

D–fortified foods available, vitamin D intake in Americans 20 years and older is far below the recommended amount of 600 to 800 IU/day (see Fig. 5.2).

Low blood levels of vitamin D appear to be widespread in studies of healthy adults and children in the United States and other countries. As many as 20% to 100% of older adults in the United States, Canada, and Europe are vitamin D deficient. In Boston, more than 50% of Hispanic and African American adolescents are deficient (Holick et al., 2011). A study by Bailey, Fulgoni, Keast, and Dwyer (2012) revealed that 90% of adults who did not use vitamin supplements failed to meet the recommended intake levels for vitamin D; even with supplement use, vitamin D intakes were low. The Endocrine Society recommends a daily supplement of 1000 to 2000 IU/day for adults as maintenance therapy; higher doses are needed to correct vitamin D deficiency (Holick et al., 2011).

Vitamin Supplements

An estimated half to two-thirds of American adults use dietary supplements, primarily in the form of multivitamins with or without minerals (Dickinson & MacKay, 2014). Supplement users tend to have better eating patterns, exercise regularly, have a healthy body weight, and avoid tobacco products compared to nonusers. Data from NHANES 2003–2006 (Bailey et al., 2012) reveal that

- Supplement use is more prevalent in older age groups than in younger adults and in each age group, usage is higher in women than men.
- Supplement use is lowest among obese and overweight individuals.
- Supplement use is highest among non-Hispanic whites and those with more than a high school education.
- Most people who take supplements use only one; however, approximately 10% of Americans take more than five dietary supplements.
- The most commonly taken vitamins are B_6, B_{12}, C, A, and E.

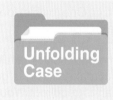

Think of Marcus. As with healthy adults, studies of children with autism taking supplements show that the children most likely to take supplements were less likely to need them, which may reflect heightened awareness of nutrition by some families in regard to both food and supplements. Is too much better than too little?

Studies show no substantial health benefits on all-cause mortality, cardiovascular disease, or cancer from the use of multivitamin supplements in well-nourished adults (Fortmann, Burda, Senger, Lin, & Whitlock, 2013). Supplements of beta-carotene, vitamin E, and possibly high doses of vitamin A are potentially harmful; other antioxidants, folic acid, B vitamins, and multivitamin and mineral supplements are ineffective at preventing chronic disease (Guallar, Stranges, Mulrow, Appel, & Miller, 2013). Evidence does not support the use of supplements by well-nourished adults.

Groups that may not qualify as "well nourished" and may therefore benefit from a multivitamin supplement include

- Dieters who consume fewer than 1200 cal/day. Even with optimal food choices, it may not be possible to consume adequate amounts of all nutrients on a low-calorie diet.
- Vegans, who eat no animal products, need supplemental vitamin B_{12} because it is found naturally only in animal products. Because vitamin B_{12} deficiency is seen in all types of vegetarians, consuming a vitamin B_{12} supplement or fortified foods is prudent regardless of the level of restriction. Vegetarians may also need vitamin D if sunlight exposure is inadequate because the only plant sources of vitamin D are some fortified margarines and some fortified cereals.
- Finicky eaters and people who eliminate one or more food groups from their typical diet. For instance, someone who cannot tolerate citrus juices because of gastric reflux may not consistently obtain adequate vitamin C without the use of a vitamin supplement.
- A large proportion of adults age 51 years and older do not consume adequate amounts of many nutrients from food alone (Sebastian, Cleveland, Goldman, & Moshfegh, 2007). Risk factors in this population include limited food budget, impaired chewing and swallowing, social isolation, physical limitations that make shopping or cooking difficult, or

BOX 5.3 Supplement Labeling Lingo

"High potency," at least to the FDA, means that at least two-thirds of the product's vitamins and minerals are provided at 100% or more of the Reference Daily Intakes.

"Advanced," "Complete," or "Maximum" formulas are not defined; manufacturers can use those terms as desired.

"Clinically proven" and "clinically tested" are not checked by any regulatory agency.

"Mature" or "50+" formulas usually have less iron and vitamin K. Although seniors do need less iron, the need for vitamin K does not decrease with aging. In fact, vitamin K may help prevent hip fractures. However, people using anticoagulants should strive for a consistent vitamin K intake.

"Women's" formulas have 18 mg of iron, which is appropriate for premenopausal women. Postmenopausal women need around 8 mg, which is the same amount of iron as men need.

"Energy" multivitamins may contain caffeine for "energy" or simply B vitamins based on the industry-promoted myth that B vitamins provide extra energy.

a decreased sense of taste leading to poor appetite. In addition, their vitamin requirements may be elevated as a result of chronic disease or as a side effect of certain medications. Low-dose multivitamin and mineral supplements can help meet recommended intake levels in the elderly when dietary selection is limited (Bernstein & Munoz, 2012).

- Alcoholics, because alcohol alters vitamin intake, absorption, metabolism, and excretion; the nutrients most profoundly affected are thiamin, riboflavin, niacin, folic acid, and pantothenic acid.
- People who are food insecure, meaning they may not always have sufficient money or other resources for food for all household members.
- People with chronic illness or chronic use of a medication that impairs nutrient absorption or increases metabolism or excretion

Choosing a Supplement

Although there is little scientific evidence to suggest that vitamin supplements can benefit the average person, there is also little evidence of harm from low-dose multivitamin or multivitamin and mineral supplements. Because vitamins work best together and in balanced proportions, a multivitamin that provides no more than 100% of the DV is usually better than single-vitamin supplements that tend to provide doses much greater than the RDA. Remember that pills are not a substitute for healthy food: "supplement" means "add to," not "replace."

The FDA requires a standardized "Supplement Facts" label on all supplements. Like the "Nutrition Facts" label, the supplement label is intended to provide consumers with better information. However, beware of label claims: Because the FDA does not closely regulate the supplement industry, manufacturers' claims may be less than reliable and not defined (Box 5.3). In fact, the term "multivitamin" does not have a standard regulatory definition. See Chapter 9 for more on dietary supplements.

How Do You Respond?

Is it better to take vitamin supplements with meals or between meals? In general, it is better to take supplements with meals because food enhances the absorption of some vitamins.

What does USP on the vitamin label mean? U.S. Pharmacopeia (USP) means the product passes tests for disintegration, dissolution, strength, and purity. It does not ensure that the supplement is safe or beneficial to health.

Is price an indication of quality? Should I buy the most expensive vitamins?
No, cost is not an indication of quality. Large retail chains are high-volume customers and can demand their own top-quality, private label supplements that are comparable to brand name varieties in content and quality. With vitamins, content and freshness are key considerations.

REVIEW CASE STUDY

Michael is a 22-year-old college student who lives off campus. Although he has a kitchen in his apartment, he has neither the time nor the interest in making his own food or stocking his own kitchen. All three of his daily meals come from fast-food restaurants. A typical day's intake is shown on the right:

- What vitamins is Michael probably lacking in his diet? What vitamins is he probably getting enough of?
- Are there better choices he could make at fast-food restaurants that would improve his vitamin intake?
- What suggestions would you make for keeping "quick" and "easy" food in his apartment that would improve his vitamin intake without being too much "bother"?
- How would you respond to this question from Michael: "Can I just take a multivitamin so I don't have to make changes in my eating habits?"

Breakfast: Two egg and bacon sandwiches on English muffins; large coffee with creamer and sugar
Lunch: Two cheeseburgers with catsup; large French fries; soft drink; cookies
Dinner: A foot-long submarine with cold cuts, cheese, mayonnaise, lettuce, tomato, onion, and pickles; bag of potato chips; soft drink
Snacks: Chocolate bar; chips and salsa; popcorn

STUDY QUESTIONS

1 When developing a teaching plan for a client who is on warfarin (Coumadin), which of the following foods would the nurse suggest the client consume a consistent intake of because of their vitamin K content?
   a. Liver, milk, and eggs
   b. Brussels sprouts, cauliflower, and spinach
   c. Fortified cereals, whole grains, and nuts
   d. Dried peas and beans, wheat germ, and seeds

2 A client asks if it is better to consume folic acid from fortified foods or from a vitamin pill. Which of the following is the nurse's best response?
   a. "It is better to consume folic acid through fortified foods because it will be better absorbed than through pill form."
   b. "It is better to consume folic acid through vitamin pills because it will be better absorbed than through fortified foods."
   c. "Fortified foods and vitamin pills have the same form of folic acid, so it does not matter which source you use because they are both well absorbed."
   d. "It is best to consume naturally rich sources of folate because that form is better absorbed than the folic acid in either fortified foods or vitamin pills."

3 Which population is at risk for combined deficiencies of thiamin, riboflavin, and niacin?
   a. Pregnant women
   b. Vegetarians
   c. Alcoholics
   d. Athletes

4 Which vitamin is given in large doses to facilitate wound and bone healing?
   a. Vitamin A
   b. Vitamin D
   c. Vitamin C
   d. Niacin

5 Which statement indicates that the client understands the instruction about using a vitamin supplement?
   a. "USP on the label guarantees safety and effectiveness."
   b. "Natural vitamins are always better for you than synthetic vitamins."
   c. "Vitamins are best absorbed on an empty stomach."
   d. "Taking a multivitamin cannot fully make up for poor food choices."

6 The client asks if taking supplements of beta-carotene will help reduce the risk of cancer. Which of the following would be the nurse's best response?
   a. "Supplements of beta-carotene may help reduce the risk of heart disease but not of cancer."
   b. "Supplements of beta-carotene have not been shown to lower the risk of cancer and may even promote cancer in certain people."
   c. "Although evidence is preliminary, taking beta-carotene supplements is safe and may prove to be effective against cancer in the future."
   d. "Natural supplements of beta-carotene are generally harmless; synthetic supplements of beta-carotene may increase cancer risk and should be avoided."

7 A client is diagnosed with pernicious anemia. What vitamin is he not absorbing?
   a. Folic acid
   b. Vitamin B_6
   c. Vitamin B_{12}
   d. Niacin

8 A client with hyperlipidemia is prescribed niacin. The client asks if he can just include more niacin-rich foods in his diet and forgo the need for niacin in pill form. Which of the following would be the nurse's best response?
   a. "The dose of niacin needed to treat hyperlipidemia is far more than can be consumed through eating a niacin-rich diet."
   b. "You can't get the therapeutic form of niacin through food."
   c. "Niacin from food is not as well absorbed as niacin from pills."
   d. "If you are able to consistently choose niacin-fortified foods in your diet, your doctor may allow you to forgo the pills and rely on dietary sources of niacin."

KEY CONCEPTS

- Vitamins do not provide energy (calories), but they are needed for metabolism of energy. Most vitamins function as coenzymes to activate enzymes.
- The body needs vitamins in small amounts (microgram or milligram quantities). Vitamins are essential in the diet because they cannot be made by the body or they are synthesized in inadequate amounts.
- Fortification and enrichment have virtually eliminated vitamin deficiencies in healthy Americans.
- It is assumed that if a variety of nutritious foods are consumed, vitamin intake will generally be adequate for most people.
- Vitamins are organic compounds that are soluble in either water or fat; their solubility determines how they are absorbed, transported through the blood, stored, and excreted.
- Vitamins A, D, E, and K are the fat-soluble vitamins. Because they are stored in liver and adipose tissue, they do not need to be consumed daily. Vitamins A and D are toxic when consumed in large quantities over a long period.
- The B-complex vitamins and vitamin C are water-soluble vitamins. Although some tissues are able to hold limited amounts of certain water-soluble vitamins, they are not generally stored in the body, so a daily intake is necessary. Because they are not stored, they are considered nontoxic; however, adverse side effects can occur from taking megadoses of certain water-soluble vitamins over a prolonged period.
- Phytonutrients are substances produced by plants to protect them from bacteria, viruses, and fungi. They add color, flavor, and aroma to foods. In the body, they impart important physiologic effects that may reduce the risk of chronic diseases.
- Not enough is known about phytonutrients to elevate them to the status of essential nutrients. Research is needed to determine which phytonutrients are protective, what quantity is optimal for health, and how they interact with other substances. Until then, the best advice is to eat a varied diet rich in fruits and vegetables.
- Antioxidant vitamins in foods are suspected of being beneficial, but high-dose supplements have not been proven to prevent disease and may disrupt nutrient balances. Long-term safety has not been established; some reports indicate that single-nutrient supplements may actually increase, not decrease, health risks.
- The 2015 Dietary Guidelines identifies vitamins A, D, E, C, and folate as shortfall vitamins. Key food groups that supply these vitamins—vegetables, fruits, whole grains, and dairy—are under consumed by the majority of Americans. Vitamin D is a public health concern because under consumption is linked to adverse health outcomes. Endogenous synthesis is negatively affected by several variables including northern latitude, winter, dark pigmented skin, the use of sunscreen, clothing, and aging. Even if a deficiency has not been diagnosed, it may be prudent for adults to take 1000 to 2000 IU of vitamin D daily.
- People older than the age of 50 years are urged to consume most of their vitamin B_{12} requirement from supplements or fortified food. Vegans need supplemental vitamin D, if exposure to sunshine is inadequate, and also supplemental vitamin B_{12}. Adequate vitamin B_{12} may be a concern for all types of vegetarians.
- It is not beneficial for well-nourished adults to take multivitamin supplements. Supplements of individual vitamins may be ineffective or potentially harmful.
- People who are not well nourished may benefit from taking a daily multivitamin, such as the elderly, dieters, finicky eaters, alcoholics, and people with chronic disease that impairs vitamin absorption, metabolism, or excretion.
- People who choose to take an all-purpose multivitamin should select one that provides 100% of the DV for vitamins with an established DV. The USP stamp ensures the quality but not safety or benefits. High-cost supplements are not necessarily superior to lower cost ones.

Check Your Knowledge Answer Key

1 **FALSE** There is no clear evidence that multivitamin supplements reduce the risk of cardiovascular disease or cancer in well-nourished adults.
2 **FALSE** Vitamins are needed to release energy from carbohydrates, protein, and fat but are not a source of energy (calories).
3 **TRUE** Vitamin D is considered a public health concern because Americans do not consume adequate amounts and underconsumption has been linked to adverse health outcomes.
4 **TRUE** Vitamins differ in their vulnerability to air, heat, light, acids, and alkalis. Proper food handling and storage, especially of fruits and vegetables, are needed to preserve vitamin content.
5 **FALSE** Cost and quality are not necessarily related.
6 **FALSE** "Natural" vitamins are not naturally better.
7 **TRUE** Under optimal conditions, such as exposing unprotected skin to the sun for several minutes, the body can make all the vitamin D it needs provided that kidney and liver functions are normal. However, sunscreen, smog, dark skin, clothing, and dense cloud cover hinder vitamin D synthesis.
8 **FALSE** Natural folate in foods is only half as available to the body as synthetic folic acid.
9 **FALSE** USP on a vitamin label means that the product passes tests that evaluate disintegration, dissolution, strength, and purity. It does not mean the product is safe. For instance, large doses of vitamin A are not safe, but they may have USP on the label.
10 **FALSE** Because fat-soluble vitamins are stored, a daily intake is not considered essential. It is recommended that water-soluble vitamins be consumed daily because they are not stored in the body.

Student Resources on thePoint®
For additional learning materials, activate the code in the front of this book at
http://thePoint.lww.com/activate

Websites

Dietary Reference Intakes from the Institute of Medicine at www.nap.edu
National Institutes of Health Office of Dietary Supplements at https://ods.od.nih.gov
Produce for Better Health Foundation at www.fruitsandveggiesmore matters.org
U.S. Department of Agriculture Nutrient Data Laboratory at https://fnic.nal.usda.gov/food-composition/usda-nutrient-data-laboratory

References

Age-Related Eye Disease Study Research Group. (2001). A randomized, placebo-controlled, clinical trial of high-dose supplementation with vitamins C and E, beta carotene, and zinc for age-related macular degeneration and vision loss: AREDS report No. 8. *Archives of Ophthalmology, 119*, 1417–1436.

American Heart Association. (2012). *Homocysteine, folic acid and cardiovascular disease.* Available at www.heart.org/HEARTORG/GettingHealthy/NutritionCenter/Homocysteine-Folic-Acid-and-Cardiovascular-Disease_UCM_305997_Article.jsp. Accessed on 9/14/12.

Armitage, J., Bowman, L., Clarke, R., Wallendszus, K., Bulbulia, R., Rahimi, K., . . . Collins, R. (2010). Effects of homocysteine-lowering with folic acid plus vitamin B12 vs placebo on mortality and major morbidity in myocardial infarction survivors. *JAMA, 303*, 2486–2492.

Bailey, R., Fulgoni, V., III, Keast, D., & Dwyer, J. (2012). Examination of vitamin intakes among US adults by dietary supplement use. *Journal of the Academy of Nutrition and Dietetics, 112*, 657.e4–663.e4.

Bergman, P., Norlin, A., Hansen, S., Rehka, R., Agerberth, B., Björkhem-Bergman, L., . . . Andersson, J. (2012). Vitamin D3 supplementation in patients with frequent respiratory tract infections: A randomised and double-blind intervention study. *BMJ Open, 2*, e001663. doi:10.1136/bmjopen-2012-001663

Bernstein, M., & Munoz, N. (2012). Position of the Academy of Nutrition and Dietetics: Food and nutrition for older adults: Promoting health and wellness. *Journal of the Academy of Nutrition and Dietetics, 112*, 1255–1277.

Bertone-Johnson, E., Powers, S., Spangler, L., Brunner, R. L., Michael, Y. L., Larson, J. C., . . . Manson, J. E. (2011). Vitamin D intake from foods and supplements and depressive symptoms in a diverse population of older women. *The American Journal of Clinical Nutrition, 94*, 1104–1112.

Bolland, M., Grey, A., Gamble, G., & Reid, I. (2011). Calcium and vitamin D supplements and health outcomes: A reanalysis of the Women's Health Initiative (WHI) limited-access data set. *The American Journal of Clinical Nutrition, 94*, 1144–1149.

Bønaa, K., Njølstad, I., Ueland, P., Schirmer, H., Tverdal, A., Steigen, T., . . . Rasmussen, K. (2006). Homocysteine lowering and cardiovascular events after acute myocardial infarction. *The New England Journal of Medicine, 354*, 1578–1588.

Breitling, L., Perna, L., Müller, H., Raum, E., Kliegel, M., & Brenner, H. (2012). Vitamin D and cognitive functioning in the elderly population in Germany. *Experimental Gerontolology, 47*, 122–127.

Dickinson, A., & MacKay, D. (2014). Health habits and other characteristics of dietary supplement users: A review. *Nutrition Journal, 13*, 14. doi:10.1186/1475-2891-13-14

Eich, M., & Kline, D. (2016). Vitamin D. Should "D" stand for deficiency? *Nutrition Dimension*, 12–17.

Elias, M., Sullivan, L., D'Agostino, R., Elias, P. K., Jacques, P. F., Selhub, J., . . . Wolf, P. A. (2005). Homocysteine and cognitive performance in the Framingham offspring study: Age is important. *American Journal of Epidemiology, 162*, 644–653.

Food and Nutrition Board, Institute of Medicine. (1997). *Dietary Reference Intakes for calcium, phosphorus, magnesium, vitamin D, and fluoride.* Washington, DC: The National Academies Press.

Food and Nutrition Board, Institute of Medicine. (1998). *Dietary Reference Intakes for thiamin, riboflavin, niacin, vitamin B6, folate, vitamin B12, pantothenic acid, biotin, and choline.* Washington, DC: The National Academies Press.

Food and Nutrition Board, Institute of Medicine. (2000). *Dietary Reference Intakes for vitamin C, vitamin E, selenium, and carotenoids.* Washington, DC: The National Academies Press.

Fortmann, S., Burda, G., Senger, C., Lin, J. S., & Whitlock, E. P. (2013). Vitamin and mineral supplements in the primary prevention of cardiovascular disease and cancer: An updated systematic evidence review for the U.S. Preventive Services Task Force. *Annals Internal Medicine, 159*, 824–834.

Fung, G., Steffan, L., Zhou, X., Harnack, L., Tang, W., Lutsey, P. L., . . . Van Horn, L. V. (2012). Vitamin D intake is inversely related to risk of developing metabolic syndrome in African American and white men and women over 20 y: The Coronary Artery Risk Development in Young Adults study. *The American Journal of Clinical Nutrition, 96*, 24–29.

Grant, W. (2011). Effect of interval between serum draw and follow-up period on relative risk of cancer incidence with respect to 25-hydroxyvitamin D level: Implications for meta-analysis and setting vitamin D guidelines. *Dermatoendocrinology, 3*, 199–204.

Guallar, E., Stranges, S., Mulrow, C., Appel, L. J., & Miller, E. R., III. (2013). Enough is enough: Stop wasting money on vitamin and mineral supplements. *Annals of Internal Medicine, 159*, 850–851.

Hasani, N., Kazemi, M., Afshar, H., Kazemi, M., & Tavakoli, M. (2015). Comparison of the effects of relaxation and vitamin B6 on emotional and physical symptoms in premenstrual syndrome. *Evidence Based Care Journal, 5*, 75–83.

Heine-Bröring, R., Winkels, R., Renkema, J., Kragt, L., van Orten-Luiten, A. C., Tigchelaar, E. F., . . . Kampman, E. (2015). Dietary supplement use and colorectal cancer risk: A systematic review and meta-analyses of prospective cohort studies. *International Journal of Cancer, 136*, 2388–2401.

Hemilä, H., & Chalker, E. (2013). Vitamin C for preventing and treating the common cold. *Cochrane Database of Systematic Reviews*, (1), CD000980. doi:10.1002/14651858.CD000980.pub4

Holick, M. (2007). Vitamin D deficiency. *The New England Journal of Medicine, 357*, 266–281.

Holick, M., Binkley, N., Bischoll-Ferrari, H., Gordon, C., Hanley, D. A., Heaney, R. P., . . . Weaver, C. M. (2011). Evaluation, treatment, and prevention of vitamin D deficiency: An Endocrine Society clinical practice guideline. *Journal of Clinical Endocrinology and Metabolism, 96*, 1911–1930.

Hollenbeck, C. (2010). The importance of being choline. *Journal of the American Dietetic Association, 110*, 1162–1165.

Hu, J., Juan, S., & Sahyoun, R. (2016). Intake and biomarkers of folate and risk of cancer morbidity in older adults, NHANES 1992-2002 with Medicare linkage. *PLoS One, 11*(2), e0148697. doi:10.1371/journal.pone.0148697

Humphrey, L., Fu, R., Rogers, K., Freeman, M., & Helfand, M. (2008). Homocysteine level and coronary heart disease incidence: A systematic review and meta-analysis. *Mayo Clinic Proceedings, 83*, 1203–1212.

Institute of Medicine. (1998). *Dietary reference intakes for thiamin, riboflavin, niacin, vitamin B6, pantothenic acid, biotin, and choline.* Washington, DC: The National Academies Press.

Institute of Medicine. (2011). *Dietary reference intakes for calcium and vitamin D.* Washington, DC: The National Academies Press.

Khaw, K., Luben, R., & Wareham, N. (2014). Serum 25-hydrosy vitamin D, mortality, and incident cardiovascular disease, respiratory disease, cancers, and fractures: A 13-y prospective population study. *The American Journal of Clinical Nutrition, 100*, 1361–1370.

Klein, E., Thompson, I., Tangen, C., Crowley, J. J., Lucia, M. S., Goodman, P. J., . . . Baker, L. H. (2011). Vitamin E and the risk of prostate cancer: The Selenium and Vitamin E Cancer Prevention Trial (SELECT). *JAMA, 306*, 1549–1556.

Lewerin, C., Jacobsson, S., Lindstedt, G., & Nilsson-Ehle, H. (2008). Serum biomarkers for atrophic gastritis and antibodies against Helicobacter pylori in the elderly: Implication for vitamin B12, folic acid and iron status and response to oral vitamin therapy. *Scandinavian Journal Gastroenterology, 43*, 1050–1056.

Lim, S., Kim, M., Choi, S., Shin, C. S., Park, K. S., Jang, H. C., . . . Meigs, J. B. (2013). Association of vitamin D deficiency with incidence of type 2 diabetes in high-risk Asian subjects. *The American Journal of Clinical Nutrition, 97*, 524–530.

Liu, Y., Yu, Z., Zhu, Z., Zhang, J., Chen, M., Tang, P., & Li, K. (2015). Vitamin and multiple-vitamin supplement intake and incidence of colorectal cancer: A meta-analysis of cohort studies. *Medical Oncology*. doi:10.1007/s12032-014-0434-5

Lonn, E., Yusuf, S., Arnold, M. J., Sheridan, P., Pogue, J., Micks, M., . . . Genest, J., Jr. (2006). Homocysteine lowering with folic acid and B vitamins in vascular disease. *The New England Journal of Medicine, 354*, 1567–1577.

McCully, L. (2007). Homocysteine, vitamins, and vascular disease prevention. *The American Journal of Clinical Nutrition, 86*, 1563S–1568S.

Medical Research Council Vitamin Study Research Group. (1991). Prevention of neural tube defects: Results of the Medical Research Council Vitamin Study. *Lancet, 338*, 131–137.

Moyer, V. (2014). Vitamin, mineral, and multivitamin supplements for the primary prevention of cardiovascular disease and cancer: U.S. Preventive Services Task Force recommendation statement. *Annals of Internal Medicine, 160*, 558–564.

Muscogiuri, G., Sorice, G., Ajjan, R., Mezza, T., Pilz, S., Prioletta, A., . . . Giaccari, A. (2012). Can vitamin D deficiency cause diabetes and cardiovascular diseases? Present evidence and future perspectives. *Nutrition, Metabolism, and Cardiovascular Diseases, 22*, 81–87.

National Institutes of Health, Office of Dietary Supplements. (2013a). *Vitamin E: Fact sheet for health professionals.* Available at https://ods.od.nih.gov/factsheets/VitaminE-HealthProfessional/#en6. Accessed on 2/14/16.

National Institutes of Health, Office of Dietary Supplements. (2013b). *Vitamin C: Fact sheet for health professionals.* Available at https://ods.od.nih.gov/factsheets/VitaminC-HealthProfessiona. Accessed on 2/16/16.

National Institutes of Health, Office of Dietary Supplements. (2014). *Vitamin D: Fact sheet for health professionals.* Available at https://ods.od.nih.gov/factsheets/VitaminD-HealthProfessional/#h3. Accessed on 2/13/16.

Nuangchamnong, N., & Niebyl, J. (2014). Doxylamine succinate-pyridoxine hydrochloride (Diclegis) for the management of nausea and vomiting in pregnancy: An overview. *International Journal of Women's Health, 6*, 401–409.

Omenn, G. S., Goodman, G. E., Thornquist, M. D., Balmes, J., Cullen, M. R., Glass, A., . . . Hammar, S. (1996). Effects of a combination of beta carotene and vitamin A on lung cancer and cardiovascular disease. *The New England Journal of Medicine, 334*, 1150–1155.

Pawlak, R., Parrott, S., Raj, S., Cullum-Dugan, D., & Lucus, D. (2013). How prevalent is vitamin B12 deficiency among vegetarians. *Nutrition Reviews, 71*, 110–117.

Pender, M. (2012). CD8 + T-cell deficiency, Epstein-Barr virus infection, vitamin D deficiency, and steps to autoimmunity: A unifying hypothesis. *Autoimmune Diseases*, doi:10.1155/2012/189096

Pludowski, P., Holick, M., Pilz, S., Wagner, C., Hollis, B. W., Grant, W. B., . . . Soni, M. (2013). Vitamin D effects on musculoskeletal health, immunity, autoimmunity, cardiovascular disease, cancer, fertility, pregnancy, dementia, and mortality—a review of recent evidence. *Autoimmunity Reviews, 12*, 976–989. doi:10.1016/j.autrev.2013.004

Ross, A., Manson, J., Abrams, S., Aloia, J. F., Brannon, P. M., & Clinton, S. K. (2011). The 2011 report on Dietary Reference Intakes for calcium and vitamin D from the Institute of Medicine: What clinicians need to know. *Journal of Clinical Endocrinology and Metabolism, 96*, 53–58.

Schöttker, B., Haug, U., Schomburg, L., Köhrle, J., Perna, L., Müller, H., . . . Brenner, H. (2013). Strong associations of 25-hydroyvitamin D concentrations with all-cause, cardiovascular, cancer, and respiratory disease mortality in a large cohort study. *The American Journal of Clinical Nutrition, 97*, 782–793.

Sebastian, R., Cleveland, L., Goldman, J., & Moshfegh, A. (2007). Older adults who use vitamin/mineral supplements differ from nonusers in nutrient intake adequacy and dietary attitudes. *Journal of the American Dietetic Association, 107*, 1322–1332.

Stabler, S. (2013). Vitamin B_{12} deficiency. *The New England Journal of Medicine, 368*, 149–160.

The Age-Related Eye Disease Study 2 Research Group. (2013). Lutein + zeaxanthin and omega-3 fatty acids for age-related macular degeneration: The Age-Related Eye Disease Study 2 (AREDS2) randomized clinical trial. *JAMA, 309*, 2005–2015.

The Alpha-Tocopherol, Beta-Carotene Cancer Prevention Study Group. (1994). The effect of vitamin D and beta carotene on the incidence of lung cancer and other cancers in small smokers. *The New England Journal of Medicine, 330*, 1029–1035.

Toole, J., Malinow, M., Chambless, L., Spence, J. D., Pettigrew, L. C., Howard, V. J., . . . Stampfer, M. (2004). Lowering homocysteine in patients with ischemic stroke to prevent recurrent stroke, myocardial infarction, and death. The Vitamin Intervention for Stroke Prevention (VISP) randomized controlled trial. *JAMA, 291*, 565–575.

U.S. Department of Health and Human Services & U.S. Department of Agriculture. (2015). *2015-2020 Dietary guidelines for Americans* (8th ed.). Available at http://health.gov/dietaryguidelines/2015/guidelines/. Accessed on 2/12/16.

Wang, L. Sesso, H., Glynn, R., Christen, W. G., Bubes, V., Manson, J. E., . . . Gaziano, J. M. (2014). Vitamin E and C supplementation and risk of cancer in men: Posttrial follow-up in the Physician's Health Study II randomized trial. *The American Journal of Clinical Nutrition, 100*, 915–923.

Watkins, R., Yamshchikov, A., Lemonovich, T., & Salata, R. (2011). The role of vitamin D deficiency in sepsis and potential therapeutic implications. *The Journal of Infection, 63*, 321–326.

Winkels, R. M., Brouwer, I. A., Siebelink, E., Katan, M. B., & Verhoef, P. (2007). Bioavailability of food folates is 80% of that of folic acid. *The American Journal of Clinical Nutrition, 85*, 465–473.

Witham, M., Nadir, M., & Struthers, A. (2009). Effect of vitamin D on blood pressure: A systematic review and meta-analysis. *Journal Hypertension, 27*, 1948–1954.

World Health Organization. (2012). Micronutrient deficiencies. Vitamin A deficiency. Available at www.who.int/nutrition/topics/vad/en/#. Accessed on 9/13/12.

Zschäbitz, S., Cheng, T., Neuhouser, M., Zheng, Y., Ray, R. M., Miller, J. W., . . . Ulrich, C. M. (2013). B vitamin intakes and incidence of colorectal cancer: Results from the Women's Health Initiative Observational Study cohort. *The American Journal of Clinical Nutrition, 97*(2), 332–343. doi:10.3945/ajcn.112.034736

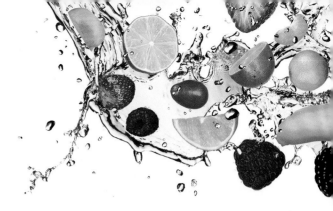

Chapter 6

Water and Minerals

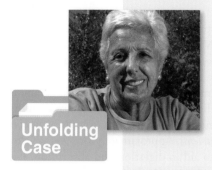

Unfolding Case

Myra Johnson

Myra is a healthy, active 83-year-old woman who is conscientious about healthy eating and exercise. She read about the many health benefits from using aloe to detox and decided to give it a try. Over a period of diligent use, she developed diarrhea but passed it off as part of the detox process. Her family took her to the emergency department when she exhibited what they thought were signs of a stroke: weakness, exhaustion, and delirium. What may be causing her symptoms?

Check Your Knowledge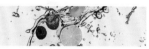

True	False		
☐	☐	1	Adults need eight 8 oz glasses of fluid daily to meet their requirement for fluid.
☐	☐	2	All minerals consumed in excess of need are excreted in the urine.
☐	☐	3	Sodium is the most plentiful mineral in the body.
☐	☐	4	Like vitamins, the mineral content of food can be destroyed by light, heat, or acids during food preparation.
☐	☐	5	Calcium supplements are a safe and effective way to ensure an adequate calcium intake.
☐	☐	6	Foods high in sodium tend to be low in potassium, and foods high in potassium tend to be low in sodium.
☐	☐	7	Major minerals are more important for health than trace minerals.
☐	☐	8	For most people, thirst is a reliable indicator of fluid needs.
☐	☐	9	Trace mineral balance is strongly influenced by interactions with other minerals and dietary factors.
☐	☐	10	A chronically low intake of calcium leads to hypocalcemia.

Learning Objectives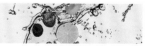

Upon completion of this chapter, you will be able to

1 Calculate a person's fluid requirement.
2 Give examples of mechanisms by which the body maintains mineral homeostasis.
3 Identify sources of minerals.
4 Discuss functions of minerals.
5 Predict potential consequences of mineral deficiencies or toxicities.
6 Describe healthy eating patterns associated with optimal mineral intake.

Water is fundamental to life. It is the single largest constituent of the human body, averaging approximately 60% of the total body weight. It is the medium in which all biochemical reactions take place. Although most people can survive 6 weeks or longer without food, death occurs in a matter of days without water.

UNDERSTANDING WATER

Water occupies essentially every space within and between body cells and is involved in virtually every body function. Water

- *Provides shape and structure to cells.* Approximately two-thirds of the body's water is located within cells (intracellular fluid). Muscle cells have a higher concentration of water (70%–75%) than fat, which is only about 25% water. Men generally have more muscle mass than women and, therefore, have a higher percentage of body water.
- *Regulates body temperature.* Because water absorbs heat slowly, the large amount of water contained in the body helps to maintain body temperature homeostasis despite fluctuations in environmental temperatures. Evaporation of water (sweat) from the skin cools the body.
- *Aids in the digestion and absorption of nutrients.* Approximately 7 to 9 L of water is secreted in the gastrointestinal (GI) tract daily to aid in digestion and absorption. Except for the approximately 100 mL of water excreted through the feces, all of the water contained in the GI secretions (saliva, gastric secretions, bile, pancreatic secretions, and intestinal mucosal secretions) is reabsorbed in the ileum and colon.
- *Transports nutrients and oxygen to cells.* By moistening the air sacs in the lungs, water allows oxygen to dissolve and move into blood for distribution throughout the body. Approximately 92% of blood plasma is water.
- *Serves as a solvent for vitamins, minerals, glucose, and amino acids.* The solvating property of water is vital for health and survival.
- *Participates in metabolic reactions.* For instance, water is used in the synthesis of hormones and enzymes.
- *Eliminates waste products.* Water helps to excrete body wastes through urine, feces, and expirations.
- *Is a major component of mucus and other lubricating fluids.* Water reduces friction in joints where bones, ligaments, and tendons come in contact with each other, and it cushions contacts between internal organs that slide over one another.

Water Balance

Water balance is the dynamic state between water output and water intake. Under normal conditions, output and intake are approximately equal (Fig. 6.1).

Water Output

On average, adults lose approximately 1750 to 3000 mL of water daily. Extreme environmental temperatures (very hot or very cold), high altitude, low humidity, and strenuous exercise increase

Figure 6.1 ▶

Water balance approximations.

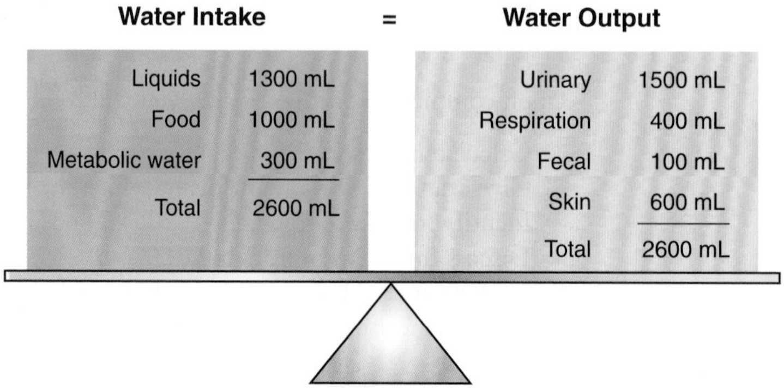

Water Intake		=	Water Output	
Liquids	1300 mL		Urinary	1500 mL
Food	1000 mL		Respiration	400 mL
Metabolic water	300 mL		Fecal	100 mL
Total	2600 mL		Skin	600 mL
			Total	2600 mL

Insensible Water Loss
immeasurable losses.

Sensible Water Loss
measurable losses.

insensible water losses from respirations and the skin. Water evaporation from the skin is also increased by prolonged exposure to heated or recirculated air, for example, during long airplane flights. **Sensible water losses** from urine and feces make up the remaining water loss. Because the body needs to excrete a minimum of 500 mL of urine daily to rid itself of metabolic wastes, the minimum daily total fluid output is approximately 1500 mL. To maintain water balance, intake should approximate output.

Water Intake

Total water intake averages about 2.5 L/day, of which approximately 80% is from fluids and 20% from solid food (Institute of Medicine [IOM], 2005). Box 6.1 describes various types of bottled water. Except for oils, almost all foods contain water, with fruits and vegetables providing the most (Fig. 6.2). The body also produces a small amount of water from normal metabolism: The catabolism of carbohydrates, protein, and fat for energy yields carbon and hydrogen atoms that combine with oxygen to form water and carbon dioxide. On average, 250 to 350 mL of **metabolic water** is produced daily, depending on total calorie intake.

Metabolic Water
water produced as a by-product from the breakdown of carbohydrates, protein, and fat for energy.

Water Recommendations

Water is an essential nutrient because the body cannot produce as much water as it needs. The Dietary Reference Intake (DRI) committee on fluid and electrolytes did not establish a Recommended Dietary Allowance (RDA) for water because of insufficient evidence linking a specific amount of water intake to health; actual requirements vary depending on diet, physical activity, environmental temperatures, and humidity.

The Adequate Intake (AI) for total water, which includes water from liquids and solids, is based on the median total water intake from U.S. food consumption survey data (IOM, 2005). For men age 19 years to older than 70 years, the AI is 3.7 L/day, which includes 3 L as fluids. For women of the same age, the AI is 2.7 L, which includes approximately 2.2 L from fluids. Similar to AIs set for other nutrients, daily intakes below the AI may not be harmful to healthy people because normal hydration is maintained over a wide range of intakes. Amounts higher than the AI are recommended for rigorous activity in hot climates. Because the body cannot store water, it should be consumed throughout the day.

BOX 6.1 **U.S. Food and Drug Administration's Standards of Identity for Common Types of Bottled Water**

- *Artesian well water* originates from a well that taps a confined aquifer and the water level must stand at some height above the top of the aquifer. An aquifer is an underground layer of rock or sand with water.
- *Mineral water* contains at least 250 ppm total dissolved solids (minerals) that are naturally present, not added.
- *Purified water* is produced by distillation, deionization, reverse osmosis, or other suitable processes to remove minerals and other solids. It may also be referred to as "distilled water" if it is produced by distillation, "deionized water" if it is produced by deionization, or "reverse osmosis water" if it was produced by reverse osmosis. Purified is not synonymous with "sterile."
- *Sparkling water* contains a "fizz" from carbon dioxide that was either present in the water when it emerged from its source or was present, removed in processing, and then replaced. Carbon dioxide levels cannot exceed the amount present in the original water. Sparkling water may be labeled as "sparkling drinking water," "sparkling mineral water," "sparkling spring water," etc. Seltzer, tonic water, and club soda are carbonated beverages; they are not types of sparkling water.
- *Spring water* comes from an underground source that flows naturally to the surface. It must be collected at the spring or through a bored hole that taps the spring underground.
- *Well water* is collected with a mechanical pump from an underground aquifer.

Source: International Bottled Water Association. *Bottled water.* Available at http://www.bottledwater.org/content/faqs#2. Accessed on 2/27/16.

Figure 6.2 ▶

Percentage of water content of various foods.

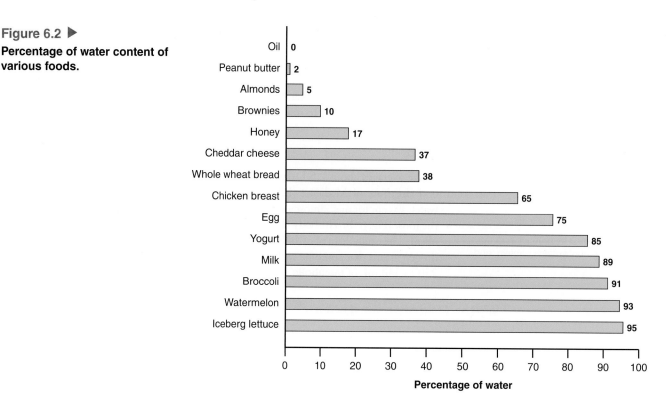

The IOM did not specify how much of total fluid intake should come specifically from water. For healthy people, the universal, age-old advice has been to drink at least eight 8-oz glasses of water daily. Although that may be excellent advice, there is little scientific evidence to support this recommendation (Valtin, 2002). For healthy people, hydration is unconsciously maintained with ad lib access to water. In healthy adults, thirst is usually a reliable indicator of water need, and fluid intake is assumed to be adequate when the color of urine produced is pale yellow. In some conditions and for some segments of the population, the sensation of thirst is blunted and may not be a reliable indicator of need. For the elderly and children, and during hot weather or strenuous exercise, drinking fluids should not be delayed until the sensation of thirst occurs because by then fluid loss is significant.

Estimating Fluid Requirements

Box 6.2 outlines several methods for estimating fluid requirements. However, according to the American Dietetic Association's Evidence Analysis Library, there are no validated equations for determining fluid needs nor is there evidence of a clinical or laboratory measure that best assesses hydration status (Academy of Nutrition and Dietetics, n.d.).

Inadequate Fluid Intake

An inadequate intake of water can lead to dehydration, characterized by impaired mental function, impaired motor control, increased body temperature during exercise, increased resting heart rate when standing or lying down, and an increased risk of life-threatening heat stroke. A net water loss of 1% to 2% of body weight causes thirst, fatigue, weakness, vague discomfort, and loss of appetite. A loss of 7% to 10% leads to dizziness, muscle spasticity, loss of balance, delirium, exhaustion, and collapse. Left untreated, dehydration ends in death.

Clinical situations in which water losses are increased—and thus water needs are elevated—include vomiting, diarrhea, fever, thermal injuries, uncontrolled diabetes, hemorrhage, certain renal disorders, and the use of drainage tubes. Intake and output records are used to assess adequacy of intake.

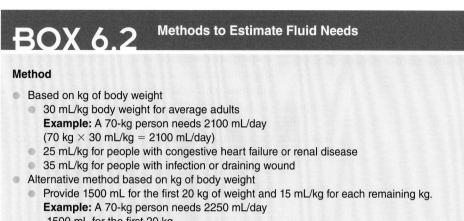

Method

- Based on kg of body weight
  - 30 mL/kg body weight for average adults
    Example: A 70-kg person needs 2100 mL/day
    (70 kg × 30 mL/kg = 2100 mL/day)
    - 25 mL/kg for people with congestive heart failure or renal disease
    - 35 mL/kg for people with infection or draining wound
- Alternative method based on kg of body weight
  - Provide 1500 mL for the first 20 kg of weight and 15 mL/kg for each remaining kg.
    Example: A 70-kg person needs 2250 mL/day
    1500 mL for the first 20 kg
    +750 mL (15 mL × 50 remaining kg)
    2250 mL/day
- Based on calories consumed
  - 1 mL/cal consumed
    Example: A person consuming 2000 cal/day needs 2000 mL/day.
    (2000 cal/day × 1 mL/cal = 2000 mL/day)
- Based on urine output
  - Urine output + 500 mL

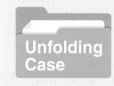

Unfolding Case

Recall Myra. She lost excessive amounts of fluid from diarrhea and is diagnosed with dehydration. Why didn't she feel thirsty as she became dehydrated?

Excessive Fluid Intake

A chronic high intake of water has not been shown to cause adverse effects in healthy people who consume a varied diet as long as intake approximates output (IOM, 2005). An excessive water intake may cause hyponatremia, but it is rare in healthy people who consume a typical diet. People most at risk include infants; psychiatric patients with excessive thirst; women who have undergone surgery using a uterine distention medium; and athletes in endurance events who drink too much water, fail to replace lost sodium, or both. Symptoms of hyponatremia include lung congestion, muscle weakness, lethargy, and confusion. Hyponatremia can progress to convulsions and prolonged coma. Death can result.

UNDERSTANDING MINERALS

Although minerals account for only about 4% of the body's total weight, they are found in all body fluids and tissues. Calcium, phosphorus, magnesium, sulfur, sodium, potassium, and chloride are considered major minerals because they are present in the body in amounts greater than 5 g (the equivalent of 1 tsp). Iron, iodine, zinc, selenium, copper, manganese, fluoride, chromium, and molybdenum are classified as trace minerals, or trace elements, because they are present in the body in amounts less than 5 g, not because they are less important than major minerals. Both groups are essential for life. As many as 30 other potentially harmful minerals are present in the body, including lead, gold, and mercury. Their presence appears to be related to environmental contamination.

General Chemistry

Unlike the energy nutrients and vitamins, minerals are **inorganic** elements that originate from the earth's crust, not from plants or animals. Minerals do not undergo digestion nor are they broken down or rearranged during metabolism. Although they combine with other elements to form salts (e.g., sodium chloride) or with organic compounds (e.g., iron in hemoglobin), they always retain their chemical identities.

Unlike vitamins, minerals are not destroyed by light, air, heat, or acids during food preparation. In fact, when food is completely burned, minerals are the ash that remains. Minerals are lost only when they leach from foods soaked in water.

General Functions

Minerals function to provide structure to body tissues and to regulate body processes such as fluid balance, acid–base balance, nerve cell transmission, muscle contraction, and vitamin, enzyme, and hormonal activities (Table 6.1).

Mineral Balance

The body has several mechanisms by which it maintains mineral balance, depending on the mineral involved, such as

- *Releasing minerals from storage for redistribution.* Some minerals can be released from storage and redistributed as needed, which is what happens when calcium is released from bones to restore normal serum calcium levels.
- *Altering rate of absorption.* For example, normally only about 10% of the iron consumed is absorbed, but the rate increases to 50% when the body is deficient in iron.
- *Altering rate of excretion.* Virtually all of the sodium consumed in the diet is absorbed. The only way the body can rid itself of excess sodium is to increase urinary sodium excretion. For most people, the higher the intake of sodium, the greater is the amount of sodium excreted in the urine. Excess potassium is also excreted in the urine.

Mineral Toxicities

Minerals that are easily excreted, such as sodium and potassium, do not accumulate to toxic levels in the body under normal circumstances. Stored minerals can produce toxicity symptoms when intake is excessive, but excessive intake is not likely to occur from eating a balanced diet.

Table 6.1   General Functions of Minerals

Functions	Examples
Provide structure	Calcium, phosphorus, and magnesium provide structure to bones and teeth. Phosphorus, potassium, iron, and sulfur provide structure to soft tissues. Sulfur is a constituent of skin, hair, and nails.
Fluid balance	Sodium, potassium, and chloride maintain fluid balance.
Acid–base balance	Sodium hydroxide and sodium bicarbonate are part of the carbonic acid–bicarbonate system that regulates blood pH. Phosphorus is involved in buffer systems that regulate kidney tubular fluids.
Nerve cell transmission and muscle contraction	Sodium and potassium are involved in transmission of nerve impulses. Calcium stimulates muscle contractions. Sodium, potassium, and magnesium stimulate muscle relaxation.
Vitamin, enzyme, and hormone activity	Cobalt is a component of vitamin B_{12}. Magnesium is a cofactor for hundreds of enzymes. Iodine is essential for the production of thyroxine. Chromium enhances the action of insulin.

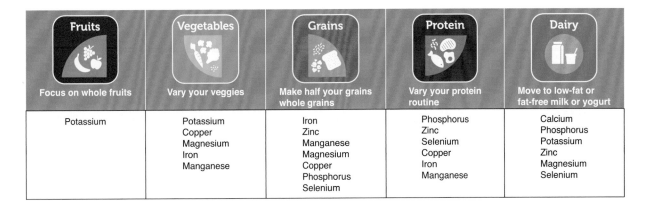

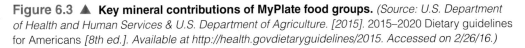

Fruits	Vegetables	Grains	Protein	Dairy
Focus on whole fruits	Vary your veggies	Make half your grains whole grains	Vary your protein routine	Move to low-fat or fat-free milk or yogurt
Potassium	Potassium Copper Magnesium Iron Manganese	Iron Zinc Manganese Magnesium Copper Phosphorus Selenium	Phosphorus Zinc Selenium Copper Iron Manganese	Calcium Phosphorus Potassium Zinc Magnesium Selenium

Figure 6.3 ▲ Key mineral contributions of MyPlate food groups. *(Source: U.S. Department of Health and Human Services & U.S. Department of Agriculture. [2015]. 2015–2020 Dietary guidelines for Americans [8th ed.]. Available at http://health.govdietaryguidelines/2015. Accessed on 2/26/16.)*

Instead, mineral toxicity is related to excessive use of mineral supplements, environmental or industrial exposure, human errors in commercial food processing, or alterations in metabolism. For instance, in 2008, the most serious selenium toxicity outbreak that has ever occurred in the United States was caused by an improperly manufactured dietary supplement that contained 200 times the labeled concentration of selenium (Morris & Crane, 2013).

Mineral Interactions

Mineral balance is influenced by hundreds of interactions that occur among minerals and between minerals and other dietary components. For instance, caffeine promotes calcium excretion, whereas vitamin D and lactose promote its absorption. Mineral status must be viewed as a function of the total diet, not just from the standpoint of the quantity consumed.

Sources of Minerals

Key minerals are found in all MyPlate food groups; items within each group vary in the amount and kind of minerals they provide (Fig. 6.3). Generally, unrefined or unprocessed foods have more minerals than refined foods. Trace mineral content varies with the content of soil from which the food originates. Within most food groups, processed foods are high in sodium and chloride. Drinking water contains varying amounts of calcium, magnesium, and other minerals; sodium is added to soften water. Fluoride may be a natural or added component of drinking water.

Mineral supplements, alone or combined with vitamins, contribute to mineral intake. As with vitamins, people who take mineral supplements have higher intakes of minerals from food than do people who do not take supplements (Bailey, Fulgoni, Keast, & Dwyer, 2011). With some minerals—namely, calcium, iron, zinc, and magnesium—supplements may contribute to potentially excessive intakes (Bailey et al., 2011).

MAJOR ELECTROLYTES

Sodium, chloride, and potassium are major minerals that are also major electrolytes in the body. Salient features for each electrolyte are presented in the following paragraphs. Table 6.2 details their recommended intakes, sources, functions, and signs and symptoms of deficiency and toxicity.

Sodium

By weight, salt (sodium chloride) is approximately 40% sodium; 1 tsp of salt (5 g) provides approximately 2300 mg of sodium. Box 6.3 describes various types of salt. It is estimated that approximately 75% of the sodium consumed in the typical American diet comes from salt or

Table 6.2 Summary of Major Electrolytes

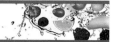

Electrolyte and Sources	Functions	Deficiency/Toxicity Signs and Symptoms
Sodium (Na) Adult AI: 19–50 y: 1.5 g 50–70 y: 1.3 g 71+ y: 1.2 g Adult UL: 2.3 g ● Processed foods; canned meat, vegetables, soups; convenience foods; restaurant and fast foods	Fluid and electrolyte balance, acid–base balance, maintains muscle irritability, regulates cell membrane permeability and nerve impulse transmission	**Deficiency** Rare, except with chronic diarrhea or vomiting and certain renal disorders; nausea, dizziness, muscle cramps, apathy **Toxicity** Hypertension, edema
Potassium (K) Adult AI: 4.7 g No UL ● Baked potato with skin, canned tomato products, sweet potatoes, soy nuts, pistachios, prunes, clams, molasses, yogurt, tomato juice, prune juice, cantaloupe, legumes, orange juice, bananas, peanuts, artichokes, fish, beef, lamb, avocados, apple juice, raisins, plantains, spinach, asparagus, kiwi-fruit, apricots, chocolate milk	Fluid and electrolyte balance, acid–base balance, nerve impulse transmission, catalyst for many metabolic reactions, involved in skeletal and cardiac muscle activity	**Deficiency** Muscular weakness, paralysis, anorexia, confusion (occurs with dehydration) **Toxicity (from supplements/drugs)** Muscular weakness, vomiting
Chloride (Cl) Adult AI: 19–50 y: 2.3 g 50–70 y: 2.0 g 71+ y: 1.8 g Adult UL: 3.6 g ● 1 tsp salt = 3600 mg Cl ● Same sources as sodium	Fluid and electrolyte balance, acid–base balance, component of hydrochloric acid in stomach	**Deficiency** Rare, may occur secondary to chronic diarrhea or vomiting and certain renal disorders: muscle cramps, anorexia, apathy **Toxicity** Normally harmless; can cause vomiting

Quick Bite Examples of sodium additives

To enhance flavor
  Sodium chloride
  Monosodium glutamate (MSG)
  Soy sauce
  Teriyaki sauce
To preserve freshness
  Brine
  Sodium sulfite (for dried fruits)
To prevent the growth of yeast and/or bacteria
  Sodium benzoate
  Sodium nitrate or sodium nitrite
  Sodium lactate
  Sodium diacetate
To prevent the growth of mold
  Sodium propionate
As an antioxidant
  Sodium erythorbate
As a sweetener
  Sodium saccharin
As a binder/thickener
  Sodium caprate
  Sodium caseinate
As a leavening agent
  Sodium bicarbonate (baking soda)
  Baking powder
As a stabilizer
  Sodium citrate
  Disodium phosphate

sodium preservatives added to foods by food manufacturers. Only 12% of total sodium intake is from sodium that occurs naturally in foods such as milk, meat, poultry, vegetables, tap water, and bottled water (IOM, 2005). Salt added during cooking or at the table accounts for the remaining sodium intake. Figure 6.4 illustrates food category sources of sodium in the U.S. population. Wide variations in sodium intake exist between cultures and between individuals within a culture, based on the amount of processed foods consumed.

As the major extracellular cation, sodium is largely responsible for regulating fluid balance. It also regulates cell permeability and the movement of fluid, electrolytes, glucose, insulin, and amino acids. Sodium is pivotal in acid–base balance, nerve transmission, and muscular irritability. Although sodium plays vital roles, under normal conditions, the amount actually needed is very small, maybe even less than 200 mg/day.

Almost 98% of all sodium consumed is absorbed; yet, humans are able to maintain homeostasis over a wide range of intakes, largely through urinary excretion. A salty meal causes a transitory increase in serum sodium, which triggers thirst. Drinking fluids dilutes the sodium in the blood to normal concentration, even though the volume of both sodium and fluid are increased. The increased volume stimulates the kidneys to excrete more sodium and fluid together to restore normal blood volume. Conversely, low blood volume or low extracellular sodium stimulates the hormone aldosterone to increase sodium reabsorption by the kidneys. In people who have minimal sweat losses, sodium intake and sodium excretion are approximately equal.

BOX 6.3 Types of Salt

- *Table salt* is a fine-grained salt from salt mines that is refined until it is pure sodium chloride. It is mainly used in cooking and at the table and may or may not contain iodine. It often contains calcium silicate to keep it free flowing.
- *Kosher salt* is a coarse-grain salt that does not contain any additives. It is used in the preparation of kosher meat according to Jewish dietary laws. Although the terms "kosher salt" and "sea salt" are often used interchangeably, kosher salt does not necessarily originate from the sea.
- *Sea salt* may be fine or coarse grained. It has a slightly different flavor than table salt due to its mineral content. Although it is often promoted as a healthier alternative to table salt, the sodium content is essentially the same. The advantage is that people may use less sea salt than table salt because of its more pronounced flavor. Examples include Mediterranean sea salt, Alaea (Hawaiian) sea salt, and Black salt—salts named after the originating sea.
- *Pickling salt* is a fine-grained salt used for making pickles and sauerkraut. It does not contain additives or anticlumping agents.
- *Specialty salts*, such as popcorn salt, come in various grains and textures and are intended for specific purposes. Generally, table salt can be substituted for these salts.
- *Seasoned salt* is a blend of salt, herbs, and other seasoning ingredients. Examples include celery salt, onion salt, and garlic salt. The actual sodium content is lower than table salt because other ingredients dilute the concentration of sodium.
- *Salt substitutes* have some or all of the sodium replaced with another mineral, such as potassium or magnesium. They are also referred to as lite salt. They may have a bitter or metallic aftertaste.
- *Rock salt* is a nonedible salt of large crystals used to deice driveways and walkways. When combined with regular ice in home ice-cream makers, it helps freeze homemade ice cream more quickly by absorbing heat.

Figure 6.4 ▶

Food category sources of sodium in the U.S. population ages 2 years and older. *(Source: U.S. Department of Health and Human Services & U.S. Department of Agriculture. [2015]. 2015–2020 Dietary guidelines for Americans [8th ed.]. Available at http://health. govdietaryguidelines/2015. Accessed on 2/22/16.)*

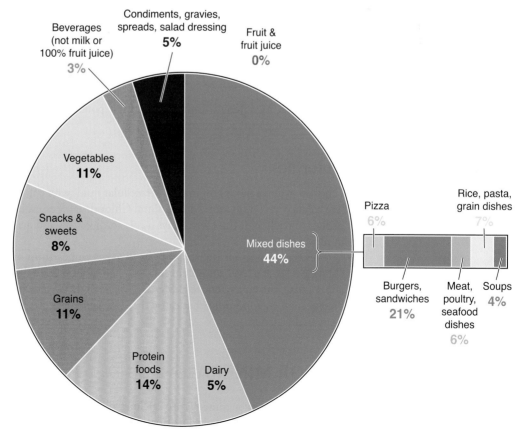

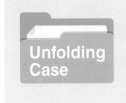

Mean sodium intake in the United States of males and females age 2 years and over exceeds recommended amounts (U.S. Department of Agriculture [USDA], Agricultural Research Service [ARS], 2014). In 2011 to 2012, mean intake of sodium among adult men and women age 20 years and older was 4218 and 2997 mg/day, respectively. These figures represent an increase over previous data reported in 2007 to 2008.

Quick Bite Average potassium content by food group

	mg K/serving
Grains (except bran or whole wheat)	35 mg/1 slice bread or ¾ cup most ready-to-eat cereals
Vegetables	0–350 mg/½ cup of most
Fruit	0–350 mg/½ cup or 1 small to medium piece fresh fruit
Milk	370 mg/cup
Meat (not including dried peas and beans)	100 mg/oz
Butter, margarine, oil	10 mg/tsp

Potassium

Most of the body's potassium is located in the cells as the major cation of the intracellular fluid. The remainder is in the extracellular fluid, where it works to maintain fluid balance, maintain acid–base balance, transmit nerve impulses, catalyze metabolic reactions, aid in carbohydrate metabolism and protein synthesis, and control skeletal muscle contractility.

Potassium is naturally present in most foods, such as fruits, vegetables, whole grains, meats, milk, and yogurt. Processed foods, such as cheeses, processed meats, breads, soups, fast foods, pastries, and sugary items, have a higher sodium-to-potassium ratio.

In healthy people with normal kidney function, a high intake of potassium does not lead to an elevated serum potassium concentration because the hormone aldosterone promotes urinary potassium excretion to keep serum levels within normal range. Therefore, an upper limit (UL) has not been set. However, when potassium excretion is impaired (e.g., secondary to diabetes, chronic kidney insufficiency, end-stage kidney disease, severe heart failure, or adrenal insufficiency), high potassium intakes can lead to hyperkalemia and life-threatening cardiac arrhythmias.

Chloride

Chloride is the major anion in the extracellular fluid, where it helps to maintain fluid and electrolyte balance in conjunction with sodium. Chloride is an essential component of hydrochloric acid in the stomach and, therefore, plays a role in digestion and acid–base balance. Its concentration in most cells is low.

Because almost all the chloride in the diet comes from salt (sodium chloride), the AI for chloride is set at a level equivalent (on a molar basis) to that of sodium. The AI for younger adults is 2.3 g/day, the equivalent to 3.8 g/day of salt or 1500 mg sodium. Sodium and chloride share dietary sources, conditions that cause them to become depleted in the body, and signs and symptoms of deficiency.

MAJOR MINERALS

The remaining major minerals are calcium, phosphorus, magnesium, and sulfur (summarized in Table 6.3); additional salient information appears in the following section.

Table 6.3 Summary of Major Minerals

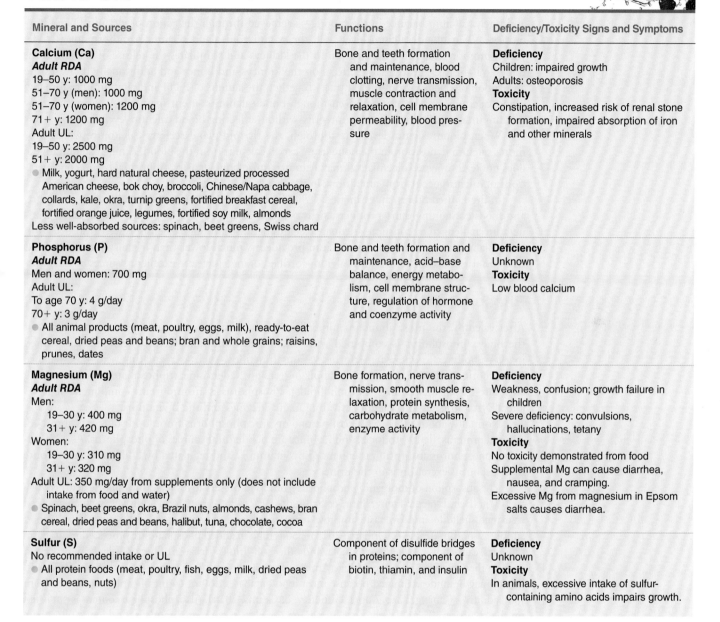

Mineral and Sources	Functions	Deficiency/Toxicity Signs and Symptoms
Calcium (Ca) *Adult RDA* 19–50 y: 1000 mg 51–70 y (men): 1000 mg 51–70 y (women): 1200 mg 71+ y: 1200 mg Adult UL: 19–50 y: 2500 mg 51+ y: 2000 mg ● Milk, yogurt, hard natural cheese, pasteurized processed American cheese, bok choy, broccoli, Chinese/Napa cabbage, collards, kale, okra, turnip greens, fortified breakfast cereal, fortified orange juice, legumes, fortified soy milk, almonds Less well-absorbed sources: spinach, beet greens, Swiss chard	Bone and teeth formation and maintenance, blood clotting, nerve transmission, muscle contraction and relaxation, cell membrane permeability, blood pressure	**Deficiency** Children: impaired growth Adults: osteoporosis **Toxicity** Constipation, increased risk of renal stone formation, impaired absorption of iron and other minerals
Phosphorus (P) *Adult RDA* Men and women: 700 mg Adult UL: To age 70 y: 4 g/day 70+ y: 3 g/day ● All animal products (meat, poultry, eggs, milk), ready-to-eat cereal, dried peas and beans; bran and whole grains; raisins, prunes, dates	Bone and teeth formation and maintenance, acid–base balance, energy metabolism, cell membrane structure, regulation of hormone and coenzyme activity	**Deficiency** Unknown **Toxicity** Low blood calcium
Magnesium (Mg) *Adult RDA* Men: 19–30 y: 400 mg 31+ y: 420 mg Women: 19–30 y: 310 mg 31+ y: 320 mg Adult UL: 350 mg/day from supplements only (does not include intake from food and water) ● Spinach, beet greens, okra, Brazil nuts, almonds, cashews, bran cereal, dried peas and beans, halibut, tuna, chocolate, cocoa	Bone formation, nerve transmission, smooth muscle relaxation, protein synthesis, carbohydrate metabolism, enzyme activity	**Deficiency** Weakness, confusion; growth failure in children Severe deficiency: convulsions, hallucinations, tetany **Toxicity** No toxicity demonstrated from food Supplemental Mg can cause diarrhea, nausea, and cramping. Excessive Mg from magnesium in Epsom salts causes diarrhea.
Sulfur (S) No recommended intake or UL ● All protein foods (meat, poultry, fish, eggs, milk, dried peas and beans, nuts)	Component of disulfide bridges in proteins; component of biotin, thiamin, and insulin	**Deficiency** Unknown **Toxicity** In animals, excessive intake of sulfur-containing amino acids impairs growth.

Calcium

Calcium is the most plentiful mineral in the body, making up about half of the body's total mineral content. Almost all of the body's calcium (99%) is found in bones and teeth, where it combines with phosphorus, magnesium, and other minerals to provide rigidity and structure. Bone tissue serves as a large, dynamic reservoir that releases calcium to maintain constant concentrations of calcium in blood, muscle, and intercellular fluids when dietary intake of calcium is inadequate. Continuous remodeling of bone occurs naturally throughout life as calcium is deposited and resorbed. The balance between bone formation and bone breakdown changes with aging. From birth through adolescence, bone formation exceeds bone breakdown. In young adults, the processes occur at approximately the same rate. Net bone loss occurs in all people after the age of about 30 years. Although an adequate calcium intake is needed to ensure bone mass is normally mineralized, an excess calcium does not lead to the creation of more bone; the amount of bone created is determined by the number and activity of osteoblasts (Reid, 2014). A dense bone mass offers protection against the inevitable net bone loss that occurs in all people after the age of about 35 years.

The remaining 1% of calcium in the body is found in plasma and other body fluids, where it has important roles in blood clotting, nerve transmission, muscle contraction and relaxation, cell membrane permeability, and the activation of certain enzymes. Calcium balance—or, more accurately, calcium balance in the blood—is achieved through the action of vitamin D and hormones. When blood calcium levels fall, the parathyroid gland secretes parathormone (PTH), which promotes calcium reabsorption in the kidneys and stimulates the release of calcium from bones. Vitamin D has the same effects on the kidneys and bones and additionally increases the absorption of calcium from the GI tract. Together, the actions of PTH and vitamin D restore low blood calcium levels to normal, even though bone calcium content may fall. A chronically low calcium intake compromises bone integrity without affecting blood calcium levels.

When blood calcium levels are too high, the thyroid gland secretes calcitonin, which promotes calcium deposition in the bone using excess calcium from the blood. A high calcium intake does not lead to hypercalcemia but may help maximize bone density. Abnormal blood concentrations of calcium occur from alterations in the secretion of PTH.

In the United States, an estimated 72% of calcium intake comes from milk, cheese, yogurt, and foods containing dairy products, such as pizza (IOM, 2011). People who avoid dairy products are challenged to consume adequate calcium because although calcium is well absorbed from some plants, the total amount of calcium provided is much lower than in dairy foods. Fortified ready-to-eat breakfast cereals and calcium-fortified orange juice are excellent sources of calcium.

Phosphorus

After calcium, the most abundant mineral in the body is phosphorus. Approximately 85% of the body's phosphorus is combined with calcium in bones and teeth. The rest is distributed in every body cell, where it performs various functions, such as regulating acid–base balance (phosphoric acid and its salts), metabolizing energy (adenosine triphosphate), and providing structure to cell membranes (phospholipids). Phosphorus is an important component of RNA and DNA and is responsible for activating many enzymes and the B vitamins.

Normally, about 40% to 60% of natural organic phosphorus from food sources is absorbed. Animal proteins, dairy products, and legumes are rich natural sources of phosphorus. As with calcium, phosphorus absorption is enhanced by vitamin D and regulated by PTH. The major route of phosphorus excretion is in the urine.

The absorption of inorganic phosphorus from food preservatives (e.g., phosphoric acid) is 90% to 100% (Bell, Draper, Tzeng, Shin, & Schmidt, 1977). Phosphate food additives—which are used to extend shelf life, improve taste, improve texture, or retain moisture—are as ubiquitous in the food supply as sodium (Calvo & Uribarri, 2013). Foods high in added phosphate are processed meat, ham, sausages, canned fish, baked goods, cola, and other soft drinks. Because of the prevalence of processed food in the American diet, the average American consumes far more phosphorus than the RDA and intake may be underestimated because most food databases do not count phosphorus derived from food additives (Chang, Lazo, Appel, Gutiérrez, & Grams, 2014). Also, phosphate content is not listed on the "Nutrition Facts" label so consumers are not able to compare brands to find lower phosphate choices. Some studies link a high phosphorous intake with increased mortality in healthy Americans (Chang et al., 2014). Additional studies are needed to determine whether the results are casual.

Magnesium

Magnesium is the fourth most abundant mineral in the body; approximately 50% of the body's magnesium content is deposited in bone with calcium and phosphorus and approximately 49% is stored in various soft tissues and muscles. Less than 1% of total magnesium is in in the blood, which is tightly regulated and not indicative of total body magnesium. The kidneys maintain magnesium balance by altering the amount excreted in the urine.

Magnesium is a cofactor for more than 300 enzymes in the body, including those involved in energy metabolism, protein synthesis, muscle and nerve function, blood glucose control, blood pressure regulation, and cell membrane transport. Studies find that supplemental magnesium lowers blood pressure but only to a small extent (Kass, Weekes, & Carpenter, 2012). Higher magnesium intakes have been linked with a lower risk of ischemic stroke (Larsson, Orsini, & Wolk, 2012) and may lower the risk of type 2 diabetes (Rodríguez-Morán, Simental, Zambrano,

& Guerrero-Romero, 2011). It has been reported that approximately 60% of Americans do not consume the recommended amount of magnesium (King, Mainous, Geesey, & Woolson, 2005), although consumption data do not include the magnesium content of water, which is significant in water classified as "hard." As much as 80% to 90% of the magnesium in food is lost in processing (de Baaij, Hoenderop, & Bindels, 2015). For instance, an average slice of white (refined) bread provides 7 mg of magnesium compared to 24 mg found in whole wheat bread.

A chronically low magnesium intake can lead to hypomagnesemia over time. Magnesium deficiency is more commonly the result of certain disorders that increase urinary excretion of magnesium, such as type 2 diabetes, or impair its absorption, such as celiac disease and small intestine bypass or resection. People who abuse alcohol are at risk of magnesium deficiency secondary to poor intake, altered absorption, and/or excess urinary excretion. Aging is associated with lower magnesium intake, decreased absorption, and increased excretion. Certain medications, such as thiazide diuretics, proton pump inhibitors, and some antibiotics, can lead to magnesium depletion (de Baaij et al., 2015).

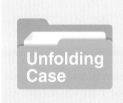

Recall Myra. Her fluid and electrolyte status was the immediate priority. However, general malabsorption of nutrients also occurred due to the diarrheal effect of the aloe. What would you tell Myra about what she should eat and how much fluid she should consume? What strategies may help her drink enough fluid given that she doesn't experience thirst?

Sulfur

Sulfur does not function independently as a nutrient, but it is a component of biotin, thiamin, and the amino acids methionine and cysteine. The proteins in skin, hair, and nails are made more rigid by the presence of sulfur.

There is neither an RDA nor an AI for sulfur, and no deficiency symptoms are known. Although food and various sources of drinking water provide significant amounts of sulfur, the major source of inorganic sulfate for humans is body protein turnover of methionine and cysteine. The need for sulfur is met when the intake of sulfur amino acids is adequate. A sulfur deficiency is likely only when protein deficiency is severe.

TRACE MINERALS

Although the presence of minerals in the body is small, their impact on health is significant. Each trace mineral has its own range over which the body can maintain homeostasis (Fig. 6.5). People who consume an adequate diet derive no further benefit from supplementing their intake with minerals and may induce a deficiency by upsetting the delicate balance that exists between minerals. Even though too little of a trace mineral can be just as deadly as too much, routine supplementation is not recommended. Factors that complicate the study of trace minerals are as follows:

- The high variability of trace mineral content of foods. The mineral content of the soil from which a food originates largely influences trace mineral content. For instance, grains, vegetables, and meat raised in South Dakota, Wyoming, New Mexico, and Utah are high in selenium, whereas foods grown in the southern states and from both coasts of the United States have much less selenium. Other factors that influence a food's trace mineral content are the quality of the water supply and food processing. Because of these factors, the trace mineral content listed in food composition tables may not represent the actual amount in a given sample.
- Food composition data are not available for all trace minerals. Food composition tables generally include data on the content of iron, zinc, manganese, selenium, and copper, but data on other trace minerals, such as iodine, chromium, and molybdenum, are not readily available.

Figure 6.5 ▶
Figure 6.5 ▶

Health effects seen over a range of trace mineral intakes.

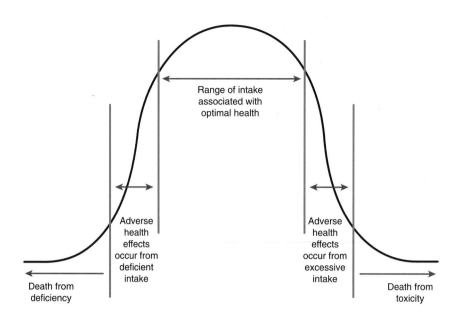

Bioavailability varies within the context of the total diet. Even when trace element intake can be estimated, the amount available to the body may be significantly less because the absorption and metabolism of individual trace elements is strongly influenced by mineral interactions and other dietary factors. An excess of one trace mineral may induce a deficiency of another. For instance, a high intake of zinc impairs copper absorption. Conversely, a deficiency of one trace mineral may potentiate toxic effects of another, as when iron deficiency increases vulnerability to lead poisoning.

Reliable and valid indicators of trace element status (e.g., measured serum levels, results of balance studies, enzyme activity determinations) are not available for all trace minerals, so assessment of trace element status is not always possible.

Table 6.4 summarizes the sources, functions, recommended intakes, and signs and symptoms of deficiency and toxicity of trace minerals that have either an RDA or AI. Additional salient features are presented in the following sections.

Iron

Approximately two-thirds of the body's 3 to 5 g of iron is contained in the heme portion of hemoglobin. Iron is also found in transferrin, the transport carrier of iron, and in enzyme systems that are active in energy metabolism. Ferritin, the storage form of iron, is located in the liver, bone marrow, and spleen.

Iron in foods exists in two forms: heme iron, found in meat, fish, and poultry, and nonheme iron, found in plants such as grains, vegetables, legumes, and nuts. The majority of iron in the diet is nonheme iron.

There is no mechanism for iron excretion so the body maintains iron balance by altering the rate of absorption. Normally, the overall rate of iron absorption in a mixed eating pattern containing both heme and nonheme iron is only 14% to 18% of total intake (Hurrell & Egli, 2010). In times of need, such as during growth, pregnancy, or iron deficiency, iron is absorbed more efficiently to boost the overall absorption rate to as high as 50%.

The bioavailability of heme and nonheme iron differs greatly. Heme iron has higher bioavailability than nonheme iron and is less affected by other dietary components. In contrast, nonheme iron absorption is impacted by numerous dietary factors. Nonheme iron absorption is enhanced when it is consumed with heme iron or vitamin C–rich foods, such as orange juice or tomatoes. Nonheme iron absorption is impaired when it is consumed at the same time as coffee, calcium, phytates (found in legumes and grains), or oxalates (found in spinach, chard). Tea is a potent inhibitor that can reduce nonheme iron absorption in a meal by 60%. However, within the context of a varied, mixed eating pattern, nonheme iron enhancers and inhibitors have very little impact on most people's iron status (National Institutes of Health [NIH], Office of Dietary Supplements [ODS], 2015). Based on

Table 6.4 Summary of Trace Minerals

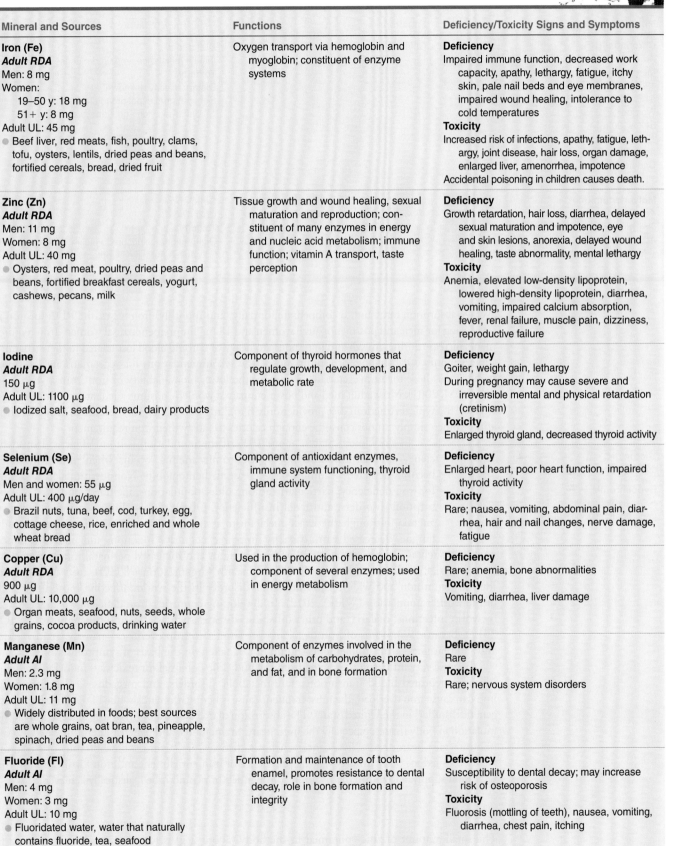

Mineral and Sources	Functions	Deficiency/Toxicity Signs and Symptoms

Iron (Fe)
Adult RDA
Men: 8 mg
Women:
   19–50 y: 18 mg
   51+ y: 8 mg
Adult UL: 45 mg
● Beef liver, red meats, fish, poultry, clams, tofu, oysters, lentils, dried peas and beans, fortified cereals, bread, dried fruit
	Oxygen transport via hemoglobin and myoglobin; constituent of enzyme systems	**Deficiency**
		Impaired immune function, decreased work capacity, apathy, lethargy, fatigue, itchy skin, pale nail beds and eye membranes, impaired wound healing, intolerance to cold temperatures
		Toxicity
		Increased risk of infections, apathy, fatigue, lethargy, joint disease, hair loss, organ damage, enlarged liver, amenorrhea, impotence
		Accidental poisoning in children causes death.

Zinc (Zn) ***Adult RDA*** Men: 11 mg Women: 8 mg Adult UL: 40 mg ● Oysters, red meat, poultry, dried peas and beans, fortified breakfast cereals, yogurt, cashews, pecans, milk	Tissue growth and wound healing, sexual maturation and reproduction; constituent of many enzymes in energy and nucleic acid metabolism; immune function; vitamin A transport, taste perception	**Deficiency** Growth retardation, hair loss, diarrhea, delayed sexual maturation and impotence, eye and skin lesions, anorexia, delayed wound healing, taste abnormality, mental lethargy **Toxicity** Anemia, elevated low-density lipoprotein, lowered high-density lipoprotein, diarrhea, vomiting, impaired calcium absorption, fever, renal failure, muscle pain, dizziness, reproductive failure
Iodine ***Adult RDA*** 150 μg Adult UL: 1100 μg ● Iodized salt, seafood, bread, dairy products	Component of thyroid hormones that regulate growth, development, and metabolic rate	**Deficiency** Goiter, weight gain, lethargy During pregnancy may cause severe and irreversible mental and physical retardation (cretinism) **Toxicity** Enlarged thyroid gland, decreased thyroid activity
Selenium (Se) ***Adult RDA*** Men and women: 55 μg Adult UL: 400 μg/day ● Brazil nuts, tuna, beef, cod, turkey, egg, cottage cheese, rice, enriched and whole wheat bread	Component of antioxidant enzymes, immune system functioning, thyroid gland activity	**Deficiency** Enlarged heart, poor heart function, impaired thyroid activity **Toxicity** Rare; nausea, vomiting, abdominal pain, diarrhea, hair and nail changes, nerve damage, fatigue
Copper (Cu) ***Adult RDA*** 900 μg Adult UL: 10,000 μg ● Organ meats, seafood, nuts, seeds, whole grains, cocoa products, drinking water	Used in the production of hemoglobin; component of several enzymes; used in energy metabolism	**Deficiency** Rare; anemia, bone abnormalities **Toxicity** Vomiting, diarrhea, liver damage
Manganese (Mn) ***Adult AI*** Men: 2.3 mg Women: 1.8 mg Adult UL: 11 mg ● Widely distributed in foods; best sources are whole grains, oat bran, tea, pineapple, spinach, dried peas and beans	Component of enzymes involved in the metabolism of carbohydrates, protein, and fat, and in bone formation	**Deficiency** Rare **Toxicity** Rare; nervous system disorders
Fluoride (Fl) ***Adult AI*** Men: 4 mg Women: 3 mg Adult UL: 10 mg ● Fluoridated water, water that naturally contains fluoride, tea, seafood	Formation and maintenance of tooth enamel, promotes resistance to dental decay, role in bone formation and integrity	**Deficiency** Susceptibility to dental decay; may increase risk of osteoporosis **Toxicity** Fluorosis (mottling of teeth), nausea, vomiting, diarrhea, chest pain, itching

(continued)

Table 6.4   Summary of Trace Minerals (continued)

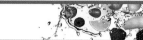

Mineral and Sources	Functions	Deficiency/Toxicity Signs and Symptoms
Chromium (Cr) *Adult AI* Men: 19–50 y: 35 μg 51+ y: 30 μg Women: 51+ y: 30 μg 19–50 y: 25 μg Adult UL: Undetermined • Broccoli, grape juice, whole grains, red wine	Cofactor for insulin	**Deficiency** Insulin resistance, impaired glucose tolerance **Toxicity** Dietary toxicity unknown Occupational exposure to chromium dust damages skin and kidneys.
Molybdenum (Mo) *Adult RDA* 45 μg Adult UL: 2000 μg • Milk, legumes, bread, grains	Component of many enzymes; works with riboflavin to incorporate iron into hemoglobin	**Deficiency** Unknown **Toxicity** Occupational exposure to molybdenum dust causes gout-like symptoms.

average absorption rates and to compensate for daily (and monthly) iron losses, the RDA for iron is set at 8 mg for men and postmenopausal women and 18 mg for premenopausal women. Iron requirements increase during growth and in response to heavy or chronic blood loss related to menstruation, surgery, injury, GI bleeding, or aspirin abuse. Iron recommendations for vegetarians are 1.8 times higher than those for nonvegetarians because of the lower bioavailability of iron from a vegetarian diet (IOM, 2001). Most adult men and postmenopausal women consume adequate amounts of iron. Because the typical American diet provides only 6 to 7 mg of iron per 1000 calories, many menstruating women simply do not consume enough calories to satisfy their iron requirement.

Microcytic
small blood cells.

Hypochromic
pale red blood cells related to the decrease in hemoglobin pigment.

In the United States, about 10% of the population is iron deficient. Iron deficiency anemia, a **microcytic**, **hypochromic** anemia, occurs when total iron stores become depleted, leading to a decrease in hemoglobin. Nonnutritional risk factors for iron deficiency, particularly among older populations, include blood loss, malabsorption disorders, and renal insufficiency. Obesity is also linked to iron deficiency anemia, although the exact mechanism is unclear. Clinical manifestations include fatigue, decreased work capacity, impaired cognitive function, and poor pregnancy outcome, such as premature delivery, low birth weight, and increased perinatal infant mortality, and maternal death. According to the World Health Organization (WHO), iron deficiency is the most common and widespread nutritional disorder in the world, affecting more than 30% of the world's population (WHO, 2012). In developing countries, iron deficiency is exacerbated by worm infections, malaria, and other infectious diseases such as HIV and tuberculosis (WHO, 2012). Because symptoms of iron deficiency are similar to iron overload—namely, apathy, lethargy, and fatigue—iron supplements should not be taken on the basis of symptoms alone.

Because very little iron is excreted from the body, the potential for toxicity is moderate to high. Although repeated blood transfusions, rare metabolic disorders, and megadoses of supplemental iron can cause iron overload, the most frequent cause is hemochromatosis, one of the most common genetic disorders in the United States. The absorption of excessive amounts of iron leads to iron accumulation in body tissues, especially the liver, heart, brain, joints, and pancreas. Left untreated, excess iron can cause heart disease, liver cancer, cirrhosis, diabetes, and arthritis. Phlebotomies or chelation are used to reduce body iron. Given the prevalence of iron enrichment and iron fortification in the U.S. food supply, a low-iron diet is not recommended nor could it be realistically achieved.

Zinc

The small amount of zinc contained in the body (about 2 g) is found in almost all cells and is especially concentrated in the eyes, bones, muscles, and prostate gland. Zinc in tissues is not available to maintain serum levels when intake is inadequate, so an adequate daily intake is necessary.

Zinc is a component of DNA and RNA and is part of more than 100 enzymes involved in protein synthesis, cell division, growth, metabolism, sexual maturation and reproduction, and the senses of taste and smell. Zinc plays important roles in immune system functioning and wound healing. Mean intake among American adults exceeds the RDA for zinc.

There is no single laboratory test that adequately measures zinc status, so zinc deficiency is not readily diagnosed. Risk factors for zinc deficiency include poor calorie intake, alcoholism, and malabsorption syndromes such as celiac disease, Crohn disease, and short bowel syndrome. Vegetarians are also at increased risk because zinc is only half as well absorbed from plants as it is from animal sources. Although overt zinc deficiency is not common in the United States, the effects of marginal intakes are poorly understood.

Iodine

Iodine is found in the muscles, the thyroid gland, the skin, the skeleton, endocrine tissues, and the bloodstream. It is an essential component of thyroxine (T_4) and triiodothyronine (T_3), the thyroid hormones responsible for regulating metabolic rate, body temperature, reproduction, growth, the synthesis of blood cells, and nerve and muscle function. It may also play a role in immune response and may have a beneficial impact on mammary dysplasia (IOM, 2001).

Most foods are naturally low in iodine. The iodine content of vegetables and grains varies with the soil content. Iodine-deficient soil around the Great Lakes was known as a "goiter belt" region in the United States. Processed foods almost always contain salt that is not iodized (NIH, ODS, 2011). Milk is naturally low in iodine but has become an important source of iodine because of the use of iodine feed supplements and iodine-containing disinfectants used to sanitize udders, milking machines, and milk tanks. However, iodine intake from dairy products may be decreasing as chlorine-based disinfectants replace iodine-containing disinfectants (Zimmermann & Boelaert, 2015). Some breads provide iodine due to the use of iodate dough conditioners. Seafood and seaweed (e.g., kelp, nori, and kombu) are a natural sources of iodine due to iodine in seawater. The United States has generally been considered iodine sufficient since table salt began to be voluntarily iodized in 1924 (Perrine, Herrick, Serdula, & Sullivan, 2010).

Although intake appears to be adequate in the United States, surveys suggest many pregnant women in both developed and developing countries have inadequate iodine intakes (Caldwell et al., 2013). At any age, the earliest clinical sign of iodine deficiency is goiter; hypothyroidism develops in severe deficiencies. Iodine deficiency during pregnancy may cause fetal neurodevelopmental deficits and growth retardation and increases infant mortality (Zimmermann, Jooste, & Panday, 2008). Cretinism, characterized by a lack of physical and mental development, can develop in the neonate born to a mother who was iodine deficient during pregnancy. Adults with iodine deficiency may have impaired mental function, reduced work productivity, and hyperthyroidism (Zimmermann & Boelaert, 2015).

Although an estimated 70% of the world's population has access to iodized salt (United Nations Children's Fund [UNICEF], 2011), an estimated 1.88 billion people still have insufficient iodine intakes (Anderson, Karumbunathan, & Zimmermann, 2012). Iodine deficiency is a major health problem because it is the most common cause of preventable mental retardation worldwide (De Benoist, McLean, Andersson, & Rogers, 2008). The effect of **goitrogens** on iodine balance is clinically insignificant except when iodine deficiency exists.

Selenium

Selenium is a component of a group of enzymes, called glutathione peroxidases, that function as antioxidants to disarm free radicals produced during normal oxygen metabolism. Selenium, as a part of more than two dozen selenoproteins, plays a role in thyroid hormone metabolism, DNA synthesis, and reproduction (Sunde, 2012). Because of selenium's antioxidant activity, researchers are studying whether it plays a role in reducing the risk of certain cancers, cardiovascular disease (CVD), and cognitive decline (NIH, ODS, 2013).

Although areas of the country with selenium-poor soil produce selenium-poor foods, mass transportation mitigates the effect on total selenium intake (IOM, 2000). Brazil nuts and seafood are the richest sources; bread, grains, meat, poultry, fish, and eggs are major sources in the typical American diet. Most Americans consume more than the RDA of selenium.

*Concept
Mastery Alert*

Few foods naturally provide iodine. Nurses should be aware that iodized salt has iodine added to it. The iodine is not naturally occurring. Seafood has naturally occurring iodine due to the iodine in sea water.

Goitrogens
thyroid antagonists found in cruciferous vegetables (e.g., cabbage, cauliflower, broccoli), soybeans, and sweet potatoes.

Selenium deficiency is rare in the United States. It is most likely to occur in people undergoing hemodialysis due to removal of selenium from the blood and poor selenium intake. People with HIV may be at risk due to diarrhea and malabsorption. Worldwide, selenium deficiency occurs in areas where the soil is selenium deficient, such as in certain areas of China (Sunde, 2012).

Copper

Copper is distributed in muscles, liver, brain, bones, kidneys, and blood. Copper is a component of several enzymes involved in hemoglobin synthesis, collagen formation, wound healing, and maintenance of nerve fibers. Copper also helps cells to use iron and plays a role in energy metabolism.

Americans typically consume adequate amounts of copper. Excess zinc intake has the potential to induce copper deficiency by impairing its absorption, but copper deficiency is rare. Supplements, not food, may cause copper toxicity, as do some genetic disorders, such as Wilson disease.

Manganese

Mean manganese intake among American adults is well above the AI, and dietary deficiencies have not been noted. Manganese toxicity is a well-known occupational hazard for miners who inhale manganese dust over a prolonged period of time, leading to central nervous system abnormalities with symptoms similar to those of Parkinson disease. There is some evidence to suggest that high manganese intake from drinking water, which may be more bioavailable than manganese from food, also produces neuromotor deficits similar to Parkinson disease.

Fluoride

Cariogenic
cavity promoting.

Fluoride promotes the mineralization of developing tooth enamel prior to tooth eruption and the remineralization of surface enamel in erupted teeth. It concentrates in plaque and saliva to inhibit the process by which **cariogenic** bacteria metabolize carbohydrates to produce acids that cause tooth decay. Fluoridation of municipal water is credited with a major decline in the prevalence and severity of dental caries in the U.S. population and is deemed one of the 10 great public health achievements of the 20th century (Centers for Disease Control and Prevention [CDC], 2013).

Fluoridation of municipal water is endorsed by the National Institute of Dental Health, the Academy of Nutrition and Dietetics, the American Medical Association, the National Cancer Institute, and the CDC. According to the CDC (2015), in 2012, 74.6% of Americans served by public water supplies had access to optimally fluoridated water to prevent tooth decay. Studies show that water fluoridation reduces tooth decay by approximately 25% over a person's lifetime (CDC, 2015). Children under the age of 8 years are susceptible to mottled tooth enamel if they ingest several times more fluoride than the recommended amount during the time of tooth enamel formation. The swallowing of fluoridated toothpaste is to blame.

Chromium

Chromium enhances the action of the hormone insulin to help regulate blood glucose levels. However, the American Diabetes Association states that there is insufficient evidence to support the use of chromium to improve glucose control in people with diabetes (Evert et al., 2013). Chromium also appears to be directly involved in the metabolism of carbohydrates, protein, and fat, but more research is needed to clarify its roles.

Even though chromium is widespread in foods, many foods provide less than 1 to 2 µg per serving. Because existing databases lack information on chromium, few food intake studies utilizing few laboratories are available to estimate usual intake. However, it appears that average intake is adequate. Unrefined foods are higher in chromium than processed foods.

Molybdenum

Molybdenum plays a role in red blood cell synthesis and is a component of several enzymes. Average American intake falls within the recommended range. Dietary deficiencies and toxicities are unknown.

Other Trace Elements

Although definitive evidence is lacking, future research may reveal that other trace elements are essential for human nutrition. However, evidence is difficult to obtain, and quantifying human need is even more formidable. In addition, as with all trace minerals, the potential for toxicity exists. Consider the following:

- Nickel, silicon, vanadium, and boron have been demonstrated to have beneficial health effects in some animals and may someday be classified as essential for humans.
- Cobalt is an essential component of vitamin B_{12}, but it is not an essential nutrient and does not have an RDA.
- It is possible that minute amounts of cadmium, lithium, tin, and even arsenic are also essential to human life.

WATER AND MINERALS IN HEALTH PROMOTION

Concerns regarding water and minerals in health promotion include making healthy beverage choices, reducing sodium intake, and consuming adequate amounts of the shortfall minerals of public health concern, namely calcium and potassium.

Choose Healthy Beverages

The *2015-2020 Dietary Guidelines for Americans* does not address water per se but recommends a shift to healthier beverage choices (U.S. Department of Health and Human Services [USDHHS] & U.S. Department of Agriculture [USDA], 2015). Beverages are often overlooked when people consider their food intake, but they are an important part of eating patterns. Beverages contribute to total water intake and account for almost 20% of total calorie intake in most eating patterns (USDHHS & USDA, 2015). Some beverages provide nutrients such as protein, vitamins, minerals, and phytonutrients; others are considered empty calories because they provide calories with few or no nutrients. When choosing beverages, the Dietary Guidelines suggest the following:

- Primary beverage selections should be either calorie-free, such as water, or provide beneficial nutrients, such a nonfat or low fat milk and 100% juice.
- Milk and juice should be consumed within the recommended amounts for the appropriate calorie level eating pattern.
- Sugar-sweetened beverages, if consumed, should be limited to amounts within overall calorie limits and limits for calories from added sugar.
- Limiting consumption of alcohol to a moderate intake or less. Moderate is defined as up to one drink per day for women and up to two drinks per day for men and only by adults of legal drinking age.
- Moderate coffee consumption (three to five 8-oz cups per day) can be part of a healthy eating pattern. In healthy adults, moderate coffee intake is not associated with an increased risk of major chronic diseases (e.g., cancer) or premature death, especially from CVD (USDHHS & USDA, 2015).
- If coffee, tea, and flavored waters are consumed, calories from cream or added sugar should fit within total calorie and added sugar limits.

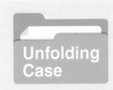

Unfolding Case

Consider Myra. Which fluids should she be encouraged to use to satisfy her fluid recommendation? Would more than 8 glass of fluid a day be excessive?

Lower Sodium Intake

Since its inception in 1980, every edition of the *Dietary Guidelines for Americans* has urged Americans to lower their sodium intake to prevent and treat hypertension, CVD, and stroke. The *2015-2020 Dietary Guidelines for Americans* quantifies the limit to 2300 mg/day for everyone 14 years and older and that people with hypertension or prehypertension limit their intake to no more than 1500 mg/day. Despite the long-standing advice to eat less sodium, intake continues to increase among all Americans age 2 years and older and exceeds the UL, making it a nutrient of public health concern (Dietary Guidelines Advisory Committee, 2015). Processed foods are the major contributor to sodium intake. Tips for reducing sodium intake appear in Box 6.4.

Scientific consensus is that average sodium intake is too high and should be lowered (USDHHS & USDA, 2015). However, intake recommendations for the general population vary. The current AI set for sodium in 2005 is 1200 to 1500 mg/day for adults and a UL of 2300 mg based on evidence showing a relationship between increased sodium intake and increased blood pressure in adults (IOM, 2005). After an updated review of evidence, the IOM issued a report in 2013 that concluded there is a positive relationship between high sodium intake and cardiovascular risks. The report also stated that there is insufficient evidence to conclude that lowering sodium to less than 2300 mg/day alters the risk of heart disease, stroke, or all-cause mortality in the general population and that evidence does not support recommendations to lower sodium intake to or below 1500 mg/day in people with diabetes, kidney disease, or heart disease. Some evidence suggests risk of adverse health outcomes is associated with sodium intake of 1500 mg/day to 2300 mg/day in these subgroups. More studies are needed to determine whether sodium intakes of 1500 to 2300 mg/day are beneficial for the general population and specific subgroups.

In June 2016, the U.S. Food and Drug Administration (FDA)-issued voluntary sodium reduction targets food manufacturers, restaurants, and food service operations (FDA, 2016). The short-term

BOX 6.4   Tips for Lowering Sodium Intake

- Know what labeling terms mean:
  - Sodium-free has less than 5 mg sodium per serving.
  - Very low sodium has less than 35 mg per serving.
  - Low sodium has 140 mg per serving.
  - Reduced or less sodium has at least 25% less sodium per serving than the traditional food.
  - Light in sodium has 50% less sodium than the traditional food.
  - Salt free has less than 5 mg of salt.
  - Unsalted or no added salt means no salt was added during processing, although the food itself may contain natural sodium.
- Avoid or limit convenience foods, such as boxed mixes, frozen dinners, and canned foods.
- Eat home-cooked meals more often.
- Eat more fresh or frozen vegetables.
- Compare labels to choose brands or varieties with the lowest amount of sodium.
- Use fresh veggies in place of pickles.
- Substitute low-sodium tuna and roasted chicken for deli meats.
- Replace sausages and hot dogs with fresh meats, such as rotisserie chicken.
- Use cheese sparingly.
- Choose nut butters with no sodium added.
- Cook rice and pasta without salt.
- Switch to pasta sauce without added salt or combine equal parts of no-salt-added tomato sauce with bottled pasta sauce.
- Choose cereals with no added salt, such as shredded wheat, puffed whole-grain cereal, and unsalted oatmeal.
- Use lower salt condiments, such as salt-free ketchup or Worcestershire sauce, vinegar, and low-sodium mayonnaise.
- Substitute homemade vinegar and oil dressing for bottled varieties.
- If you use canned vegetables, drain away liquid and rinse thoroughly.
- Limit salty snacks.
- Instead of salt, season food with spices, herbs, lemon, vinegar, or salt-free seasonings.

goal is to reduce the current average adult sodium intake of 3400 to 3000 mg/day within 2 years. The 10-year sodium reduction target is a further lowering to 2300 mg/day. The targets cover almost 150 food categories and are intended to complement existing efforts by the food industry to reduce sodium in foods.

Although lowering sodium is unarguably beneficial for people with hypertension, the benefit—or risk—of lowering intake for the general population is hotly debated and not likely to be resolved soon (Bayer, Johns, & Galea, 2012). Prospective cohort studies have shown inconsistent associations between sodium intake and rates of cardiovascular events and death in the general population (Aburto et al., 2013; Graudal, Jürgens, Baslund, & Alderman, 2014). In contrast, Cook, Appel, and Whelton (2014) suggested that paradoxical findings on the adverse effects of consuming less than 2300 mg/day of sodium may be due to suboptimal measurement of sodium and potential biases. They conclude that results of the Trials of Hypertension Prevention (TOHP) trial support the benefits of reducing sodium to 1500 to 2300 mg/day for the majority of the population. Similarly, many expert advisory groups conclude that evidence supports the public health value of reducing sodium intake in the general population (FDA, 2016). Because an ideal sodium intake assessment tool is unknown, the sodium controversy is not likely to end soon (Wolfram, 2016).

Shortfall Minerals

Because Americans on average have low intakes of vegetables, fruits, and dairy, certain minerals are consumed in less than recommended amounts, namely, potassium, magnesium, and calcium. Iron is also under consumed by adolescent girls and women ages 19 to 50 years old (USDHHS & USDA, 2015). Figure 6.6 illustrates mean intake of these nutrients expressed

Figure 6.6 ▶

Mean intake of shortfall minerals as a percentage of the dietary reference intakes in adult men and women aged 20 and older. *(Source: U.S. Department of Agriculture & Agricultural Research Service. [2014]. Nutrition intakes from food: Mean amounts consumed per individual, by gender and age. What We Eat in America, NHANES 2011-2012. Available at www.ars.usda.gov/bc/bhnrcfsrg. Accessed on 1/22/16.)*

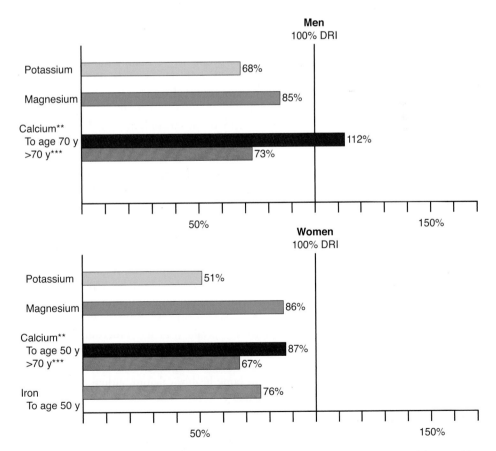

* Daily Reference Intakes are Recommended Dietary Allowances for magnesium, calcium, and iron, and an Adequate Intake for potassium.

** RDA increases in men >70 and women >50.

*** Based on mean intake specific to age 70+ older.

as a percentage of the DRIs. Calcium and potassium are of particular public health concern because shortages of these minerals are associated with adverse health effects. Eating a variety of nutrient-dense items within each group is advocated to help ensure nutritional adequacy.

- Eat the recommended amounts of fruits, vegetables, and dairy. This will provide adequate calcium and boost potassium and magnesium intakes.
- To ensure adequate potassium, not only should the amount of fruit, vegetables, and dairy intake be adequate, choices within those groups should also include foods that are high in potassium, such as baked potato with the skin, prune juice, sweet potato baked in the skin, salmon, orange juice, yogurt, legumes, banana, and tomato products.
- Shift to more whole grains in place of refined grains. Whole grains, particularly the bran, provide more magnesium and trace minerals than refined grains.
- Women and adolescent girls should consume heme iron found in lean meats, poultry, and seafood because it is more readily absorbed by the body. Absorption of nonheme sources of iron, such as fortified cereals, legumes, and dark green vegetables, is enhanced when consumed at the same time as a source of vitamin C such as tomatoes or orange juice.

Calcium

Lifestyle choices, including nutrition and exercise, influence 20% to 40% of adult peak bone mass (Weaver et al., 2016). Consuming adequate amounts of calcium, vitamin D, and phosphorus are critical for optimum bone health. Entering adulthood with peak bone mass and strength may help reduce the risk of osteoporosis or low bone mass later in life.

Low bone mineral density and osteoporosis are common in the United States, especially in older adults (Dietary Guidelines Advisory Committee, 2015). Studies suggest as many as 50% of women and up to 25% of men over the age of 50 years will break a bone due to osteoporosis (National Osteoporosis Foundation, n.d.). Fractures are a major cause of morbidity and mortality in the elderly: 20% of people who sustain a hip fracture die within the first year, and 60% who survive a hip fracture still need assistance to walk 1 year later (National Osteoporosis Foundation, n.d.). An inadequate intake of calcium has long been regarded as one of the modifiable risk factors for osteoporosis; however, some studies show little evidence of a relationship between calcium intake and bone density or the rate of bone loss (Reid, Bristow, & Bolland, 2015). The estimated low levels of calcium intake in various age and gender groups place many Americans at risk for suboptimal bone health.

Experts recommend calcium requirements be met from food sources. Calcium recommendations are 1000 mg/day for men 50 to 70 years old and 1200 mg/day for women 51 years and older and men 71 years and older. Supplemental calcium is recommended only if an adequate dietary intake cannot be achieved (Cosman et al., 2014). There is no evidence that consuming amounts of calcium higher than the recommendation enhances bone strength; both too little and too much calcium may have adverse health effects.

Generally, three daily servings of milk, yogurt, or cheese plus nondairy sources of calcium are needed to ensure an adequate calcium intake. Milk is a "nearly perfect" source because it contains vitamin D and lactose, which promote calcium absorption. People who are lactose intolerant can obtain calcium from lactose-reduced milk, acidophilus milk, lactose-free yogurt; hard cheeses; and low-oxalate green vegetables, such as broccoli, bok choy, collard greens, and kale. Significant amounts of calcium can be found in calcium-fortified foods, such as fruit juices, tomato juice, and ready-to-eat breakfast cereals.

In addition to bone health, calcium, either alone or with vitamin D, may impact chronic disease risk, particularly

- *Colorectal cancer.* Considerable evidence exists that milk intake may reduce the risk of colorectal cancer (Aune et al., 2012). A meta-analysis of prospective observational studies found that a high intake of calcium from either dietary or supplemental calcium is associated with a decrease risk of colorectal cancer and the benefit may continue even beyond an intake of 1000 mg/day (Keum, Aune, Greenwood, Ju, &

Giovannucci, 2014). Longer duration randomized controlled trials are needed to confirm the benefit of calcium. It is important to note that the efficacy of calcium in lowering the risk of colorectal cancer is dependent on adequate vitamin D status (Peterlik, Kállay, & Cross, 2013).

- *Prostate cancer.* High dietary intake of calcium has been identified as a probable cause of prostate cancer, although the underlying mechanism is unclear (Rowland, Schwartz, John, & Ingles, 2012). A systematic review and meta-analysis of cohort studies found that high intakes of dairy products, but not supplemental or nondairy calcium, may increase total prostate cancer risk, suggesting that other components in dairy products rather than calcium, raise prostate cancer risk (Aune et al., 2015). Additional studies are needed.
- *Weight loss.* Some studies suggest calcium may promote weight loss, perhaps by stimulating fat break down or by impairing fat absorption from the GI tract. However, a meta-analysis of randomized controlled trials showed that increasing calcium intake from supplements or dairy foods is not an effective weight loss strategy in adults, although three servings of dairy may promote fat loss on weight loss diets in the short term (Booth, Huggins, Wattanapenpailboon, & Nowson, 2015).

Calcium Supplements

Calcium supplements have long been prescribed to prevent or treat osteoporosis, particularly in postmenopausal women; however, a number of studies have found that calcium supplement use, with or without vitamin D, may increase the risk of cardiovascular events (Bolland et al., 2008; Bolland, Grey, Avenell, Gamble, & Reid, 2011; Reid et al., 2015). Most experts agree that calcium be obtained from food instead of supplements (Reid, 2014). Dietary calcium has not been linked to the adverse effects of supplements probably because the concentration of calcium from food is much less and it is more slowly absorbed from the GI tract due to the presence of protein and fat in food. Furthermore, some studies found that calcium supplements produce only a small, initial, and nonprogressive increase in bone density that is unlikely to result in a clinically significant decrease in fracture risk (Tai, Leung, Grey, Reid, & Bolland, 2015).

Potassium

The AI for potassium is set at a level believed necessary to maintain lower blood pressure levels, lessen the adverse effects of high sodium intake on blood pressure, reduce the risk of kidney stones, and possibly reduce bone loss. Indeed, moderate potassium deficiency, which typically occurs without hypokalemia, is characterized by increased blood pressure, increased salt sensitivity, increased risk of kidney stones, and increased bone turnover (IOM, 2005). Most American adults consume only half to two-thirds of the recommended potassium intake (USDA, ARS, 2014).

Although potassium plays a role in blood pressure, the exact mechanism is not well understood. A meta-analysis of randomized controlled and cohort studies showed that an increased potassium intake lowers systolic pressure in people with hypertension but not in normotensive people (Aburto et al., 2013). Evidence suggests that altered sodium and potassium balance may play a key role in hypertension (Zhang et al., 2013) and that when people have an increased intake of potassium, a high sodium intake is not associated with higher blood pressure (Rodrigues et al., 2014).

Although there is not enough evidence to support dietary potassium specifically to lower blood pressure, dietary patterns shown to lower high blood pressure, namely, the Dietary Approaches to Stop Hypertension (DASH) diet, provide ample potassium (Appel et al., 1997). The DASH diet is rich in fruits, vegetables, low-fat dairy products, and whole grains; moderate in poultry, fish, and nuts; and low in fat, red meat, and added sugar. Its blood pressure–lowering effect likely comes from a combination of factors, including its high content of potassium, calcium, and magnesium.

How Do You Respond?

Do zinc lozenges cure the common cold? Systematic review and meta-analysis of randomized, placebo-controlled trials show that oral zinc taken within 24 hours of the onset of common cold symptoms significantly reduces both the duration and severity of symptoms (Science, Johnstone, Roth, Guyatt, & Loeb, 2012; Singh & Das, 2011). Side effects were common, with bad taste and nausea reported most frequently. Prolonged high serum levels of zinc can suppress copper and iron absorption; long-term effects of zinc used prophylactically are not known. In 2009, the FDA advised consumers to stop using specific zinc-containing intranasal products based on numerous reports linking their use to a loss of the sense of smell, which in some cases has been long-lasting or permanent. A general recommendation for using zinc to treat a cold cannot be made until more research is conducted to identify the optimal dosage, formulation, and duration of treatment.

Does chlorine in drinking water cause cancer? When organic matter is present in water, chlorine reacts with it to form a by-product called trihalomethane (THM). If THM forms, it is in such small quantities that it is not a cancer risk. The benefits of chlorine in preventing outbreaks of cholera, hepatitis, and other diseases far outweigh the negligible effects of THM.

What are chelated minerals? A chelated mineral is surrounded by an amino acid to protect it from other food components such as oxalates and phytates that can bind to the mineral and prevent it from being absorbed. Chelated minerals are probably not worth the added expense because chelated calcium is absorbed 5% to 10% better than ordinary calcium but costs about 5 times more.

REVIEW CASE STUDY

Bill is a 45-year-old bachelor who eats a grab-and-go breakfast, eats all of his lunches out, and has takeout or "something easy" for dinner. Bill's doctor is concerned that his blood pressure is progressively rising with every office visit and has advised him to "cut out the salt" to lower his sodium intake. Bill rarely uses salt from a salt shaker and is unsure what else he can do to lower his sodium intake. A typical day's intake is shown on the right:

- What foods did Bill eat yesterday that were high in sodium? What foods were relatively low in sodium? What would be better choices for him when eating out? How could he lower his sodium intake while still relying on "something easy" when he prepares food at home?
- Knowing that potassium may help blunt the effect of a high sodium intake on blood pressure, what foods would you recommend he add to his diet that would increase his potassium intake?
- In overweight people, weight loss helps lower high blood pressure. Bill is "a little heavy." What changes/substitutions would help him lose weight?

Breakfast: Black coffee; two jelly doughnuts
Midmorning snack: Black coffee; cookies
Lunch: Two fast-food tacos with tortilla chips and salsa or a 6-in cold cut submarine with potato chips; cola
Midafternoon snack: candy bar
Dinner: If takeout, Chinese food or pizza; if "something easy," boxed macaroni and cheese with a couple of hot dogs, canned soup with a cold cut sandwich, or frozen TV dinners
Dessert: Instant pudding or ice cream or candy bars
Evening snacks: Cereal and milk or potato chips and dip

STUDY QUESTIONS

1   A healthy, young adult client asks how much water he should drink daily. Which of the following would be the nurse's best response?
   a. "The old adage is true: Drink eight 8-oz glasses of water daily."
   b. "Drink to satisfy thirst and you will consume adequate fluid."
   c. "You can't overconsume water, so drink as much as you can spread out over the course of the day."
   d. "It is actually not necessary to drink water at all. It is equally healthy to meet your fluid requirement with sugar-free soft drinks."

2   When developing a teaching plan for a client who is lactose intolerant, which of the following foods would the nurse suggest as sources of calcium the client could tolerate?
   a. Cheddar cheese, bok choy, broccoli
   b. Spinach, beet greens, skim milk
   c. Poultry, meat, eggs
   d. Whole grains, nuts, and cocoa

3   A client with osteoporosis was advised to drink 3 glasses of milk daily to increase her calcium intake. She wants to know why she just can't take calcium supplements. The nurse's best response is
   a. "Calcium supplements are a better idea than drinking more milk because milk provides calories. Just be sure to take the doses spread out over 3 meals."
   b. "Calcium supplements should be avoided because they raise blood levels of calcium to an unhealthy level."
   c. "Calcium is best obtained from foods, not pills, and fat-free milk is one of the best options."
   d. "It is hard to consume enough calcium through pill form only."

4   Which of the following recommendations would be most effective at increasing potassium intake?
   a. Choose enriched grains in place of whole grains.
   b. Eat more fruits and vegetables.
   c. Eat more seafood and poultry in place of red meat.
   d. Because there are few good dietary sources of potassium, it is best obtained by taking potassium supplements.

5   A client asks why eating less sodium is important for healthy people. The nurse's best response is
   a. "Low-sodium diets tend to be low in fat and therefore may reduce the risk of heart disease."
   b. "Low-sodium diets are only effective at preventing high blood pressure, not lowering existing high blood pressure, so the time to implement a low-sodium diet is when you are healthy."
   c. "There is a positive relationship between higher sodium intake and the risk of high blood pressure; lowering sodium intake may help prevent or delay high blood pressure."
   d. "Low-sodium diets are inherently low in calories and help people lose weight, which can help prevent a variety of chronic diseases."

6   Which of the following recommendations would be most effective at helping a client maximize iron absorption?
   a. Drink orange juice when you eat iron-fortified breakfast cereal.
   b. Avoid drinking coffee when you eat red meat.
   c. Drink milk with all meals.
   d. Eat dried peas and beans in place of red meat.

7   A client says he never adds salt to any foods that his wife serves, so he believes he is consuming a low-sodium diet. Which of the following is the nurse's best response?
   a. "If you don't add salt to any of your foods, you are probably eating a low-sodium diet. Continue with that strategy."
   b. "Even though you aren't adding salt to food at the table, your wife is probably salting food as she cooks. She should stop doing that."
   c. "Lots of foods are naturally high in sodium, such as milk and meat; in addition to not using a salt shaker, you must also limit foods that are naturally high in sodium."
   d. "The major sources of sodium are processed and convenience foods. Limiting their intake makes the biggest impact on overall sodium intake."

8   What should you tell the client about taking mineral supplements?
   a. "Most Americans are deficient in minerals, so it is wise to take a multimineral supplement."
   b. "Like water-soluble vitamins, if you consume more minerals than your body needs, you will excrete them in the urine, so do not worry about taking in too much."
   c. "If you do not have a mineral deficiency, taking supplements can lead to a potentially excessive intake that can cause adverse health effects."
   d. "Mineral deficiencies do not exist in the United States, so you do not need to waste your money on them."

KEY CONCEPTS

- Because water is involved in almost every body function, is not stored, and is excreted daily, it is more vital to life than food.
- Under normal conditions, water intake equals water output to maintain water balance. In most healthy people, thirst is a reliable indicator of need.
- The body's need for water is influenced by many variables, including activity, climate, and health. A general guideline is to consume 1.0 mL of fluid per calorie consumed, with a minimum of 1500 mL/day.
- Minerals are inorganic substances that cannot be broken down and rearranged in the body.
- Mineral toxicities are not likely to occur from diet alone. They are most often related to excessive use of mineral supplements, environmental exposure, or alterations in metabolism.
- Depending on the mineral involved, the body can maintain mineral balance by altering the rate of absorption, altering the rate of excretion, or releasing minerals from storage when needed.
- The absorption of many minerals is influenced by mineral–mineral interactions. Too much of one mineral may promote a deficiency of another mineral.
- Sodium, potassium, and chloride are electrolytes because they carry electrical charges when they are dissolved in solution.
- Macrominerals are needed in relatively large amounts and are found in the body in quantities greater than 5 g. Trace minerals are needed in very small amounts and are found in the body in amounts less than 5 g.
- Approximately 75% of sodium consumed in the average American diet is from processed food. Virtually all Americans consume more than the UL for sodium.
- The potassium content of the diet tends to decrease as the sodium content increases, largely because high-sodium processed foods tend to be low in potassium.
- Many American adults consume less than the RDA for calcium. Milk and yogurt are the richest sources of calcium, and their vitamin D and lactose content promote its absorption.
- Phosphorus is pervasive in foods and is also widely used in food additives to extend shelf life, enhance flavor, or improve quality characteristics. Americans consume more than they need.

- Although most Americans consume less than the RDA for magnesium, overt deficiency symptoms are rare and occur only secondary to certain diseases such as protein malnutrition and alcoholism.
- Trace minerals are not less important than major minerals; "trace" refers to the small amount normally found and needed in the body.
- The typical American diet supplies only 6 to 7 mg of iron per 1000 calories, so menstruating females typically do not eat enough calories to meet their RDA of 18 mg. Iron deficiency anemia is one of the most common nutritional deficiencies in the world.
- Americans generally consume adequate amounts of zinc. A regular intake is necessary because zinc in tissues cannot be released to maintain normal blood levels.
- The natural iodine content of most foods is low. Iodized salt, dairy products, and breads provide added iodine. Processed foods are often made with salt that is not iodized. People living in the United States are generally considered to have sufficient iodine intake.
- Selenium is a component of substances that act as antioxidants. It is being studied for its potential to decrease the risk of CVD, neurodegenerative diseases, and certain cancers.
- Fluoridated water has dramatically reduced the prevalence and severity of cavities in the U.S. population. Bottled water may not be fluoridated.
- Dietary calcium is the preferred method for achieving calcium requirements; supplements are used only when necessary because they may increase health risks, such as risk of CVD.
- A high potassium intake may blunt the effect of a high sodium intake. Americans are urged to increase their potassium intake by eating more fruits and vegetables. Meat, fish, whole grains, and legumes are also sources of potassium, but potassium is less well absorbed from them than the potassium in fruits and vegetables.
- Americans are urged to reduce their intake of sodium because of its potential role in the development of hypertension.

Check Your Knowledge Answer Key

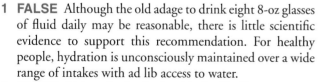

1 **FALSE** Although the old adage to drink eight 8-oz glasses of fluid daily may be reasonable, there is little scientific evidence to support this recommendation. For healthy people, hydration is unconsciously maintained over a wide range of intakes with ad lib access to water.

2 **FALSE** Although the body rids itself of some excess minerals such as sodium and potassium through urinary excretion, homeostasis of other minerals is achieved by adjusting the rate of mineral absorption (e.g., iron, calcium).

3 **FALSE** Calcium is the most plentiful mineral in the body. For most Americans, sodium is the most abundant mineral in the diet.

4 **FALSE** Unlike vitamins, minerals are inorganic elements that are not digested nor are they destroyed by light, heat, or acids during food preparation.

5 **FALSE** People are urged to get their nutrients from food rather than supplements. Recent studies suggest calcium supplements, with or without vitamin D, may increase the risk of cardiovascular events.

6 TRUE Foods high in sodium tend to be low in potassium (e.g., processed foods like frozen entrees), and foods high in potassium tend to be low in sodium (e.g., fresh vegetables and whole grains).

7 FALSE The "major" and "trace" descriptions refer to the relative quantity of the mineral found in the body, not to its importance in maintaining health.

8 TRUE For most people, thirst is a reliable indicator of fluid needs. Exceptions are the elderly, children, and during hot weather or strenuous exercise.

9 TRUE Trace mineral balance is a function not only of the quantity of the element consumed but also of the presence of other trace minerals and dietary factors. For instance, nonheme iron absorption is impaired by tea but enhanced by orange juice.

10 FALSE A chronically low intake of calcium compromises the density and strength of bones but does not lead to hypocalcemia. Serum levels of calcium are maintained within normal range regardless of calcium intake at the expense of calcium in bones.

Student Resources on thePoint®
For additional learning materials, activate the code in the front of this book at
http://thePoint.lww.com/activate

Websites

National Dairy Council at www.nationaldairycouncil.org

National Academy of Sciences, Institute of Medicine for Reference Dietary Intakes at www.nap.edu

National Institutes of Health, Office of Dietary Supplements https://ods.od.nih.gov/

Nutrient sources at USDA National Nutrient Database for Standard Reference, Release 28, at http://www.ars.usda.gov/Services/docs.htm?docid=8964

National Osteoporosis Foundation at http://nof.org/

References

Aburto, N., Hanson, S., Gutierrez, H., Hooper, L., Elliott, P., & Cappuccio, F. P. (2013). Effect of increased potassium intake on cardiovascular risk factors and disease: Systematic review and meta-analyses. *BMJ, 346*, f1378. doi:10.1136/bmj.f1378

Academy of Nutrition and Dietetics. (n.d.). *Nutrition care manual. Methods for estimating fluid requirements.* Available at https://www.nutritioncaremanual.org/topic.cfm?ncm_toc_id=255307. Accessed on 1/18/16.

Anderson, M., Karumbunathan, V., & Zimmermann, M. (2012). Global iodine status in 2011 and trends over the past decade. *The Journal of Nutrition, 142*, 744–750.

Appel, L., Moore, T., Obarzanek, E., Vollmer, W. M., Svetkey, L. P., Sacks, F. M., . . . Karanja, N. (1997). A clinical trial of the effects of dietary patterns on blood pressure. *The New England Journal of Medicine, 336*, 1117–1124.

Aune, D., Lau, R., Chan, D., Vieira, R., Greenwood, D., Kampman, E., & Norat, T. (2012). Dairy products and colorectal cancer risk: A systematic review and meta-analysis of cohort studies. *Annals of Oncology, 23*, 37–45.

Aune, D., Navarro Rosenblatt, D. A., Chan, D. S., Vieira, A. R., Vieira, R., Greenwood, D. C., . . . Norat, T. (2015). Dairy products, calcium, and prostate cancer risk: A systematic review and meta-analysis of cohort studies. *The American Journal of Clinical Nutrition, 101*, 87–117. doi:10.3945/ajcn.113.067157

Bailey, R., Fulgoni, V., Keast, D., & Dwyer, J. (2011). Dietary supplement use is associated with higher intakes of minerals from food sources. *The American Journal of Clinical Nutrition, 94*, 1376–1381.

Bayer, R., Johns, D., & Galea, S. (2012). Salt and public health: Contested science and the challenge of evidence-based decision making. *Health Affairs, 31*, 2738–2746.

Bell, R., Draper, J., Tzeng, D., Shin, H. K., & Schmidt, G. R. (1977). Physiological responses of human adult to foods containing phosphate additives. *The Journal of Nutrition, 107*, 45–50.

Bolland, M., Barber, P., Doughty, R., Mason, B., Horne, A., Ames, R., . . . Reid, I. R. (2008). Vascular events in healthy older women receiving calcium supplementation: Randomized controlled trial. *BMJ, 336*, 262–266.

Bolland, M., Grey, A., Avenell, A., Gamble, G. D., & Reid, I. R. (2011). Calcium supplements with or without vitamin D and risk of cardiovascular events: Reanalysis of the Women's Health Initiative limited access dataset and meta-analysis. *BMJ, 342*, d2040.

Booth, A., Huggins, C., Wattanapenpailboon, N., & Nowson, C. (2015). Effect of increasing dietary calcium through supplements and dairy food on body weight and body composition: A meta-analysis of randomised controlled trials. *The British Journal of Nutrition, 114*, 1013–1026.

Caldwell, K., Pan, Y., Mortensen, M. E., Makhmudov, A., Merrill, L., & Moye, J. (2013). Iodine status in pregnant women in the National Children's Study and in U.S. women (15–44 years), National Health and Nutrition Examination Survey 2005–2010. *Thyroid, 23*, 927–937.

Calvo, M., & Uribarri, J. (2013). Public health impact of dietary phosphorus excess on bone and cardiovascular health in the general population. *The American Journal of Clinical Nutrition, 98*, 6–15.

Centers for Disease Control and Prevention. (2013). *Ten great public health achievements in the 20th century.* Available at http://www.cdc.gov/about/history/tengpha.htm. Accessed on 8/23/16.

Centers for Disease Control and Prevention. (2015). *Community water fluoridation.* Available at http://www.cdc.gov/fluoridation/. Accessed on 2/22/16.

Chang, A., Lazo, M., Appel, L., Gutiérrez, O. M., & Grams, M. E. (2014). High dietary phosphorus intake is associated with all-cause mortality: Results from NHANES III. *The American Journal of Clinical Nutrition, 99*, 320–327.

Cook, N., Appel, L., & Whelton, P. (2014). Lower levels of sodium intake and reduced cardiovascular risk. *Circulation, 129*, 981–989. doi:10.1161/CIRCULATIONAHA.113.006032

Cosman, F., de Beur, S., LeBoff, M., Lewiecki, E. M., Tanner, B., Randall, S., & Lindsay, R. (2014). Clinician's guide to prevention and treatment of osteoporosis. *Osteoporosis International, 25*, 2359–2381.

de Baaij, J., Hoenderop, J., & Bindels, R. (2015). Magnesium in man: Implications for health and disease. *Physiological Reviews, 95*, 1–46. doi:10.1152/physrev.00012.2014

De Benoist, B., McLean, E., Andersson, M., & Rogers, L. (2008). Iodine deficiency in 2007: Global progress since 2003. *Food and Nutrition Bulletin, 29*, 195–202.

Dietary Guidelines Advisory Committee. (2015). *Scientific report of the 2015 Dietary Guidelines Advisory Committee.* Available at http://health.gov/dietaryguidelines/2015-scientific-report/. Accessed on 2/22/16.

Evert, A., Boucher, J., Cypress, M., Dunbar, S. A., Franz, M. J., Mayer-Davis, E. J., . . . Yancy, W. S., Jr. (2013). Nutrition therapy recommendations for the management of adults with diabetes. *Diabetes Care, 36*, 3821–3842.

Graudal, N., Jürgens, S., Baslund, B., & Alderman, M. (2014). Compared with usual sodium intake, low- and excessive sodium diets are associated with increased mortality: A meta-analysis. *American Journal of Hypertension, 27*, 1129–1137.

Hurrell, R., & Egli, I. (2010). Iron bioavailability and dietary reference values. *American Journal of Hypertension, 91*, 1461S–1467S.

Institute of Medicine. (2000). *Dietary reference intakes for vitamin C, vitamin E, selenium, and carotenoids.* Washington, DC: National Academy Press.

Institute of Medicine. (2001). *Dietary reference intakes for vitamin A, vitamin K, arsenic, boron, chromium, copper, iodine, iron, manganese, molybdenum, nickel, silicon, vanadium, and zinc.* Washington, DC: National Academy Press.

Institute of Medicine. (2005). *Dietary reference intakes for water, potassium, sodium, chloride, and sulfate.* Available at http://www.nap.edu/catalog.php?record_id=10925#. Accessed on 9/25/12.

Institute of Medicine. (2011). *Dietary Reference Intakes for calcium and vitamin D.* Available at http://www.nap.edu. Accessed on 2/17/12.

Institute of Medicine. (2013). *Sodium intake in populations: Assessment of evidence.* Washington, DC: The National Academies Press.

Kass, L., Weekes, J., & Carpenter, L. (2012). Effect of magnesium supplementation on blood pressure: A meta-analysis. *European Journal of Clinical Nutrition, 66*, 411–418.

Keum, N., Aune, D., Greenwood, D., Ju, W., & Giovannucci, E. L. (2014). Calcium intake and colorectal cancer risk: Dose-response meta-analysis of prospective observational studies. *International Journal of Cancer, 135*, 1940–1948.

King, D., Mainous, A., III, Geesey, M., & Woolson, R. (2005). Dietary magnesium and C-reactive protein levels. *Journal of the American College of Nutrition, 24*, 166–171.

Larsson, S., Orsini, N., & Wolk, A. (2012). Dietary magnesium intake and risk of stroke: A meta-analysis of prospective studies. *Journal of the American College of Nutrition, 95*, 362–366.

Morris, J., & Crane, S. (2013). Selenium toxicity from a misformulated dietary supplement, adverse health effects, and the temporal response in the nail biologic monitor. *Nutrients, 5*, 1024–1057. doi:10.3390/nu5041024

National Institutes of Health, Office of Dietary Supplements. (2011). *Iodine: Fact sheet for health professionals.* Available at https://ods.od.nih.gov/factsheets/Iodine-HealthProfessional/. Accessed on 2/21/16.

National Institutes of Health, Office of Dietary Supplements. (2013). *Selenium: Dietary supplement fact sheet.* Available at https://ods.od.nih.gov/factsheets/Selenium-HealthProfessional/#en5. Accessed on 2/22/16.

National Institutes of Health, Office of Dietary Supplements. (2015). *Iron: Dietary supplement fact sheet.* Available at https://ods.od.nih.gov/factsheets/Iron-HealthProfessional/. Accessed on 2/21/16.

National Osteoporosis Foundation. (n.d.). *Debunking the myths.* Available at http://nof.org/learns. Accessed on 2/26/16.

Perrine, C., Herrick, K., Serdula, M., & Sullivan, K. (2010). Some subgroups of reproductive age women in the United States may be at risk for iodine deficiency. *The Journal of Nutrition, 140*, 1489–1494.

Peterlik, M., Kállay, E., & Cross, H. (2013). Calcium nutrition and extracellular calcium sensing: Relevance for the pathogenesis of osteoporosis, cancer and cardiovascular diseases. *Nutrients, 5*, 302–327. doi:10.3390/nu5010302

Reid, I. (2014). Should we prescribe calcium supplements for osteoporosis prevention? *Journal of Bone Metabolism, 21*, 21–28.

Reid, I., Bristow, S., & Bolland, M. (2015). Cardiovascular complications of calcium supplements. *Journal of Cellular Biochemistry, 116*, 494–501.

Rodrigues, S., Baldo, M., Machado, R., Forechi, L., Molina Mdel, C., & Mill, J. G. (2014). High potassium intake blunts the effect of elevated sodium intake on blood pressure levels. *Journal of the American Society of Hypertension, 8*, 232–238.

Rodríguez-Morán, M., Simental, L., Zambrano, G., & Guerrero-Romero, F. (2011). The role of magnesium in type 2 diabetes: A brief based-clinical review. *Magnesium Research, 24*, 156–162.

Rowland, G., Schwartz, G., John, E., & Ingles, S. (2012). Calcium intake and prostate cancer among African Americans: Effect modification by vitamin D receptor calcium absorption genotype. *Journal of Bone and Mineral Research, 27*, 187–194.

Science, M., Johnstone, J., Roth, D., Guyatt, G., & Loeb, M. (2012). Zinc for the treatment of the common cold: A systematic review and meta-analysis of randomized controlled trials. *Canadian Medical Association Journal, 184*, E551–E561.

Singh, M., & Das, R. (2011). Zinc for the common cold. *Cochrane Database of Systematic Reviews, (2)*, CD001364.

Sunde, R. A. (2012). Selenium. In A. C. Ross, B. Caballero, R. J. Cousins, K. L. Tucker, T. R. Ziegler (Eds.), *Modern nutrition in health and disease* (11th ed., pp. 225–237). Philadelphia, PA: Lippincott Williams & Wilkins.

Tai, V., Leung, W., Grey, A., Reid, I. R., & Bolland, M. J. (2015). Calcium intake and bone mineral density: Systematic review and meta-analysis. *BMJ, 351*, h4183. doi:10.1136/bmj.h4183

United Nations Children's Fund. (2011). *The state of the world's children 2011: Adolescence: An age of opportunity.* New York, NY: Author.

U.S. Department of Agriculture, Agricultural Research Service. (2014). *Nutrient intakes from food: Mean amounts consumed per individual, by gender and age. What we eat in America, NHANES 2011–2012.* Available at www.ars.usda.gov/ba/bhnrc/fsrg. Accessed on 1/22/16.

U.S. Department of Health and Human Services & U.S. Department of Agriculture. (2015). *2015-2020 Dietary guidelines for Americans* (8th ed.). Available at www.health.gov/dietaryguidelines/2015. Accessed on 1/7/16.

U.S. Food and Drug Administration. (2009). *Warnings on three Zicam intranasal zinc products.* Available at http://www.fda.gov/ForConsumers/ConsumerUpdates/ucm166931.htm. Accessed on 2/21/16.

U.S. Food and Drug Administration. (2016). *Draft guidance for industry: Voluntary sodium reduction goals: Target mean and upper bound concentrations for sodium in commercially processed, packaged, and prepared foods.* Available at http://www.fda.gov/Food/GuidanceRegulation/GuidanceDocumentsRegulatoryInformation/ucm494732.htm. Accessed on 8/26/16.

Valtin, H. (2002). "Drink at least eight glasses of water a day." Really? Is there scientific evidence for "8 × 8"? *American Journal of Physiology. Regulatory, Integrative and Comparative Physiology, 283*, R993–R1004.

Weaver, C., Gordon, C., Janz, K., Kalkwarf, H. J., Lappe, J. M., Lewis, R., . . . Zemel, B. S. (2016). The National Osteoporosis Foundation's position statement on peak bone mass development and lifestyle factors: A systematic review and implementation recommendations. *Osteoporosis International, 27*, 1281–1386. doi:10.1007.s00198-015-3440-3

Wolfram, T. (2016). A big sodium debate. *Food & Nutrition, 5*, 18–19.

World Health Organization. (2012). *Micronutrient deficiencies: Iron deficiency anaemia.* Available at www.who.int/nutrition/topics/ida/en/index.html. Accessed on 9/26/12.

Zhang, Z., Cogswell, M., Gillespie, C., Fang, J., Loustalot, F., Dai, S., . . . Yang, Q. (2013). Association between usual sodium and potassium intake and blood pressure and hypertension among U.S. adults: NHANES 2005-2010. *PLoS One, 8*(1), e75289. doi:10.1371/journal.pone.0075289

Zimmermann, M., & Boelaert, K. (2015). Iodine deficiency and thyroid disorders. *Lancet. Diabetes & Endocrinology, 3,* 286–295.

Zimmermann, M., Jooste, P., & Pandav, C. (2008). Iodine-deficiency disorders. *Lancet, 372,* 1251–1262.

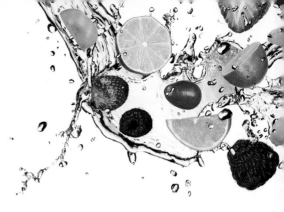

Chapter 7   Energy Balance

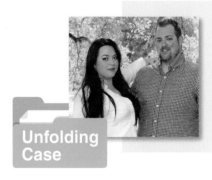

Unfolding Case

Kyla and Garrett Wilkinson

Kyla and Garrett are 25 years old and have been married 6 months. Since then, she has gained 10 to 15 pounds and he has gained 40 pounds, which they attribute to eating dinner out three to four times a week and getting takeout the other days of the week. They are shocked at how quickly "things got out of control" and want to adopt a healthier lifestyle before embarking on parenthood.

Check Your Knowledge

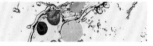

True	False		
☐	☐	**1**	A food that is high in "energy" is high in calories.
☐	☐	**2**	A pound of body fat is equivalent to 3500 calories.
☐	☐	**3**	People shaped like "apples" are at greater health risk than people shaped like "pears."
☐	☐	**4**	The formulas to calculate body mass index (BMI) are different for men and women.
☐	☐	**5**	Calorie-dense foods provide a relatively high amount of calories with low levels of vitamins, minerals, and other beneficial substances.
☐	☐	**6**	The majority of calories expended daily by most Americans are spent on basal needs.
☐	☐	**7**	Building muscle increases metabolic rate.
☐	☐	**8**	To reap health benefits, you must participate in continuous activity for at least 30 minutes.
☐	☐	**9**	Sitting too much may be a health risk even when physical activity goals are met.
☐	☐	**10**	An effective strategy for limiting calorie intake is to limit food and beverages high in added sugar and solid fat.

Learning Objectives

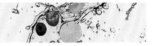

Upon completion of this chapter, you will be able to

1 Estimate an individual's total calorie requirements.
2 Determine an individual's BMI.
3 Evaluate weight status based on BMI.
4 Assess a person's waist circumference.
5 Compare the terms "nutrient density" and "calorie density."
6 Evaluate a person's usual activity level based on Dietary Guidelines recommendations.

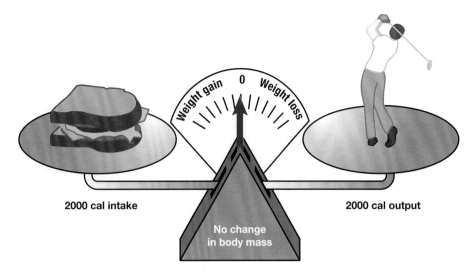

Figure 7.1 ▲ A state of energy balance: Calorie intake is equal to calorie output.

The state of energy balance is the relationship between the amount of energy (calories) consumed and the amount of energy (calories) expended. When calorie intake and output are balanced—that is, approximately the same over time—body weight is stable (Fig. 7.1). A positive energy balance occurs when calorie intake exceeds calorie output, whether the imbalance is caused by overeating, low activity, or both (Fig. 7.2). Over time, the calories consumed in excess of need contribute to weight gain. Because a pound of body fat is equivalent to 3500 calories, a surplus of 500 cal/day over a 7-day period can result in a 1-pound weight gain. Conversely, a negative calorie balance occurs when calorie output exceeds intake, whether the imbalance is from decreasing calorie intake, increasing PA, or (preferably) both (Fig. 7.3).

This chapter discusses energy intake, energy output, and how total calorie requirements are estimated. Methods of evaluating body weight are presented. Energy in health promotion focuses on the *2015-2020 Dietary Guidelines for Americans* recommendations for weight management and physical activity.

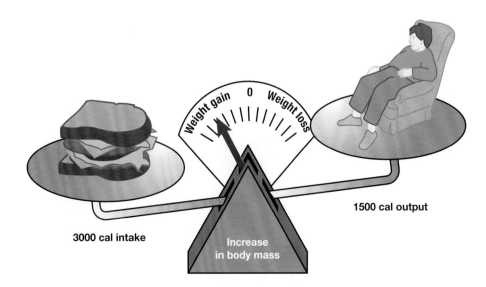

Figure 7.2 ▲ A positive energy balance: Calorie intake is greater than calorie output.

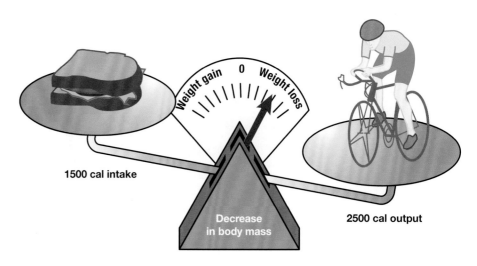

Figure 7.3 ▲ **A negative energy balance: Calorie intake is less than calorie output.**

ENERGY INTAKE

Calorie
unit by which energy is measured; the amount of heat needed to raise the temperature of 1 kg of water by 1°C. Technically, calorie is actually kilocalorie or kcal.

Technically, a **calorie** is the amount of energy required to raise the temperature of 1 kg of water by 1°C. In nutrition, calories are the measure of the amount of energy in a food or used by the body to fuel activity. Energy balance is a function of calorie intake versus calorie output (Fig. 7.4).

Carbohydrates, protein, fat, and alcohol provide calories. The total number of calories in a food or eating pattern can be estimated by multiplying total grams of these nutrients by the appropriate calories per gram—namely, 4 cal/g for carbohydrates and protein, 9 cal/g for fat, and 7 cal/g for alcohol.

In practice, "counting calories"—whether manually, online, or with a mobile phone app—is an imprecise process dependent on knowing accurate portion sizes of all foods consumed and the exact nutritional composition of each item, neither of which conditions is easily met. Even when all food consumed is measured, the nutrient values available in food composition databases represent *average* not *actual* nutrition content based on analysis of a number of food samples.

An imprecise but easy way to estimate calorie intake is to estimate or count the number of servings from each food group a person consumes. Using a standard reference, such as Food Lists for Weight Management (American Diabetes Association & Academy of Nutrition and Dietetics, 2014), the number of servings from each group is multiplied by the average amount of calories in a serving (Table 7.1). The sum of from all food groups provides an approximation

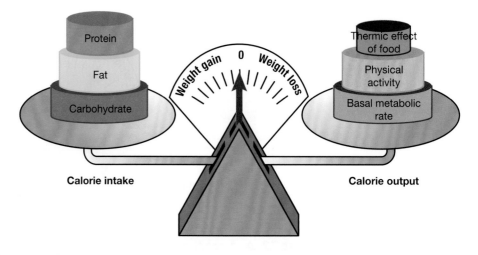

Figure 7.4 ▲ **Sources of calorie intake and calorie expenditure.**

Table 7.1 Calories by Food Lists

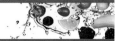

Food Group	Representative Serving Size	Average Calories per Serving
Starch (breads, grains, cereals, starchy vegetables, dried peas and beans)	1 oz bread	80
Fruits	1 small fresh fruit, ½ cup canned or frozen fruit	60
Milk	1 cup	
Skim or 1%		100
2%		120
Whole		160
Nonstarchy vegetables	½ cup cooked or 1 cup raw	25
Protein foods	1 oz	
Plant-based protein		Varies
Lean		45
Medium fat		75
High fat		100
Fat/oils	1 tsp butter or margarine	45

For example:

Number of servings consumed	calories per serving	calories consumed per food group
6 grains	80	480
4 fruit	60	240
5 vegetables	25	125
2½ cup nonfat milk	80	200
6 oz medium-fat protein	75	450
3 tsp oils	45	135
Total calories per day		1630

Source: American Diabetes Association & Academy of Nutrition and Dietetics. (2014). *Choose your foods: Food Lists for weight management.* Alexandria, VA: American Diabetes Association.

of total calories consumed. However, representative foods within each of the Food Lists groups are generally free of added fat or sugar. For instance, items such as onion rings, cheesecake, and sugar-sweetened beverages are not part of those food groups. It is easy to underestimate calorie intake if the actual foods consumed are higher in caloric density.

The drawback of counting calories by any method is that appropriate calories are only one aspect of a healthy eating pattern; nutritional adequacy is not guaranteed. For instance, an individual can eat the appropriate number of calories, but if the calories come from burgers and fries and not fruits, vegetables, whole grains, or dairy, the pattern is not healthy even though it is calorie appropriate.

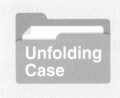

Unfolding Case

Recall Kyla and Garrett. A food record would help identify the types, amounts, and pattern of food they eat so that a strategy to improve intake can be formulated. What other factors need to be assessed before recommending changes to their intake?

ENERGY EXPENDITURE

The body uses energy for involuntary activities and purposeful PA. The thermic effect of food is another category of energy expenditure, although in practice it is often disregarded. The total of these expenditures represents an estimate of the number of calories a person expends in a day (Box 7.1).

Basal Metabolism

Basal Metabolic Rate (BMR) or Basal Energy Expenditure (BEE)
the amount of calories expended in a 24-hour period to fuel the involuntary activities of the body at rest and after a 12-hour fast.

Resting Metabolic Rate (RMR) or Resting Energy Expenditure (REE)
the amount of calories expended in a 24-hour period to fuel the involuntary activities of the body at rest. RMR does not adhere to the criterion of a 12-hour fast, so it is slightly higher than BEE because it includes energy spent on digesting, absorbing, and metabolizing food.

Basal metabolism is the amount of calories required to fuel the involuntary activities of the body at rest after a 12-hour fast. These involuntary activities include maintaining body temperature and muscle tone, producing and releasing secretions, propelling the gastrointestinal tract, inflating the lungs, and beating the heart. For most people, the **basal metabolic rate (BMR)** or **basal energy expenditure (BEE)** accounts for approximately 60% to 70% of total calories expended. The less active a person is, the greater is the proportion of calories used for BEE. The term "BEE" is often used interchangeably with **resting metabolic rate (RMR)** or **resting energy expenditure (REE)** even though they are slightly different measures.

One imprecise, rule-of-thumb guideline for estimating BMR is to multiply healthy weight (in pounds) by 10 for women and 11 for men. For example, a 130-pound woman expends approximately 1300 cal/day on BMR (130 pounds × 10 cal/pound = 1300 calories). When actual weight exceeds healthy weight, an "adjusted" weight of halfway between healthy and actual can be used. For instance, if healthy weight is 130 pounds, but actual weight is 170 pounds, 150 pounds would be the "adjusted" weight for estimating basal calories. Methods used to determine BMR and total calorie requirements in the clinical setting are discussed in Chapter 16.

A drawback of using a rule-of-thumb method for determining BMR is that it is based only on weight; it does not account for other variables that affect metabolic rate, such as body composition. Lean tissue (muscle mass) contributes to a higher metabolic rate than fat tissue. Therefore, people with more muscle mass have higher metabolic rates than do people with proportionately

BOX 7.1   Estimating Total Energy Expenditure

1. **Estimate basal metabolic rate (BMR)**

   Multiply your healthy weight (in pounds) by 10 for women or 11 for men. If you are overweight, multiply by the average weight within your healthy weight range.

   _____ (weight in pounds) × _____ = _____ calories for BMR

2. **Estimate total calories according to usual activity level**
   Choose the category that describes your usual activities and then multiply BMR by the appropriate percentage.

   _____ (calories for BMR) × _____% = calories spent on activity

Sedentary: mostly sitting, driving, sleeping, standing, reading, typing, and other low-intensity activities	20
Light activity: light exercise such as walking not more than 2 hours/day	30
Moderate activity: moderate exercise such as heavy housework, gardening, and very little sitting	40
High activity: active in physical sports or a labor-intensive occupation such as construction work	50

3. **Add BMR calories and physical activity calories**

   _____ calories for BMR + _____ calories spent on activity = _____ estimate of total expended daily (imprecise estimate of thermic effect of food is generally not included).

Table 7.2	Factors that Affect Basal Metabolic Rate (BMR)

Variables	Effect on Metabolism
Age	Loss of lean body mass with age lowers BMR.
Growth	The formation of new tissue, as seen in children and during pregnancy, increases BMR.
Stresses	Stresses, such as infection and many diseases, raise BMR.
Thyroid hormones: tetraiodothyronine (thyroxine, or T_4) and triiodothyronine (T_3)	An oversecretion of thyroid hormones (hyperthyroidism) speeds up BMR; undersecretion of thyroid hormones (hypothyroidism) lowers BMR. The change may be as great as 50%.
Fever	BMR increases 7% for each degree Fahrenheit above 98.6.
Height	When considering two people of the same gender who weigh the same, the taller one has a higher BMR than the shorter one because of a larger surface area.
Extreme environmental temperatures	Very hot and very cold environmental temperatures increase the BMR because the body expends more energy to regulate its own temperature.
Starvation, fasting, and malnutrition	Part of the decline in BMR that occurs with these conditions is attributed to the loss of lean body tissue. Hormonal changes may contribute to the decrease in metabolic rate.
Weight loss from calorie deficits	With smaller body mass, less energy is required to fuel metabolism.
Smoking	Nicotine increases BMR.
Caffeine	Increases BMR
Certain drugs, such as barbiturates, narcotics, and muscle relaxants	Decrease BMR
Sleep, paralysis	Decrease BMR

more fat tissue. This explains why men, who have a greater proportion of muscle, have higher metabolic rates than women, who have a greater proportion of fat. Conversely, the loss of lean tissue that usually occurs with aging is one reason why calorie requirements decrease as people get older. Other factors that affect BMR appear in Table 7.2.

Physical Activity

Physical activity (PA), or voluntary muscular activity, generally accounts for approximately 30% of total calories used, although it may be as low as 20% in sedentary people and as high as 50% in people who are very active. The actual amount of energy expended on PA depends on the intensity and duration of the activity and the weight of the person performing the activity. The more intense and longer the activity, the greater is the amount of calories burned. Heavier people, who have more weight to move, use more energy than lighter people to perform the same activity. A rule-of-thumb method for estimating daily calories expended on PA is to calculate the percentage increase above BMR on the basis of estimated intensity of usual daily activities (Box 7.1). Estimating calorie expenditure from PA is easily obtained by wearing a device created to track activity and other functions, such as sleep, heart rate, calorie intake, and calorie output. Using algorithms and sensors, such as temperature sensors and optical sensors, trackers measure motion which is then converted into steps and activity; from there, calories and sleep quality are estimated. Apps present the data after more fine-tuning with algorithms. Due to differences in sensors and algorithms, reported statistics vary among individual devices even when the same data is used. Mobile phones have similar built-in sensors that pedometer-like apps can use to estimate activity. Tracking devices provide an estimate, not an actual reading.

Thermic Effect of Food

Thermic Effect of Food
an estimation of the amount of energy
required to digest, absorb, transport,
metabolize, and store nutrients.

The **thermic effect of food** is another category of energy expenditure that represents the calories spent on processing food. In a normal mixed diet, the thermal effect of food is estimated to be about 10% of the total calorie intake. For instance, people who consume 1800 cal/day use about 180 calories to process their food. The actual number of calories spent varies with the composition of food eaten, the frequency of eating, and the size of meals consumed. Although it represents an actual and legitimate use of calories, the thermic effect of food in practice is often disregarded when calorie requirements are estimated because it constitutes such a small amount of energy and is imprecisely estimated.

Estimating Total Energy Expenditure

Total calorie needs can be imprecisely estimated by using predictive equations, of which more than 200 have been published. The following are different approaches for estimating calorie needs; all yield estimates, not precise measurements.

- Add the results of the rule-of-thumb methods described earlier for estimating BMR and calories spent on activity (Box 7.1).
- Use a simple formula of calories per kilogram of body weight, such as 25 to 30 cal/kg, which is often used for nonobese adults. This formula is adjusted upward or downward based on the client's age, weight, or activity level.
- Use a standard reference that lists estimated daily calorie needs based on gender, age, and activity. Table 7.3 lists estimated daily calorie needs.

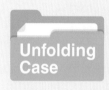

Unfolding Case

Think of Kyla and Garrett. They want to lose weight and they also want to eat healthy. Often, people forget about health and just concentrate on calories and weight. Although their estimated calories as sedentary 25-year-olds are 2000 calories for Kyla and 2400 calories for Garrett, they do not want to count calories or measure serving sizes. What strategies can they use to eat a healthy, calorie-appropriate eating pattern that will promote weight loss without actually counting calories?

EVALUATING WEIGHT STATUS

From a health perspective, healthy or desirable weight is that which is statistically correlated to good health. But the relationship between body weight and good health is more complicated than simply the number on the scale. For instance, although increased body weight is a risk factor for type 2 diabetes, actual risk is more accurately related to the quantity and distribution of body fat (Després, 2012). However, methods to accurately assess quantity of body fat and its distribution are not readily available or cost-effective (Hsu, Araneta, Kanaya, Chiang, & Fujimoto, 2015). Therefore, the most widely used tool to assess risk for obesity-related diseases is to evaluate weight for height because it is economical and practical in clinical settings and epidemiological studies (Hsu et al., 2015).

Body Mass Index

Ideal Body Weight
the formula given here is a universally used standard in clinical practice to quickly estimate a person's reasonable weight based on height, even though this and all other methods are not absolute.

Historically, a quick and easy method of calculating **ideal body weight** and evaluating weight for height is the Hamwi method (Table 7.4). However, since the early 1980s, weight status has been assessed by body mass index (BMI). BMI is calculated by dividing weight in kilograms by height in meters squared (kg/m^2). Nomograms and tables that plot height and weight to determine BMI eliminate complicated mathematical calculations (Table 7.5). Established cutoffs identify overweight as BMI ≥ 25 and obese as BMI ≥ 30, which are based on the rationale that adults with a BMI ≥ 25

Table 7.3	Estimated Calorie Needs per Day by Age, Gender, and Physical Activity Level					

| | Male | | | Female* | | |
Activity Level**	Sedentary	Moderately Active	Active	Sedentary	Moderately Active	Active
Age (years)						
2	1000	1000	1000	1000	1000	1000
3	1200	1400	1400	1000	1200	1400
4	1200	1400	1600	1200	1400	1400
5	1200	1400	1600	1200	1400	1600
6	1400	1600	1800	1200	1400	1600
7	1400	1600	1800	1200	1600	1800
8	1400	1600	2000	1400	1600	1800
9	1600	1800	2000	1400	1600	1800
10	1600	1800	2200	1400	1800	2000
11	1800	2000	2200	1600	1800	2000
12	1800	2200	2400	1600	2000	2200
13	2000	2200	2600	1600	2000	2200
14	2000	2400	2800	1800	2000	2400
15	2200	2600	3000	1800	2000	2400
16	2400	2800	3200	1800	2000	2400
17	2400	2800	3200	1800	2000	2400
18	2400	2800	3200	1800	2000	2400
19–20	2600	2800	3000	2000	2200	2400
21–25	2400	2800	3000	2000	2200	2400
26–30	2400	2600	3000	1800	2000	2400
31–35	2400	2600	3000	1800	2000	2200
36–40	2400	2600	2800	1800	2000	2200
41–45	2200	2600	2800	1800	2000	2200
46–50	2200	2400	2800	1800	2000	2200
51–55	2200	2400	2800	1600	1800	2200
56–60	2200	2400	2600	1600	1800	2200
61–65	2000	2400	2600	1600	1800	2000
66–70	2000	2200	2600	1600	1800	2000
71–75	2000	2200	2600	1600	1800	2000
76+	2000	2200	2400	1600	1800	2000

Estimated amounts of calories*** needed to maintain calorie balance for various gender and age groups at three different levels of physical activity. The estimates are rounded to the nearest 200 calories for assignment to a USDA Food Pattern. An individual's calorie needs may be higher or lower than these average estimates.

*Estimates for females do not include women who are pregnant or breastfeeding.

**Sedentary means a lifestyle that includes only the light physical activity associated with typical day-to-day life. Moderately active means a lifestyle that includes physical activity equivalent to walking about 1.5 to 3 miles per day at 3 to 4 miles per hour, in addition to the light physical activity associated with typical day-to-day life. Active means a lifestyle that includes physical activity equivalent to walking more than 3 miles per day at 3 to 4 miles per hour, in addition to the light physical activity associated with typical day-to-day life.

***Based on estimated energy requirements (EER) equations, using reference heights (average) and reference weights (healthy) for each age–gender group. For children and adolescents, reference height and weight vary. For adults, the reference man is 5 ft 10 in tall and weighs 154 pounds. The reference woman is 5 ft 4 in tall and weighs 126 pounds. EER equations are from the Institute of Medicine. (2002). Dietary reference intakes for energy, carbohydrate, fiber, fat, fatty acids, cholesterol, protein, and amino acids. Washington, DC: The National Academies Press.

Source: U.S. Department of Health and Human Services & U.S. Department of Agriculture. (2015). Dietary guidelines for Americans (8th ed.). Available at www.health .gov/dietaryguidelines/2015/guidelines. Accessed on 3/14/16.

Table 7.4   Evaluating Weight

Standard	Calculation	Interpretation
Percentage of "ideal" body weight as determined by the Hamwi method (% IBW)	Hamwi method calculation Women: Allow 100 pounds for the first 5 ft of height; add 5 pounds for each additional inch. Men: Allow 106 pounds for the first 5 ft of height: add 6 pounds for each additional inch	• ≤69% severe malnutrition • 70%–79% moderate malnutrition • 80%–89% mild malnutrition • 90%–110% within normal range • 110%–119% overweight • ≥120% obese • ≥200% morbidly obese
Body mass index (BMI)	For men and women: weight in kg ÷ height in meters squared	• ≤18.5 may ↑ health risk • 18.5–24.9 healthy weight • 25–29.9 overweight • 30–34.9 obesity class 1 • 35–39.9 obesity class 2 • ≥40 obesity class 3

Table 7.5   Body Mass Index

	Normal						Overweight					Obese					
BMI	19	20	21	22	23	24	25	26	27	28	29	30	31	32	33	34	35
Height (inches)								Body Weight (pounds)									
58	91	96	100	105	110	115	119	124	129	134	138	143	148	153	158	162	167
59	94	99	104	109	114	119	124	128	133	138	143	148	153	158	163	168	173
60	97	102	107	112	118	123	128	133	138	143	148	153	158	163	168	174	179
61	100	106	111	116	122	127	132	137	143	148	153	158	164	169	174	180	185
62	104	109	115	120	126	131	136	142	147	153	158	164	169	175	180	186	191
63	107	113	118	124	130	135	141	146	152	158	163	169	175	180	186	191	197
64	110	116	122	128	134	140	145	151	157	163	169	174	180	186	192	197	204
65	114	120	126	132	138	144	150	156	162	168	174	180	186	192	198	204	210
66	118	124	130	136	142	148	155	161	167	173	179	186	192	198	204	210	216
67	121	127	134	140	146	153	159	166	172	178	185	191	198	204	211	217	223
68	125	131	138	144	151	158	164	171	177	184	190	197	203	210	216	223	230
69	128	135	142	149	155	162	169	176	182	189	196	203	209	216	223	230	236
70	132	139	146	153	160	167	174	181	188	195	202	209	216	222	229	236	243
71	136	143	150	157	165	172	179	186	193	200	208	215	222	229	236	243	250
72	140	147	154	162	169	177	184	191	199	206	213	221	228	235	242	250	258
73	144	151	159	166	174	182	189	197	204	212	219	227	235	242	250	257	265
74	148	155	163	171	179	186	194	202	210	218	225	233	241	249	256	264	272
75	152	160	168	176	184	192	200	208	216	224	232	240	248	256	264	272	279
76	156	164	172	180	189	197	205	213	221	230	238	246	254	263	271	279	287

Source: Adapted from U.S. Department of Health and Human Services. (1998). *Clinical guidelines on the identification, evaluation, and treatment of overweight and obesity in adults: The evidence report*. Rockville, MD: Author.

have increased risks of both morbidity and mortality (National Institutes of Health, 1998). Those risks include coronary heart disease, hypertension, hypercholesterolemia, type 2 diabetes, and other diseases.

Despite its widespread use as a screening tool, BMI is not without controversy. For instance, the BMI levels that define overweight and obesity are somewhat arbitrary because the relationship between increasing weight and risk of disease is continuous. Also, BMI does not take gender into account nor body composition; a lean athlete may have well-developed muscle mass and little fat tissue, yet if his BMI is high, he would fall under the designation of overweight or obese. Conversely, an elderly person may have a normal BMI and be deemed "healthy" despite a low percentage of muscle mass masked by a high amount of body fat. Also, BMI cannot distinguish the location of body fat distribution.

Evidence that health risks such as diabetes begin at lower BMI cutoffs for some ethnic groups has led to an international debate over whether cutoff points for overweight and obesity should be lower for Asians than other ethnic groups (Low, Chin, Ma, Heng, & Deurenberg-Yap, 2009). Some Asian countries have lowered their recommended cutoff points. In China, the recommended BMI cutoff points are 24 for overweight and 28 for obesity (Bei-Fan et al., 2002). In India, overweight is defined as a BMI of 23 (Misra et al., 2009). The American Diabetes Association recommends testing for diabetes be considered for all Asian American adults who have a BMI ≥23 (Hsu et al., 2015).

							Extreme Obesity											
36	37	38	39	40	41	42	43	44	45	46	47	48	49	50	51	52	53	54
							Body Weight (pounds)											
172	177	181	186	191	196	201	205	210	215	220	224	229	234	239	244	248	253	258
178	183	188	193	198	203	208	212	217	222	227	232	237	242	247	252	257	262	267
184	189	194	199	204	209	215	220	225	230	235	240	245	250	255	261	266	271	276
190	195	201	206	211	217	222	227	232	238	243	248	254	259	264	269	275	280	285
196	202	207	213	218	224	229	235	240	246	251	256	262	267	273	278	284	289	295
203	208	214	220	225	231	237	242	248	254	259	265	270	278	282	287	293	299	304
209	215	221	227	232	238	244	250	256	262	267	273	279	285	291	296	302	308	314
216	222	228	234	240	246	252	258	264	270	276	282	288	294	300	306	312	318	324
223	229	235	241	247	253	260	266	272	278	284	291	297	303	309	315	322	328	334
230	236	242	249	255	261	268	274	280	287	293	299	306	312	319	325	331	338	344
236	243	249	256	262	269	276	282	289	295	302	308	315	322	328	335	341	348	354
243	250	257	263	270	277	284	291	297	304	311	318	324	331	338	345	351	358	365
250	257	264	271	278	285	292	299	306	313	320	327	334	341	348	355	362	369	376
257	265	272	279	286	293	301	308	315	322	329	338	343	351	358	365	372	379	386
265	272	279	287	294	302	309	316	324	331	338	346	353	361	368	375	383	390	397
272	280	288	295	302	310	318	325	333	340	348	355	363	371	378	386	393	401	408
280	287	295	303	311	319	326	334	342	350	358	365	373	381	389	396	404	412	420
287	295	303	311	319	327	335	343	351	359	367	375	383	391	399	407	415	423	431
295	304	312	320	328	336	344	353	361	369	377	385	394	402	410	418	426	435	443

Figure 7.5 ▶
Pear shape versus apple shape.

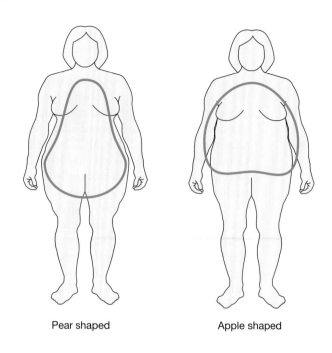

Pear shaped   Apple shaped

Body Fat Distribution

Overwhelming evidence shows that central obesity, as opposed to total obesity assessed by BMI, is associated with the most health risks including diabetes, hypertension, stroke, dyslipidemia, and cardiovascular disease (Ashwell & Gibson, 2014). As far back as the 1940s, researchers noted that a central type fat distribution, commonly referred to as an apple shape, posed greater health risks than when fat was deposited peripherally, or a pear shape (Fig. 7.5). Within the last few decades, there has been general agreement that the health risks, predominately cardiovascular disease and diabetes, are more accurately determined by assessing the relative distribution of excess fat rather than by total fat amount (World Health Organization, 1998).

Waist circumference and waist-to-hip ratio (WHR) have been proposed as screening tools for identifying central obesity. The current waist circumference recognized as central or abdominal obesity in the United States is 40 in or more for men and 35 in or more for women (Alberti et al., 2009). As with BMI, ethnic groups differ in regard to where risk begins in relation to waist circumference.

More recently, WHR has been suggested as a better screening tool than both waist circumference and BMI for cardiometabolic risk factors such as hypertension, diabetes, dyslipidemia, metabolic syndrome, and cardiovascular disease (Ashwell, Gunn, & Gibson, 2012). A study by Ashwell and Gibson (2014) found WHR to be an easy and practical tool that is a good predictor for morbidity and mortality in all ethnic groups. The suggested cutoff value of 0.5 translates to the practical advice of "keep your waist to less than half your height," which the authors suggest can be cheaply and easily determined by a single piece of string.

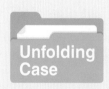
Unfolding Case

Recall Kyla and Garrett. Kyla is 5 ft 5 in tall, currently weighs 150 pounds, and has a waist size of 31 in. Garrett is 6 ft tall, currently weighs 210 pounds, and has a waist size of 36 in. Evaluate their BMI, waist circumference, and WHR.

ENERGY BALANCE IN HEALTH PROMOTION

Energy in health promotion means attaining and maintaining healthy body weight. Healthy body weight is achieved by balancing calorie intake with calorie expenditure. Appropriate calories, PA, and sitting time are discussed in the following sections.

BOX 7.2 — Life Cycle Considerations Regarding Weight

- In children and adolescents, calorie intake must be sufficient to support normal growth and development without promoting excess weight. Overweight and obese children and adolescents should make healthier food choices and increase activity to maintain or reduce their rate of weight gain as linear growth occurs to reduce BMI percentile to a healthier range (USDHHS & USDA, 2015).
- Before becoming pregnant, women should attain and maintain a healthy weight.
- Pregnant women should gain the appropriate amount of weight throughout the course of pregnancy.
- Obese adults should change their eating and activity patterns to prevent additional weight gain and/or promote weight loss.
- Overweight adults should not gain additional weight; those with one or more cardiovascular risk factors, such as hypertension or dyslipidemia, should change their eating and activity patterns to lose weight.
- Overweight or obese adults ages 65 years and older should not gain additional weight. Older obese adults with cardiovascular risk factors can experience improved quality of life and lower risk of chronic disease and disability by achieving intentional weight loss.

Appropriate Calories

The first guideline of the *2015-2020 Dietary Guidelines for Americans* is to "Follow a healthy eating pattern across the lifespan." Expanding upon that, the guideline continues with "choose a healthy eating pattern at an appropriate calorie level" (U.S. Department of Health and Human Services [USDHHS] & U.S. Department of Agriculture [USDA], 2015). An "appropriate" calorie level is one in which the individual is able to attain and maintain healthy weight, achieve an adequate nutrient intake, and reduce the risk of chronic disease.

Table 7.3 can be used as a reference to choose a reasonable calorie level based on age, gender, and activity; the appropriateness of the calorie level is determined by monitoring body weight. Life cycle considerations are highlighted in Box 7.2.

Growing evidence suggests that calorie for calorie, some foods may be more likely to cause weight gain than others and that some foods may be protective against weight gain when their intake is increased (Mozaffarian et al., 2015). High glycemic carbohydrates and red and processed meats are associated with weight gain, whereas an increase in wholesome food intake is associated with relative weight loss over time.

Nutrient Density

Choosing nutrient-dense foods within all food groups helps ensure nutrient needs are met without exceeding calorie limits. Nutrient-dense foods are those that provide significant amounts of nutrients and other beneficial substances relative to the amount of calories provided with little or no solid fats, added sugars, and refined grains. Nutrient-dense items include fruit, vegetables, whole grains, legumes, nuts, low-fat and fat-free dairy, eggs, and lean proteins that are prepared without added solid fats, sugars, refined starches, and sodium. Substituting these healthy choices for calorie-dense items, such as regular soft drinks, most desserts, fried foods, full-fat dairy products, high-fat meat, alcohol, and most fast foods, lowers calorie intake while increasing nutrient intake (Box 7.3). Note that the emphasis is on healthy and wholesome choices, not commercially prepared "junk" foods that have been modified to be "fat free" or "sugar free." Those labels may give the impression that the food is

Quick Bite

Foods most positively associated with weight gain

Potatoes
White bread
White rice
Low-fiber breakfast cereals
Sweets/desserts
Sugar-sweetened beverages
Red and processed meats

Foods associated with weight loss over time when intake is increased

Vegetables
Whole grains
Fruits
Nuts
Legumes
Fish
Yogurt

Source: Smith, J., Hou, T., Ludwig, D., Rimm, E. B., Willett, W., Hu, F. B., & Mozaffarian, D. (2015). Changes in intake of protein foods, carbohydrate amount and quality, and long-term weight change: Results from 3 prospective cohorts. *The American Journal of Clinical Nutrition*, *101*, 1216–1224; and Mozaffarian, D., Hao, T., Rimm, E., Willett, W. C., & Hu, F. B. (2011). Changes in diet and lifestyle and long-term weight gain in women and men. *The New England Journal of Medicine*, *364*, 2392–2404.

BOX 7.3   Steps to a Healthier Weight

Making Nutrient-Dense Food Choices

Here are some foods that contain extra calories from solid fats and added sugars and some "smarter" replacements. Choices on the right side are more nutrient dense—lower in solid fats and added sugars. Try these new ideas instead of your usual choices. This guide gives sample ideas; it is not a complete list. Use the "Nutrition Facts" label to help identify more alternatives.

Instead of . . .	Replace with . . .
Milk Group	
Sweetened fruit yogurt	Plain fat-free yogurt with fresh fruit or vanilla flavoring
Whole milk	Low-fat or fat-free milk
Natural or processed cheese	Low-fat or reduced-fat cheese
Protein Foods	
Beef (corned beef, prime cuts of beef, short ribs, 85% lean or lower ground beef)	Beef round steaks and roasts (eye of round, top round), top sirloin, top loin, 90% lean or higher ground beef
Chicken legs with skin	Chicken breast without skin
Lunch meats (such as bologna)	Low-fat lunch meats (95%–97% fat free)
Hot dogs (regular)	Hot dogs (lower fat)
Bacon or sausage	Canadian bacon or lean ham
Refried beans	Cooked or canned kidney or pinto beans
Grain Group	
Granola	Reduced-fat granola
Sweetened cereals	Unsweetened cereals with cut-up fruit
Pasta with cheese sauce	Pasta with vegetables (primavera)
Pasta with white sauce (alfredo)	Pasta with red sauce (marinara)
Croissants or pastries	Toast or bread (try whole-grain types)
Fruit Group	
Apple or berry pie	Fresh apple or berries
Sweetened applesauce	Unsweetened applesauce
Canned fruit packed in syrup	Canned fruit packed in juice or "lite" syrup
Vegetable Group	
Deep-fried French fries	Oven-baked French fries
Baked potato with cheese sauce	Baked potato with salsa
Fried vegetables	Steamed or roasted vegetables
Solid Fats	
Cream cheese	Light or fat-free cream cheese
Sour cream	Plain low-fat or fat-free yogurt
Regular margarine or butter	Light-spread margarines, diet margarine
Added Sugars	
Sugar-sweetened soft drinks	Seltzer mixed with 100% fruit juice
Sweetened tea or drinks	Unsweetened tea or water
Syrup on pancakes or French toast	Unsweetened applesauce or berries as a topping
Candy, cookies, cake, or pastry	Fresh or dried fruit
Sugar in recipes	Experiment with reducing amount and adding spices (cinnamon, nutmeg, etc.)

Source: ChooseMyPlate.gov. U.S. Department of Agriculture.

also "calorie free," but that is not necessarily true. Fat-free milk is a good choice because milk is a fundamentally healthy food made healthier by the elimination of fat. In contrast, fat-free cookies are still cookies—"treats" made with sugar and refined flour—not an inherently healthy food. In both cases, these fat-free foods still contain calories from protein and carbohydrates.

Plate Method

One strategy to help achieve nutrient density and overall balance is to use the "plate method" of meal planning for lunch and dinner where ½ of the plate is filled with vegetables or both fruits and vegetables, ¼ with whole grains, and ¼ with protein. Fruit and dairy can accompany the meal. SuperTracker (www.choosemyplate.gov) offers ideas for implementing healthy changes and can help plan, analyze, and monitor eating patterns and PA.

Portion Control

Choosing appropriate portion sizes is vital to keep from exceeding calorie limits. Over the last 20 years, portion sizes have grown in restaurants (Table 7.6) (Young & Nestle, 2003) and at home as the size of dinnerware increased (Wansink, 2006). For instance, it has been shown that young children request almost twice as much cereal to eat when given a larger bowl compared to a smaller bowl; older children ate 52% more when given a larger bowl (Wansink, van Ittersum, & Payne, 2014).

Over time, excessive portion sizes distort peoples' perception of how much food is "normal" or necessary and leads to an increase in the amount of food eaten in a single eating occasion (Wansink & van Ittersum, 2007). "Portion distortion" appears to be a widespread problem not linked to income, education, hunger, or body weight (Wansink & van Ittersum, 2007). Even overconsumption of healthy food can lead to a positive calorie balance and weight gain over time.

According to Wansink and van Ittersum (2007), telling people to remind themselves not to overeat is not the answer; changing the environment that led to large portion sizes is easier. For instance, a study by Van Kleef, Shimizu, and Wansink (2013) found that smaller sized portions of common snack foods satisfied participant's ratings of hunger and craving similar to portions 5 to 10 times larger—with considerably fewer calories. Strategies to make food less accessible and less visible include

- Switching to smaller plates, bowls, and glasses
- Buying smaller packages of food at the grocery store; forgo the jumbo size
- Buying prepackaged, portion-controlled items, such as 100-calorie packs
- Storing food out of sight
- Ordering smaller portions at restaurants
- Filling a doggie bag before beginning to eat

Table 7.6	Portion Distortion: A Comparison Between Portion Sizes 20 Years Ago and Today	
	20 Years Ago	**Today**
Bagel	3 in diameter 140 calories	6 in diameter 350 calories
Blueberry muffin	1.5 oz 210 calories	5 oz 500 calories
Chicken Caesar salad	1½ cups 390 calories	3½ cups 790 calories
Coffee	8 oz with whole milk and sugar 45 calories	16 oz with whole milk and mocha syrup 350 calories
French fries	2.4 oz 210 calories	6.9 oz 610 calories
Soda	6.5 oz 85 calories	20 oz 250 calories
Spaghetti with meatballs	1 cup pasta with sauce and 3 meatballs 500 calories	2 cups pasta with sauce and 3 large meatballs 1025 calories
Popcorn	5 cups 270 calories	11 cups 630 calories

Source: U.S. Department of Health and Human Services, National Heart Lung and Blood Institute, National Institutes of Health. (2015). *Portion distortion.* Available at http://www.nhlbi.nih.gov/health/educational/wecan/eat-right/portion-distortion .htm. Accessed on 3/14/16.

Physical Activity

Another key recommendation of the *2015-2020 Dietary Guidelines for Americans* is to meet the *Physical Activity Guidelines for Americans* (USDHHS, 2008). PA is noted to be one of the most important things individuals can do to improve their health. Strong evidence shows that regular PA helps maintain healthy weight, prevent excessive weight gain, and lose weight when combined with a healthy eating pattern that is lower in calories (USDHHS & USDA, 2015). Strong evidence also shows that regular PA lowers the risk of early death, coronary heart disease, stroke, hypertension, dyslipidemia, type 2 diabetes, breast and colon cancer, and metabolic syndrome. Regular physical fitness also improves depression and prevents falls.

The *2008 Physical Activity Guidelines for Americans* (USDHHS, 2008) urge all adults to avoid inactivity (Table 7.7). Although any exercise is better than none, the benefits of increasing activity are dose dependent and occur along a continuum. A minimum of 2 hours and 30 minutes per week of moderate-intensity aerobic activity is recommended to gain substantial health benefits. For more extensive health benefits, 5 hours per week of moderate-intensity aerobic activity are suggested. Additional benefits are obtained with even higher amounts of aerobic activity. Tips for increasing activity appear in Box 7.4. Exercising with the support of others helps maintain motivation.

Table 7.7	**2008 Physical Activity Guidelines for Americans Summary** 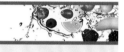

Key Guidelines for Adults

- All adults should avoid inactivity. Some physical activity is better than none, and adults who participate in any amount of physical activity gain some health benefits.
- For substantial health benefits, adults should do at least 150 minutes (2 hours and 30 minutes) a week of moderate-intensity* or 75 minutes (1 hour and 15 minutes) a week of vigorous-intensity** aerobic physical activity, or an equivalent combination of moderate- and vigorous-intensity aerobic activity. Aerobic activity should be performed in episodes of at least 10 minutes, and, preferably, it should be spread throughout the week.
- For additional and more extensive health benefits, adults should increase their aerobic physical activity to 300 minutes (5 hours) a week of moderate-intensity or 150 minutes a week of vigorous-intensity aerobic physical activity, or an equivalent combination of moderate- and vigorous-intensity activity. Additional health benefits are gained by engaging in physical activity beyond this amount.
- Adults should also do muscle-strengthening activities[†] that are moderate or high intensity and involve all major muscle groups on 2 or more days a week, as these activities provide additional health benefits.

Key Guidelines for Older Adults

The Key Guidelines for Adults also apply to older adults. In addition, the following guidelines are just for older adults:
- When older adults cannot do 150 minutes of moderate-intensity aerobic activity a week because of chronic conditions, they should be as physically active as their abilities and conditions allow.
- Older adults should do exercises that maintain or improve balance if they are at risk of falling.
- Older adults should determine their level of effort for physical activity relative to their level of fitness.
- Older adults with chronic conditions should understand whether and how their conditions affect their ability to do regular physical activity safely.

*Moderate-intensity physical activity: aerobic activity that increases a person's heart rate and breathing to some extent. On a scale relative to a person's capacity, moderate-intensity activity is usually a 5 or 6 on a 0 to 10 scale. Brisk walking, dancing, swimming, or bicycling on a level terrain are examples.
**Vigorous-intensity physical activity: aerobic activity that greatly increases a person's heart rate and breathing. On a scale relative to a person's capacity, vigorous-intensity activity is usually a 7 or 8 on a 0 to 10 scale. Jogging, singles tennis, swimming continuous laps, or bicycling uphill are examples.
†Muscle-strengthening activity: physical activity including exercise that increases skeletal muscle strength, power, endurance, and mass. It includes strength training, resistance training, and muscular strength and endurance exercises.
Source: U.S. Department of Health and Human Services. (2008). *2008 Physical activity guidelines for Americans.* Washington, DC: U.S. Department of Health and Human Services. Available at http://www.health.gov/paguidelines. Accessed on 3/11/16.

Concept Mastery Alert

Although exercise should be spread across the week if possible, muscle-strengthening activities for recently ill clients who need to increase their physical activity to prevent further deterioration should be undertaken at least twice a week.

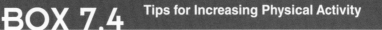

BOX 7.4 Tips for Increasing Physical Activity

- **Find something enjoyable.** The best chance of success comes from choosing a physical activity (PA) that is enjoyable to the individual. The best activity or exercise is one that is performed, not just contemplated.
- **Use the buddy system.** Committing to an exercise program or increased PA with a friend makes the activity less of a chore and helps to sustain motivation.
- **Spread activity over the entire day if desired.** This recommendation is particularly important for people who "don't have time to exercise." Many people find it easier to fit three 10-minute activity periods into a busy lifestyle than to find 30 uninterrupted minutes to dedicate to activity.
- **Start slowly and gradually increase activity.** For people who have been inactive, it is prudent to start with only a few minutes of daily activity, such as walking, and gradually increase the frequency, duration, and then intensity. People with existing health problems such as diabetes, heart disease, and hypertension should consult a physician before beginning a PA program, as should all men older than 40 years and all women older than 50 years.
- **Move more.** Just moving more can make a cumulative difference in activity. Take the stairs instead of the elevator, park at the far end of the parking lot, walk around while talking on the portable phone, walk instead of driving short distances, or play golf without a golf cart or caddy, or fidget.
- **Track it.** Just as people tend to underestimate the amount of food they eat, people usually overestimate the amount of PA they perform. Monitoring PA provides objective data for evaluating progress.

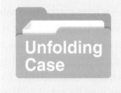

Unfolding Case

Think of Kyla and Garrett. They admit that they get hungry after doing cardio at the gym and may be sabotaging themselves by eating too much afterward. What would you suggest they consume after working out if they cannot wait until the next meal to eat?

In addition to regular aerobic exercises, muscle-strengthening activities that involve all major muscle groups are recommended on 2 or more days a week. Muscle-strengthening activities, which include strength training, resistance training, and strength and endurance exercises, build muscle, which helps to raise metabolic rate and increase the likelihood of weight loss and body fat loss. In both men and women, resistance training exercise can effectively counteract the loss of muscle mass and strength related to aging (Leenders et al., 2013)—and thus increase BMR. Changes in body composition—more muscle, less fat—are positive outcomes of muscle-strengthening activities that are not reflected on the scale, as are improved bone density and decreased risk of osteoporosis.

Sitting Time

Although not all studies show that sitting time is associated with all-cause mortality risk (Pulsford, Stamatakis, Britton, Brunner, & Hillsdon, 2015), emerging evidence suggests that the more time spent sitting, the greater the risk of weight gain (Mozaffarian, Hao, Rimm, Willett, & Hu, 2011), obesity (Hu, Li, Colditz, Willett, & Manson, 2003), type 2 diabetes (Grøntved & Hu, 2011), cardiovascular disease (Wijndaele et al., 2011), and all-cause mortality (Biswas et al., 2015)—independent of moderate to vigorous activity. Studies show that prolonged sitting suppresses lipase and insulin activity in muscles, leading to metabolic abnormalities (Bergouignan, Rudwill, Simon, & Blanc, 2011) and that interrupting prolonged sitting with regular activity breaks is more effective than continuous PA at decreasing postprandial blood glucose and insulin levels (Peddie et al., 2013). Too much overall sitting time may be as important a health risk as too little PA. Strategies to reduce sedentary activity include limiting television viewing and replacing television time with more physically active pursuits.

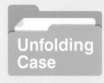

Consider Kyla and Garrett. They should be encouraged to add two to three resistance training sessions per week to their PA routine to build muscle, which will increase metabolic rate and may promote weight loss through increased calorie expenditure. In addition to the cardio exercise they are already doing, what other PA recommendations may be helpful?

How Do You Respond?

Do calories eaten at night promote weight gain? Emerging evidence demonstrates a relationship between the timing of food intake and weight loss success. When overweight and obese women with metabolic syndrome were given a weight loss diet of 1400 calories, those who ate a large breakfast (700 calories) had greater weight loss and reduction in waist circumference than those who ate 700 calories for dinner (Jakubowicz, Barnea, Wainstein, & Froy, 2013). The large breakfast group also had lower fasting glucose and insulin levels and lower serum triglycerides, lower total cholesterol, and higher high-density lipoprotein (HDL) cholesterol. Likewise, a weight loss study found that participants who ate their biggest meal later in the day lost less weight and had a slower rate of weight loss than those whose largest meal was earlier in the day (Garaulet et al., 2013). Eating a large percentage of calories earlier instead of later in the day may be a useful strategy for promoting weight loss and managing and metabolic syndrome.

Which diet is best for losing weight—a low-carbohydrate diet or a low-fat diet?
In 2013, The American College of Cardiology/American Heart Association Task Force on Practice Guidelines and The Obesity Society examined evidence-based literature and concluded that weight loss is similar with all types of diets (e.g., low carbohydrate vs. low fat) as long as the diets achieved the same calorie restriction (Jensen et al., 2014). However, although weight loss may be the same cardiovascular risk markers may be greatly different based on the metabolic status of the individual. Controlled studies have shown that although low-carbohydrate and low-fat diets result in similar weight loss and lowering of fasting glucose levels, low-carbohydrate diets are more beneficial in terms of glycemic variability, serum triglyceride and HDL levels, and blood pressure and may prevent further complications of type 2 diabetes in those who already have type 2 diabetes (Tay et al., 2015). So although weight loss is similar between isocaloric low-carbohydrate and low-fat diets, low-carbohydrate diets may offer more overall improvements in health. More research is needed to determine if manipulating the macronutrient content of a diet can delay or prevent type 2 diabetes in people who are at risk (Apovian, 2015).

REVIEW CASE STUDY

Tonya is 5 ft 3 in tall, weighs 151 pounds, and is 38 years old. Her waist circumference is 37 in. As a receptionist for a law firm and mother of two socially active children, her life is busy but sedentary. She simply does not have the time or energy to stay with an exercise program after working all day and caring for her children. She would like to lose about 20 pounds but knows "dieting" doesn't work for her—all the diets she has tried in the past have left her hungry and feeling deprived. Losing weight has taken on greater importance since her doctor told her that both her blood pressure and glucose level are at "borderline" high levels.

- What is her BMI? Assess her weight based on BMI.
- Estimate her total calorie requirements using the rule-of-thumb method of calculating BMR and adding calories for

a sedentary lifestyle. How does it compare to the level of calories recommended in Table 7.3 for a woman of her age and sedentary lifestyle? Which calorie level do you think is most accurate? Why?
- How many calories would she need to eat to lose 1 pound of weight per week if her activity level stays the same? Two pounds per week? Is a 2-pound weight loss per week a reasonable goal?
- To help her avoid feeling hungry while eating fewer calories, what foods would you recommend she consume more of? She knows she should drink fewer soft drinks. What advice would you give her to help her do that?

STUDY QUESTIONS

1 For most Americans, the largest percentage of their total calories expended daily is from
a. PA
b. Thermal effect of food
c. Basal energy expenditure
d. Sitting

2 The nurse knows her instructions about portion control have been effective when the client verbalizes she will
a. Prepare a doggie bag after she feels she is full enough while eating out
b. Use a smaller dinner plate
c. Be careful not to overfill her cereal bowl when she serves herself from the large, family-sized box
d. Remind herself not to overeat

3 A client asks how she can speed up her metabolism. The best response is
a. "You can't. Metabolic rate is genetically determined."
b. "Ask your doctor to check your thyroid hormone levels. Taking thyroid hormone will stimulate metabolism."
c. "Include resistance training in your exercise program because adding muscle tissue will increase metabolic rate."
d. "Eat fewer calories because that will stimulate metabolic rate."

4 How much weight will a person lose in a week if he eats 500 fewer cal/day than he needs and increases his exercise expenditure by 500 cal/day?
a. 1 pound/week
b. 2 pounds/week
c. 3 pounds/week
d. There isn't enough information provided to estimate weekly weight loss.

5 Using a simple formula based on calories, how many calories per day would a healthy-weight adult who weighs 70 kg need?
a. 2350 to 2800 calories
b. 2100 to 2350 calories
c. 1750 to 2100 calories
d. 1400 to 1750 calories

6 Waist circumference is an indicator of
a. Percentage of body fat
b. Abdominal fat content
c. The ratio of body fat to muscle mass
d. BMI

7 Which of the following substitutions results in a healthier choice?
a. Eye of round steak instead of beef short rib
b. Refried beans instead of cooked or canned pinto beans
c. Natural cheese instead of low-fat cheese
d. Baked potato with cheese sauce instead of baked potato with salsa

8 A BMI of 26 is classified as
a. Normal
b. Overweight
c. Class 1 obesity
d. Class 2 obesity

KEY CONCEPTS

- Calories are a measure of energy. The body obtains calories from carbohydrates, protein, fat, and alcohol.
- Basal metabolism refers to the calories used to conduct the involuntary activities of the body, such as beating the heart and inflating the lungs. For most Americans, basal metabolism accounts for approximately 60% to 70% of total daily calories used.
- The sum of calories spent on basal metabolism and PA represent a person's total calorie expenditure.
- The thermic effect of food is the cost of digesting, absorbing, and metabolizing food. At about 10% of total calories consumed, it is a small part of total energy requirements and is often not factored into the total energy equation.
- Estimated calorie needs per day are based on gender, age, and PA level. Sedentary adult women need approximately 1600 to 2000 cal/day, and sedentary adult men need 2000 to 2600 cal/day.

- Desirable weight is defined as weight for height that is statistically correlated to good health.
- BMI is the most widely used method of evaluating weight status, but it does not account for how weight is distributed. Overweight is defined as a BMI of 25 to 29.9; obesity is defined as a BMI of 30 or higher.
- Waist circumference is a tool to assess for central obesity. "Apples" (people with upper body obesity) have more health risks than "pears" (people with lower body obesity).
- WHR is a good predictor or morbidity and mortality among all ethnic groups. The ratio should be less than 0.5.
- Virtually all health agencies urge people to attain and maintain healthy body weight.
- The *2015-2020 Dietary Guidelines for Americans* urge Americans to consume a healthy eating pattern within an appropriate calorie level.

- Important concepts inherent in choosing an appropriate calorie level healthy eating pattern include variety, nutrient density, and portion control. Portion sizes have grown over the last two decades, and people often overestimate how much food they really need. Portion control is facilitated by eating less at restaurants, using smaller dinner plates, and buying prepackaged, portion-controlled foods.

- The vast majority of Americans do not get the recommended amount of PA. The benefits of PA are dose dependent.
- Exercise leads to only modest weight loss if calories are not also restricted. In the long term, exercise promotes weight loss by promoting fat loss and preventing loss of muscle, which contributes to metabolic rate.
- Too much sitting time may be as great a health risk as too little PA.

Check Your Knowledge Answer Key

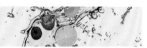

1 **TRUE** Calorie is a unit of measure pertaining to energy in foods. Thus, a food that is high in "energy" is high in calories.
2 **TRUE** One pound of body fat is equivalent to 3500 calories. In theory, to lose 1 pound of weight per week, a daily deficit of 500 calories for 7 days is necessary, whether from eating less, doing more, or both.
3 **TRUE** People of either gender with a high distribution of abdominal fat ("apples") have a greater health risk than people with excess fat in the hips and thighs ("pears").
4 **FALSE** The formulas to calculate BMI are used for either men or women.
5 **TRUE** Calorie-dense foods have relatively high levels of calories for the amount of nutrients they provide.
6 **TRUE** On average, basal metabolism accounts for 60% to 70% of total calories expended in a day. Active people use a smaller percentage of total calories on BMR.

7 **TRUE** Building muscle speeds metabolic rate because lean tissue is metabolically active compared with fat tissue, which is relatively inert and requires few calories to exist.
8 **FALSE** Activity does not need to be sustained for any given duration to provide health benefits. Snippets of activity accumulated over the entire day can provide the same health benefits as one exercise session of the same total length of time.
9 **TRUE** Sitting too much, even if PA goals are met, is a health risk.
10 **TRUE** Foods with added sugar and solid fat have greater calorie density than foods prepared without added sugar and solid fat, making them more nutrient dense. Focusing on nutrient-dense foods can help control calorie intake.

Student Resources on the Point®
For additional learning materials, activate the code in the front of this book at
http://thePoint.lww.com/activate

Websites

2015-2020 Dietary Guidelines for Americans at http://health.gov/dietaryguidelines/2015/guidelines/

American College of Sports Medicine at www.acsm.org

American Council on Exercise at www.acefitness.org

Calculate your own BEE at http://www-users.med.cornell.edu/~spon/picu/calc/beecalc.htm

National Institute of Diabetes and Digestive and Kidney Diseases, Weight-control Information Network at http://www.niddk.nih.gov/health-information/health-communication-programs/win/Pages/community-groups-organizations.aspx

President's Council on Physical Fitness and Sports at www.fitness.gov

References

Alberti, K., Eckel, R., Grundy, S., Zimmet, P. Z., Cleeman, J. I., Donato, K. A., . . . Smith, S. C., Jr. (2009). Harmonizing the metabolic syndrome: A joint interim statement of the International Diabetes Federation Task Force on Epidemiology and Prevention; National Heart, Lung, and Blood Institute: American Heart Association; World Heart Federation; International Atherosclerosis Society; and International Association for the Study of Obesity. *Circulation, 120,* 1640–1645.

American Diabetes Association & Academy of Nutrition and Dietetics. (2014). *Choose your foods: Food Lists for weight management.* Alexandria, VA: American Diabetes Association.

Apovian, C. (2015). The low-fat, low-carb debate and the theory of relativity. *The American Journal of Clinical Nutrition, 102,* 719–720.

Ashwell, M., & Gibson, S. (2014). A proposal for a primary screening tool: "Keep your waist circumference to less than half your height." *BMC Medicine, 12,* 207. doi:10.1186/s12916-014-0207-1

Ashwell, M., Gunn, P., & Gibson, S. (2012). Waist-to-height ratio is a better screening tool than waist circumference and BMI for adult cardiometabolic risk factors: Systematic review and meta-analysis. *Obesity Reviews, 13,* 275–286.

Bei-Fan, Z., & Cooperative Meta-Analysis Group of Working Group on Obesity in China. (2002). Predictive values of body mass index and waist circumference for risk factors of certain related diseases in

Chinese adults: Study on optimal cut-off points of body mass index and waist circumference in Chinese adults. *Asia Pacific Journal of Clinical Nutrition, 11*(Suppl. 8), S685–S693.

Bergouignan, A., Rudwill, F., Simon, C., & Blanc, S. (2011). Physical inactivity as the culprit of metabolic inflexibility: Evidence from bed-rest studies. *Journal of Applied Physiology, 111*, 1201–1210.

Biswas, A., Oh, P., Faulkner, G., Bajaj, R. R., Silver, M. A., Mitchell, M. S., & Alter, D. A. (2015). Sedentary time and its association with risk for disease incidence, mortality, and hospitalization in adults: A systematic review and meta-analysis. *Annals of Internal Medicine, 162*, 123–132.

Després, J. (2012). Body fat distribution and risk of cardiovascular disease: An update. *Circulation, 126*, 1301–1313.

Garaulet, M., Gómez-Abellán, P., Alburquerque-Béjar, J., Lee, Y. C., Ordovás, J. M., & Scheer, F. A. (2013). Timing of food intake predicts weight loss effectiveness. *International Journal of Obesity, 37*, 604–611.

Grøntved, A., & Hu, F. (2011). Television viewing and risk of type 2 diabetes, cardiovascular disease, and all-cause mortality: A meta-analysis. *JAMA, 305*, 2448–2455.

Hsu, W., Araneta, M., Kanaya, A., Chiang, J., & Fujimoto, W. (2015). BMI cut points to identify at-risk Asian Americans for type 2 diabetes screening. *Diabetes Care, 38*, 150–158.

Hu, F. B., Li, T., Colditz, G., Willett, W. C., & Manson, J. E. (2003). Television watching and other sedentary behaviors in relation to risk of obesity and type 2 diabetes mellitus in women. *JAMA, 289*, 1785–1791.

Jakubowicz, D., Barnea, M., Wainstein, J., & Froy, O. (2013). High caloric intake at breakfast vs. dinner differentially influences weight loss of overweight and obese women. *Obesity, 21*, 2504–2512.

Jensen, M., Ryan, D., Apovian, C., Ard, J. D., Comuzzie, A. G., Donato, K. A., . . . Yanovski, S. Z. (2014). 2013 AHA/ACC/TOS guideline for the management of overweight and obesity in adults: A report of the American College of Cardiology/American Heart Association Task Force on Practice Guidelines and The Obesity Society. *Journal of the American College of Cardiology, 63*(25, Pt. B), 2985–3023.

Leenders, M., Verdijk, L., van der Hoeven, L., van Kranenburg, J., Nilwik, R., & van Loon, L. J. (2013). Elderly men and women benefit equally from prolonged resistance-type exercise training. *The Journals of Gerontology. Series A: Biological Sciences and Medical Sciences, 68*, 769–779.

Low, S., Chin, M. C., Ma, S., Heng, D., & Deurenberg-Yap, M. (2009). Rationale for redefining obesity in Asians. *Annals of the Academy of Medicine, Singapore, 38*, 66–69.

Misra, A., Chowbey, P., Makkar, B. M., Vikram, N. K., Wasir, J. S., Chadha, D., . . . Munjal, Y. P. (2009). Consensus statement for diagnosis of obesity, abdominal obesity and the metabolic syndrome for Asian Indians and recommendations for physical activity, medical and surgical management. *The Journal of the Association of Physicians of India, 57*, 163–170.

Mozaffarian, D., Benjamin, E., Go, A. S., Arnett, D., Blaha, M. J., Cushman, M., . . . Turner, M. B. (2015). Heart disease and stroke statistics—2016 update: A report from the American Heart Association. *Circulation, 133*, e38–e360. doi:10.1161/CIR.0000000000000350

Mozaffarian, D., Hao, T., Rimm, E., Willett, W. C., & Hu, F. B. (2011). Changes in diet and lifestyle and long-term weight gain in women and men. *The New England Journal of Medicine, 364*, 2392–2404.

National Institutes of Health. (1998). Clinical guidelines on the identification, evaluation, and treatment of overweight and obesity in adults—the evidence report. *Obesity Research, 6*(Suppl. 2), 51S–209S.

Peddie, M., Bone, J., Rehrer, N., Skeaff, C. M., Gray, A. R., & Perry, T. L. (2013). Breaking prolonged sitting reduces postprandial glycemia in healthy, normal-weight adults: A randomized crossover trial. *The American Journal of Clinical Nutrition, 98*, 358–366.

Pulsford, R., Stamatakis, E., Britton, A., Brunner, E. J., & Hillsdon, M. (2015). Associations of sitting behaviours with all-cause mortality over a 16-year follow-up: The Whitehall II study. *International Journal of Epidemiology, 44*, 1909–1916.

Smith, J., Hou, T., Ludwig, D., Rimm, E. B., Willett, W., Hu, F. B., & Mozaffarian, D. (2015). Changes in intake of protein foods, carbohydrate amount and quality, and long-term weight change: Results from 3 prospective cohorts. *The American Journal of Clinical Nutrition, 101*, 1216–1224.

Tay, J., Luscombe-Marsh, N., Thompson, C., Noakes, M., Buckley, J. D., Wittert, G. A., . . . Brinkworth, G. D. (2015). Comparison of low- and high-carbohydrate diets for type 2 diabetes management: A randomized trial. *The American Journal of Clinical Nutrition, 102*, 780–790.

U.S. Department of Health and Human Services. (2008). *Physical activity guidelines for Americans*. Washington, DC: U.S. Department of Health and Human Services. Available at www.health.gov/paguidelines. Accessed on 3/12/16.

U.S. Department of Health and Human Services & U.S. Department of Agriculture. (2015). *2015-2020 Dietary guidelines for Americans* (8th ed.). Available at http://health.gov/dietaryguidelines/2015/guidelines/. Accessed on 3/14/16.

Van Kleef, E., Shimizu, M., & Wansink, B. (2013). Just a bite: Considerably smaller snack portions satisfy delayed hunger and craving. *Food Quality and Preference, 27*, 96–100.

Wansink, B. (2006). *Mindless eating: Why we eat more than we think*. New York, NY: Bantam Dell.

Wansink, B., & van Ittersum, K. (2007). Portion size me: Downsizing our consumption norms. *Journal of the American Dietetic Association, 107*, 1103–1106.

Wansink, B., van Ittersum, K., & Payne, C. (2014). Larger bowl size increases the amount of cereal children request, consume, and waste. *The Journal of Pediatrics, 164*, 323–326.

Wijndaele, K., Brage, S., Besson, H., Khaw, K. T., Sharp, S. J., Luben, R., . . . Ekelund, U. (2011). Television viewing and incident cardiovascular disease: Prospective associations and mediation analysis in the EPIC Norfolk Study. *PLoS One, 6*, e20058.

World Health Organization. (1998). *Obesity: Preventing and managing the global epidemic. Report of a WHO consultation on obesity, Geneva 3–5 June 1997*. Geneva, Switzerland: Author.

Young, L., & Nestle, M. (2003). Expanding portion sizes in the US marketplace: Implications for nutritional counseling. *Journal of the American Dietetic Association, 103*, 231–234.

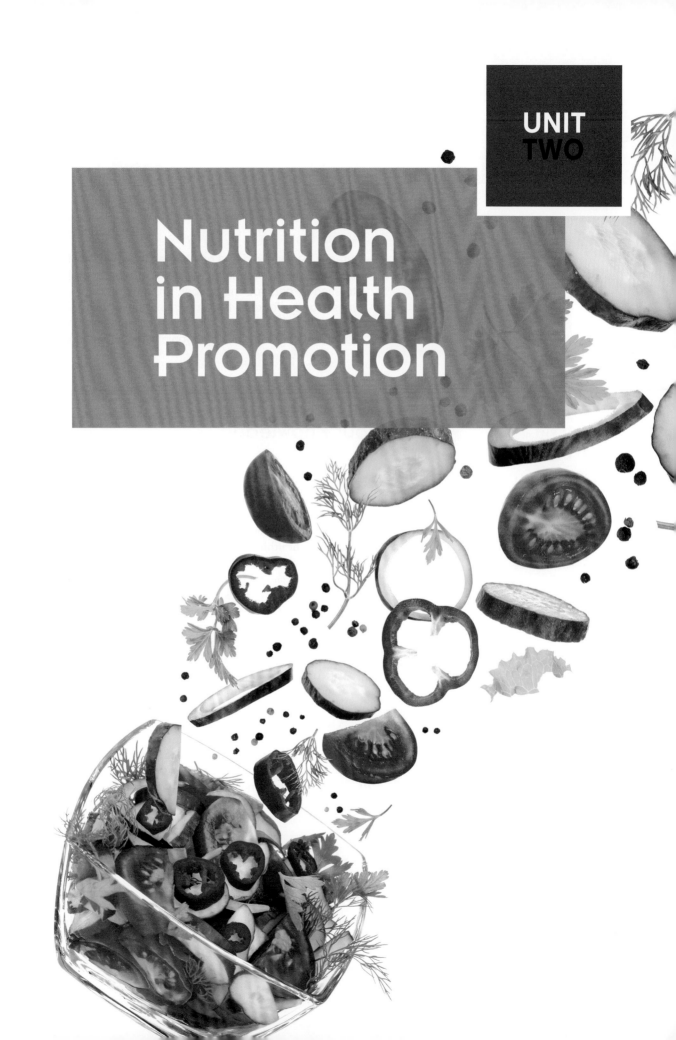

Nutrition in Health Promotion

Chapter 8

Guidelines for Healthy Eating

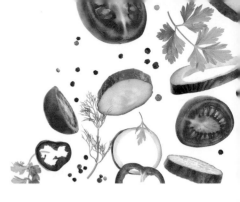

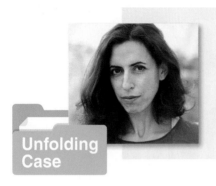

Unfolding Case

Aurea Espada

Aurea is 30 years old and has battled ulcerative colitis for more than 10 years. Medication helps keep her in remission, but when she is stressed or eats too much fiber, she has diarrhea, which is sometimes bloody. To keep her gut calm, she avoids fruits, vegetables, and whole grains. She worries that her diet lacks healthy foods and that she is at greater risk of chronic disease because of it.

Check Your Knowledge

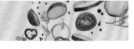

True	False		
☐	☐	**1**	The Recommended Dietary Allowances (RDAs) are intended for healthy people only.
☐	☐	**2**	The Dietary Reference Intakes (DRIs) are useful to teach people how to choose a healthier diet.
☐	☐	**3**	The Tolerable Upper Intake Level (UL) is the optimal level of nutrients that people should try to consume.
☐	☐	**4**	All nutrients have an established RDA.
☐	☐	**5**	The *Dietary Guidelines for Americans* are intended to help people attain and maintain a healthy weight, reduce the risk of chronic disease, and promote wellness in Americans 2 years of age and older.
☐	☐	**6**	A Mediterranean-style eating pattern is named the single preferred eating pattern because it reflects the *Dietary Guidelines for Americans*.
☐	☐	**7**	A food that is nutrient dense has a high amount of calories for the amount of nutrients it supplies.
☐	☐	**8**	A serving is the amount of food usually consumed at one time.
☐	☐	**9**	The MyPlate graphic features a dinner plate with ½ the plate devoted to meat, ¼ devoted to vegetables, and ¼ devoted to grains with milk and fruit served alongside.
☐	☐	**10**	The American Cancer Society and the American Heart Association both recommend a plant-based diet to reduce the risk of chronic disease.

Learning Objectives

Upon completion of this chapter, you will be able to

1 Describe the four sets of standards that compose the Dietary Reference Intakes.
2 Explain what the Recommended Dietary Allowances represent.
3 Summarize the *2015-2020 Dietary Guidelines for Americans*.
4 Give examples of nutrient-dense foods.

5 Describe how the Healthy U.S.-Style Eating Pattern differs from a typical American eating pattern.

6 Describe how the Healthy U.S.-Style Eating Pattern differs from the Healthy Mediterranean-Style Eating Pattern and the Healthy Vegetarian Eating Pattern.

7 Compare nutrition recommendations from the American Heart Association, the American Cancer Society, and the American Institute for Cancer Research.

Who determines how much of each nutrient people need and how much is too much? What is the right combination and proportion of foods that must be consumed in order to be healthy? This chapter covers nutrient needs and how they translate into food and eating patterns. Topics include the *Dietary Guidelines for Americans* and its companion tool MyPlate, a comparison of guidelines issued by leading health agencies, and a sampling of guidelines and graphics from other countries.

DIETARY REFERENCE INTAKES

Dietary Reference Intakes (DRIs)
a set of four nutrient-based reference values used to plan and evaluate diets.

Recommended Dietary Allowances (RDAs)
the average daily dietary intake level sufficient to meet the nutrient requirement of 97% to 98% of healthy individuals in a particular life stage and gender group.

In the early 1990s, Canadian scientists and the Food and Nutrition Board of the Institute of Medicine embarked on a comprehensive, multiyear project to update and expand nutrient intake recommendations. Based on the results of thousands of research studies, nutrition experts produced a series of in-depth reports featuring a new set of references called **Dietary Reference Intakes (DRIs)** that estimate nutrient needs for healthy people. The reports are summarized in *Dietary Reference Intakes: The Essential Guide to Nutrient Requirements* (Institute of Medicine, 2006). Recommendations are made for vitamins, minerals, carbohydrates, protein, fat, cholesterol, fiber, electrolytes, and water. The DRIs is a group name for four separate reference sets:

- **Recommended Dietary Allowances (RDAs)**
- Estimated Average Requirement
- Adequate Intake
- Tolerable Upper Intake Level

Each of these reference values has a specific purpose and represents a different level of intake (Fig. 8.1). Nutrients have either an RDA or an Adequate Intake; not all nutrients have an established Tolerable Upper Intake Level (Table 8.1). Each reference value is viewed as an average daily intake over time, at least 1 week for most nutrients. Summary tables of the DRIs appear in Appendices 1, 2, and 3. Additional reference values include Acceptable Macronutrient Distribution Ranges and an Estimated Energy Requirement.

DRIs are used by scientists and nutritionists who work in research or academic settings and by dietitians who plan menus for specific populations, such as elderly, schools, prisons, hospitals, nursing homes, and military feeding programs. They are also used to assess the adequacy of an individual's intake by comparing estimated intake with estimated requirements. Keep in mind that

Figure 8.1 ▶
Representation of DRI along a continuum of intake.

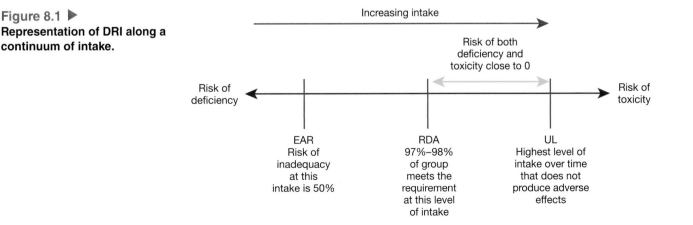

Table 8.1	Standards Applied to Each Nutrient for People Age 1 Year and Older		
Nutrient	**RDA**	**AI**	**UL***
Total water		✓	
Macronutrients			
Carbohydrate	✓		
Fiber		✓	
Linoleic acid		✓	
Alpha-linolenic acid		✓	
Protein	✓		
Fat-soluble vitamins			
Vitamin A	✓		✓
Vitamin D	✓		✓
Vitamin E	✓		✓
Vitamin K		✓	
Water-soluble vitamins			
Thiamin	✓		
Riboflavin	✓		
Niacin	✓		✓
Vitamin B_6	✓		✓
Folate	✓		✓
Vitamin B_{12}	✓		
Pantothenic acid		✓	
Biotin		✓	
Choline		✓	
Vitamin C	✓		
Elements			
Calcium	✓		✓
Chromium		✓	
Copper	✓		✓
Fluoride		✓	✓
Iodine	✓		✓
Iron	✓		✓
Magnesium	✓		✓
Manganese		✓	✓
Molybdenum	✓		✓
Phosphorus	✓		✓
Selenium	✓		✓
Zinc	✓		✓
Potassium		✓	
Sodium		✓	✓
Chloride		✓	✓

*An Upper Intake Level (UL) has also been established for boron and nickel even though neither nutrient has a Recommended Dietary Allowance (RDA) or Adequate Intake (AI).

obtaining a reliable estimate of a person's actual intake is difficult due to reporting errors, flaws in estimating portion sizes, and day-to-day variation in food intake. Unless a person has participated in a nutrient requirement study, it is impossible to quantify exact nutrient requirements for an individual. Because consumers eat food and not nutrients, the DRIs are not suited to teaching people how to make healthy choices.

Recommended Dietary Allowances

The RDAs represent the average daily recommended intake to meet the nutrient requirements of 97% to 98% of healthy individuals by life stage and gender. The recommendations are based on specific criteria indicators for estimating requirements, such as plasma and serum nutrient concentrations, and are set high enough to account for daily variations in intake. When estimating the nutritional needs of people with health disorders, health professionals use the RDAs as a starting point and adjust the values according to the individual's need.

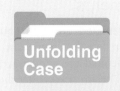

Think of Aurea. During periods of exacerbation, her nutrient needs increase related to impaired nutrient absorption secondary to inflammation and diarrhea. The RDA and other DRI references are intended for healthy people only and thus may not reflect Aurea's actual needs during periods of exacerbation. Unfortunately, evidence-based diet recommendations do not exist for patients with inflammatory bowel disease other than to follow a healthy and varied diet. How can she achieve that goal given her food intolerances? Would she benefit from a multivitamin and mineral supplement? What nutrients and nonnutrient substances are not found in multivitamin and mineral supplements that are also important for health?

Estimated Average Requirement

Estimated Average Requirement (EAR)
the nutrient intake estimated to meet the requirement of half of the healthy individuals in a particular life stage and gender group.

Estimated Average Requirement (EAR) values are used to determine RDA values; they are not used as a stand-alone reference. The EAR is the amount of a nutrient that is estimated to meet the requirement of half of healthy people in a lifestyle or gender group. "Average" actually means *median*. By definition, the EAR exceeds the requirements of half of the group and falls below the requirements of the other half. The EAR is not based solely on the prevention of nutrient deficiencies but includes consideration for reducing the risk of chronic disease and takes into account the bioavailability of the nutrient—that is, how its absorption is affected by other food components.

Adequate Intake

Adequate Intake (AI)
an intake level thought to meet or exceed the requirement of almost all members of a life stage and gender group. An AI is set when there are insufficient data to define an RDA.

An **Adequate Intake (AI)** is set when an RDA cannot be determined due to lack of sufficient data on requirements. It is a recommended average daily intake level thought to meet or exceed the needs of virtually all members of a life stage or gender group based on observed or experimentally determined estimates of nutrient intake by groups of healthy people. The primary purpose of the AI is as a goal for the nutrient intake of individuals. This is similar to the use of the RDA except that the RDA is expected to meet the needs of almost all healthy people, while in the case of an AI, it is not known what percentage of people are covered.

Tolerable Upper Intake Level

Tolerable Upper Intake Level (UL)
the highest average daily intake level of a nutrient likely to pose no danger to most individuals in the group.

The **Tolerable Upper Intake Level (UL)** is the highest level of average daily nutrient intake that is likely to pose no risk of adverse health effects to almost all individuals in the general population. It is not intended to be a recommended level of intake; there is no benefit in consuming amounts greater than the RDA or AI.

Acceptable Macronutrient Distribution Ranges

Acceptable Macronutrient Distribution Ranges (AMDRs)
an intake range as a percentage of total calories for energy nutrients.

The **Acceptable Macronutrient Distribution Ranges (AMDRs)** are broad ranges for each energy nutrient, expressed as a percentage of total calories consumed. These ranges are associated with reduced risk of chronic disease and are such that an AI of all nutrients can be obtained. Over time, intakes above or below this range may increase the risk of chronic disease or deficiency, respectively. The AMDRs for adults are as follows:

	% Total Calories Consumed
Carbohydrate	45–65
Protein	10–35
Fat	20–35
Linoleic acid (*n*-6)	5–10
Alpha-linolenic acid (*n*-3)	0.6–1.2

Estimated Energy Requirements

Estimated Energy Requirements (EERs) level of calorie intake estimated to maintain weight in normal-weight individuals based on age, gender, height, weight, and activity.

Similar to the EAR, the **Estimated Energy Requirements (EERs)** are defined as the dietary energy intake predicted to maintain energy balance in healthy, normal-weight individuals of a defined age, gender, weight, height, and level of physical activity consistent with good health. Exceeding the EER may produce weight gain. See Chapter 7 for more on determining energy needs.

FROM NUTRIENTS TO FOOD: HEALTHY EATING

Healthy eating guidelines translate the science of nutrient needs into evidence-based recommendations for eating patterns to meet those needs. A healthy eating pattern not only provides adequate amounts of all essential nutrients but also helps people attain and maintain healthy body weight, promotes overall health, and reduces the risk of chronic disease. Prominent characteristics of healthy eating patterns are the following:

- Variety—in the color of fruits and vegetables, the selections within each group, and methods of cooking
- Balance—all food groups are included in reasonable proportions
- Moderation—limited amounts of saturated fat, added sugars, and sodium; moderate amounts of alcohol and coffee if adults so choose
- Individually appropriate—calorically, culturally, personally, and economically
- No foods are prohibited

Dietary Guidelines for Americans

The *Dietary Guidelines for Americans* (DGA), published jointly every 5 years since 1980 by the U.S. Department of Health and Human Services (USDHHS) and the U.S. Department of Agriculture (USDA), are a report containing nutritional and dietary information and guidelines for the general public. It serves as the federal policy on nutrition, dictating how education, communication, and food assistance programs are conducted by the government. They are evidence-based recommendations designed for professionals to help people ages 2 years and older consume a healthy, nutritionally adequate diet.

As the science of nutrition has evolved, so have the DGA; the 2015–2020 version focuses on healthy eating patterns as a whole rather than individual components such as food groups and nutrients. This shift in focus is in recognition of the interactive and potentially cumulative effects food components can have on health (USDHHS & USDA, 2015). A focus on eating patterns is supported by results of studies that examine the relationship between eating patterns, health, and risk of disease. The 2015–2020 DGA contain five overarching guidelines that encourage healthy eating patterns that are proposed as a framework rather than a rigid requirement. Key recommendations are included to help Americans implement the guidelines in their entirety. Americans are urged to make gradual changes in their eating patterns by shifting their food choices to higher quality selections. The guidelines and recommendations are featured in Box 8.1.

To illustrate how the guidelines and recommendations translate into types and amounts of food, the DGA feature three styles of different healthy eating patterns. Within each style, there are 12 different calorie levels, ranging from 1000 to 3200 calories in 200-calorie increments. This wide range of calorie levels is intended to meet the needs of individuals across the lifespan. Each style lists recommended amounts of food within each food group for each calorie level. Table 8.2 compares each of the styles at 1600- and 2000-calorie levels. The styles are summarized in the following sections.

Healthy U.S.-Style Eating Pattern

This pattern is based on the types and proportions of foods Americans typically consume but in nutrient-dense forms and appropriate amounts. The most notable difference from the typical

---

BOX 8.1 **2015–2020 Dietary Guidelines for Americans**

The Guidelines

1. Follow a healthy eating pattern across the lifespan. All food and beverage choices matter. Choose a healthy eating pattern at an appropriate calorie level to help achieve and maintain a healthy body weight, support nutrient adequacy, and reduce the risk of chronic disease.
2. Focus on variety, nutrient density, and amount. To meet nutrient needs within calorie limits, choose a variety of nutrient-dense foods across and within all food groups in recommended amounts.
3. Limit calories from added sugars and saturated fats and reduce sodium intake. Consume an eating pattern low in added sugars, saturated fats, and sodium. Cut back on foods and beverages higher in these components to amounts that fit within healthy eating patterns.
4. Shift to healthier food and beverage choices. Choose nutrient-dense foods and beverages across and within all food groups in place of less healthy choices. Consider cultural and personal preferences to make these shifts easier to accomplish and maintain.
5. Support healthy eating patterns for all. Everyone has a role in helping to create and support healthy eating patterns in multiple settings nationwide, from home to school to work to communities.

Key Recommendations

Consume a healthy eating pattern that accounts for all foods and beverages within an appropriate calorie level.

A Healthy Eating Pattern Includes

- A variety of vegetables from all of the subgroups—dark green, red and orange, legumes (beans and peas), starchy, and other
- Fruits, especially whole fruits
- Grains, at least half of which are whole grains
- Fat-free or low-fat dairy, including milk, yogurt, cheese, and/ or fortified soy beverages
- A variety of protein foods, including seafood, lean meats and poultry, eggs, legumes (beans and peas), and nuts, seeds, and soy products
- Oils

A Healthy Eating Pattern Limits

- Saturated fats and *trans* fats, added sugars, and sodium

Key recommendations that are quantitative are provided for several components of the diet that should be limited. These components are of particular public health concern in the United States, and the specified limits can help individuals achieve healthy eating patterns within calorie limits:

- Consume less than 10% of calories per day from added sugars.
- Consume less than 10% of calories per day from saturated fats.
- Consume less than 2,300 mg per day of sodium.
- If alcohol is consumed, it should be consumed in moderation— up to 1 drink per day for women and up to 2 drinks per day for men—and only by adults of legal drinking age.

Source: U.S. Department of Health and Human Services & U.S. Department of Agriculture. (2015). *2015-2020 Dietary guidelines for Americans* (8th ed.). Available at http://health.gov/dietaryguidelines/2015/guidelines/. Accessed on 3/15/16.

American pattern is the reduction of meat and poultry. Although this style is designed to meet the nutritional needs of almost all healthy people, the amounts of vitamin D, vitamin E, potassium, and choline are marginal or less than the RDA or AI for many or all age and gender groups. Of these nutrients, low intakes of potassium and vitamin D are of most concern.

Healthy Mediterranean-Style Eating Pattern

This pattern modifies the Healthy U.S.-Style Eating Pattern to more closely resemble a traditional Mediterranean diet. Because there is not a single defined standard Mediterranean diet, this eating pattern is based on the food intakes of groups of people studied who displayed positive health outcomes related to a Mediterranean-type diet. A traditional Mediterranean diet is higher in unsaturated fat than a typical American diet, but because the Healthy U.S.-Style Eating Pattern was designed to incorporate more oils, the Healthy Mediterranean-Style Eating Pattern features the same amount of oil as the U.S.-style pattern. However, it is higher in fruits and seafood and contains less dairy. It is comparable to the U.S. pattern in nutrient content except that it is lower in calcium and vitamin D related to lower amounts of dairy.

Healthy Vegetarian Eating Pattern

This pattern is a modified Healthy U.S.-Style Eating Pattern made to resemble eating patterns reported by self-identified vegetarians. This pattern differs in that eggs are included but meat,

Table 8.2	1600- and 2000-Calorie Levels for the Healthy U.S.-Style Eating Pattern, Healthy Mediterranean-Style Eating Pattern, and the Healthy Vegetarian Eating Pattern					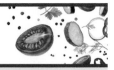
	Healthy U.S.-Style Eating Pattern		Healthy Mediterranean-Style Eating Pattern		Healthy Vegetarian Eating Pattern	
Calorie level of pattern	1600	2000	1600	2000	1600	2000
Daily Amount of Food from Each Group (vegetable and protein foods subgroup amounts are per week)						
Vegetables	2 c-eq	2½ c-eq	2 c-eq	2½ c-eq	2 c-eq	2½ c-eq
Dark green vegetables (c-eq/wk)	1½	1½	1½	1½	1½	1½
Red and orange vegetables (c-eq/wk)	4	5½	4	5½	4	5½
Legumes (c-eq/wk)	1	1½	1	1½	1	1½
Starchy vegetables (c-eq/wk)	4	5	4	5	4	5
Other vegetables (c-eq/wk)	3½	4	3½	4	3½	4
Fruits	1½ c-eq	2 c-eq	2 c-eq	2½ c-eq	1½ c-eq	2 c-eq
Grains	5 oz-eq	6 oz-eq	5 oz-eq	6 oz-eq	5½ oz-eq	6½ oz-eq
Whole grains (oz-eq/d)	3	3	3	3	3	3½
Refined grains (oz-eq/d)	2	3	2	3	2½	3
Dairy	3 c-eq	3 c-eq	2 c-eq	2 c-eq	3 c-eq	3 c-eq
Protein foods	5 oz-eq	5½ oz-eq	5½ oz-eq	6½ oz-eq	2½ oz-eq	3½ oz-eq
Seafood (oz-eq/wk)	8	8	11	15		
Meats, poultry, eggs (oz-eq/wk)	23	26	23	26	3 egg oz-eq/wk	3 egg oz-eq/wk
Nuts, seeds, soy products (oz-eq/wk)	4	5	4	5	6 nuts and seeds (oz-eq/wk)	7 nuts and seeds (oz-eq/wk)
					6 soy products (oz-eq/wk)	8 soy products (oz-eq/wk)
Legumes (oz-eq/wk)					4	6
Oils (g)	22	27	22	27	22	27
Limit on calories for other uses, calories (% of calories)	130 (8%)	270 (14%)	140 (9%)	260 (13%)	180 (11%)	290 (15%)

All foods are assumed to be in nutrient-dense forms, lean or low-fat, and prepared without added fats, sugars, refined starches, or salt.

poultry, and seafood are excluded. Soy products, legumes, nuts and seeds, and whole grains are provided in higher amounts, and the limit of calories for other uses is slightly higher compared to the Healthy U.S.-Style Eating Pattern. Dairy, like eggs, are included because they are consumed by the majority of vegetarians studied. Because of the differences in foods included, this style is slightly higher in calcium and fiber and provides less vitamin D than the U.S.-Style Pattern.

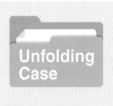

Unfolding Case

Consider Aurea. She excludes fruits, vegetables, and whole grains from her eating pattern to avoid aggravating her bowel. Is this necessary, or are some fruits, vegetables, and whole grains lower in fiber and therefore possibly easier for her to tolerate? Would her tolerance improve with smaller portions consumed more often?

Underlying Concepts of Healthy Eating

Inherent in all three styles of healthy eating patterns is an emphasis on choosing nutrient-dense foods and portion control to avoid exceeding calorie limits. Each pattern limits calories for other uses and promotes variety.

Quick Bite

This amount . . .	Looks like . . .
1 cup cooked vegetables	a woman's tight fist
1 baked potato	a computer mouse
3 oz of meat or chicken	deck of cards
2 tbsp of peanut butter or hummus	a ping-pong ball
1 ½ oz of cheese	regular size dice
1 oz of nuts	a scant average adult woman's handful
½ cup cooked pasta, rice, or cereal	½ baseball
1 medium-sized piece of fruit	a tennis ball
1 tbsp margarine, butter, mayonnaise, or oil	a poker chip

Source: Patritto, L. (2013). Estimate food portions with handy, everyday items. Available at http://msue.anr.msu.edu/news/estimate_food_portions_with_handy_everyday_items. Accessed on 11/17/16.

Serving Size
the amount of food "officially" recommended, for example, ½ cup of pasta.

Portion Size
the amount of food usually consumed at one time (e.g., 3 cups of spaghetti served as a restaurant entrée).

Nutrient Density

At each calorie level, the amount of food recommended in each eating pattern is based on the assumption that all foods are chosen in their most nutrient-dense form; that is, the leanest possible variety made with no added sugars, fats, refined starches, or salt. For instance, whole milk is not made with added fat, but it is not the leanest possible variety of milk, so eating patterns are based on the assumption that fat-free milk will be chosen. Selecting the healthiest food choices from each food group is vital for achieving appropriate calorie and nutrient recommendations.

Even when it is carefully planned, an eating plan may not provide optimal amounts of all nutrients if the food has been improperly stored or overly processed. Food generally begins to lose its nutrients the moment harvesting or processing begins; the more done to a food before it is eaten, the greater the loss of naturally present nutrients. Heat, light, air, soaking in water, mechanical injury, dry storage, and acidic or alkaline food processing ingredients can hasten nutrient losses. Vitamins, minerals, and fibers are particularly vulnerable to the effects of food processing. Tips to retain the nutrient value of foods are featured in Box 8.2.

Portion Sizes

Just as the quality of foods chosen influences total calorie intake, so does the quantity. Eating patterns specify daily amounts from each food group in "ounce-equivalents" or "cup-equivalents" with examples of equivalents provided for each group. Total oils recommended per day are in grams. Although these measures are more specific than the previously used terms of serving, which consumers often confused with portion, it is still a matter of estimating how much food is consumed. Using common objects is an excellent way to convey the concept of normal **serving sizes**. Strategies to help downsize **portion sizes** include using smaller dinnerware at home and using a tall slender glass instead of a short wide one.

BOX 8.2 Tips for Retaining the Nutrient Value of Foods

- Don't buy produce that is damaged or wilted or that has been improperly stored. Produce picked when fully ripe is higher in nutrients than produce picked when green.
- Refrigerate most fruits and vegetables immediately to slow enzyme activity and retain nutrients.
- Keep produce in the refrigerator crisper or in moisture-proof bags.
- Wash, don't soak, produce to avoid leaching nutrients.
- Avoid peeling and paring vegetables before cooking because a valuable layer of nutrients is stored directly beneath the skin. If necessary, scrape or pare as thin a layer as possible.
- Avoid cutting produce into small pieces: The more surface area exposed, the greater the nutrient loss.
- Prepare vegetables as close to serving time as possible to avoid excessive exposure to light and air. Don't thaw frozen vegetables before cooking.
- Eat some fruits and vegetables raw.
- Cook produce in as little water as possible to avoid leaching vitamins. Stir fry, steam, microwave, or pressure cook vegetables to retain nutrients. If water is used in cooking, save it and use it as stock for soups, gravies, or sauces.
- Shorten cooking time as much as possible. Cook vegetables to the tender crunchy, rather than to the mushy, stage of doneness; cover the pan to retain heat; and preheat the pan or water before adding foods to speed heating time.
- Cook only as many vegetables as are needed at a time because reheating causes considerable loss of vitamins.

Quick Bite

A comparison between 1-oz grain equivalent *serving* and a typical American *portion*

	Amount that qualifies as 1-oz grain equivalent	Common portion size eaten
Bagel	1 in mini bagel	1 large bagel = 4 ounce-equivalents
Bread	1 regular slice	2 slices = 2 ounce-equivalents
Pancakes	1 (4½ in diameter)	3 (4½ in diameter) = 3 ounce-equivalents
Popcorn	3 cups, popped	100-calorie bag, popped = 2 once-equivalents
Rice or	½ cup cooked	1 cup cooked = pasta 2 ounce-equivalents
Tortillas	1 small (6 in)	1 large (12 in) = 4 ounce-equivalents

Source: www.ChooseMyPlate.gov.

Limit on Calories for Other Uses

If all food choices are in nutrient-dense forms, a small number of calories remain within the overall calorie limit of the eating patterns; this is identified as "limit on calories for other uses" in the eating patterns and is expressed in both calories and in percentage of total calories (USDHHS & USDA, 2015). These limits are low at 8% to 19% of total calories, and for most Americans, the allowance is toward the lower end of this range. Calories up to the specified limit can be used for added sugars, added refined starches, solid fats, alcohol, or to eat more than the recommended amount of food in a food group. However, the overall eating pattern should also be within the recommended limit of less than 10% of calories from added sugars and less than 10% of calories from saturated fats.

Variety

Choosing a variety of foods within each food group helps ensure that the more than 40 known essential nutrients are consumed in adequate amounts based on the rationale that some nutrients, such as iron, calcium, vitamin C, and vitamin A, are concentrated in a few foods. For instance, choosing a variety of vegetables, such as carrots, broccoli, tomatoes, and garbanzo beans, helps ensure adequate nutrient intake because each has a different composition and nutrient profile. Conversely, choosing a variety of refined grains (e.g., white bread, white pasta, hamburger bun) does little to ensure nutritional adequacy because, although they are each different foods, their nutrient profile is remarkably similar.

Concept Mastery Alert

When providing an explanation of MyPlate, the nurse should note that it is a graphic of a place setting with a quarter of the plate devoted to grains and one-half devoted to fruits and vegetables. MyPlate covers all aspects of the diet and reflects a philosophy that nutrient needs should be met through food as much as possible.

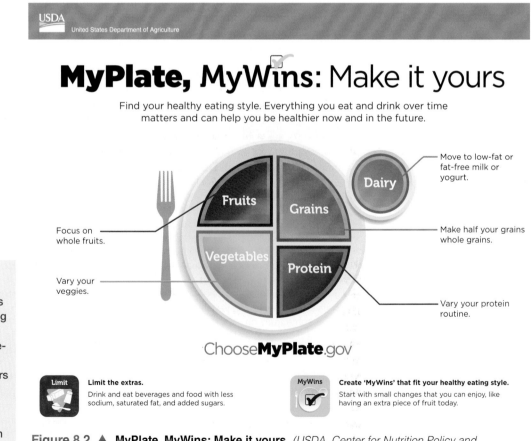

Figure 8.2 ▲ **MyPlate, MyWins: Make it yours.** *(USDA, Center for Nutrition Policy and Promotion. [2016]. Available at www.choosemyplate.gov)*

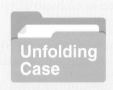

Recall Aurea. She may be able to achieve variety in fruits and vegetables; for instance, certain items in the vegetable sub-groups of dark green (raw chopped spinach), red (tomato), orange (carrot juice), and other (zucchini) are low in fiber. However, she may not be able to tolerate legumes or many whole grains. How do you respond to her frustration about having to adhere to a restrictive eating pattern?

MyPlate

In early 2011, MyPlate replaced MyPyramid as the new graphic by which the DGA are translated into food choices for healthy individuals older than 2 years. It features a place setting with half of the dinner plate devoted to fruits and vegetables, ¼ to protein foods, and ¼ to grains; dairy accompanies the plate (Fig. 8.2) (USDA, Center for Nutrition Policy and Promotion, 2016). Daily food group targets for a 2000-calorie plan translate the MyPlate concept into food group recommendations (Fig. 8.3). Consistent with the DGA, it is based on the philosophy that nutrient needs, to the greatest extent possible, should be met through food, not supplements. It urges Americans to make healthier choices within the context of their own

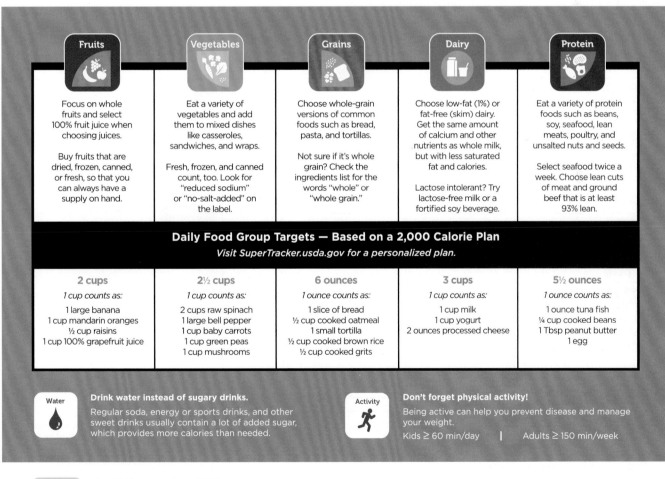

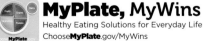

Figure 8.3 ▲ **Daily food group targets based on a 2000-calorie plan.** *(USDA, Center for Nutrition Policy and Promotion [2016]. Available at www.choosemyplate.gov)*

preferences, culture, traditions, and budget to evolve to a healthy eating style that encompasses these main points:

- Everything you eat and drink matters—focus on variety, amount, and nutrition.
- Choose foods and beverages with less saturated fat, sodium, and added sugars.
- Start with small changes.

ChooseMyPlate.gov includes a wealth of information, including details about each of the food groups, their nutritional value and health benefits, and specific tips for improving intake. Online tools include SuperTracker to help plan, analyze, and monitor food intake and physical activity as well as to track weight, personal goals, and group challenges. Users can download a daily checklist to track their intake according to the food group targets for their calorie allowance (Fig. 8.4). Consistent with the healthy eating pattern styles featured in the DGA, daily food plans are available from 1000 to 3200 calories in 200-calorie increments. Other tools include a body mass index (BMI) calculator and interactive quizzes. Tip sheets, recipes, menus, food safety information, suggestions for eating on a budget, and MyPlate videos are also featured. Users can choose a specific audience such as for children, students, adults, and professionals. The MyPlate graphic is available in 20 languages, including Spanish (Fig. 8.5). A "Physical Activity" tab addresses the importance of exercise, how much is recommended, and tips for how to become more physically active. Users can also sign up for e-mail updates.

MyPlate Daily Checklist

Write down the foods you ate today and track your daily MyPlate, MyWins!

Food group targets for a 2,000 calorie* pattern are:

		Write your food choices for each food group	Did you reach your target?
Fruits	**2 cups** 1 cup of fruits counts as • 1 cup raw or cooked fruit; or • 1/2 cup dried fruit; or • 1 cup 100% fruit juice.	_____ _____ _____	Y N
Vegetables	**2 1/2 cups** 1 cup vegetables counts as • 1 cup raw or cooked vegetables; or • 2 cups leafy salad greens; or • 1 cup 100% vegetable juice.	_____ _____ _____	Y N
Grains	**6 ounce equivalents** 1 ounce of grains counts as • 1 slice bread; or • 1 ounce ready-to-eat cereal; or • 1/2 cup cooked rice, pasta, or cereal.	_____ _____ _____	Y N
Protein	**5 1/2 ounce equivalents** 1 ounce of protein counts as • 1 ounce lean meat, poultry, or seafood; or • 1 egg; or • 1 Tbsp peanut butter; or • 1/4 cup cooked beans or peas; or • 1/2 ounce nuts or seeds.	_____ _____ _____	Y N
Dairy	**3 cups** 1 cup of dairy counts as • 1 cup milk; or • 1 cup yogurt; or • 1 cup fortified soy beverage; or • 1 1/2 ounces natural cheese or 2 ounces processed cheese.	_____ _____ _____	Y N

Limit:
- Sodium to **2,300 milligrams** a day.
- Saturated fat to **22 grams** a day.
- Added sugars to **50 grams** a day.

Y   N

Be active your way:
Adults:
- Be physically active at least 2 1/2 hours per week.

Children 6 to 17 years old:
- Move at least **60 minutes** every day.

Y   N

* This 2,000 calorie pattern is only an estimate of your needs. Monitor your body weight and adjust your calories if needed.

MyWins   Track your MyPlate, MyWins

_____
_____
_____

Center for Nutrition Policy and Promotion
January 2016
USDA is an equal opportunity provider and employer.

Figure 8.4 ▲ MyPlate 2000-Calorie Daily Checklist. *(USDA, Center for Nutrition Policy and Promotion. [2016]. Available at www.choosemyplate.gov)*

Figure 8.5 ▶ MyPlate graphic in Spanish. *(USDA, Center for Nutrition Policy and Promotion. [2016]. Available at www.choosemyplate.gov)*

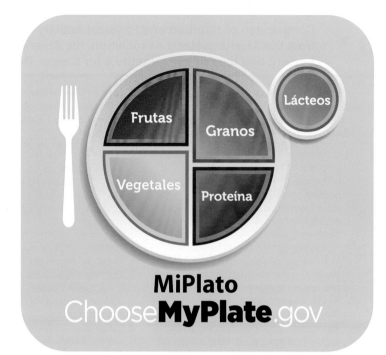

Recommended Patterns Versus Typical Intake

Despite the wealth of nutrition information available to consumers, there is a large gap between what Americans eat and what is recommended. Food trends show that (USDHHS & USDA, 2015)

- Approximately 75% of the population does not eat enough vegetables, fruits, dairy, and oils.
- More than 50% of the population meet or exceed total grain and total protein but do not eat enough whole grains and lack variety in protein choices.
- Most Americans eat too much added sugar, saturated fat, and sodium.
- Many people consume too many calories.

However, the International Food Information Council Foundation's 2015 Food and Health Survey found that 55% of American adults polled are trying to take some control over the healthfulness of their diet and their level of physical activity and that 82% are trying to eat more fruits and vegetables (International Food Information Council Foundation, 2015). Other positive changes were also identified (Box 8.3). Not surprising, most people say they respond more favorably to messages about what *to* eat instead of what *not* to eat.

BOX 8.3   2015 Health and Diet Survey Results

From March 13 to March 26, 2015, 1007 Americans ages 18 to 80 years, chosen to represent the demographics of the United States, were surveyed about their attitudes toward food safety, nutrition, and health:

91% thought about the healthfulness of their diet in the last year, and 94% thought about the amount of physical activity they get.

84% are actively trying to maintain or lose weight.

55% who rate their health as very good or excellent are overweight or obese.

42% know at least something about the MyPlate graphic.

76% are trying to cut calories by drinking water or low- and no-calorie beverages.

70% are eating more whole grains.

69% are eating less of foods high in added sugar.

78% would rather hear what to eat instead of what not to eat.

27% see sugars as the calorie source most likely to cause weight gain.

Source: International Food Information Council Foundation. *Food & Health Survey 2015.* Available at http://www.foodinsight.org/2015-food-health-survey-consumer-research. Accessed on 3/20/16.

| Table 8.3 | Comparison of Nutrition and Physical Activity Recommendations from the American Heart Association, the American Cancer Society, and the American Institute for Cancer Research |

Criteria	American Heart Association/American College of Cardiology Guidelines on Lifestyle Management to Reduce Cardiovascular Risk*	American Cancer Society Guidelines on Nutrition and Physical Activity for Cancer Prevention†	American Institute for Cancer Research Recommendations for Cancer Prevention‡
Nutrition	• Consume an eating pattern that emphasizes the intake of vegetables, fruits, and whole grains; includes low-fat dairy products, poultry, fish, legumes, nontropical vegetable oils, and nuts; and limits the intake of sweets, sugar-sweetened beverages, and red meats. • This eating pattern should be adapted to the individual's calorie requirements, personal and cultural food preferences, and nutrition therapy for other medical conditions (including diabetes). • This pattern can be achieved by following such plans as the Dietary Approaches to Stop Hypertension (DASH) pattern, the USDA Food Pattern, or the American Heart Association (AHA) diet. • Limit saturated fat to 5%–6% of total calories. • Reduce the percentage of calories from trans fat. • For adults who would benefit from blood pressure lowering: Limit sodium intake to no more than 2400 mg/day. A further reduction to 1500 mg/day can result in greater reduction in blood pressure. Even without achieving these goals, reducing sodium intake by 1000 mg/day will lower blood pressure. Combine the DASH eating pattern with a lower sodium intake.	• Achieve and maintain healthy weight throughout life. • Be as lean as possible without being underweight. • Avoid excess weight gain at all ages. • Consume a healthy diet with an emphasis on plant foods. Choose foods and beverages in amounts that help you achieve and maintain a healthy weight. • Limit consumption of processed and red meats. • Eat at least 2½ cups of vegetables and fruits each day. • Choose whole grains instead of refined grains. • If you drink alcoholic beverages, limit consumption. • Drink no more than 1 drink per day for women or 2 drinks per day for men.	• Be as lean as possible without being underweight. • Avoid sugary drinks. Limit consumption of energy-dense foods. • Eat more of a variety of vegetables, fruits, whole grains, and legumes such as beans. • Limit consumption of red meats (such as beef, pork, and lamb) and avoid processed meats. • If consumed at all, limit daily alcoholic drinks to 2 for men and 1 for women. • Limit consumption of salty foods and foods processed with salt (sodium). • Don't use supplements to protect against cancer.

Physical activity	• Adults should engage in aerobic physical activity 3–4 times per week, lasting 40 minutes per session, of moderate- to vigorous-intensity physical activity to improve cholesterol levels and lower blood pressure.	• Adopt a physically active lifestyle.
		• Adults: Get at least 150 minutes or more of moderate-intensity or 75 minutes of vigorous-intensity activity, or an equivalent combination, preferably spread throughout the week.
		  • Limit sedentary behavior such as sitting and watching television.
		  • Doing some physical activity above usual activities, no matter what one's level of activity, can provide many health benefits.
			• Be physically active for at least 30 minutes each day. Limit sedentary habits.

*Eckel, R., Jakicic, J., Ard, J., de Jesus, J. M., Houston Miller, N., Hubbard, V., . . . Tomaselli, G. F. (2014). 2013 American Heart Association/American College of Cardiology Guideline on Lifestyle Management to Reduce Cardiovascular Risk: A report of the American College of Cardiology/American Heart Association Task Force of Practice Guidelines. *Circulation, 129*(25, Suppl. 2), S76–S99. doi:10.1161/01.cir.0000437740.48606.dl
†Kushi, L., Doyle, C., McCullough, M., Rock, C. L., Demark-Wahnefried, W., Bandera, E. V., . . . Gansler, T. (2012). American Cancer Society guidelines on nutrition and physical activity for cancer prevention. Reducing the risk of cancer with healthy food choices and physical activity. *CA: A Cancer Journal for Clinicians, 62,* 30–67.
‡World Cancer Research Fund & American Institute for Cancer Research. *Recommendations for cancer prevention.* Available at http://www.aicr.org/reduce-your-cancer-risk/recommendations-for-cancer-prevention/. Accessed on 3/18/16.

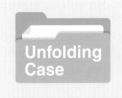

Think of Aurea. Studies suggest that probiotics may have a complementary role in treating and preventing flares of ulcerative colitis and other inflammatory bowel disorders (Chibbar & Dieleman, 2015). Which probiotic foods would you recommend she add to her diet? Are probiotics in pill form as beneficial as those from food?

Recommendations from Health Agencies

Many health agencies publish guidelines or recommendations for healthy eating including the American Heart Association (Eckel et al., 2014), the American Cancer Society (Kushi et al., 2012), and the American Institute for Cancer Research (World Cancer Research Fund & American Institute for Cancer Research, 2007) (Table 8.3). The recommendations are similar to each other and to the DGA. Common recommendations are to attain healthy weight, choose a nutrient-dense eating pattern, and become more physically active.

Guidelines and Graphics in Other Countries

Cultural differences in communicating symbolism and other cultural norms influence the shape of food guides in other countries. Similar to MyPlate, a circle or dinner plate with each section depicting relative proportion to the total diet is used by many countries, including the United Kingdom (Fig. 8.6), Germany, and Mexico. Korea and China use a pagoda shape,

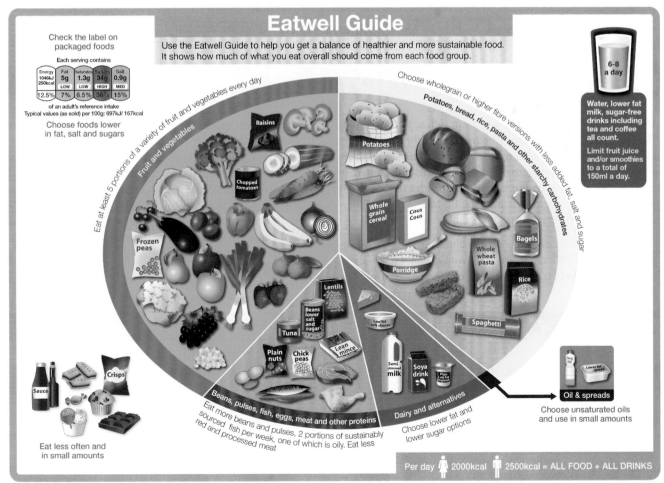

Figure 8.6 ▲ Great Britain's Eatwell Guide: The Balance of Good Health Food Standards Agency (United Kingdom).

the Bahamas uses a goat-skin drum divided into different food groups, and Canada uses a rainbow shape.

Despite the differences in the shape of the graphics, the core recommendations are consistently similar: Eat plenty of grains, vegetables, and fruit; limit fat, saturated fat, and sugars; eat a variety of foods; and eat to balance intake with activity.

How Do You Respond?

Which foods are "good"? Which foods are "bad"? Instead of thinking of individual foods as good or bad, consider how a food fits within the context of the total intake. For instance, broccoli is among the best plant foods available, yet if someone ate only broccoli all day long, it would not be "good" because it does not supply adequate amounts of all essential nutrients for health. What matters is how often a particular food is eaten, the amount eaten, and overall calorie and nutrient balance. If most of a person's intake is of nutrient-dense foods, small amounts of less nutritious choices can fit into the eating pattern without wreaking havoc as long as total calorie intake is appropriate. The keys to fitting in less-than-healthful foods are to eat them *infrequently, in small amounts, and in the context of an otherwise healthy eating pattern.*

How can I eat whole grains if I don't like whole wheat bread? Just as there are no good or bad foods, there is not one particular food you must eat to be healthy or one particular food you must never eat to be healthy. Instead of whole wheat bread, consider whole wheat bagels or tortillas for sandwiches and wraps. Whole grains also can be consumed as cereals (e.g., oatmeal, shredded wheat), side dishes (e.g., quinoa, brown rice), and even snacks (e.g., popcorn).

REVIEW CASE STUDY

Andrew wants to eat healthier and went online to learn about MyPlate. He came away overwhelmed at all the information and was turned off by reading about ounces and cups—concepts that are unfamiliar to him. He is clearly interested in changing his food habits but is stuck on the idea that that isn't possible unless he weighs and measures his food. He is wondering if eating healthier is worth the trouble.

- How would you encourage him to approach the goal of eating healthier? What information would you gather about his usual intake? His willingness to change? How would you use MyPlate to help him make better choices without overwhelming him?
- Andrew's girlfriend thinks he is not consuming enough vitamin C. Andrew is worried that he will develop scurvy. Can you assume that he is at risk for scurvy if he isn't consuming the RDA for vitamin C? Why may his girlfriend's assessment be inaccurate? How can you determine if Andrew isn't consuming enough vitamin C? What would you tell Andrew to calm his fears?

STUDY QUESTIONS

1 The greatest percentage of calories in the diet should come from
   a. Carbohydrates
   b. Protein
   c. Fat
   d. Either carbohydrate or protein

2 The DGA recommend Americans
   a. Eliminate their intake of refined grains
   b. Reduce their intake of seafood
   c. Limit added sugars to less than 10% of total calories
   d. Eat calorically dense foods

3 "Moderate" alcohol consumption is
   a. Three to four drinks per week for women, six to eight drinks per week for men
   b. Up to one drink per day for both men and women
   c. Up to one drink per day for women, up to two drinks per day for men
   d. Up to two drinks per day for women, up to three drinks per day for men

4 The nurse knows her instructions about grain equivalents have been understood when the client verbalizes that one grain equivalent is equal to
   a. One slice of bread
   b. Two cups of ready-to-eat cereal
   c. One cup of cooked pasta
   d. One cup of cooked rice

5 A client states that there is no way he can eat all the vegetables recommended in his MyPlate plan. Which of the following would be the nurse's best response?
   a. "If you can't eat all the vegetables, make up for the difference by eating more fruit."
   b. "Be sure you take a daily multivitamin to provide the nutrients that may be missing from your diet."
   c. "Set a goal of eating larger quantities of the vegetable servings you currently eat and gradually increase the servings and variety as you become more skillful in adding vegetables to your diet."
   d. "No one can. The recommendations are only a guide. Just eat what you can."

6 The nurse knows her instructions about portion sizes have been effective when the client verbalizes that ½ cup cooked cereal looks like
   a. A ½ baseball
   b. An adult handful
   c. A ping-pong ball
   d. A softball

7 Which of the following items is not nutrient dense?
   a. Whole milk
   b. Whole wheat bread
   c. Orange juice
   d. Steamed broccoli

8 Compared to a healthy U.S.-style eating pattern, a Mediterranean-style eating plan is higher in
   a. Vegetables and whole grains
   b. Seafood and fruits
   c. Olive oil and dairy
   d. Nuts and vegetables

KEY CONCEPTS

- The DRIs are the accepted reference of nutrient needs and recommendations intended for healthy people. They serve as the basis for creating nutrition education programs, planning diets for groups of people, setting standards for food assistance programs and nutrition labeling, and assessing the adequacy of the food supply. The DRIs are a set of reference values: the RDAs, EARs, AIs, and ULs. Individual nutrients do not have each of these reference values; a nutrient has an EAR plus either an RDA or an AI. ULs are not established for all nutrients.

- The DRIs are primarily for professional use because they deal with quantities of nutrients as opposed to amounts of food.

- The RDAs are amounts of essential nutrients considered adequate to meet the nutritional needs of 97% to 98% of healthy people in a gender or life stage group. The AIs are similar to the RDA, but it is not known what percentages of people are meeting nutritional needs by consuming the AI.

- UL is the highest intake of a nutrient over time that does not pose a risk. There is no benefit to consuming amounts between the RDA and UL of a nutrient.

- The DGA are guidelines and recommendations intended to help the public choose eating patterns that promote health, reduce the risk of chronic disease, and help them attain and maintain healthy weight. They are revised every 5 years.

- The Guidelines are to follow a healthy eating pattern across the lifespan; focus on variety, nutrient density, and amount; limit calories from added sugars and saturated fats and reduce sodium intake; shift to healthier food and beverage choices; and support healthy eating patterns for all. Key recommendations within the DGA describe what foods are included in a healthy eating pattern, which components should be eaten in limited quantities, and urge people to meet the Physical Activity Guidelines for Americans.

- DGA features three healthy style eating patterns to illustrate how the guidelines and recommendations translate into food across 12 different calorie levels, from 1000 to 3200 calories. The patterns are a Healthy U.S.-style, Mediterranean-style, and Vegetarian-style.

- Common characteristics of all three eating patterns are the concepts of nutrient density, portion control, limit of calories for other uses, and variety.

- MyPlate is the newest generation of graphic to illustrate the DGA. The graphic features a dinner plate with ½ devoted to fruits and vegetables, ¼ to protein, and ¼ to grains with dairy alongside.

- An abundance of online resources and tools are available at ChooseMyPlate.gov to help consumers learn about nutrition, implement changes, and track their progress.

- Despite the wealth of nutrition information available, the typical American diet falls short of recommendations: not enough fruits, vegetables, dairy, oils, whole grains, and seafood; lack of variety from the protein group; and too much added sugar, saturated fat, sodium, and calories.

- The American Heart Association, American Cancer Society, and the American Institute for Cancer Research nutrition and lifestyle recommendations all recommend Americans manage their weight, become more physically active, and eat a more plant-based eating pattern.

- Circles, a rainbow, a pagoda, and a plate are used as food graphics in other countries. Worldwide, food guides consistently recommend a high intake of whole grains, fruits, and vegetables.

Check Your Knowledge Answer Key
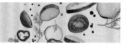

1 **TRUE** The RDAs are intended for healthy people and also people at risk of chronic disease.
2 **FALSE** The DRIs are most often used by dietitians to plan and evaluate menus and by researchers studying nutrition. Because they focus on nutrients, not foods, they are of limited value in teaching people how to choose healthy diets.
3 **FALSE** The UL is the highest intake of a nutrient that does not produce any adverse effects. There is no advantage in consuming amounts greater than the RDA.
4 **FALSE** Not all nutrients have an RDA. When an RDA cannot be determined because there is not enough evidence to determine a requirement, an AI is established. It is not known what percentage of people will obtain an AI by meeting the AI for a nutrient.
5 **TRUE** The DGA are intended to help people attain and maintain a healthy weight, reduce the risk of chronic disease, and promote wellness in Americans 2 years of age and older.

6 **FALSE** A Mediterranean-style eating pattern is suggested as one of three healthy eating styles that Americans can adopt to eat healthier. The other two are the Healthy U.S.-Style Eating Pattern, which is patterned after a typical American intake, and a Healthy Vegetarian Eating Pattern. All styles reflect the DGA.
7 **FALSE** A food that is nutrient dense has a high amount of nutrients for the amount of calories in supplies.
8 **FALSE** A portion is the amount of food usually consumed at one time. A serving is the official recommended amount of food.
9 **FALSE** The MyPlate graphic features a dinner plate with ½ of the plate devoted to fruits and vegetables, ¼ to protein, and ¼ to grains with dairy served alongside.
10 **TRUE** Both the American Cancer Society and American Heart Association recommend a plant-based diet to reduce the risk of chronic disease.

Student Resources on thePoint®
For additional learning materials, activate the code in the front of this book at
http://thePoint.lww.com/activate

Websites

2015-2020 Dietary Guidelines for Americans at http://health.gov/dietaryguidelines/2015/guidelines/
American Cancer Society Guidelines on Nutrition and Physical Activity for Cancer Prevention at http://www.cancer.org/healthy/eathealthygetactive/acsguidelinesonnutritionphysicalactivityforcancerprevention/index
American Heart Association's Healthy Eating at http://www.heart.org/HEARTORG/HealthyLiving/HealthyEating/Healthy-Eating_UCM_001188_SubHomePage.jsp
American Institute for Cancer Research Recommendations for Cancer Prevention at http://www.aicr.org/research/research_science_expert_report.html
Dietary Guidelines from Around the World at https://fnic.nal.usda.gov/professional-and-career-resources/ethnic-and-cultural-resources/dietary-guidelines-around-world
Dietary Reference Intakes from the National Academy Press are found at www.nap.edu
MyPlate at ChooseMyPlate.gov
The 2015 Food & Health Survey: Consumer Attitudes toward Food Safety, Nutrition & Health at http://www.foodinsight.org/2015-food-health-survey-consumer-research

References

Chibbar, R., & Dieleman, L. (2015). Probiotics in the management of ulcerative colitis. *Journal of Clinical Gastroenterology, 49*(Suppl. 1), S50–S55.
Eckel, R., Jakicic, J., Ard, J., Hubbard, V., de Jesus, J. M., Lee, I. M., . . . Yanovski, S. Z. (2014). 2013 AHA/ACC guideline on lifestyle management to reduce cardiovascular risk: A report of the American College of Cardiology/American Heart Association Task Force of Practice Guidelines. *Circulation, 129*(25, Suppl. 2), S76–S99. doi:10.1161/01.cir.0000437740.48606.d1
Institute of Medicine. (2006). *Dietary reference intakes: The essential guide to nutrient requirements.* Washington, DC: The National Academies Press.
International Food Information Council Foundation. *Food & Health Survey 2015.* Available at http://www.foodinsight.org/2015-food-health-survey-consumer-research. Accessed on 3/20/16.
Kushi, L., Doyle, C., McCullough, M., Rock, C. L., Demark-Wahnefried, W., Bandera, E. V., . . . Gansler, T. (2012). American Cancer Society guidelines on nutrition and physical activity for cancer prevention. Reducing the risk of cancer with healthy food choices and physical activity. *CA: A Cancer Journal for Clinicians, 62,* 30–67.
U.S. Department of Agriculture, Center for Nutrition Policy and Promotion. (2016). *MyPlate.* Available at www.choosemyplate.gov. Accessed on 10/11/12.
U.S. Department of Health and Human Services & U.S. Department of Agriculture. (2015). *2015-2020 Dietary guidelines for Americans* (8th ed.). Available at http://health.gov/dietaryguidelines/2015/guidelines/. Accessed on 3/14/16.
World Cancer Research Fund & American Institute for Cancer Research. (2007). *Food, nutrition, physical activity, and the prevention of cancer: A global perspective.* Washington, DC: American Institute for Cancer Research.

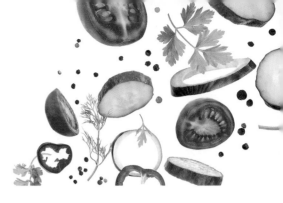

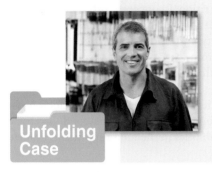

Unfolding Case

Paul Youngblood

Paul is a 58-year-old single man with mild developmental and cognitive impairments who has lived with his mother for his entire life. He has held the same part-time entry level position at a local hardware store for 40 years. His mother's recent death means he will be living independently for the first time in his life. He has no life skills pertaining to shopping or cooking because his mother always took care of that.

Check Your Knowledge

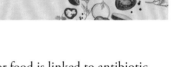

True	False		
☐	☐	**1**	Overuse of antibiotics in animals raised for food is linked to antibiotic-resistant infections in humans.
☐	☐	**2**	The newly revised "Nutrition Facts" label includes the % Daily Value for added sugars.
☐	☐	**3**	The % Daily Value listed on the "Nutrition Facts" label is based on a 2000-calorie diet.
☐	☐	**4**	Structure/function claims that appear on food labels are accurate and reliable.
☐	☐	**5**	Supplement manufacturers must prove that their products are safe and effective before they can be marketed.
☐	☐	**6**	Supplement manufacturers must list potential side effects on the label.
☐	☐	**7**	Organically grown foods are significantly more nutritious for you than their conventionally raised counterparts.
☐	☐	**8**	Bacteria cause the majority of foodborne illnesses.
☐	☐	**9**	Genetically modified food is to be consumed with caution.
☐	☐	**10**	Irradiated food may contain small amounts of radioactive substances.

Learning Objectives

Upon completion of this chapter, you will be able to

1. Analyze a nutrition or health claim for credibility.
2. Explain how the new changes to the "Nutrition Facts" label will help consumers make better food choices.
3. Compare how the regulation and marketing of dietary supplements differ from regulation and marketing of drugs.
4. Advise clients of questions to consider before using a supplement.

5 Give examples of natural and manufactured functional foods.
6 Interpret labeling on organic products.
7 Discuss the benefits and disadvantages of consuming organic foods.
8 Teach clients about the four simple steps to keep food safe.
9 Debate whether genetically modified food is safe.
10 Explain the reason why some foods are irradiated.

Functional Foods
commonly (not legally) defined as foods that provide health benefits beyond basic nutrition.

Food Irradiation
treatment of food with approved levels of ionizing radiation for a prescribed period of time and a controlled dose to destroy bacteria and parasites that would otherwise cause foodborne illness.

The proliferation of cyberspace information—and misinformation—gives millions of Americans ready access to nutritional concepts. Advances in food technology have brought us **functional foods**, bioengineering, and **food irradiation** as well as new questions about food safety and optimal nutrition. The ever-evolving science of nutrition has progressed from three square meals a day and a well-rounded diet to MyPlate. This is an era that presents old and new challenges for health professionals.

This chapter focuses on a variety of consumer issues, including nutrition misinformation, food labels, dietary supplements, functional food, organic foods, foodborne illnesses, biotechnology, antibiotics in the food supply, and irradiation.

CONSUMER INFORMATION AND MISINFORMATION

Quick Bite

When asked to identify their top two to three sources of information about food and food safety, consumers cited the following (International Food Information Council [IFIC], 2015a):

Personal health-care professional	70%
Friends/family	34%
U.S. government agencies	26%
A food expert on TV	24%
Health, food, and nutrition bloggers	24%
Farmer	18%
Food company or manufacturer	7%

Quick Bite

Red flags or "buzz words" signaling that a health or nutrient claim may be fraudulent include the following:

Breakthrough
Easy
Enzymatic process
Discovered in Europe
New
Mysterious
Quick
Secret
Absolutely safe
Miraculous cure
Ancient formula
All natural
Exclusive formula
Scientifically proven

The role of food has shifted from simply a means to prevent deficiency diseases to a tool for optimizing health, preventing chronic disease, and delaying aging. Several factors are driving this "food as medicine" paradigm, including

- Consumers' interest in managing their own health
- Increasing age of the population
- Escalating health-care costs
- Technologic advances, such as biotechnology
- The obesity epidemic
- Evidence-based science that links healthy eating patterns to a reduced risk of chronic disease

Combating Misinformation

Nutrition misinformation abounds. "Breaking news" stories may be little more than "spin" (a favorable slant) or incomplete coverage of preliminary results from scientific studies, which are often discounted later as more research is completed. The distinction between correlation and causation may be blurred, and inappropriate conclusions may be made from study results. Features or articles that fail to identify how much or little of a food should be eaten, how often it should be eaten, or to whom the advice applies do not give consumers enough information to appropriately judge what the study means to them personally. Other types of media inaccuracy include generalizing a study to a broader population than was actually studied and overstating the size of the effect. And although the information available on the Internet is vast, there are no regulatory safeguards in place to ensure that the information is accurate. Junk science coexists with legitimate data. It is the responsibility of each individual consumer to evaluate the reliability of information (Box 9.1).

Many people treat nutrition as a belief system rather than a science, formulating opinions in response to emotional appeals rather than scientific evidence. Others assume that anything that appears in print form (e.g., in a book, magazine, or newspaper)

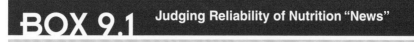

BOX 9.1 Judging Reliability of Nutrition "News"

Who is promoting the message? Anyone who stands to benefit economically by promoting a food, supplement, or diet is not likely to be an objective resource.

What is the message? Generally, if it sounds too good to be true, it usually is.

When was the study conducted, the results published, or the website updated? Even seemingly legitimate information can become quickly outdated.

Where was the study conducted? Was the site a reputable research institution or an impressive-sounding but unknown facility? Internet addresses ending in .edu (educational institutions), .org (organizations), or .gov (government agencies) are more credible than those ending in .com (commercial), whose main objective may be to sell a product.

Why was the article written—to further the reader's awareness and knowledge or to sell or promote a product? Question objectivity when the author or site has a financial interest.

is accurate and not everyone recognizes the shortcomings of the Internet. If clients' beliefs are unsupported but harmless, you may risk alienating them for no reason by trying to convince them they're misinformed. Determine how much of an emotional investment the client has in believing harmless misinformation. Be aware that casual or judgmental dismissal of misinformation can cause clients to become defensive and distrustful; clients may conclude that you are not as up-to-date as they are about nutrition, and they may reject you as a credible reference.

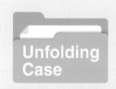

Unfolding Case

Recall Paul. He is used to treating himself to fast-food meals and eating what food mom buys—without thought about nutrition and health. He is not capable of applying critical thinking to news about nutrition but in his eagerness to please, is easily directed. What points should a learning plan include to enable Paul to purchase and prepare food for himself?

Food Labels

Food labels provide a wealth of information consumers can use to make better food choices. Information provided on a label includes "Nutrition Facts" and an ingredient list; nutrient content claims, health claims, and structure/function claims may also be found.

Nutrition Facts

The "Nutrition Facts" panel has been required on food labels since 1993. With the exception of the addition of trans fat content in 2006, the original "Nutrition Facts" label was unchanged since its inception. In spring of 2016, the U.S. Food and Drug Administration (FDA) finalized approval of an updated "Nutrition Facts" panel that reflects current dietary recommendations, national survey data, and evidence on the role of eating patterns in health promotion and disease prevention (FDA, 2016a, 2016b). Most manufacturers will be required to use the new label by July 26, 2018. Figure 9.1 features the original "Nutrition Facts" label and the new version. Changes are summarized below.

Greater Understanding of Nutrition Science

To reflect what is currently known about nutrition and health, the new "Nutrition Facts" label

Percent Daily Value (%DV)
Amount of nutrients to consume, or not exceed, which is used on both food and dietary supplement labels. The %DV refers to the percentage of the nutrient in one serving of food based on a 2000-calorie diet. The label indicates what percentage of the daily goal a serving of food contributes.

- Requires declaration of added sugars in grams and as the **percent daily value (%DV)**, based on the recommendation that the daily intake of calories from added sugars not exceed 10% of total calories consumed. Added sugars were previously not included.
- Updates the DVs for sodium, dietary fiber, and vitamin D based on newer scientific evidence

Original

Revised

1. Servings per container in larger bold type

2. Serving sizes updated to reflect how much people typically eat at one time

3. Calories in larger bold type

4. % Daily Values updated

5. New: Added sugars included

6. Change in vitamins and minerals required to reflect nutrients that, when deficient, are associated with risk of chronic disease

7. Actual amounts of nutrients declared

8. The footnote better explains the % Daily Value

Figure 9.1 ▲ "Nutrition Facts" label. *(Source: U.S. Food and Drug Administration. [2016a]. Changes to the Nutrition Facts label. Available at http://www.fda.gov/food/guidanceregulation /guidancedocumentsregulatoryinformation/labelingnutrition/ucm385663.htm. Accessed on 9/19/16.)*

- Requires the actual gram amount and %DV of potassium and vitamin D on the label because they are nutrients of public health significance. Iron and calcium content will continue to be required. Vitamin A and C content will not be required because deficiencies of these nutrients in the general population are not common.
- Removes "calories from fat" based on evidence that the type of fat consumed is more important than total fat intake

Updated Serving Sizes and New Requirements for Certain Package Sizes

To reflect how people currently eat and drink the new label

- Updates serving sizes to correspond to the amount people actually eat now, not what was typically consumed in the early 1990s. By law, serving sizes must be based on amounts people eat, not what the "should" eat. For instance, the reference amount for a serving of soda is changing from 8 to 12 oz.
- Requires that packaged foods, including beverages, that are typically consumed in one sitting be labeled as a single serving; therefore, calories and nutrient information will be for the entire package. For instance, a 20-oz soft drink, typically consumed in one sitting, will be labeled as one serving, not more than one serving.
- Requires "dual column" labels on certain larger packages that could be consumed in either one or multiple sittings, such as a 24-oz bottle of soft drink or a pint of ice cream. One column is per serving and one per package.

Refreshed Design

In order to ensure consumers have access to information they need to make informed decisions, the label has been redesigned. Changes to the design include

- The iconic looks of the label remain but with subtle changes. The font size will increase for calories, servings per container, and serving size.
- The number of calories and the serving size declaration will be in bold type to emphasize their importance in public health concerns such as obesity, diabetes, and cardiovascular disease.

- In addition to the %DV, the gram amounts of required vitamins and minerals are included. Declaring the gram amount for other vitamins and minerals is voluntary.
- An updated footnote more clearly explains the meaning of the %DV. It will read "The % Daily Value tells you how much a nutrient in a serving of food contributes to a daily diet. 2000 calories a day is used for general advice."

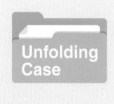

Unfolding Case

Think of Paul. He has never thought about nutrition, never been in charge of taking care of himself or a household. He is overweight and takes five medications for blood pressure. What points about the "Nutrition Facts" label are important for Paul to learn?

Nutrient Content Claims
label descriptions of the amount of a nutrient or substance provided in a food or beverage.

Health Claim
a statement that describes a relationship between a food, food substance, or dietary supplement ingredient and a reduced risk of disease or a disease-related condition.

Structure/Function Claims
statements identifying relationships between nutrients or dietary ingredients and a body function.

Ingredient List

Ingredients are listed in descending order by weight. The further down the list an item appears, the less of that ingredient is in the product. This information gives the consumer a relative idea of how much of each ingredient is in a product but not the proportion. Manufacturers are required to clearly state if a food product contains any ingredients that contain protein from the eight major food allergens: milk, eggs, fish, crustacean shellfish, tree nuts, peanuts, wheat, and soybeans.

FDA-Allowed Claims

The FDA allows three types of claims on food and dietary supplement labels: **nutrient content claims**, **health claims**, and **structure/function claims**.

Nutrient Content Claims

Terms such as "low," "free," and "high" describe the level of a nutrient or substance in a food. The terms are legally defined and so they are reliable and valid. Nutrient claims may also compare the level of a nutrient to that of comparable food with terms such as "more," "reduced," or "light." Box 9.2 defines the terms used in nutrient claims.

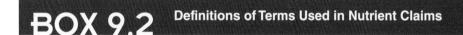

BOX 9.2 Definitions of Terms Used in Nutrient Claims

Free means the product contains virtually none of that nutrient. "Free" can refer to calories, sugar, sodium, salt, fat, saturated fat, and cholesterol.

Low means there is a small enough amount of a nutrient that the product can be used frequently without concern about exceeding dietary recommendations. Low sodium, low calorie, low fat, low saturated fat, and low cholesterol are all defined as to the amount allowed per serving. For instance, to be labeled low cholesterol, a product must have no more than 20 mg cholesterol per serving.

Very low refers to sodium only. The product cannot have more than 35 mg sodium per serving.

Reduced or less means the product has at least a 25% reduction in a nutrient compared to the regular product.

Light or lite means the product has fewer calories than a comparable product or 50% of the fat found in a comparable product.

Good source means the product provides 10% to 19% of the daily value for a nutrient.

High, rich in, or excellent source means the product has at least 20% of the daily value for a nutrient.

More means the product has at least 10% more of a desirable nutrient than does a comparable product.

Lean refers to meat or poultry products with less than 10 g fat, less than 4 g saturated fat, and less than 95 mg cholesterol per standardized serving and per 100 g.

Extra lean refers to meat or poultry products with less than 5 g fat, less than 2 g saturated fat, and less than 95 mg cholesterol per standardized serving and per 100 g.

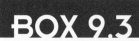

BOX 9.3 — Examples of Approved Unqualified Health Claims that Are Supported by Significant Scientific Agreement

Cancer Risk

- Dietary fat
- Fruits and vegetables
- Fiber-containing grain products

Coronary Heart Disease Risk

- Saturated fat and cholesterol
- Fruits, vegetables, and grain products that contain fiber, particularly soluble fiber
- Plant sterol/stanol esters
- Soluble fiber, such as that found in whole oats and psyllium seed husk
- Soy protein

Useful in Not Promoting Dental Caries

- Dietary noncariogenic carbohydrate sweeteners (e.g., sugar alcohols such as xylitol and sorbitol and the nonnutritive sweetener sucralose)

Hypertension Risk

- Sodium

Neural Tube Defect Risk

- Folate

Osteoporosis Risk

- Calcium
- Calcium and vitamin D

Unqualified Health Claim
A type of health claim supported by significant scientific agreement.

Daily Values (DVs)
are reference values established by the FDA for use on food labels. For some nutrients (e.g., sodium), they are amounts that should not be exceeded; for others (e.g., fiber), they are amounts to strive toward. For nutrient intakes that are based on the percentage of calories consumed, 2000 calories is the standard used.

Qualified Health Claim
A type of health claim that must be qualified by a statement that specifies the degree of scientific evidence that supports it. These claims are based on the weight of evidence but are not considered to be backed by significant scientific agreement.

Health Claims

A health claim proposes a relationship between a food or substance in a food and a disease or health-related condition. There are two types of health claims; they differ in the degree of scientific evidence that supports the claim. **Unqualified health claims**, also known as "authorized health claims," are supported by significant scientific agreement (SSA) among experts who have examined the evidence (Box 9.3). Foods that make one of these claims also meet other requirements: (1) They do not exceed specific levels for total fat, saturated fat, cholesterol, and sodium and (2) they contain at least 10% of the **Daily Values (DVs)** (before supplementation) for any one or all of the following: protein, dietary fiber, vitamin A, vitamin C, calcium, and iron. Additional health claim criteria are specific for the claim made. For instance, the claim regarding calcium and osteoporosis is only allowed on foods that have at least 20% DV for calcium. These claims are referred to as unqualified health claims because they do not require a qualifying statement about the strength of evidence supporting the claim.

The FDA allows certain **qualified health claims** when the relationship between food, a food component, and a supplement is not strong enough to meet SSA or published authoritative standards. Specific FDA-approved labeling language must be used for qualified health claims, and companies must petition the FDA for prior written permission to make a qualified health claim. The weakest claim is as follows: "Very limited and preliminary scientific research suggests [health claim]. The FDA concludes that there is little scientific evidence supporting this claim." Examples of qualified health claims are listed in Box 9.4.

Structure/Function Claims

Structure/function claims offer the possibility that a food may improve or support body function, which is a fine distinction from the approved health claims that relate a food or nutrient to a disease. An example of a disease claim needing approval is "suppresses appetite to treat obesity,"

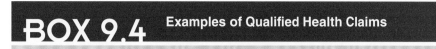

BOX 9.4   Examples of Qualified Health Claims

Cancer Risk

- Green tea
- Selenium
- Antioxidant vitamins
- Tomatoes and/or tomato sauce (prostate, ovarian, gastric, and pancreatic cancers)

Cardiovascular Disease Risk

- Nuts
- Walnuts
- Monounsaturated fatty acids from olive oil
- Omega-3 fatty acids
- B vitamins
- Unsaturated fatty acids from canola oil
- Corn oil

Hypertension Risk (and Pregnancy-Induced Hypertension and Preeclampsia)

- Calcium

whereas a function claim that does not need approval is "suppresses appetite to aid weight loss." These structure claims had previously been used primarily by supplement manufacturers with the disclaimer that "These statements have not been evaluated by the FDA. This product is not intended to diagnose, treat, cure, or prevent any disease." Structure/function claims are now appearing on food labels and do not require a disclaimer. Unlike health claims that can only appear on foods that meet other nutritional criteria (e.g., they cannot be high in fat, cholesterol, sodium), structure/function claims can appear on "junk" foods. Structure/function claims do not require FDA approval, so there may be no evidence to support the claim. See Box 9.5 for structure/function claims that do not need prior approval.

Industry-Originated Labeling

Over the last decade, many food manufacturers and retailers have added a variety of nutrition symbols and rating systems to the front of food packages to show how nutritious they are. For instance, the American Heart Association Heart-Check utilizes a single symbol to guide consumers toward heart healthy choices. The Whole Grain Council's Whole Grain Stamp is a front-of-package symbol used to indicate the presence of a food group or ingredient. Although intended to simplify choices for consumers, having too many types of front-of-package labels may actually increase confusion.

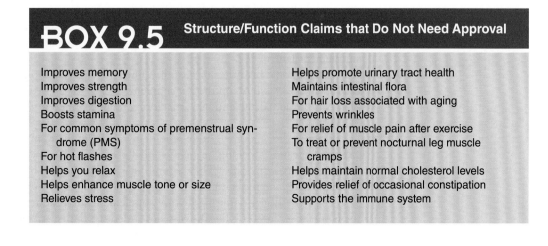

BOX 9.5   Structure/Function Claims that Do Not Need Approval

Improves memory	Helps promote urinary tract health
Improves strength	Maintains intestinal flora
Improves digestion	For hair loss associated with aging
Boosts stamina	Prevents wrinkles
For common symptoms of premenstrual syndrome (PMS)	For relief of muscle pain after exercise
For hot flashes	To treat or prevent nocturnal leg muscle cramps
Helps you relax	Helps maintain normal cholesterol levels
Helps enhance muscle tone or size	Provides relief of occasional constipation
Relieves stress	Supports the immune system

Figure 9.2 ▶
Facts Up Front.

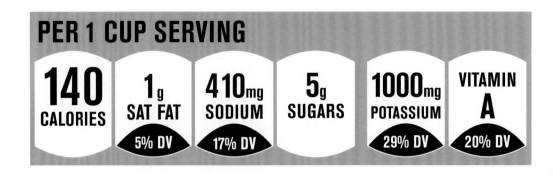

The Grocery Manufacturers Association and Food Marketing Institute have created Nutrition Keys, a voluntary front-of-package labeling initiative known as Facts Up Front. In a standardized format, four basic icons provide information from the "Nutrition Facts" panel on calories, saturated fat, sodium, and sugar. All four basic icons must appear. Some products may add up to two optional icons of nutrients that have positive health benefits—namely, potassium, fiber, protein, vitamin A, vitamin C, vitamin D, calcium, and iron (Fig. 9.2). Smaller packages may limit the icon to just calories. The icon began appearing in the marketplace in late 2011. Facts Up Front is a complement to the "Nutrition Facts" label, not a replacement for it.

The FDA views the Nutrition Keys basic icons (calories, saturated fat, sodium, and total sugar content) and optional icons as nutrient content claims subject to all FDA requirements and regulations. However, the FDA intends to exercise enforcement discretion in regard to certain aspects of nutrition labeling regulations to facilitate implementation of the Nutrition Keys program in an effort to provide consumers ready access to nutrient content information (FDA, 2015).

CONSUMER-RELATED INTERESTS AND CONCERNS

As knowledge of nutrition in health and disease continues to grow, consumers interested in self-directed care look to food and nutrition-related strategies to ensure health and wellness. Some of those strategies may include using dietary supplements, choosing functional foods, and opting for organic foods. Consumer concerns include foodborne illness, biotechnology, antibiotics, and irradiation.

Dietary Supplements

Herbal Supplements
supplements from plants or parts of plants used to alleviate health problems or promote wellness.

Dietary supplements represent a broad range of products that contain one or more dietary ingredients, including vitamins and minerals; specialty supplements, such as amino acids, omega-3 fatty acids, fiber, and probiotics; **herbal supplements**, such as cranberry, garlic, and Echinacea; and sports nutrition/weight management supplements, such as whey protein, energy drinks, and hydration drinks. They are intended to *add to* (supplement) the diets of some people, not to replace a healthy diet. Supplements are taken by mouth as a capsule, tablet, lozenge, liquid, or tea. Labeling laws require the front label to state that the product is a dietary supplement. Figure 9.3 depicts a supplement label.

The National Institutes of Health, Office of Dietary Supplements (2016) estimates Americans spent $36.7 billion on dietary supplements in 2014. The top 10 selling herbal dietary supplements in food, drug, and mass marketing retail channels in the United States are summarized in Table 9.1.

Whereas the functions and requirements of vitamins and minerals are fairly well understood, scientific research is lacking for many herbal products. Many people mistakenly believe "natural" is synonymous with "safe." They assume that herbs must be harmless because they come from flowers, leaves, and seeds. In truth, herbs are not guaranteed to be safe or effective.

The FDA began requiring dietary supplements be produced using current good manufacturing practices in 2007. For the first time, identity, purity, strength, and composition of dietary

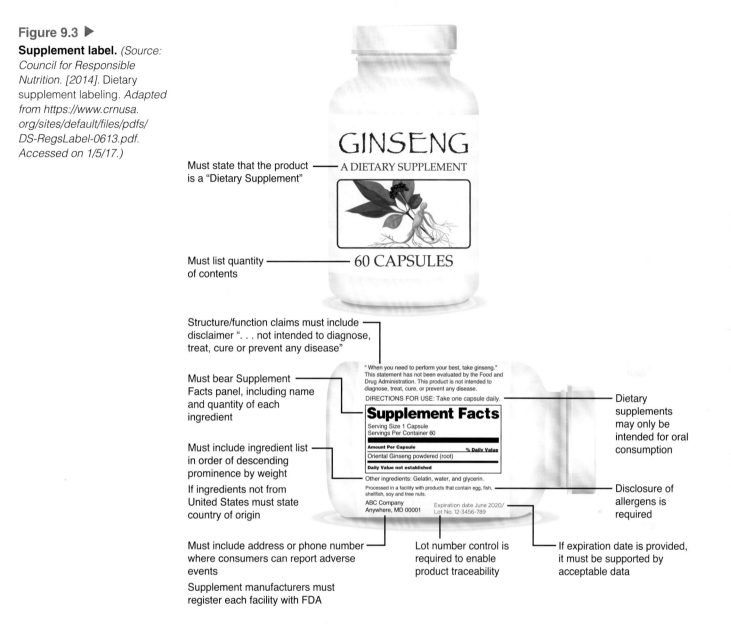

Figure 9.3 ▶

Supplement label. *(Source: Council for Responsible Nutrition. [2014]. Dietary supplement labeling. Adapted from https://www.crnusa. org/sites/default/files/pdfs/ DS-RegsLabel-0613.pdf. Accessed on 1/5/17.)*

supplements were required to be accurately reflected on the label. This was a significant step in protecting consumers by ensuring supplements

- Meet quality standards for manufacturing processes
- Are free of contaminants or impurities such as natural toxins, bacteria, pesticides, glass, lead, or other substances
- Are manufactured to ensure identity, purity, strength, and composition
- Have an accurate listing of ingredients

Supplement Regulation

In their medicinal sense, herbs are technically unapproved drugs; approximately 30% of drugs used today originated from plants (e.g., paclitaxel, aspirin, digoxin). In the United States, dietary supplements are regulated by the FDA as *foods*, which means they do not have to meet the same standards as drugs and over-the-counter medications. Supplements differ greatly from conventional drugs in how they are marketed and regulated.

Safety and Effectiveness Are Not Proven

Before a drug can be marketed, the FDA must authorize its use based on the results of clinical studies performed to determine safety, effectiveness, possible interactions with other substances, and

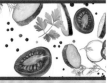

Table 9.1	2012 Top 10 Selling Herbal Supplements in the United States*: What Science Says and Possible Side Effects and Cautions†	
Herb	**What Science Says**	**Side Effects and Cautions**
Cranberry	Some evidence that it may help prevent urinary tract infections; has not been found to effectively treat urinary tract infections May help impair the ability of *Helicobacter pylori* to live in the stomach May help reduce dental plaque	Appears safe; excessive intake could cause gastrointestinal (GI) upset or diarrhea Some indications that it should be used cautiously by people on anticoagulants, medications that affect the liver, and aspirin
Garlic	Some evidence suggests it may slightly reduce serum cholesterol levels and also slow the development of atherosclerosis. May lower blood pressure, especially in people with hypertension No clinical trials have examined the effect of garlic on lowering cancer risk.	Safe for most adults Side effects include breath and body odor, heartburn, GI upset, and allergic reactions; side effects are more common with raw garlic May increase prothrombin time and enhance the effects and adverse effects of anticoagulant and antiplatelet medications Interferes with the effectiveness of saquinavir, a drug to treat HIV
Saw palmetto	Has not been found to reduce urinary symptoms associated with benign prostatic hypertrophy or any other conditions	Well tolerated; may cause stomach discomfort in some
Soy	Daily intake may slightly lower low-density lipoprotein (LDL) cholesterol. May reduce hot flashes in postmenopausal women but study results are inconsistent Not enough evidence to determine if it is effective for any other health issues	Is considered safe for most people when used as a food or taken for short periods of time as a supplement The safety of long-term use of soy isoflavones has not been established. Its role in breast cancer risk is uncertain.
Ginkgo biloba	Not effective in lowering the overall incidence of dementia and Alzheimer disease in the elderly Has not shown significant benefit for intermittent claudication Conflicting evidence that it helps tinnitus	Side effects may include headache, nausea, GI upset, diarrhea, dizziness, or allergic skin reactions. May increase bleeding risk Rats and mice given a specific ginkgo extract for up to 2 years developed tumors; research is needed to determine whether ginkgo affects cancer risk in people.
Milk thistle	Small clinical trials evaluating its efficacy in protecting and promoting the growth of liver cells, fighting oxidation, and inhibiting inflammation have been mixed and two rigorously designed studies found no benefit.	Well tolerated May cause allergic reaction in people allergic to plants in the daisy family (ragweed, chrysanthemums, marigolds, daisies) May lower blood glucose levels; should be used with caution by people with diabetes or hypoglycemia
Black cohosh	Results are mixed on whether it effectively relieves menopausal symptoms. A National Center for Complementary and Integrative Health (NCCIH)-funded study found it did not relieve hot flashes and night sweats in perimenopausal or postmenopausal women when used alone or in combination with other herbs.	Experts suggest women should stop using black cohosh and consult a health-care provider if they have a liver disorder or develop symptoms of impaired liver function. Although there are reports of hepatitis and liver failure in women using black cohosh, it is not certain that black cohosh is to blame. In general, studies evaluating it for menopausal symptoms have not found serious side effects. It is not known whether it is safe for women who have had hormone-sensitive conditions, such as breast cancer.

Concept Mastery Alert

For clients with metabolic disorders who are on drugs to control that disorder, including drugs that lower cholesterol and blood pressure, as well as treat diabetes and heart disease, herbal supplements (such as cranberry) with few or no drug/supplement interactions are recommended. Supplements such as ginseng, St. John's wort, and ginkgo biloba all have significant interaction potential.

Table 9.1	2012 Top 10 Selling Herbal Supplements in the United States*: What Science Says and Possible Side Effects and Cautions† (continued)	
Herb	**What Science Says**	**Side Effects and Cautions**
Echinacea	Results of studies on whether it can prevent or treat upper respiratory tract infections are mixed.	Mostly well tolerated; GI side effects are most common. May cause allergic reaction in people allergic to plants in the daisy family (ragweed, chrysanthemums, marigolds, daisies) and those with asthma or a genetic tendency toward allergic reactions
St. John's wort	Has not been found to be more effective than placebo in treating minor depression or major depression of moderate severity	Interacts with numerous medications, including antidepressants, birth control pills, cyclosporine, digoxin, indinavir, antiseizure medications, and warfarin and related anticoagulants May cause increased sensitivity to sunlight; may also cause anxiety, dry mouth, dizziness, GI symptoms, fatigue, headache, or sexual dysfunction
Ginseng	Some studies show it may lower blood glucose; other studies suggest possible beneficial effects on immune function. Research results do not conclusively support health claims associated with ginseng.	Likely safe when taken by mouth for a short period of time May cause headaches, sleep problems, and GI problems diarrhea Asian ginseng can cause allergic reactions.

*Lindstrom, A., Ooyen, C., Lynch, M. E., & Blumenthal, M. (2013). Herb supplement sales increase 5.5% in 2012: Herbal supplement sales rise for 9th consecutive year; turmeric sales jump 40% in natural channel. *HerbalGram, 99,* 60–65. Available at http://cms.herbalgram.org/herbalgram/issue99/hg99-mktrpt.html. Accessed on 3/25/16.
†National Center for Complementary and Integrative Health, National Institutes of Health. *Herbs at a glance.* Available at https://nccih.nih.gov/health/herbsataglance.htm. Accessed on 3/25/16.

appropriate doses. In contrast, the regulations regarding dietary supplements are lax. Supplement ingredients sold in the United States before October 15, 1994, are assumed to be safe and so do not require FDA review for safety before they are marketed. Dietary supplement manufacturers that want to market a **new dietary ingredient** must submit information to the FDA that supports their conclusion that *reasonable* evidence exists that the product is safe for human consumption. Manufacturers do not have to *prove* to the FDA that dietary supplements are safe or effective; however, they are not supposed to market unsafe or ineffective products and are required to report all serious dietary supplement adverse events to the FDA.

New Dietary Ingredient
supplement ingredient not marketed in the United States before October 15, 1994.

Once a product is marketed, the responsibility lies with the FDA to prove danger rather than with the manufacturer to prove safety. They do this through adverse event monitoring and research. When the FDA determines that a supplement is unsafe, it issues a consumer advisory discouraging its use. Only one supplement, ephedra, has actually been banned by the FDA in an unprecedented move that resulted from a 7-year review of tens of thousands of public comments and peer-reviewed scientific literature on the safety of ephedra. Despite the ban, consumers are still able to buy ephedra.

Strength Is Not Standardized

Standardization
a manufacturing process that ensures product consistency from batch to batch.

Dietary supplements are not required to be standardized in the United States. In fact, there is no legal definition of **standardization** as it applies to supplements, so the concentration of active compounds in different batches of supposedly identical plant material can vary greatly. The difference in concentration may be related to several factors such as the variety of plant used and the part of the plant used (e.g., the stems or leaves).

Dosages Are Not Standardized

Recommended dosages vary among manufacturers because there is no premarket testing to determine optimum dosage or maximum safe dosage. Other than the manufacturers' responsibility to ensure safety, there are no regulations that limit a "serving size" of any supplement.

Claims on Packaging Do Not Require FDA Approval

Although dietary supplements cannot claim to be used for the diagnosis, treatment, cure, or prevention of disease, they can be labeled with statements explaining their purported effect on the structure or function of the human body (e.g., "alleviates fatigue") or their role in promoting well-being (e.g., "improves mood"). These statements do not require FDA approval, but the label must include the following disclaimer: "This statement has not been evaluated by the FDA. This product is not intended to diagnose, treat, cure, or prevent any disease."

Warnings Are Not Required

Unlike drugs, supplements are not required to carry warning labels about potential side effects, adverse effects, or supplement–drug interactions. There are also no advisories about who should not use the product.

Supplements Are Self-Prescribed

A major concern with self-medication is that consumers may misdiagnose their condition or forsake effective conventional medical care to treat themselves "naturally." Another problem with self-medicating is that patients may not inform their physicians about their use of herbs, so side effects and herb–drug interactions go undiagnosed and unreported.

Advice for Supplement Users

Clients who choose to use supplements should

- Ask critical questions beforehand, such as whether there is any scientific evidence to support the use of the product or if there are any potential adverse side effects associated with its use.
- Check with the FDA website for consumer advisories on supplements to avoid.
- Discuss supplement use with the physician.
- Take only single supplement products and keep the dose small to prevent and manage adverse side effects and supplement–drug interactions.
- Take supplements at different times from prescribed medications to help reduce the potential for supplement–drug interactions.
- Discontinue supplements immediately if adverse side effects or supplement–drug interactions occur.
- Avoid herbs and other botanical supplements if they are pregnant or lactating women or children under the age of 6 years.

Functional Foods

Functional foods are one of the fastest growing segments of the food industry. The term has no legal meaning in the United States; it is currently a marketing, not regulatory, term. In reality, all food is in essence "functional" in that it provides calories and nutrients necessary to sustain life; however, functional food is generally considered a food or food component that provides health benefits beyond basic nutrition. The Academy of Nutrition and Dietetics defines functional foods as "whole foods along with fortified, enriched, or enhanced foods that have a potentially beneficial effect on health when consumed as part of a varied diet on a regular basis at effective levels" (Crowe & Francis, 2013). Functional foods may be natural (Table 9.2) or manufactured.

Manufactured functional foods are a blend of food and pharmacy ("phoods") in which food has one or more functional ingredients added, such as vitamins, minerals, phytochemicals, or herbs. They differ from nutraceuticals, which are substances derived from foods that are used in the medicinal form of pills, capsules, or liquids for physiological benefit. Like supplements, once functional foods are marketed, adverse effects are brought to light only if consumers alert the FDA to suspected problems.

Quick Bite **Examples of manufactured functional foods**

Plant sterols added to
  Granola bars
  Bread
  Yogurt
  Margarine

Omega-3 fatty acids added to
  Ice cream   Orange juice
  Organic milk   Yogurt
  Peanut butter   Baby food

Probiotics added to
  Yogurt   Cheese
  Cereal   Juice

Table 9.2 Natural Functional Foods

Food	Active Ingredient	Potential Health Benefits
Berries: strawberries, cranberries, blueberries, raspberries, black berries	Anthocyanins	May reduce the risk of Alzheimer disease through anti-inflammatory and antioxidant properties
Soy foods	Soy protein	Lower total and low-density lipoprotein (LDL) cholesterol, may inhibit tumor growth
Oats	Soluble fiber (beta-glucan)	Lower total and LDL cholesterol
Fatty fish	Omega-3 fatty acids	Lower triglycerides, lower heart disease, lower cardiac deaths, and lower fatal and nonfatal heart attacks
Purple grape juice or red wine	Resveratrol	Decrease platelet aggregation
Cranberry juice	Proanthocyanidins	Reduces bacteriuria
Green tea	Catechins	Reduces the risk of certain cancers, such as breast and prostate
Tomatoes and tomato products	Lycopene	Reduce the risk of prostate, ovarian, gastric, and pancreatic cancer
Yogurt and fermented dairy products	Probiotics	Promote gastrointestinal health
Nuts	Monounsaturated fatty acids and vitamin E	Reduce the risk of cardiovascular disease
Citrus fruits	Flavanones	Neutralize free radicals; promote cellular antioxidant defenses
Cruciferous vegetables (e.g., broccoli, cauliflower, cabbage)	Sulforaphane	Reduce the risk of certain types of cancer
Garlic, onions, leeks, scallions	Sulfur compounds	Lower total and LDL cholesterol; may promote healthy immune function
Orange, red, and dark green fruits and vegetables	Beta-carotene	Neutralize free radicals, which may damage cells; may inhibit cancer growth; may improve immune response
Spinach, kale, collard greens	Lutein	Lower risk of age-related macular degeneration

Source: International Food Information Council Foundation. (2015). *Functional foods fact sheet: Antioxidants.* Available at http://www.foodinsight.org/Functional_Foods _Fact_Sheet_Antioxidants. Accessed on 3/29/16; American Institute for Cancer Research. *Phytochemicals: The cancer fighters in the foods we eat.* Available at http://www.aicr.org/reduce-your-cancer-risk/diet/elements_phytochemicals.html. Accessed on 3/29/16.

As scientific evidence mounts in the role of specific nutrients or food substances in preventing chronic diseases such as heart disease, cancer, diabetes, hypertension, and osteoporosis, it is likely that more foods will be considered functional and the supply of manufactured functional foods will expand exponentially. Natural functional foods—namely, fruits, vegetables, nuts, whole grains, and fatty fish—are the foundation of a healthy eating plan. Manufactured functional foods should be viewed as an option to optimize a healthy eating plan, not as a "magic bullet" to compensate for poor food choices.

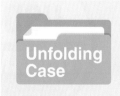

Recall Paul. He heard about functional foods but has been unable to find them labeled as such in the grocery store. What do you tell Paul about natural and manufactured functional foods?

Organically Grown Foods

Organic
in a chemical sense, organic means carbon containing. Generally, organic refers to living organisms; as such, all foods are technically organic.

Sales of **organic** food and beverages in the United States have grown from $1 billion in 1990 to over $39 billion in 2014, representing approximately 5% of total food sales (Organic Trade Association, 2015). An estimated 30% of consumers regularly buy foods labeled as "organic" (IFIC, 2015a). Fresh fruits and vegetables have been the top selling category of organically grown food since retail sale of organic food began more than 30 years ago (U.S. Department of Agriculture [USDA], Economic Research Service [ERS], 2014). In 2012, produce accounted for 43% of organic food sales, followed by dairy (15%), and packaged/prepared foods (11%). Meat, fish, and poultry represented only 3% of total organic sales. Consumers have the impression that organic vegetables and fruits are safer, more nutritious, and healthier—ideas promoted by the organic food industry, its advocates, food marketers, and even some physicians and scientists (Tarver, 2012).

Organic foods are grown without synthetic fertilizers and pesticides. Instead, "natural" products, such as manure, compost, and other organic wastes, are used to fertilize crops, and chemicals that occur naturally in the environment, such as sulfur, nicotine, and copper, may be used as pesticides. Insects that do not harm a particular crop may be used to control other insects known to cause crop damage. Crop rotation, tillage, and cover crops are used to manage soil. Food irradiation, sewage sludge, and bioengineered plants cannot be used.

> **Organically Grown or Organically Produced**
> foods produced with little or no synthetic fertilizers or pesticides (e.g., plants) and no antibiotics or hormones (e.g., livestock).

Regulations are also in place for raising organically grown livestock. **Organically produced** feed must be used for a specified period of time toward the end of gestation; animals may be given vitamin and mineral supplements, but the use of growth hormones (GHs) and antibiotics is prohibited; and animals treated with medication cannot be sold as organic.

The USDA ensures that the production, processing, and certification of **organically grown** foods adhere to strict national standards and that organic labeling meets criteria that define the four official organic categories (Table 9.3). Most consumers assume that produce sold at local farmers' markets is grown locally and is organic, but neither is necessarily true.

Organic food is usually more expensive because of higher production costs, greater losses, and smaller yields. For instance, a gallon of organic milk typically costs twice as much as a

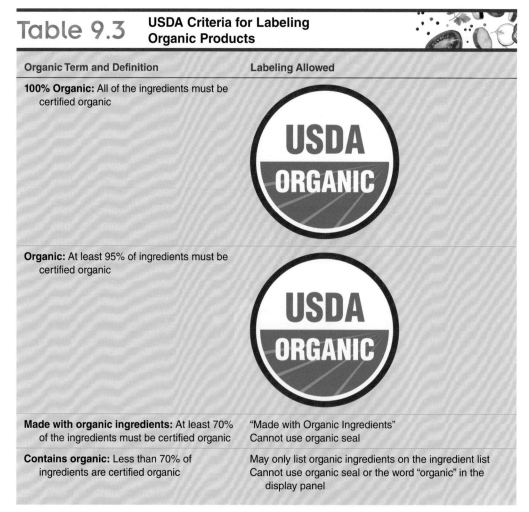

Table 9.3	USDA Criteria for Labeling Organic Products
Organic Term and Definition	**Labeling Allowed**
100% Organic: All of the ingredients must be certified organic	
Organic: At least 95% of ingredients must be certified organic	
Made with organic ingredients: At least 70% of the ingredients must be certified organic	"Made with Organic Ingredients" Cannot use organic seal
Contains organic: Less than 70% of ingredients are certified organic	May only list organic ingredients on the ingredient list Cannot use organic seal or the word "organic" in the display panel

Source: U.S. Department of Agriculture. (2012). *Labeling organic products.* Available at https://www.ams.usda.gov/sites/default/files/media/Labeling%20Organic%20Products.pdf. Accessed on 3/26/16.

gallon of store brand or name brand milk. However, not all organic foods are appreciably more expensive than their conventional counterparts, such as oranges, grapes, and bread.

Are organically produced foods more nutritious or safer than their conventionally raised counterparts? Key points summarized in an American Academy of Pediatrics report intended to help pediatricians advise their patients about organic and conventional food choices are as follows (Forman & Silverstein, 2012):

- There are minimal nutritional differences between organic and conventional produce; however, it is difficult to reliably measure differences because variables such as maturity of the produce and soil characteristics are difficult to control. Sound evidence shows organic produce has more vitamin C and phosphorus than conventional foods, but there is no evidence that this is clinically relevant.
- Organic diets unequivocally expose consumers to fewer pesticides associated with human disease; however, it is not certain that lower exposure is clinically meaningful. Large prospective cohort studies are needed to assess the relationship between pesticide exposure in conventional foods and human disease.
- Organic animals have the potential to reduce antibiotic resistant infections in humans.
- There are no clinically relevant differences between organic and conventional milk, including nutritional content. There is no evidence that conventional milk contains significantly higher amounts of bovine GH, which is given to cows to increase milk production. Whatever GH is present in milk is digested in the human GI tract.
- Organic products are usually more expensive, but as organic farming practices advance, the differences in price may be lowered.

Pediatricians were advised to first and foremost encourage patients and their families to consume a healthy eating pattern rich in fruits, vegetables, whole grains, and low-fat or fat-free dairy (Forman & Silverstein, 2012). For families concerned about pesticides, the Environmental Working Group (EWG) is suggested as a reliable resource. Each year, the EWG compiles a list of the "Dirty Dozen" and the "Clean 15," which identify fruits and vegetables with the most and least levels of pesticides, respectively (EWG, 2015) (Table 9.4). However, their methodology and interpretation

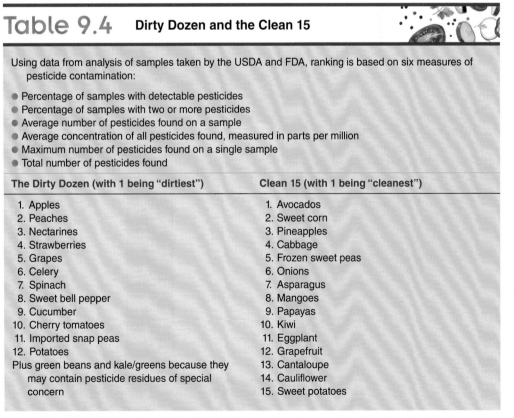

Table 9.4   Dirty Dozen and the Clean 15

Using data from analysis of samples taken by the USDA and FDA, ranking is based on six measures of pesticide contamination:

- Percentage of samples with detectable pesticides
- Percentage of samples with two or more pesticides
- Average number of pesticides found on a sample
- Average concentration of all pesticides found, measured in parts per million
- Maximum number of pesticides found on a single sample
- Total number of pesticides found

The Dirty Dozen (with 1 being "dirtiest")	Clean 15 (with 1 being "cleanest")
1. Apples	1. Avocados
2. Peaches	2. Sweet corn
3. Nectarines	3. Pineapples
4. Strawberries	4. Cabbage
5. Grapes	5. Frozen sweet peas
6. Celery	6. Onions
7. Spinach	7. Asparagus
8. Sweet bell pepper	8. Mangoes
9. Cucumber	9. Papayas
10. Cherry tomatoes	10. Kiwi
11. Imported snap peas	11. Eggplant
12. Potatoes	12. Grapefruit
Plus green beans and kale/greens because they may contain pesticide residues of special concern	13. Cantaloupe
	14. Cauliflower
	15. Sweet potatoes

Source: Environmental Working Group. (2015). *EWG's 2015 shopper's guide to pesticides in produce.* Available at http://www.ewg.org/foodnews/summary.php. Accessed on 3/26/16.

of residue findings are not without controversy. A study by Winter and Katz (2011) found that exposure to detected pesticides on the Dirty Dozen posed negligible risks to consumers and that replacing the Dirty Dozen with organically grown varieties did not result in any appreciable reduction of consumer risk. For instance, in 75% of the pesticide/food combinations studied, they found consumer exposure estimates more than 1 million times *lower* than doses given to laboratory animals continuously over their lifetimes that do not show adverse effects (Winter, 2011). An example cited in a fact sheet by the IFIC (2015b) says that "a child could consume over 1500 servings of strawberries in one day without any adverse health effects from pesticide residues, even if the strawberries have the maximum pesticide residue level identified by the FDA or USDA." Despite the controversy regarding the risks of pesticide residues in food, both sides agree that the benefits of eating a diet rich in fruits and vegetables outweigh any potential risks of pesticide exposure (EWG, 2015).

Whether produce is grown organically or conventionally, thoroughly rinsing all fruits and vegetables under running water and discarding the outer leaves, where appropriate, are recommended to reduce exposure to natural dangers such as bacteria and man-made risks such as chemical residues.

Foodborne Illness

Foodborne Illness
an illness transmitted to humans via food.

More than one-third of Americans believe that **foodborne illness** from bacteria is the most important food safety issues today (IFIC, 2015a). The Centers for Disease Control and Prevention (CDC) estimates that every year, approximately 48 million Americans experience a foodborne illness, resulting in 128,000 hospitalizations and 3000 deaths (CDC, 2014). Eight known pathogens account for the vast majority of those estimates (Table 9.5). Although more than half of foodborne illnesses are caused by viruses, the majority of deaths are attributed to bacteria (Fig. 9.4).

The microorganisms that cause foodborne illness are found widely in nature and are transmitted to people from within food (e.g., meat and fish), from on food (e.g., eggshell or vegetables), from unsafe water, or from human or animal feces. Any uncooked food that is handled by someone who is ill poses a risk. Results from a study that estimated foodborne illnesses, hospitalizations, and deaths attributed to food commodities found that (Painter et al., 2013)

- Nearly half of all foodborne illnesses were linked to produce with leafy greens implicated most often. The pathogen was often norovirus.
- Dairy were the most common source of foodborne illnesses that lead to hospitalization. Leafy vegetables and poultry were the second and third sources, respectively.
- Contaminated poultry is blamed for the most deaths: 19% of fatal cases. *Listeria* and *Salmonella* infections are most often to blame.

Figure 9.4 ▶

Top five pathogens contributing to domestically acquired foodborne illness, hospitalizations, and deaths each year. *(Source: Centers for Disease Control and Prevention, [2014]. Available at www.cdc.gov. Accessed on 3/27/16.)*

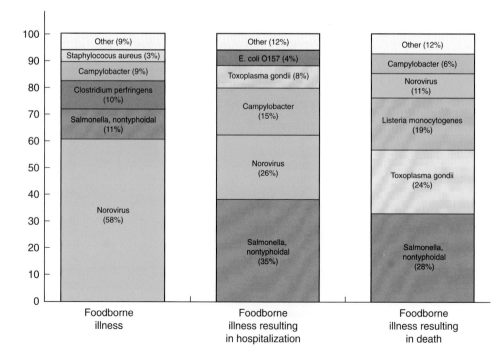

Table 9.5		**Top Pathogens Contributing to Domestically Acquired Foodborne Illnesses, Hospitalizations, and Death in the United States**			
Pathogen	**Type of Pathogen**	**Common Food Vehicles**	**Onset**	**Symptoms**	**Other**
Norovirus (food poisoning; viral gastroenteritis)	Virus	Fruits, vegetables, meat, and salads prepared or handled by infected person; oysters from contaminated water	24–48 hours	Explosive and projectile vomiting, watery diarrhea, cramps, headache, mild fever, muscle aches	Leading cause of viral diarrhea in the United States Environmentally hardy; also transferred from person to person and from contact with surfaces Very contagious Severe illness is rare
Salmonella species (salmonellosis)	Bacteria	Raw and undercooked eggs, poultry, meats, milk and dairy products; fresh produce, including raw sprouts (alfalfa, bean); shrimp; sauces; and salad dressings	6–72 hours	Nausea, vomiting, cramps, fever, diarrhea, headache Arthritic symptoms may occur 3–4 weeks after onset of acute symptoms.	Can be fatal Incidence is increasing in the United States
Clostridium perfringens (perfringens food poisoning)	Bacteria	Meat, poultry, stuffing, gravy, and cooked foods held or stored at inappropriate temperatures	16 hours	Intense abdominal cramps, diarrhea, headache, the chills	The "cafeteria germ," associated with steam table foods not kept hot enough Illness usually over within 24 hours
Campylobacter jejuni (campylobacter enteritis)	Bacteria	Unpasteurized milk and cheeses made from it; undercooked poultry, raw beef, unchlorinated water	2–5 days	Gastroenteritis; diarrhea, fever, abdominal cramps, vomiting	Small percentage develops severe complications, such as bacteremia, meningitis, hepatitis, pancreatitis, and Guillain-Barré syndrome.
Staphylococcus aureus (staphylococcal food poisoning)	Bacteria	Meat and meat products; custard- or cream-filled baked goods, sandwich fillings; poultry and egg products; salad made of egg, tuna, chicken, potato, and macaroni	1–7 hours	Severe nausea, vomiting, diarrhea, abdominal cramps	Of healthy people, 50% are carriers. Most frequently found in the nose, throat, on skin and hair, and in infected boils, pimples, cuts, and burns. Frequently transmitted to foods by human carriers
Escherichia coli (*E. coli* 0157-H7; hemorrhagic colitis, hemolytic-uremic syndrome)	Bacteria	Undercooked beef, especially ground beef; raw milk; unpasteurized fruit juice and cider; alfalfa and radish sprouts; plant foods fertilized with raw manure or irrigated with contaminated water	2–5 days	Severe abdominal cramps and diarrhea Hemorrhagic colitis may lead to hemolytic-uremic syndrome (severe anemia and renal failure).	
Listeria monocytogenes (listeriosis)	Bacteria	Raw milk, deli-type salads, processed meats, soft cheese, undercooked poultry, ice cream, raw vegetables, raw and cooked poultry	2 days to 3 weeks; severe form may have incubation period of 3 days to 3 months	Healthy people may have no or mild symptoms. Sudden fever, headache, backache, occasional abdominal pain, and diarrhea Septicemia and meningitis may lead to death. One-third of confirmed cases in pregnant women may end in spontaneous abortion or stillbirth; infants born alive may have bacteremia and meningitis.	This bacterium thrives in cold temperatures and appears to be able to survive short-term pasteurization. Mortality from listeric meningitis may be as high as 70%.

(continued)

Table 9.5	Top Pathogens Contributing to Domestically Acquired Foodborne Illnesses, Hospitalizations, and Death in the United States (continued)				
Pathogen	**Type of Pathogen**	**Common Food Vehicles**	**Onset**	**Symptoms**	**Other**
Toxoplasma gondii	Parasite	Raw or undercooked meats (e.g., pork, lamb, wild game), untreated water from rivers or ponds; contact with cat, rat, rodent, or bird feces (e.g., handling cats, cleaning cat litter box, gardening); shellfish, raw or undercooked clams and oysters	1–3 weeks	Swollen glands, fever, muscle aches CNS disorders, such as mental retardation and visual impairments, in children	Especially dangerous to pregnant women; may cause stillbirth, miscarriage; can pass to fetus More than 60 million Americans may be infected with *T. gondii* but are asymptomatic because the immune system prevents illness caused by the parasite.

Source: U.S. Food and Drug Administration. (2012). *The bad bug book: Handbook of foodborne pathogenic microorganisms and natural toxins* (2nd ed.). Available at http://www.fda.gov/downloads/Food/FoodSafety/FoodborneIllness/FoodborneIllnessFoodbornePathogensNaturalToxins/BadBugBook/UCM297627.pdf. Accessed on 3/26/16.

All food categories were involved in outbreaks, but the frequency varies for each category. The most common symptoms of foodborne illness may be mistaken for the flu—diarrhea, nausea, vomiting, fever, abdominal pain, and headaches. Most cases are self-limiting and run their course within a few days. Symptoms that warrant medical attention include bloody diarrhea (possible *Escherichia coli* 0157:H7 infection), a stiff neck with severe headache and fever (possible meningitis related to *Listeria*), excessive diarrhea or vomiting (possible life-threatening dehydration), and any symptoms that persist for more than 3 days. Infants, pregnant women, the elderly, and people with compromised immune systems (e.g., people with AIDS or cancer, organ transplant recipients, people taking corticosteroids) are particularly vulnerable to the effects of foodborne illness.

The major cause of foodborne illnesses is unsanitary food handling. To reduce the risk of contamination, proper personal hygiene and handwashing must be practiced by all food handlers. Steps must be taken to prevent cross-contamination between raw and cooked foods and through food handlers. Because heat kills most bacteria, thorough cooking of meat and fish is vital, as is pasteurization of all milk products. Adequate refrigeration inhibits the growth of bacteria. Figure 9.5 depicts the four simple steps to keep food safe, promoted by the Fight BAC! (as in bacteria) campaign of the Partnership for Food Safety Education. See the Partnership for Food Safety Education website for additional food safety tips.

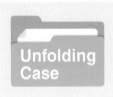

Consider Paul. Paul is very proud of his cooking accomplishment—a big pot of homemade chili. You learn that he keeps it on the stove all the time and just heats it up when it is time for lunch and dinner so he doesn't have to wash the pan. What points would you include in teaching Paul about food safety?

Food Biotechnology
a process that involves taking a gene with a desirable trait from one plant and inserting it into another with the goal of changing one or more of its characteristics; also called genetically engineered food.

Food Biotechnology

Food biotechnology, also referred to as "genetically engineered" or "genetically modified organisms (GMOs)," combines plant science with genetics to improve food. Genes associated with desirable characteristics are moved from one plant to another—a quicker and more precise version of old-fashioned crossbreeding,

Figure 9.5 ▶
Fight BAC! infographic.
(Source: Partnership for Food Safety Education. [n.d.]. The core four practices. Available at http://www.fightbac.org /food-safety-basics/the-core -four-practices/. Accessed on 11/17/16.)

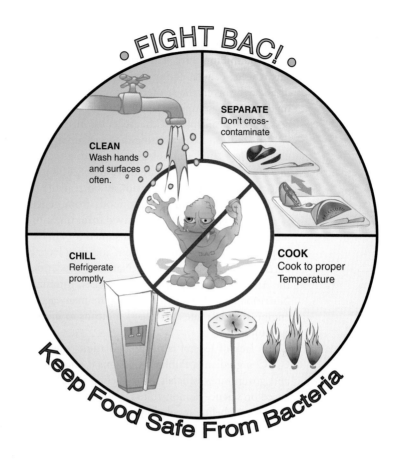

which still may take 5 to 7 years or longer to accomplish. The positive results are numerous and varied:

- *Healthier crops and greater yields.* Some plants are genetically modified to increase their resistance to plant viruses and other diseases; this means they can be raised using fewer pesticides to help reduce production costs and environmental residues. Genetically modified crops are estimated to have reduced chemical pesticide use by 37% and increase crop yields by 22% (International Service for the Acquisition of Agri-Biotech Applications [ISAAA], 2014).

- *Greater resistance to severe weather,* which reduces crop losses and increases year-round availability of fresh crops. One example is a biotech drought-tolerant corn.

- *Longer shelf life and increased freshness.* Plants can be made to ripen more slowly, staying fresher longer—a big plus for transportation.

- *Higher nutritional value.* Plants can be genetically modified to contain more vitamins, minerals, or protein, or less fat. For instance Golden Rice has been genetically engineered to be rich in beta-carotene, the precursor of vitamin A. A study by Tang et al. (2012) found Golden Rice to be as effective as pure beta-carotene in oil and better than beta-carotene in spinach at providing vitamin A to children. They concluded that Golden Rice may help prevent vitamin A deficiency in rice-consuming populations, such as China.

- *Healthier composition.* For instance, innate potato has been approved for use in the United States. It has lower levels of acrylamide, a potential carcinogen in humans produced when potatoes are cooked at high temperatures (ISAAA, 2014).

- *Better flavor.* Genetic modification has produced sweeter melons and sweeter strawberries.

- *Improved characteristics.* An example is celery without strings.

- *New food varieties through crossbreeding.* Broccoflower (a blend of broccoli and cauliflower) and tangelos (a tangerine–grapefruit hybrid) are examples.

- *Potential to alleviate world hunger.* Greater yields of stronger crops with enhanced nutritional value benefit consumers worldwide.

In 2014, biotechnology continued to grow globally for the 19th consecutive year of commercialization with 18 million farmers in 28 countries planting more than 447 million acres of crops (ISAAA, 2014). The United States is the leading producer of biotech crops with more than 180 million acres. The primary crops grown in the United States are corn, cotton, soybeans, sugar beets, canola, squash, papaya, and alfalfa. Ninety-three percent of all the corn and 94% of all soybeans in the United States are grown using biotechnology (ISAAA, 2014). Ingredients made from these top crops, such as soybean oil, corn oil, and corn syrup, are pervasive in processed foods available in U.S. grocery stores such as cereals, frozen pizza, hot dogs, and soft drinks.

In addition to permeating the food supply, biotechnology has provided breakthrough health-care products and technologies, beginning with FDA approval of recombinant human insulin in 1982. Currently, there are more than 250 biotechnology health-care products, tests, and vaccines available, many for previously untreatable diseases (Biotechnology Industry Organization, 2010). The FDA requires that foods from genetically engineered plants meet that same food safety requirements as foods derived from traditionally bred plants. Foods produced through biotechnology have been widely consumed for almost 20 years with no evidence of harm, including in pregnant women and children, and they have been found to be as healthful as their counterparts (IFIC, 2016). The U.S. National Academies of Science, the World Health Organization, the American Society of Plant Biologists, International Food Technologists, and the Academy of Nutrition and Dietetics are among the many agencies that support the responsible use of genetic engineering as a safe and effective means to improve food security and reduce negative effects of agriculture.

A lack of federal labeling regulations leaves consumers unable to identify foods containing GMO ingredients. Public campaigns by non-GMO advocates have convinced many consumers and government officials that labeling of GMO ingredients is necessary, often with arguments based on science demonstrated to be unsound (Fahlgren et al., 2016). Several states have enacted their own labeling regulations, and in summer of 2016, a bill was signed into law that requires a federal labeling standard for foods containing GMO ingredients. The USDA has 2 years to write the rules. In the meantime, many national food manufacturers are voluntarily disclosing on the label that their products contain genetically engineered ingredients.

Antibiotics in the Food Supply

In recent years, there have been more kilograms of antibiotics sold in the United States for food-producing animals such as hogs, cattle, and poultry than for people (FDA, 2014). Antibiotics are appropriately used to treat animals with infections. However, they were often routinely given in low doses to healthy animals for the purpose of promoting growth or preventing disease in crowded, unhygienic living conditions. The widespread use of antibiotics in animals contributes to the emergence of antibiotic-resistant bacteria which can be transmitted to humans through the food supply and can cause antibiotic-resistant infections (Fig. 9.6). As of January 2017, new federal regulations prohibit the use of antibiotics in healthy animals for the purpose of promoting weight gain and require a veterinarian's approval before using antibiotics that are important for human health.

Fueled by concerns about personal health, the environment, animal welfare, taste, and quality consumer demand for animal products produced without the routine use of antibiotics is growing, particularly for poultry (Natural Resources Defense Council, 2015). In response to consumer demands, McDonalds announced in early 2015 that within 2 years, it will only serve chicken raised without the use of medically important antibiotics. Tyson Foods, the nation's largest chicken processor, announced that by September 2017, it will not use human antibiotics to raise chickens in its U.S. operations. Elevation Burger, Panera Bread, Chick-Fil-A, and Chipotle are restaurants that are leading the industry in featuring antibiotic-free animal products. For consumers, products labeled *Organic*, *No Antibiotics/Raised without Antibiotics*, and *American Grassfed Certified* mean the animal was never given antibiotics.

Food Irradiation

To many consumers, the term *irradiated food* conjures up visions of radioactive fallout. In truth, irradiation is a safe and effective technology that can prevent many foodborne illnesses by reducing or

Figure 9.6 ▶

Antibiotic resistance from the farm to the table.
(Source: Centers for Disease Control and Prevention. [n.d.]. Antibiotic resistance from the farm to the table. Available at http://www.cdc.gov/foodsafety /challenges/from-farm-to-table .html. Accessed on 11/17/16.)

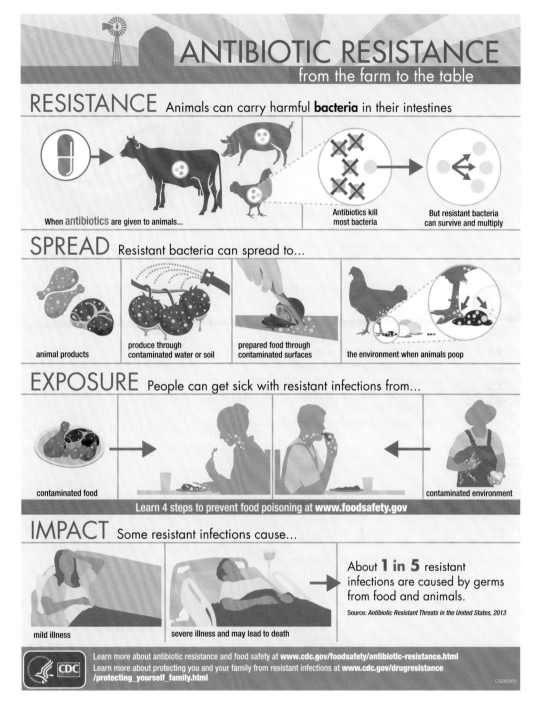

eliminating pathogens, controlling insects, or killing parasites. Irradiation also reduces food losses from infestation, contamination, and spoilage.

Irradiation does not use heat; it is sometimes referred to as "electronic pasteurization." Bacteria, mold, fungi, and insects are destroyed as radiant energy, such as gamma rays, electron beams, and x-rays, pass through the food. A small amount of new compounds are formed that are similar to the changes seen in food as it is cooked, pasteurized, frozen, or otherwise prepared. Except for a slight decrease in thiamin, the nutrient losses are less than or about the same as losses caused by cooking and freezing. Because irradiation kills any living cells that may be contained in the food, such as in seeds or potatoes, shelf life may be prolonged. For instance, irradiated potatoes do not sprout during storage. However, irradiation does not hide spoilage or eliminate the need for safe food handling; irradiated food can still become contaminated through cross-contamination.

Figure 9.7 ▶

Radura: international symbol for irradiation.

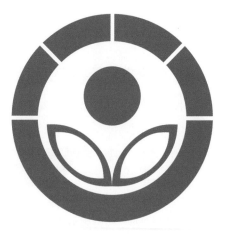

Irradiation is the most extensively studied food-processing technique available in the world and is used by more than 50 countries on more than 60 products (Institute of Food Science and Technology, 2015). The FDA first approved the use of radiation in 1963 and is responsible for establishing the maximum radiation dose allowed on foods. Approximately, one-third of the total foods irradiated in the United States are spices; the other top items are fresh produce, ground beef, and pet treats (Institute of Food Science and Technology, 2015). Federal law requires irradiated food to be labeled with the international symbol, the radura (Fig. 9.7), and state "Treated with irradiation" or "Treated by irradiation." Research on irradiation as a part of an overall system of ensuring food safety is ongoing.

Quick Bite

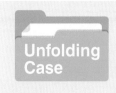

Foods allowed to be irradiated in the United States include

Wheat and wheat flour to control mold
White potatoes to inhibit sprouting
Pork to kill trichina parasites
Fresh produce to control insects
Iceberg lettuce and spinach to kill bacteria
Many spices and dry vegetable seasonings for sterilization
Fresh red meat and poultry to reduce bacterial pathogens

Unfolding Case

Think of Paul. He watched a documentary on irradiated food and is convinced he will get cancer if he eats any of it. How can Paul avoid irradiated food?

How Do You Respond?

Is grass-fed beef better than grain-fed beef? The nutritional difference between grass-fed and grain-fed beef is slight. Grass-fed beef is slightly lower in calories and total fat and slightly higher in protein (Vogliano et al., 2015). Actually, all cattle start their lives eating grass; grains are added to the diet when grazing is not adequate to meet the animals' needs. Although there is little difference in the nutritional value of grass-fed versus grain-fed beef, there is a difference in environmental impact. Grass-fed cattle gain weight slower and thus take longer to reach slaughter weight. Because they are alive longer than grain-fed cattle, they produce more methane gas during their lives. In addition, grass is lower in digestibility than grain, leaving more fiber available for microbiota that produces methane.

Can you prevent foodborne illness by washing produce? Although washing produce—even varieties that you peel—is recommended, it cannot guarantee food safety. For instance, it is difficult to remove sticky bacteria from leafy greens like spinach. Even "triple" washed or thoroughly washed ready-to-eat bags of spinach, lettuce, and mixed greens may be contaminated with bacteria because the cleaning process using chlorinated water kills only 90% to 95% of microbes when performed correctly. And with other produce, such as melon, mango, or apple, if bacteria have migrated to the inside of the fruit, such as traveling through the apple core to the interior, washing will not remove it. Safe food handling at home is important but cannot guarantee safety.

REVIEW CASE STUDY

Maria is 52 years old, has a normal body mass index (BMI), and does not have any health problems. She prides herself on being "into" holistic treatments and goes to the doctor only when her attempts to treat herself fail. She occasionally takes one aspirin a day because she has heard that it can prevent heart attacks. She tries to eat a healthy diet and uses supplements to give her added protection against chronic diseases, especially heart disease, which runs in her family. Currently, she takes ginkgo biloba to prevent memory loss, garlic to prevent heart disease, and fish oil supplements to keep her blood thin. She routinely drinks omega-3–fortified orange juice and organic milk. She attributes the bruises on her legs to being clumsy. She is thinking about adding vitamin E to her regimen because she heard it may also lower the risk of heart disease. She is thinking about discontinuing her use of garlic pills and fish oil supplements and instead eating more garlic and fish in her diet.

- What are the dangers of her present regimen? What may be responsible for the bruising she is experiencing?
- What would you tell Maria about the use of supplements in general? About the types and combination of supplements she is currently using? What specific changes would you suggest she make?
- What would you tell her about using omega-3–fortified milk and juice?
- Is it safer for her to eat more garlic and fish instead of taking them as supplements? Is it as "effective" as taking them as supplements? Could she "overdose" on garlic and fish oil from food?
- What questions would you ask about her diet to see if there are any improvements in her eating habits she could make to reduce the risk of heart disease?

STUDY QUESTIONS

1 Which statement indicates that the client needs further instruction about reading nutrition labels?
  a. "The %DV is based on a 2000-calorie eating pattern."
  b. "The %DV represents the percentage of calories in that food from each energy-yielding nutrient."
  c. "The dual column labels show information per serving and per package.
  d. "The serving size listed on the label is based on how much people actually eat, not on what they should be eating."

2 The client asks if a tea that claims to "improve memory" really works. Which of the following would be the nurse's best response?
  a. "If the tea claims to improve memory, it has been tested and proven effective at improving memory."
  b. "Claims on food labels are not regulated by law and cannot be trusted."
  c. "Function claims like 'improve memory' can be used on labels without supporting proof that they are accurate."
  d. "That type of claim is illegal and should not appear on any food label."

3 Which statement about supplements is accurate?
  a. "All supplements must be tested for safety and effectiveness before they can be marketed."
  b. "Supplement dosages are standardized."
  c. "Proper handling of supplement ingredients is required by law."
  d. "Warnings about potential side effects or interactions must be stated on the packaging."

4 Which supplement should be used with caution by people taking anticoagulants?
  a. Echinacea
  b. St. John's wort
  c. Cranberry
  d. Garlic

5 A client asks how she can minimize her risk of foodborne illness. Which of the following should the nurse include in the response as the best way to reduce the risk? Select all that apply.
  a. "Wash your hands before and after handling food."
  b. "Rely on organically grown foods as much as possible."
  c. "Cook foods thoroughly."
  d. "Avoid cross-contamination by using separate surfaces for meats and foods that will be eaten raw."

6 The best response to a client's question about whether organic food is worth the extra cost is
  a. "Is there anything more important to spend money on than your health?"
  b. "There is no difference in pesticide levels and nutritional value of organically grown foods compared to conventional foods."
  c. "Buying organic foods is an individual decision; some may have more nutritional value than their conventional counterparts, and they do have lower pesticide levels."
  d. "It is worth it to buy organic produce but not organic meats."

7   A client asks how she can avoid meat and poultry that are given antibiotics. The nurse's best response is
   a. "Meat and poultry labeled as 'organic' cannot be given antibiotics."
   b. "There is no way to avoid meat and poultry that have been given antibiotics."
   c. "Buy meat and poultry labeled as 'natural' or 'all natural.'"
   d. "Buy meat and poultry labeled as 'American Humane Association.'"

8   A client asks how she can avoid buying foods that are genetically engineered. The nurse's best response is
   a. "Foods labeled as 'organic' cannot be genetically engineered."
   b. "There is no way to avoid genetically engineered foods."
   c. "Buy foods that have the radura symbol on them; they cannot be genetically engineered."
   d. "Buy foods labelled as 'natural' because they cannot be genetically engineered."

KEY CONCEPTS

- The field of nutrition is rapidly changing and growing. New challenges in nutrition stem from advances in food technology, the explosion of information available on the Internet, and the concept of food as medicine.
- To judge the validity and reliability of nutrition "news," ask who, what, when, where, and why. Beware of claims that sound too good to be true, quick fixes, and recommendations that are intended to help sell a product.
- Nutrition misinformation is everywhere and can be difficult to refute in a client who is convinced that what he or she knows is accurate.
- The "Nutrition Facts" label is intended to provide consumers with reliable and useful information to help avoid nutritional excesses such as calories, saturated fat, trans fat, added sugars, and sodium.
- The "Nutrition Facts" label is being revised to reflect updated dietary recommendations, current national survey data, and evidence on the role of eating patterns in health promotion and disease prevention. Serving sizes will be updated to correspond to the amounts people typically eat. Serving size and calories will be more prominent. Added sugars, vitamin D, and potassium will be new additions.
- The %DV listed on food labels for fat, saturated fat, carbohydrate, added sugars, and dietary fiber is based on a 2000-calorie eating pattern. The %DV for these nutrients underestimates the contribution in eating patterns containing fewer than 2000 calories.
- Ingredients are listed in order of descending weight.
- Unqualified health claims on food labels are based on SSA and include statements such as "calcium may help prevent osteoporosis" and "low sodium may help prevent high blood pressure."
- Qualified health claims are supported by scientific evidence but do not meet the standard for SSA. Examples of qualified health claims include the role of nuts in reducing cardiovascular disease risk and the role of green tea in reducing cancer risk.
- Structure/function claims, such as "improves mood," "relieves stress," and "for hot flashes," can be used without FDA approval and do not have to carry a disclaimer.
- A dietary supplement is a product (other than tobacco) intended to supplement the diet and that contains one or more of the following: vitamins, minerals, herbs, amino acids, or any combination of these ingredients.
- Dietary supplements are regulated by the FDA like food; proof of their safety and effectiveness is not required before marketing. When a dietary supplement is deemed to be unsafe by the FDA, consumer advisories are issued and the manufacturer is requested, not ordered, to stop selling the product. As such, harmful supplements may remain on the market.
- People choosing to use supplements should first check with the FDA for consumer advisories and consult with their physicians. Many supplements can render certain drugs ineffective or potentiate the effectiveness of drugs.
- Pregnant and lactating women and children under the age of 6 years should not use dietary supplements.
- Functional foods contain substances that appear to enhance health beyond their basic nutritional value. Incorporating more natural functional foods into the diet is prudent; the use of manufactured functional foods may be healthful but cannot compensate for poor overall food choices.
- There is a lack of strong evidence in the literature that organically grown foods are nutritionally superior to their conventionally grown counterparts. Because of production costs, higher losses, and lower yields, they are generally more expensive than other foods. However, organic produce consistently has lower levels of pesticides, and organic meats cannot be given antibiotics.
- The majority of foodborne illnesses are caused by norovirus; the majority of foodborne illness–related deaths are attributed to bacteria. Other causes of foodborne illness are parasites, molds, and unknown causes.
- The foods most commonly causing foodborne illness are those that are eaten raw or undercooked, such as fresh fruits and vegetables, raw meat and shellfish, undercooked poultry and eggs, and unpasteurized milk and fruit juices. Improper food handling, such as inadequate cooking and poor personal hygiene, is the major cause of foodborne illness.
- Food biotechnology uses genetic modification to improve the characteristics of a food. Biotechnology has created plant foods that are more resistant to disease, stay fresher longer,

have higher nutritional value, or are more resistant to severe weather. The FDA considers biotechnology safe. However, due to public pressure, a federal bill has been passed that requires a federal labeling standard for foods containing GMO ingredients. The USDA has 2 years to write the rules.
- Routine use of antibiotics in healthy animals to promote growth or prevent infection has been linked to antibiotic resistance that can be passed to humans through the food

supply. New federal regulations prohibit the use of antibiotics in healthy animals for the purpose of promoting weight gain.
- Irradiation is used to reduce or eliminate pathogens that can cause foodborne illness. The food remains uncooked and completely free of any radiation residues. Strict regulations and ongoing research protect consumers from potential risks regarding irradiation.

Check Your Knowledge Answer Key

1 **TRUE** Overuse of antibiotics in animals raised for food is linked to antibiotic-resistant infections in humans.
2 **TRUE** The new "Nutrition Facts" label includes the %DV for added sugars for the first time since the inception of the label.
3 **TRUE** The %DVs for fat, saturated fat, carbohydrate, added sugars, and fiber listed on the "Nutrition Facts" label are based on a 2000-calorie diet. The values are not accurate percentages for anyone who eats more or less than 2000 cal/day. The %DV for other nutrients, such as cholesterol and sodium, are based on daily reference values that are constant for all adults regardless of total calorie intake.
4 **FALSE** Structure/function claims are not regulated by the FDA; their use does not require prior approval nor is a disclaimer necessary.
5 **FALSE** Supplement manufacturers do not have to prove safety or effectiveness before marketing a product,

although they are not supposed to sell dangerous or ineffective products.
6 **FALSE** Warning labels about potential side effects or supplement–drug interactions are not required, nor is a statement regarding who should *not* use the product such as pregnant and lactating women, children under 6 years of age, or people with certain chronic illnesses.
7 **FALSE** The nutritional differences between an organic and conventionally grown produce are minimal, although it is difficult to reliably measure the differences due to variability of confounding factors, such as ripeness at the time of harvest.
8 **FALSE** Norovirus is responsible for an estimated 58% of all foodborne illnesses.
9 **FALSE** There is no evidence in harm from consuming genetically modified foods, including among pregnant women and children.
10 **FALSE** Irradiated food is completely free of radiation residues.

Student Resources on thePoint®
For additional learning materials, activate the code in the front of this book at
http://thePoint.lww.com/activate

Websites

Reliable nutrition information
Academy of Nutrition and Dietetics at www.eatright.org
American Cancer Society at www.cancer.org
American Diabetes Association at www.diabetes.org
Cancer Net, National Cancer Institute, National Institutes of Health at www.nci.nih.gov
New Wellness Consumer Health Information at www.netwellness.org
Center for Science in the Public Interest at www.cspinet.org
Health On the Net Foundation at www.hon.ch
International Food Information Council at www.ific.org
Mayo Clinic at www.mayohealth.org
National Council Against Health Fraud, Inc. at www.ncahf.org
National Heart, Lung, and Blood Institute, National Institutes of Health at www.nhlbi.nih.gov

Nutrition.gov at www.nutrition.gov
Office of Disease Prevention and Health Promotion at http://health.gov
PubMed, National Library of Medicine at www.ncbi.nlm.nih.gov/Pubmed/
U.S. Department of Agriculture Food and Nutrition Information Center at fnic.nal.usda.gov
U.S. Department of Health and Human Services Healthfinder at www.healthfinder.gov
U.S. Food and Drug Administration Center for Food Safety and Applied Nutrition at www.fda.gov/AboutFDA/CentersOffices/OfficeofFoods/CFSAN/default.htm

Supplement information
National Center for Complementary and Alternative Medicine Clearinghouse provides information on complementary and alternative medication at www.nccam.nih.gov
Office of Dietary Supplements (ODS) of the National Institutes of Health at http://ods.od.nih.gov/

U.S. Food and Drug Administration Center for Food Safety and Applied Nutrition at www.fda.gov/AboutFDA/CentersOffices/OfficeofFoods/CFSAN/default.htm. Check out "Tips for the Savvy Supplement User: Making Informed Decisions and Evaluating Information."

Food safety
International Food Information Council at www.ific.org
Partnership for Food Safety Education at www.fightbac.org
U.S. Food and Drug Administration at www.fda.gov

References

Biotechnology Industry Organization. (2010). *Healing, fueling, feeding: How biotechnology is enriching your life.* Available at https://www.bio.org/articles/healing-fueling-feeding-how-biotechnology-enriching-your-life. Accessed on 3/29/16.

Centers for Disease Control and Prevention. (2014). *Estimating foodborne illness: An overview.* Available at http://www.cdc.gov/foodborneburden/estimates-overview. Accessed on 3/27/16.

Crowe, K., & Francis, C. (2013). *Position of the academy of nutrition and dietetics: Functional foods. Journal of the Academy of Nutrition and Dietetics, 113,* 1096–1103.

Fahlgren, N., Bart, R., Herrara-Estrella, L., Rellán-Álvarez, R., Chitwood, D. H., & Dinneny, J. R. (2016). Plant scientists: GM technology is safe. *Science, 351,* 824.

Forman, J., & Silverstein, J. (2012). Organic foods: Health and environmental advantages and disadvantages. *Pediatrics, 130,* e1406–1405. doi:10.1542/peds.2012-2579

Institute of Food Science and Technology. (2015). *Food irradiation.* Available at http://www.ifst.org/knowledge-centre/information-statements/food-irradiation. Accessed on 3/28/16.

International Food Information Council. (2015a). *The 2015 Food & Health Survey: Consumer attitudes toward food safety, nutrition & health.* Available at http://www.foodinsight.org/2015-food-health-survey-consumer-research. Accessed on 3/26/16.

International Food Information Council. (2015b). *Pesticides and food: What you need to know.* Available at http://www.foodinsight.org/sites/default/files/Pesticide%20and%20Food%20Factsheet.pdf. Accessed on 3/29/16.

International Food Information Council. (2016). *No matter the food, ingredients product with biotechnology are as safe as "non-GMO."* Available at http://www.foodinsight.org/biotech-gmo-ingredients-safe-infant-formula. Accessed on 3/28/16.

International Service for the Acquisition of Agri-Biotech Applications. (2014). *ISAAA Brief 49-2014: Executive summary.* Available at http://www.isaaa.org/resources/publications/briefs/49/executivesummary/default.asp. Accessed on 3/27/16.

National Institutes of Health, Office of Dietary Supplements. (2016). *Multivitamin/mineral supplements.* Available at https://ods.od.nih.gov/factsheets/MVMS-HealthProfessional/. Accessed on 3/28/16.

Natural Resources Defense Council. (2015). *Going mainstream: Meat and poultry raised without routine antibiotics use.* Available at http://www.nrdc.org/food/files/antibiotic-free-meats-CS.pdf. Accessed on 3/28/16.

Organic Trade Association. (2015). *There's more to organic than meets the eye.* Available at http://ota.com/sites/default/files/indexed_files/PolicyConference2015_Infographic_8.5x11_1a_0.pdf. Accessed on 3/26/16.

Painter, J., Hoekstra, R., Ayers, T., Tauxe, R., Braden, C. R., Angulo, F. J., & Griffin, P. M. (2013). Attribution of foodborne illnesses, hospitalizations, and deaths to food commodities by using outbreak data, United States, 1998-2008. *Emerging Infectious Diseases, 19,* 407–415. doi:10.3201/eid1903.111866

Tang, G., Hu, Y., Yin, S-A., Wang, Y., Dallal, G. E., Grusak, M. A., & Russell, R. M. (2012). β-Carotene in Golden Rice is as good as β-carotene in oil at providing vitamin A to children. *American Journal of Clinical Nutrition, 96,* 658–664.

Tarver, T. (2012). Is the pathway to health organic? *Food Technology, 66,* 27–33.

U.S. Department of Agriculture, Economic Research Service. (2014). *Organic market overview.* Available at http://www.ers.usda.gov/topics/natural-resources-environment/organic-agriculture/organic-market-overview.aspx. Accessed on 3/26/16.

U.S. Food and Drug Administration. (2014). *Summary report on antimicrobials sold or distributed for use in food-producing animals.* Available at www.fda.gov/downloads/ForIndustry/UserFees/AnimalDrugUserFeeActADUFA/UCM338170.pdf. Accessed on 11/17/16.

U.S. Food and Drug Administration. (2015). *Letter of enforcement discretion to GMA/FMI re "Facts up Front."* Available at http://www.fda.gov/Food/IngredientsPackagingLabeling/LabelingNutrition/ucm302720.htm. Accessed on 9/18/16.

U.S. Food and Drug Administration. (2016a). *Changes to the Nutrition Facts label.* Available at http://www.fda.gov/food/guidanceregulation/guidancedocumentsregulatoryinformation/labelingnutrition/ucm385663.htm. Accessed on 9/19/16.

U.S. Food and Drug Administration. (2016b). *FDA modernizes Nutrition Facts label for packaged foods.* Available at www.fda.gov/NewsEvents/Newsroom/PressAnnouncements/ucm502182.htm. Accessed on 5/21/16.

Vogliano, C., Brown, K., Miller, A., Gree-Burgeson, D., Copenhaver, A. A., & Schmidt, J. (2015). Plentiful, nutrient-dense food for the world: a guide for registered dietitian nutritionists. *Journal of the Academy of Nutrition and Dietetics, 115,* 2014–2018.

Winter, C. (2011). *Expert perspective: Eat your fruits and veggies and don't fear the "dirty" rhetoric.* Available at http://www.foodinsight.org/Newsletter/Detail.aspx?topic=Expert_Perspective_Eat_Your_and_Veggies_and_Don_t_Fear_the_Dirty_Rhetoric. Accessed on 10/19/12.

Winter, C., & Katz, J. (2011). Dietary exposure to pesticide residues from commodities alleged to contain the highest contamination levels. *Journal of Toxicology, 2011,* 589674.

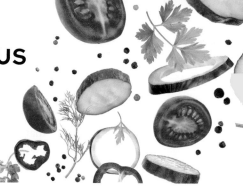

Chapter 10

Cultural and Religious Influences on Food and Nutrition

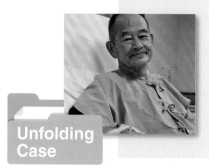

Unfolding Case

Phouvong Chanthavong

Phouvong is a 61-year-old man who immigrated with his wife and two daughters to the United States from Laos at the age of 35 years. He does not speak English, but his daughters are bilingual. He has just been admitted to the hospital for pneumonia where it was discovered he also has type 2 diabetes.

Check Your Knowledge

True	False		
☐	☐	**1**	Religion tends to have a greater impact on food choices than culture does.
☐	☐	**2**	Race and ethnicity are synonymous with culture.
☐	☐	**3**	Core foods tend to be complex carbohydrates, such as cereal grains, starchy tubers, and starchy vegetables.
☐	☐	**4**	Both Hinduism and Buddhism promote vegetarianism.
☐	☐	**5**	The hot–cold theory of health and diet refers to the temperature of the food eaten.
☐	☐	**6**	First-generation Americans tend to adhere more closely to their cultural food patterns than subsequent generations.
☐	☐	**7**	For many ethnic groups who move to the United States, breakfast and lunch are more likely than dinner to be composed of new "American" foods.
☐	☐	**8**	Food prepared away from home tends to increase a person's intake of calories, sodium, added sugar, and saturated and solid fat.
☐	☐	**9**	Dietary acculturation always produces unhealthy changes in eating.
☐	☐	**10**	Like restaurant food, the portion sizes listed on convenience meals are much larger than they should be.

Learning Objectives

Upon completion of this chapter, you will be able to

1 Debate the value of using convenience foods to prepare home-cooked meals.
2 Select the healthiest choices from a restaurant menu.
3 Give examples of how culture influences food choices.
4 Explain the general ways in which people's food choices change as they become acculturated to a new area.
5 Contrast American cultural values with those of traditional cultures.
6 Give examples of questions that may aid in the understanding of a person's cultural food pattern.
7 Summarize dietary laws followed by major world religions.

Based on Maslow's hierarchy of needs, food and nutrition rank on the same level as air in the basic necessities of life. Obviously, death eventually occurs without food. But unlike air, food does so much more than simply sustain life. Food is loaded with personal, social, and cultural meanings that define our food values, beliefs, and customs. That food nourishes the mind as well as the body broadens nutrition to an art as well as a science. Nutrition is not simply a matter of food or no food but rather a question of what kind, how much, how often, and why. Merging want with need and pleasure with health are keys to nourishing body, mind, and soul.

Culture
encompasses the total way of life of a particular population or community at a given time.

This chapter discusses what America eats and the impact of **culture** on food choices. Traditional food practices of major cultural subgroups in the United States are presented, as are religious food practices.

AMERICAN CUISINE

Foodway
an all-encompassing term that refers to all aspects of food including what is edible, the role of certain foods in the diet, how food is prepared, the use of foods, the number and timing of daily meals, how food is eaten, and health beliefs related to food.

American cuisine is a rich and complex melting pot of foods and cooking methods that have been adapted and adopted from cuisines brought to the United States by immigrants. Early settlers from northern and southern Europe came with their own established **foodway** that changed in response to what was available in the New World. Native Americans made significant contributions to American cuisine by introducing items such as corn, squash, beans, cranberries, and maple syrup. Later, West African slaves brought okra, watermelon, black-eyed peas, and taro and influenced the regional cuisine in the Southeastern United States with fried, boiled, and roasted dishes made with pork and pork fat. Likewise, American Southwest cuisine was shaped by flavors and ingredients brought across the border by Mexican Indians and Spanish settlers.

In the early 1850s, the first wave of Chinese immigrants came to the United States to join the gold rush. They brought stir-fry, a novel cooking method, and new foods such as egg rolls, fried rice, and spare ribs. The first wave of Italian immigrants arrived around 1880, and although they were unable to replicate their native foods, they utilized the available ingredients to create Americanized versions of lasagna, manicotti, veal parmigiana, and meatballs. Today, Italian food is mainstream American fare.

The influx of immigrants continued, and cuisines from around the globe melded. Today, it is difficult to determine which foods are truly American and which are an adaptation from other cultures. Swiss steak, Russian dressing, and chili con carne are American inventions. And although ethnic restaurants and ethnic foods sections in grocery stores offer distinct fare, cross-cultural food creations, such as Tex-Mex wontons and tofu lasagna, reaffirm the ongoing melting pot nature of American cuisine.

Although a "typical American diet" is difficult to define, Box 10.1 offers a snapshot view of what and how America eats. Driven by expediency and ease, convenience foods and restaurant-sourced meals (either dine in or takeout) are a driving force in current food trends.

BOX 10.1 Snapshot View of What and How America Eats

- More than 80% of our meals are prepared at home.
- Bananas are the most purchased fresh fruit, followed by apples, grapes, strawberries, and oranges.
- Tomatoes are the most purchased vegetable, followed by potatoes, onions, carrots, bell peppers, and broccoli.
- The average number of in-between meal snacks eaten daily per person is 2.6.
- 41% of adults eat three or more snacks daily.
- 79% of all restaurant meals are from fast-food outlets.
- Pizza is the most popular fast-food item ordered for dinner.
- 42% of women take calorie counts on the menu into account when ordering at a restaurant; 29% of men do.

Sources: Parade. (2014). *What American eats: Our exclusive survey on the nation's changing tastes.* Available at http://parade.com/334779/parade/what-america-eats-our-exclusive-survey-on-the-nations-changing-tastes/. Accessed on 4/1/16; and Sloan, A. (2016). What, when, and where America eats. *Food Technology, 70,* 23–35.

Quick Bite Examples of convenience items with a positive impact on nutrition

Fresh fruits and vegetables from the salad bar
Frozen juice concentrate
Washed spinach
Prewashed and cut vegetables
Complete salad kits
Plain frozen vegetables
Fresh sushi
Whole-grain rolls from the bakery section
Jarred spaghetti sauce
Prepared hummus
Rotisserie chickens
Lean delicatessen meats

Food Prepared at Home

During an average week, American consumers eat dinner at home 5.7 times (Sloan, 2016). Generally, food prepared at home is healthier than food obtained away from home (Virudachalam, Long, Harhay, Polsky, & Feudtner, 2014). Lower household wealth and education attainment are associated with a higher likelihood of either always or never cooking dinner at home; wealthier, more educated households were more likely to sometimes cook dinner at home (Virudachalam et al., 2014).

Fifty-eight percent of the main dishes made at home are made from scratch or made with fresh ingredients (Parade, 2014). Most people who prepare meals at home either very often or occasionally incorporate convenience items, such as pre-prepared and/or frozen ingredients to make from scratch cooking easier and quicker. Generally, the more convenient the meal is, the greater the impact all around on time, budget, and nutritional value. Frozen complete or nearly complete meals or boxed "helper" type entrées earn their designation as "convenient" but cost more than "from-scratch" items, lack that "homemade" taste, tend to be high in sodium, and the 1- to 2-cup portion sizes listed on the label may leave many people hungry. See Box 10.2 for tips on balancing convenience with nutrition.

A relatively new and growing option for preparing food at home is to use a meal kit delivery service. Consumers choose from a list of available meals online and receive the recipe and all the ingredients in the proper portions delivered to their door. Salt, pepper, and oil may be the only additional ingredients needed. These services are attractive to people who do not have the time for or interest in meal planning and food selection and they enable people to try new cuisines without investing in exotic ingredients such as a bottle of a spice when only a fraction of a teaspoon is needed. Meal kits tend to get favorable reviews for taste, variety, freshness, and convenience and eliminate waste from leftovers. On the downside, they are more expensive than traditionally prepared meals, the sodium content tends to be high, and not all delivery services provide nutrition information on their recipe cards.

Food Cooked Away from Home

Data from 2012 show that 43.1% of food spending was on food away from home (FAFH), which has risen steadily from 25.9% in 1970 (U.S. Department of Agriculture [USDA], Economic

---

BOX 10.2   Tips for Balancing Convenience with Nutrition

Read the label to comparison shop. Calories, fat, saturated fat, and sodium can vary greatly among different brands of similar items. A rule-of-thumb guideline is to limit sodium to less than 800 mg and fat to no more than 10 to 13 g in a meal that provides 300 to 400 calories.

Look for "healthy" on the label. The government allows "healthy" on the label of meals or entrées that limit sodium to 140 mg/100 g of food. And "healthy" foods must also provide 3 g or less of total fat or 1 g of saturated fat per 100 g of food. They are a better choice than the products not labeled "healthy" yet may still lack adequate fiber.

Add additional ingredients to "stretch" the meal. For instance, adding a bag of frozen vegetables, a can of tomatoes, or a can of garbanzo or black beans provides nutrients and increases volume.

Add healthy side dishes. A convenience "meal" that provides 300 to 400 calories may leave many people hungry. Adding quick and easy side dishes, such as bagged salad mixes, raw vegetables, whole-grain rolls, an instant cup of soup, or piece of fresh fruit, can greatly increase nutritional and satiety values.

Adjust the seasoning when possible. Some frozen meal solutions contain a separate seasoning packet; using half satisfies taste while cutting sodium.

Research Service [ERS], 2014). Although eating out may be easy and quick, diet quality suffers. Meals and snacks based on food prepared away from home contain more calories per eating occasion than home-prepared food (USDA, ERS, 2014). A study by Todd, Mancino, and Lin (2010) found that for the average adult, eating one meal of FAFH increases daily calorie intake by 134 calories. In addition, FAFH decreases the number of servings of fruit, vegetables, whole grains, and dairy per 1000 calories consumed; and fiber, calcium, and iron intakes decline. Conversely, FAFH increases sodium per 1000 calories and the percentage of calories from saturated fat, solid fat, alcohol, and added sugar. Because eating out has evolved from a special treat to a regular event, planning and menu savvy are needed to ensure that eating out is consistent with, not contradictory to, eating healthy. Tips for eating healthy while eating out appear in Box 10.3. "Best bet" choices from various ethnic restaurants are listed in Box 10.4.

Another category of food cooked away from home is prepared meals from the grocery store. Prepared food is a $29-billion-a-year business and is growing twice as fast as overall grocery store sales (Hobson, 2016). The trend in buying prepared items began with the desire for convenience;

BOX 10.3 Tips for Eating Healthy While Eating Out

Plan Ahead

- Choose the restaurant carefully so you know there are reasonable choices available.
- Check online or call ahead to inquire about menu selections. This is an especially important strategy when the location is not a matter of choice but, rather, a requirement such as for business luncheons or conferences. It may be possible to make a special request ahead of time.

Don't Arrive Starving

- People become much less discriminating in their food choices when they are hungry.
- Eating a small, high-fiber snack an hour or so before going out to dinner, such as whole wheat crackers with peanut butter or a piece of fresh fruit with milk, can take the edge off hunger without bankrupting healthy eating.

Balance the Rest of the Day

- When eating out *is* an occasion, such as for a birthday or anniversary celebration, make healthier choices the rest of the day to compensate for a planned indulgence.

Practice Portion Control

- Order the smallest size meat available.
- Create a doggie bag before eating; if you wait until the end of the meal, there may not be any left.
- Order regular size, not biggie size or super size.
- Order a la carte. Is a value meal a "better value" if it undermines your attempt to eat healthily?
- Order a half portion when available.
- Order two (carefully chosen) appetizers in place of an entrée, or order an appetizer and split an entrée with a companion.

Know the Terminology

Calorie-laden words to watch out for include:
- Buttered
- Battered

- Breaded
- Deep fried
- Au gratin
- Creamy
- Crispy
- Alfredo
- Bisque
- Hollandaise
- Parmigiana
- Béarnaise
- En croute
- Escalloped
- French fried
- Pan fried
- Rich
- Sautéed
- With gravy, with mayonnaise, with cheese

Less fatty terms are baked, braised, broiled, cooked in its own juice, grilled, lightly sautéed, poached, roasted, and steamed.

Beware of Hidden Fats, Such as

- High-fat meats
- Nuts
- Cream and full-fat milk
- Full-fat salad dressings and mayonnaise
- Sauces and gravies

Make Special Requests

- Order sauces and gravies "on the side."
- Ask that lower fat items be substituted for high-fat items (e.g., a baked potato instead of French fries).
- Substitute brown rice for white rice.
- Request an alternate cooking method (e.g., broiled instead of fried).

BOX 10.4 Best Bet Choices from Fast-Food and Ethnic Restaurants

Fast Foods

English muffins or bagels with spreads on the side
Butter, margarine, or syrups on the side—not added to food
Baked potato—plain or with reduced-fat or fat-free dressings or salsa
Pretzels or baked chips
Regular, small, or junior sizes
Ketchup, mustard, relish, BBQ sauce, and fresh vegetables as toppings
Grilled chicken sandwiches without "special sauce"
Veggie burger
Small roast beef on roll
Fruit 'n yogurt parfait
Lean, 6-in subs on whole-grain rolls
Side salads with reduced-fat or fat-free dressings
Salads with grilled chicken
Low-fat or nonfat milk
Fresh fruit
Specialty coffees with skim milk

Salad Bars

Dark, leafy greens
Plain raw vegetables
Chickpeas, kidney beans, peas
Low-fat cottage cheese
Hard-cooked egg
Fresh fruit
Lean ham, turkey
Reduced-fat or fat-free dressings

Pizza

Thin crust
Vegetables: onions, spinach, tomatoes, broccoli, mushrooms, peppers
Lean meats: Canadian bacon, ham, grilled chicken, shrimp, crab meat
Half-cheese pizza
Salad as a side dish

Buffet

Survey the buffet before beginning.
Use a small plate.
Pile food no thicker than a deck of cards.
Practice the "plate method": one-quarter meat, three-quarters plants.

Mexican

Sauces: salsa, mole, picante, enchilada, pico de gallo
Guacamole and sour cream on the side
Black bean soup, gazpacho
Soft, nonfried tortillas as in bean burritos or enchiladas
Refried beans (without lard)
Arroz con pollo (chicken with rice)
Grilled meat, fish, or chicken
Steamed vegetables
Soft-shell chicken or veggie tacos
A la carte or half entrée
Fajitas: chicken, seafood, vegetable, beef
Flan (usually a small portion)

Chinese

Hot-and-sour soup, wonton soup
Chicken chow mein
Chicken or beef chop suey
Szechuan dishes
Shrimp with garlic sauce
Stir-fried and teriyaki dishes
Noodles: lo mein, chow fun, Singapore noodles
Steamed rice instead of fried
Steamed spring rolls
Tofu
Steamed dumplings and other dim sum instead of egg rolls
Fortune cookies
Use chopsticks
No monosodium glutamate (MSG)

Italian

Minestrone
Garden salad; vinegar and oil dressing
Breadsticks, bruschetta, Italian bread
Sauces: red clam, marinara, wine, cacciatore, fra diavolo, marsala
Shrimp, veal, chicken without breading
Choose vegetables for a side dish instead of pasta or potatoes
Limit "unlimited" bread or breadsticks
Italian ice or fruit

Indian

Raw vegetable salads, Mulligatawny soup (lentil soup)
Tandoori meats
Condiments: fruits and vegetable chutneys, raita (cucumber and yogurt sauce)
Lentil and chickpea curries
Chicken and vegetables
Chicken rice pilaf
Basmati rice
Naan (bread baked in tandoori oven)
Dal

Japanese

Boiled green soybeans, miso soup, bean soups
Sushi—cooked varieties include imitation crab, cooked shrimp, scrambled egg
Most combinations of grilled meats or seafood
Teriyaki chicken or seafood
Steamed rice, rice noodles
Green tea

Greek

Lentil soup
Greek salad, tabouli
Chicken, lamb, pork souvlaki salad or sandwich
Shish kebabs
Pita bread
Make a meal of appetizers: baba ghanoush (smoked eggplant), hummus (mashed chickpeas), dolma (stuffed grape leaves), and tabouli (cracked wheat salad). Olive oil is often poured on the baba ghanoush, hummus, and other foods, so ask for it on the side.

its growth is fueled by consumers' perception that prepared food is fresher and healthier than take out dinners or **convenience foods** from the frozen food aisle. However, the "fresh" food may not actually be made on premises, sodium content is often high, serving sizes are not suggested so it is easy to over buy and overeat, and items are generally much more expensive than making the item at home.

THE EFFECT OF CULTURE

Quick Bite Culture

- Has an inherent value system that defines what is "normal"
- Is learned, not instinctive
- Is passed from generation to generation
- Has an unconscious influence on its members
- Resists change but is not static

Culture has a profound and unconscious effect on food choices. Yet, within all cultures, individuals or groups of individuals may behave differently from the socially standardized foodway because of age, gender, state of health, household structure, or socioeconomic status. Race, ethnicity, and geographic region are often inaccurately assumed to be synonymous with culture. This misconception leads to stereotypic grouping, such as assuming that all Jews adhere to orthodox food laws or that all Southerners eat sausage, biscuits, and gravy. **Subgroups** within a culture display a

Subgroups
unique cultural groups that exists within a dominant culture.

unique range of cultural characteristics that affect food intake and nutritional status. What is edible, the role of food, how food is prepared, the symbolic use of food, and when and how food is eaten are among the many characteristics defined by culture.

Culture Defines What Is Edible

Edible
foods that are part of an individual's diet.

Inedible
foods that are usually poisonous or taboo.

Culture determines what is **edible** and what is **inedible**. To be labeled a food, an item must be readily available, safe, and nutritious enough to support reproduction. However, cultures do not define as edible all sources of nutrients that meet those criteria. For instance, in the United States, horsemeat, insects, and dog meat are not considered food, even though they meet the food criteria. Culture overrides flavor in determining what is offensive or unacceptable. For example, you may like a food (e.g., rattlesnake) until you know what it is; this reflects disliking the *idea* of the food rather than the actual food itself. An unconscious food selection decision process appears in Figure 10.1.

The Role of Certain Foods in the Diet

Every culture has a ranking for its foods that is influenced by cost and availability. Major food categories include core foods, secondary foods, and peripheral, or occasional, foods.

Core Foods

Core Foods
the important and consistently eaten foods that form the foundation of the diet; they are the dietary staples.

Core foods provide a significant source of calories and are regularly included in the diet, usually on a daily basis. Core foods are typically complex carbohydrates, such as cereal grains (rice, wheat, millet, corn), starchy tubers (potatoes, yams, taro, cassava), and starchy vegetables (plantain or green bananas). In much of the world, high-fat, energy-dense diets have replaced traditional diets high in complex carbohydrates (Caprio et al., 2008).

Unfolding Case

Consider Phouvong. A core food in his eating pattern is sticky rice, a type of rice referred to as glutinous because it is glue-like or sticky, not because it contains gluten. Through an interpreter, the nurse learns Phouvong eats a traditional Laotian eating pattern and will not eat American food. The only food he eats that is not prepared by his wife is food prepared by other Laotians in his tightly knit community. What information would be important to obtain in order to meet his nutritional needs in a culturally appropriate manner?

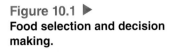

Figure 10.1 ▶
Food selection and decision making.

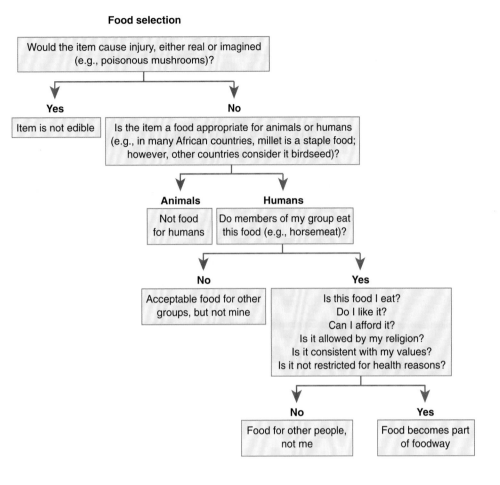

Secondary Foods

> **Secondary Foods**
> foods that are widespread in the diet but not eaten consistently.

Foods widely consumed, but not on a daily basis, are considered **secondary foods**, such as vegetables, legumes, nuts, fish, eggs, and meats. Secondary foods used by a culture vary with availability. For instance, the types of legumes used in Chinese culture include mung beans and soybeans, whereas those used in Latin American culture include black beans and pinto beans.

Peripheral Foods

> **Peripheral, or Occasional, Foods**
> foods that are infrequently consumed.

Peripheral, or occasional, foods, eaten sporadically, are typically based on an individual's preferences, not cultural norms. They may be foods that are reserved for special occasions, not readily available, or not generally well tolerated, as is the case with milk among Asian Americans.

How Food Is Prepared

Traditional methods of preparation vary between and within cultural groups. For instance, vegetables often are stir-fried in Asian cultures but boiled in Hispanic cultures. What is deemed a healthy cooking method in the United States, such as baking and grilling, may be seen by other groups as causing an undesirable change in the nature of the food (Carr, 2012). Traditional seasonings also vary among cultures and may be the distinguishing feature between one culture's foods and another's (Table 10.1). The choice of seasonings varies among geographic regions and between seasons, based on availability. With home-prepared meals, seasonings are adjusted to suit the family's preferences.

Table 10.1   Examples of Seasonings Used by Various Cultures

Cultural Group	Distinguishing Flavors
Asian Indian	Garam masala (curry blend of coriander, cumin, fenugreek, turmeric, black pepper, cayenne, cloves, cardamom, and chili peppers), mint, saffron, mustard, fennel, cinnamon
Brazilian (Bahia)	Chili peppers, dried shrimp, ginger root, palm oil
Chinese	Soy sauce, rice wine, ginger root
French	Butter, cream, wine, bouquet garni (tarragon, thyme, bay leaf)
German	Sour cream, vinegar, dill, mustard, black pepper
Greek	Lemon, onions, garlic, oregano, olive oil
Italian	Tomato, garlic, basil, oregano, olive oil
Japanese	Soy sauce, sugar, rice wine vinegar
Korean	Soy sauce, garlic, ginger root, black pepper, scallions, chili peppers, sesame seeds or oil
Mexican	Tomatoes, onions, chili peppers, cumin
Puerto Rican	Sofrito (seasoning sauce of tomatoes, onions, garlic, bell peppers, cilantro, capers, pimento, annatto seeds, and lard)
Thai	Fermented fish sauce, coconut milk, chili peppers, garlic, ginger root, lemon grass, tamarind

Source: Kittler, P., Sucher, K., & Nahikian-Nelms, M. (2012). *Food and culture* (6th ed.). Belmont, CA: Wadsworth Cengage Learning.

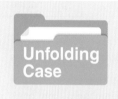

Unfolding Case

Recall Phouvong. A Laotian comfort food is pho, a beef broth–based soup that is made by boiling the broth and then adding sliced raw beef with the idea that the broth cooks the meat. His wife is smuggling pho, sticky rice, and a variety of other foods into the hospital because he will not eat American food. His wife has been hiding the food in his bedside table to avoid getting in trouble. What should the nurse do?

Symbolic Use of Foods

Each culture has food customs and bestows symbolism on certain foods. Custom determines what foods are served as meals versus snacks and what foods are considered feminine versus masculine. Symbolically, food can be used to express love, to reward or punish, to display piety, to express moral sentiments, to demonstrate belongingness to a group, or to proclaim the separateness of a group. On a personal level, food may be used inappropriately to relieve anxiety, reduce stress, ease loneliness, or to substitute for sex. Culture also determines which foods are used in celebration and which provide comfort. People who move to other cultures may retain their own cultural comfort foods as a link with the past.

When and How Food Is Eaten

All cultures eat at least once a day. Some may eat five or more meals each day. Dinner may start at 6 PM in Australia or 7 to 9 PM in Kenya. A Lebanese custom is to arrive anytime when invited for dinner, even as early as 9 or 10 AM. Food may be eaten with chopsticks, a knife and fork, or fingers. In the United States, bad manners in eating may be associated with animal behavior, as in "He eats like a pig," "She chews like a cow," or "Don't wolf down your food."

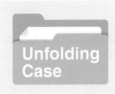

Unfolding Case

Think of Phouvong. He eats sticky rice with his hands, dipping it in fish paste or pho. What measures can you take to help minimize Phouvong's risk of foodborne illness?

Cultural Values

Cultural values define desirable and undesirable personal and public behavior and social interaction. Understanding the client's cultural values and their impact on health and food choices facilitates cross-cultural nutrition care. Table 10.2 highlights the contrast between selected American cultural values and values of more traditional cultures.

Health Beliefs

Each culture has a unique point of view on life, health, and illness, and the meaning of each in society (Kittler, Sucher, & Nahikian-Nelms, 2012). Almost all cultures define certain foods that promote wellness, cure disease, or impart medicinal properties. For instance, hot oregano tea seasoned with salt is used to treat an upset stomach in Vietnamese culture. A South Asian belief is that ghee (clarified butter) is soothing and gives strength, which may make it hard for some South Asian people to accept that ghee is not good for health, despite its high fat and calorie content (Carr, 2012). Some cultures define foods that create equilibrium within the body and soul (Kittler et al., 2012). Culture also shapes body image. In the United States, "you can never be too thin," and thinness, particularly in women, is equated with beauty and status. Overweight and

Table 10.2 A Contrast of Cultural Values

American Values	Traditional Values	Potential Considerations of Traditional Values
Personal control Individuals believe they have personal control over their future.	**Fate** Individuals may have an external locus of control, believing that what happens to them as out of their control and that their personal habits have little or no effect.	Patients may not consider themselves active participants in their own healing but rather recipients.
Individualism Interests and needs of the individual have preference over those of the group.	**Group welfare** The needs of the group (family) are valued over the needs of the individual; decisions may be left up to the head of the family.	Establish close rapport with the patient by asking about the family; make family feel welcome. Involve family in planning. Emphasize the good of the entire family rather than individual benefits.
Time dominates "Being on time" and "not wasting time" are virtues.	**Human interaction dominates** Personal interaction is more important than time management.	Expediency and efficiency may be counterproductive. Pause while talking. Avoid interruptions.
Informality Informality is viewed as a sign of friendliness.	**Formality** Informality may be equated with disrespect.	Use a formal tone, especially with older people.
Directness Honest, open communication is considered effective communication.	**Indirectness** Straightforwardness may be rude or too personal.	It may be appropriate to avoid eye contact. Talking in the third person, such as "someone who wants to eat less sodium may choose fresh vegetables over canned" is valued over "you should. . . ." Asking questions may be considered disrespectful; ask questions judiciously.

obesity may be viewed as a character flaw. Conversely, thinness has historically been a risk factor for poor health or associated with poverty. In many cultures today, including those of some Africans, Mexicans, American Indians, and Caribbean Islanders, being overweight is a sign of health, beauty, and prosperity (Kittler et al., 2012). To some people, "healthy eating" is synonymous with eating large quantities of food rather than making more nutritious food choices. Questions that may aid in the understanding of health beliefs include the following (Eggenberger, Grassley, & Restrepo, 2006):

- What does it mean to be healthy?
- What do you do to keep healthy?
- What do you teach your children about health?
- What health practices do you engage in that differ from what your ancestors did?
- What do you think makes a person sick?
- When a person is sick, do you think they are in control of making themselves better?
- What do you do when you are sick?
- Who helps you when you are sick?
- Have you been to a folk healer or used folk medicine when you are sick?
- Where do you get health information?

Dietary Acculturation

Dietary Acculturation
the process that occurs as members of a minority group adopt the eating patterns and food choices of the host country.

Acculturation
the process that occurs as people who move to a different cultural area adopt the beliefs, values, attitudes, and behaviors of the dominant culture; not limited to immigrants but affects anyone (to varying degrees) who moves from one community to another.

Dietary acculturation occurs when eating patterns of immigrants change to resemble those of the host country. In the United States, **acculturation** is linked to increased risk of chronic disease and obesity; however, its effect on diet quality is inconsistent (Sofianou, Fung, & Tucker, 2011). For instance, a study by Batis, Hernandez-Barrera, Barquera, Rivera, and Popkin (2011) found that dietary acculturation in Mexican Americans leads not only to some positive changes, such as higher intakes of low-fat meat and fish, high-fiber bread, and low-fat milk, but also to some negative effects, such as higher intakes of saturated fat, sugar, dessert, salty snacks, pizza, and French fries. Likewise, studies show that acculturation in Asian Americans causes an increase in the intake of grains, dairy products, fruits, and vegetables but also of fat and sweets (Lv & Carson, 2004; Satia et al., 2001). Clearly, acculturation is a highly complex, dynamic, multidimensional process that is impacted by a variety of personal, cultural, and environmental factors (Satia, 2009). Associations of acculturation with diet are often inconsistent and do not fit an expected pattern (Satia, 2009).

Generally, food habits are one of the last behaviors people change through acculturation, possibly because eating is done in the privacy of the home, not in full view of the majority culture. Usually, first-generation Americans adhere more closely to cultural food patterns and have at least one native meal daily (Brown, 2005). They may cling to traditional foods to affirm their cultural identity. Second-generation Americans do not have the direct native connection and may follow cultural patterns only on holidays and at family gatherings, or they may give up ethnic foods but retain traditional methods of preparation. Children tend to adopt new ways quickly as they learn from other children at school. Points to keep in mind regarding dietary acculturation appear in Box 10.5.

Interrelated changes in food choices that occur as part of acculturation are as follows:

- *New foods are added to the diet.* Status, economics, information, taste, and exposure are some of the reasons why new foods are added to the diet. Eating "American" food may symbolize status and make people feel more connected to their new culture. Frequently, new foods are added because they are relatively inexpensive and widely available.
- *Some traditional foods are replaced by new foods.* This often occurs because traditional foods may be difficult to find, are too expensive, or have lengthy preparation times. For many ethnic groups who move to the United States, breakfast and lunch are most likely to be composed of convenient American foods, whereas traditional foods are retained for the major dinner meal, which has greater emotional significance.
- *Some traditional foods are rejected.* To become more like their peers, children and adolescents are more likely than older adults to reject traditional foods. Traditional foods

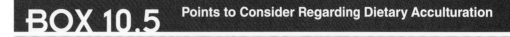

BOX 10.5 **Points to Consider Regarding Dietary Acculturation**

- Generally with acculturation, the intake of sweets and fats increases, neither of which has a positive effect on health.
- Because dietary acculturation is most likely to change food choices for breakfast and lunch rather than dinner, focus on promoting healthy "American" food choices for those meals.
- Portion control is a better option than advising someone to eliminate an important native food from their diet. Lower fat or lower sodium options, when available, may also be an acceptable option for the client. Although giving up soy sauce may not be an option for a Chinese American, using a reduced-sodium version may be doable.
- It is essential to determine how often a food is consumed in order to determine the potential impact of that food. For instance, lard is unimportant in the context of the total diet if it is used in cooking only on special occasions.
- Don't assume the client knows what American foods are considered healthy.
- Suggest fruits and vegetables that are similar in texture to those that are familiar but unavailable to the client.

may also be rejected because of an increased awareness of the role of nutrition in the development of chronic diseases. For instance, one reason why Indians who have resided in the United States for a relatively long period tend to eat significantly less ghee (clarified butter served with rice or spread on Indian breads) may be that they are trying to decrease their intake of saturated fat.

Understanding Acculturation

It is important to understand acculturation so that interventions to promote healthy food choices can be tailored to be culturally and individually appropriate. Ideally, clients will retain healthy traditional food practices, adopt healthy new food behaviors, and avoid forming less healthy American dietary habits. Although first-generation citizens usually need help choosing American replacements for their native foods, second-generation citizens may need help selecting healthy American foods.

To be effective in encouraging clients to make healthier food choices, health-care professionals must possess specific knowledge about food habits, preferences, and practices among the cultural and ethnic groups they see in their practice (Goody & Drago, 2009). Questions that may aid in the understanding of food habits include the following:

- What traditional foods do you eat daily?
- What are your favorite foods?
- What foods do you eat on holidays or special occasions?
- What traditional foods do you no longer eat?
- What new foods do you eat? Remember that new immigrants may not know the name of American foods.
- What prompted you to eat these new foods?
- Do you regularly eat new foods?
- What foods do you eat to keep you healthy?
- What natural herbs or home remedies do you use?
- What foods do you avoid to prevent illness?
- Do you balance some foods with other foods?
- Are there foods you will not eat? Is it because of personal preference, cultural norms, or religious mandate?
- Do you have enough food to eat each day?
- For hospitalized clients: Are there any special customs or religious practices you want performed before or after a meal?

Suggestions for conducting effective cross-cultural nutrition counseling are listed in Box 10.6.

BOX 10.6   Suggestions for Conducting Effective Cross-Cultural Nutrition Counseling

- Establish rapport; respect cultural differences.
- Be knowledgeable about cultural food habits and health beliefs.
- Relevant guidance must include advice on traditional foods and preparation methods to retain or reduce.
- Use culturally appropriate verbal and nonverbal communication.
- Determine the primary written and spoken language used in the client's home.
- Use trained interpreters when necessary.
- Determine whether the client prefers direct or indirect communication.
- Pare down information to only what the client needs to know.
- Emphasize the positive food practices of traditional health beliefs and food customs.
- Explain medical reasons for recommended changes.
- Provide written material only after determining reading ability.
- Communicate consistent messages.

TRADITIONAL DIETS OF SELECTED CULTURAL SUBGROUPS IN THE UNITED STATES

The U.S. Census Bureau (2015) projects that by the year 2044, more than half of all Americans will belong to a minority group. The nutritional implication of this shift in cultural predominance is that cultural competence will become increasingly important to nursing care. Nutrition information that is technically correct but culturally inappropriate does not produce behavior change. Cultural competence facilitates nutrition care consistent with the individual's attitudes, beliefs, and values.

The minimum categories for data on race and ethnicity as determined by the U.S. Office of Management and Budget (1997) are

- American Indian or Alaska Native: people having origins in any of the original peoples of North and South America, including Central America, who maintain tribal affiliation or community attachment
- Asian: people having origins in any of the original peoples of the Far East, Southeast Asia, or the Indian subcontinent, including China, India, Pakistan, Thailand, Vietnam
- Black or African American: people having origins in any of the black racial groups of Africa
- Hispanic or Latino: people of Cuban, Mexican, Puerto Rican, South or Central American, or other Spanish culture or origin, regardless of race, "Spanish origin" can be used in addition to Hispanic or Latino
- Native Hawaiian or Other Pacific Islander: people having origins in any of the original peoples of Hawaii, Guam, Samoa, or other Pacific Islands
- White: people having origins in any of the original peoples of Europe, the Middle East, or North Africa

Each of these categories has multiple, diverse subgroups. For instance, the category of Native Americans comprises more than 575 federally recognized tribes and more than 300 other tribes, each with their own language and culture (Kagawa-Singer, Dadia, Yu, & Surbone, 2010). In addition, multiracial individuals represent a growing population.

Three major cultural subgroups in the United States are highlighted in the following sections. A summary of health statistics by cultural group appears in Table 10.3. Although generalizations can be made about traditional eating practices and dietary changes related to acculturation, actual food choices vary greatly within a subgroup on the basis of national, regional, ethnic, and individual differences.

African Americans

According to the U.S. Census Bureau, 13.2% of the population in 2014 was Black or African American alone (U.S. Census Bureau, 2014). The majority of African Americans can trace their ancestors to West Africa, although some have immigrated from the Caribbean, Central

Table 10.3   Summary of Health Statistics by Cultural Group

Health Indicators	Asian or Pacific Islander Americans	Black or African Non-Hispanic Americans	Hispanic or Latino Americans	White Non-Hispanic Americans
% of people all ages in fair or poor health	7%	13.5%	9.6%	9.4%
Obesity in people ≥20 years old				
Males	11.2%	37.5%	39.0%	33.6%
Females	11.9%	56.9%	45.7%	33.5%
Hypertension in people ≥18 years old				
Men	26.5%	40.8%	25.4%	29.4%
Women	23.5%	41.5%	26.2%	26.57%
Leading causes of death	Cancer Heart disease Stroke	Heart disease Cancer Stroke	Cancer Heart disease Accidents	Heart disease Cancer Chronic lower respiratory disease
Infant deaths/1000 live births	4.07	11.11	5	5.06

Sources: Centers for Disease Control and Prevention, National Center for Health Statistics. (n.d.). *FactStats—statistics by topic*. Available at http://www.cdc.gov/nchs /fastats/default.htm. Accessed on 3/31/16; Centers for Disease Control and Prevention, National Center for Health Statistics. (2015). *Prevalence of obesity among adults and youth: United States, 2011-2014*. Available at http://www.cdc.gov/nchs/data/databriefs/db219.htm. Accessed on 3/31/16; and Centers for Disease Control and Prevention, National Center for Health Statistics. (2012). Hypertension among adults in the US, 2009-2010. Available at http://www.cdc.gov/nchs/data/databriefs /db107.htm. Accessed on 3/31/16.

America, and East African countries. Because most are many generations away from their original homeland, much of their native heritage has been assimilated, lost, or modified.

Traditional Food Practices

"Soul food" describes traditional Southern African American foods and cooking techniques that evolved from West African, slave, and postabolition cuisine. Many soul food customs and practices are shared by white Americans in the Southern United States, particularly those of lower socioeconomic status or living in rural areas (Kulkarni, 2004).

Traditional soul foods tend to be high in fat, cholesterol, and sodium and low in protective nutrients, such as potassium (fruits and vegetables), fiber (whole grains and vegetables), and calcium (milk, cheese, and yogurt). Corn and corn products (grits and cornmeal) are the primary grain. Meats are often breaded and fried. A variety of beef and pork cuts are consumed, as are poultry, oxtail, tripe, and tongue. Table 10.4 highlights traditional soul foods and the impact of acculturation on food choices.

Although soul food has become a symbol of African American identity and African heritage, today, African Americans' food habits usually reflect their current socioeconomic status, geographic location, and work schedule more than their African or Southern heritage (Kittler et al., 2012). Soul food may be reserved for special occasions and holidays.

Health Beliefs

The health beliefs and practices of some African Americans are a blend of traditional African concepts as well as those encountered through early contact with both Native Americans and Whites (Kittler et al., 2012). Some African Americans believe that ill health is due to bad luck or fate. Home remedies and natural therapies may be frequently used.

Nutrition-Related Health Problems

African Americans score just slightly below the national population average on the Healthy Eating Index (HEI), a tool developed by the USDA Center for Nutrition Policy and Promotion

Table 10.4   Traditional Soul Foods and the Effects of Acculturation

Food Group	Foods Commonly Consumed	Effects of Acculturation
Grains	Rice, grits, cornbread, biscuits, muffins, dry and cooked cereals, macaroni	Substitution of commercially made bread for homemade biscuits
Vegetables	Green leafy vegetables (collard, mustard, turnip, and dandelion greens), kale, spinach, and pokeweed are collectively known as "greens" Corn, sweet and white potatoes	Vegetable intake remains low and is based on availability; greens remain popular.
Fruit	Apples, bananas, berries, peaches, and watermelon, based on availability	Fruit intake remains low and is based on availability.
Milk	Whole milk (commonly referred to as "sweet milk") and buttermilk	Greater consumption of milk, at least among blacks living in urban areas
Meat and beans	A variety of beef, pork, poultry, and fish; oxtail, tripe, tongue Dried beans (pinto, navy, lima, butter, kidney); fresh or dried peas (black-eyed, field, green, crowder, butter); beans with pork; succotash (corn with lima beans)	Packaged and luncheon meats are popular; intake of fatty meats, such as sausage and bacon, is high.
Fats	Butter, lard, bacon, fatback, salt pork, meat drippings, vegetable shortening	
Beverages	Coffee, fruit drinks, fruit wine, soft drinks, tea	

Source: Kittler, P., Sucher, K., & Nahikian-Nelms, M. (2012). *Food and culture* (6th ed.). Belmont, CA: Wadsworth Cengage Learning.

that measures dietary factors, such as the intake of total fat, saturated fat, cholesterol, and sodium as well as dietary variety (Ervin, 2011). In a study that examined dietary quality by race and ethnicity, African Americans had lower intakes of vegetables, whole grains, and milk than whites and higher scores for saturated fat and sodium (Hiza, Casavale, Guenther, & Davis, 2013). African Americans have a high prevalence of obesity, particularly in African American women who have the highest prevalence of adult obesity in the United States. These women also have lower life expectancy and higher rates of chronic diseases than the general population (James, Pobee, Oxidine, Brown, & Joshi, 2012). African American women are less likely to participate in weight loss programs and tend to have low success when they do perhaps because most weight-loss programs ignore culturally influenced factors such as body image, beauty, and traditions (James et al., 2012). Studies have shown that, in general, African Americans accept or are comfortable with larger body sizes (Boyington et al., 2008) and may also feel less guilty about overeating (Satia, 2009). African American women are half as likely to consider themselves overweight or obese compared to their white counterparts. A study by James et al. (2012) found that African American women defined healthy weight as "when your jeans fit right," overweight was "just of few pounds over where you want to be," and obesity was "when you're like 300 pounds and even 600 pounds." African American women need help in assessing their weight in terms of health risks.

The percentage of African Americans whose health is fair or poor is greater than in any other ethnic group as is infant mortality. African Americans are almost twice as likely as whites to be diagnosed with diabetes and are more likely to suffer diabetes complications, such as end-stage renal disease and lower extremity amputations (Office of Minority Health [OMH], 2014b). They are also more likely to have high blood pressure and less likely to have it under control.

Hispanic/Latino Americans

Hispanic/Latino Americans are a diverse group differing in native language, customs, history, and foodways. According to 2014 U.S. Census Bureau population estimates, approximately 17.4% of the U.S. population are Hispanic or Latino (U.S. Census Bureau, 2014). Mexicans are the largest subgroup at 63% of the Hispanic American population.

Traditional Food Practices

The traditional Mexican diet, influenced by Spanish and Native American cultures, is generally a low-fat, high-fiber diet rich in complex carbohydrates and vegetable proteins, with an emphasis on corn, corn products, beans, and rice. Tortillas are a staple and may be consumed at every meal. Pork, goat, and poultry are the most used animal proteins; they are usually served ground or chopped as part of a mixed dish. Vegetables are also rarely served separately; they are incorporated into soups, rice, pasta, and tortilla-based dishes. Milk is not widely used, and lactose intolerance is common. Table 10.5 highlights traditional Mexican food practices and the impact of acculturation.

Health Beliefs

Spiritual and religious beliefs greatly influence health and illness practices, which result from a blend of European folk medicine introduced from Spain and Native American rituals. Health is viewed as a gift from God, and illness may be due to bad luck or as a punishment from God for sin (Kittler et al., 2012). That illness is inevitable and to be endured is more likely to be a belief among women born in Mexico than in women of Mexican descent who are born in the United States (Eggenberger et al., 2006). Certain foods may be considered "cold" or "hot" for healing purposes. Herbs used during illness include mint tea, chamomile tea, and cinnamon. Prayer is appropriate for all illnesses, and lighting of candles on behalf of a sick person is common (Kittler et al., 2012). Extended and nuclear families are highly valued and relied on for intergenerational help (Eggenberger et al., 2006).

Nutrition-Related Health Problems

A study of diet quality showed that, compared to whites, Hispanics had higher scores for fruit, dark green and orange vegetables, legumes, saturated fat, and sodium, and lower scores for whole

Table 10.5 Traditional Mexican Foods and the Effects of Acculturation

Food Group	Foods Commonly Consumed	Effects of Acculturation
Grains	Corn, rice	Rice eaten as part of a mixed dish with vegetables decreases; intake of plain rice increases. Flour tortillas are used more often than corn tortillas. Intake of white bread and sweetened cereals increases.
Vegetables	Cactus, calabaza criolla (green pumpkin), chili peppers, corn, jicama, lettuce, onions, peas, plantains, potatoes, squash, tomatillos, tomatoes, yams, yucca	Intake of most vegetables decreases.
Fruit	Avocados, bananas, carambola, cherimoya, coconut, passion fruit, guava, lemons, limes, mangoes, melon, oranges, papaya, pineapple, strawberries	Intake of bananas, apples, oranges, orange juice, and cantaloupe remains relatively constant.
Milk	Goat and cow's milk (whole is preferred), evaporated milk, café con leche, hot chocolate, cheese	Milk intake increases related to its use with a new food, such as ready-to-eat breakfast cereal; whole milk is replaced with low-fat or nonfat milk.
Meat and beans	Beef, goat, pork, chicken, turkey, shrimp, eggs Legumes: black beans, chickpeas, kidney beans, pinto beans	Red meat intake increases. Legume intake falls. Intake of traditional meat and vegetable preparations declines drastically.
Fats	Butter, lard, Mexican cream	Butter, margarine, and salad dressing intake increases related to introduction of cooked vegetables and salads.
Beverages	Fruit-based beverage	Severe decline in fruit-based beverage consumption; increased use of highly sweetened drinks (e.g., Kool-Aid, soft drinks) and caffeinated beverages Alcohol intake increases.

Source: Kittler, P., Sucher, K., & Nahikian-Nelms, M. (2012). *Food and culture* (6th ed.). Belmont, CA: Wadsworth Cengage Learning.

grains, milk, and oils (Hiza et al., 2013). Studies on Mexico-born Americans show that the intake of fiber, fruit, legumes, and vegetables decreases with duration of residence in the United States, whereas consumption of processed foods, refined carbohydrates, and added sugars increases (Sofianou et al., 2011). Acculturation also changes food consumption behaviors, such as increases in eating out, eating at fast-food outlets, and eating salty snacks, which contribute to higher fat and sodium intakes and a decrease in diet quality (Ayala, Baquero, & Klinger, 2008). English-speaking Hispanics tend to spend less time on meal preparation than Spanish-speaking Hispanics (Langellier, Brookmeyer, Wang, & Glik, 2015). Promoting home meal preparation and improving the quality, variety, and prices of prepared foods available in food outlets where Latinos shop are strategies to improve eating patterns.

Hispanics have a high prevalence of obesity; the majority of studies show the rate of obesity in Latinos rises with acculturation (Oza-Frank & Cunningham, 2010). Although acculturation has a detrimental effect on diet quality and obesity, its association with type 2 diabetes is inconsistent (Pérez-Escamilla, 2011). One reason may be that acculturation is associated with greater access to health care, such as diabetic screening and timely intervention when indicated. Another possibility is that acculturation is positively associated with higher socioeconomic position and more leisure time physical activity (Fitzgerald, 2010). Still, diabetes is one of the leading causes of death among Hispanics (OMH, 2015). Other significant health conditions and risk factors that impact Hispanic health include asthma, chronic obstructive pulmonary disease, HIV/AIDS, suicide, and liver disease (OMH, 2015).

Asian Americans

The term "Asian Americans" encompasses a diverse population originating from at least 37 different ethnic groups; Pacific Islander includes about 25 nationalities (Kagawa-Singer et al., 2010). Asian Americans account for approximately 5% of the nation's population, and Chinese, alone or in any combination, is the largest Asian American subgroup in the United States (Hoeffel, Rastogi, Kim, & Shahid, 2012). Two dietary commonalities exist between these diverse cultures: (1) emphasis on rice and vegetables with relatively little meat and (2) cooking techniques that include meticulous attention to preparing ingredients before cooking. Chinese food practices and health and nutrition status are described in the following section.

Traditional Food Practices

Traditional Chinese foods and the effect of acculturation are highlighted in Table 10.6. Grains are the foundation of the traditional diet—predominately rice in southern China and wheat, in the

Table 10.6   Traditional Chinese Foods and the Effects of Acculturation

Food Group	Foods Commonly Consumed	Effects of Acculturation
Grains	Rice, wheat, buckwheat, corn, millet, sorghum	Rice remains a staple, but the intake of wheat bread and cereals increases.
Vegetables	Amaranth, asparagus, bamboo shoots, bean sprouts, bitter melon, cassava, cauliflower, celery, bok choy, napa cabbage, chili peppers, Chinese broccoli, Chinese long beans, eggplant, flat beans, garlic, lily root, dried and fresh mushrooms, okra, onions, seaweed, spinach, taro	Raw vegetable and salad intake increases. Traditional vegetables are replaced by more commonly available ones.
Fruit	Apples, bananas, coconut, dates, figs, kumquats, lime, litchi, mango, oranges, passion fruit, pineapple, pomegranates, tangerines, watermelon	Intake of temperate fruits increases (e.g., apples, grapes, pears, peaches).
Milk	Cow's milk, buffalo milk	Milk, ice cream, and cheese intake increases.
Meat and beans	Almost all sources of protein are eaten.	Intake of meat and ethnic dishes increases.
Fats	Butter, lard, corn oil, peanut oil, sesame oil, soybean oil, suet	Fat intake increases as fast-food intake increases.
Beverages	Tea (southern China), soup (northern China), wine, beer	

Source: Kittler, P., Sucher, K., & Nahikian-Nelms, M. (2012). *Food and culture* (6th ed.). Belmont, CA: Wadsworth Cengage Learning.

form of noodles, dumplings, pancakes, and steamed bread, in northern China. A variety of vegetables are used extensively; other foods commonly consumed include sea vegetables, nuts, seeds, beans, soy foods, vegetable and nut oils, herbs and spices, tea, wine, and beer. A variety of animal proteins are consumed; the use of fish and seafood depends on availability. Most Chinese food is cooked; the exception is fresh fruit, which is eaten infrequently. Few dairy products are consumed because lactose intolerance is common. Calcium is provided by tofu, small fish (bones are eaten), and soups made with bones that have been partially dissolved by vinegar in making stock. Sodium intake is generally assumed to be high because of traditional food preservation methods (salting and drying) and condiments (e.g., soy sauce).

Health Beliefs

Asian cultures believe that health and illness are related to the balance between yin and yang forces in the body. Yin represents female, cold, and darkness; yang represents male, hot, and light. Digested foods turn into air that is either yin or yang. Diseases caused by yin forces are treated with yang foods, and diseases caused by yang forces are treated with yin foods. Pregnancy is considered a yang or "hot" condition, so women following traditional practices during pregnancy eat yin foods such as most fruits and vegetables, seaweed, cold drinks, juices, and rice water. Yang foods include chicken, meat, pig's feet, meat broth, nuts, fried food, coffee, and spices. The hot–cold theory of foods and illness also exists in Puerto Rico and Mexico, but the food designations are not universal within or across cultures.

Nutrition-Related Health Problems

The traditional Chinese diet is low in fat and dairy products and high in complex carbohydrates and sodium (Kittler et al., 2012). With acculturation, the diet becomes higher in fat, protein, sugar, and cholesterol.

Asian American women have the highest life expectancy of all ethnic groups in the United States at 85.8 years and are the group with the lowest percentage of people in fair or poor health. Life expectancy varies among Asian subgroups: Filipino women 81.5 years, Japanese women 84.5 years, and Chinese women 86.1 years (OMH, 2014a). Asian Americans have the lowest prevalence of obesity among cultural groups in the United States. However, weight gain over time has been shown to be more harmful in Asians than in other ethnic groups: For every 11 pounds gained during adulthood, the risk of type 2 diabetes increased by 84% (Shai et al., 2006). Other studies have found that at the same body mass index (BMI), Asians are at higher risk of hypertension and cardiovascular disease than whites (Wen et al., 2009). One possible explanation is that at any given BMI, Asians have a greater percentage of body fat than whites (Deurenberg, Deurenberg-Yap, & Guricci, 2002).

Cancer is the leading cause of death among Asian Americans. Asian/Pacific Islander men are 40% less likely to have prostate cancer than white men, but they are 60% more likely to have stomach cancer. Asian/Pacific Islander women are 30% less likely to have breast cancer than white women but are almost three times as likely to have stomach cancer (OMH, 2014a).

Negative factors that may impact their health include infrequent medical visits for fear of deportation, language/cultural barriers, and lack of health insurance. Asian Americans have a high prevalence of chronic obstructive pulmonary disease, hepatitis B, HIV/AIDS, smoking, tuberculosis, and liver disease (OMH, 2014a).

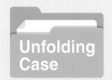

Recall Phouvong. His BMI is 24.5. Although that is considered "healthy," risk of type 2 diabetes starts at a lower BMI in Asians than among other cultural groups. Attaining a BMI of less than 23 will help control his type 2 diabetes. Options to promote weight loss are to change the foods consumed, change the amounts, and/or increase activity. Which option (or options) would you recommend for Phouvong? How will you convey information given the language barrier?

Unfolding Case

FOOD AND RELIGION

Religion tends to have a greater impact on food habits than nationality or culture does (e.g., Orthodox Jews follow **kosher** dietary laws regardless of their national origin). However, religious food practices vary significantly even among denominations of the same faith. National variations also exist. How closely an individual follows dietary laws is based on his or her degree of orthodoxy. An overview of religious food practices follows. Table 10.7 outlines major features of various religious dietary laws.

Christianity

The three primary branches of Christianity are Roman Catholicism, Eastern Orthodox Christianity, and Protestantism. Dietary practices vary from none to explicit.

- Roman Catholics do not eat meat on Ash Wednesday or on Fridays of Lent. Food and beverages are avoided for 1 hour before communion is taken. Devout Catholics observe several fast days during the year.
- Eastern Orthodox Christians observe numerous feast and fast days throughout the year.

The only denominations in the Protestant faith with dietary laws are the Mormons (Church of Jesus Christ of Latter-Day Saints) and Seventh-Day Adventists.

- Mormons do not use coffee, tea, alcohol, or tobacco. Followers are encouraged to limit meats and consume mostly grains. Some Mormons fast 1 day a month.
- Most Seventh-Day Adventists are lacto-ovo vegetarians; those who do eat meat avoid pork. Overeating is avoided, and coffee, tea, and alcohol are prohibited. An interval of 5 to 6 hours between meals is recommended with no snacking between meals. Water is consumed before and after meals. Strong seasonings, such as pepper and mustard, are avoided.

Judaism

In the United States, there are three main Jewish denominations: Orthodox, Conservative, and Reform. Hasidic Jews are a sect within the Orthodox. These groups differ in their interpretation of the precepts of Judaism. Orthodox Jews believe that the laws are the direct commandments of God, so they adhere strictly to dietary laws. Reform Jews follow the moral law but may selectively follow other laws; for instance, they may not follow any religious dietary laws. Conservative Jews

Table 10.7   Summary of Dietary Laws of Selected Religions

	Orthodox Judaism	Islam	Hinduism	Buddhism
Meat	Cannot be eaten with dairy products		Beef is prohibited.	Avoided by the most devout
Pork and pork products	Prohibited	Prohibited	Avoided by the most devout	Avoided by the most devout
Lacto-ovo vegetarianism			Encouraged	Practiced by many
Seafood	Only fish with fins and scales are allowed.		Restricted	Avoided by the most devout
Alcohol		Prohibited	Avoided by the most devout	
Coffee/tea		Strongly discouraged		
Ritual slaughter of animals	Yes	Yes		
Moderation		Practiced		Practiced
Partial or total fasting	Practiced	Practiced	Practiced	Practiced

Sources: Minority Nurse. (2013a). *Hindu dietary practices: Feeding the body, mind and soul.* Available at http://minorityhnurse.com/?s=Hindu+dietary=practices. Accessed on 1/5/17. Minority Nurse. (2013b). *Meeting Jewish and Muslim patient's dietary needs.* Available at http://minorityhnurse.com/?s=Jewish+dietary+practices. Accessed on 1/5/17. ElGindy, G. (2013). *Understanding Buddhist patient's dietary needs.* Available at http://minorityhnurse.com/understanding-buddhist-patients-dietary-needs/. Accessed on 1/5/17.

fall between the other two groups in their beliefs and adherence to the laws. They may follow the Jewish dietary laws at home but take a more liberal attitude on social occasions. Because Jews have diverse backgrounds and nationalities, their food practices vary widely.

The kashrut (or kashruth) is the list of dietary laws adhered to by Orthodox Jews. Because the laws are rigid, Orthodox Jews rarely eat outside the home except at homes or restaurants with kosher kitchens. The laws focus on three major issues:

- Kosher animals are allowed, which include cattle, sheep, goats, chicken, turkey, goose, and certain ducks. Nonkosher animals include birds of prey, pork, fish without scales or fins (e.g., shrimp, lobster), catfish, swordfish, underwater mammals, reptiles, or egg yolk containing any blood.
- Blood is not allowed. Animals must be slaughtered under the supervision of a rabbi or other authorized person to ensure blood is properly removed.
- Meat and poultry cannot be consumed at the same meal as milk and dairy products. Dairy products are not allowed within 1 to 6 hours after eating meat or poultry, depending on the individual's ethnic tradition. Meat and poultry cannot be eaten for 30 minutes after dairy products have been consumed. **Pareve** is a classification of food that contains neither dairy nor meat ingredients. Margarine-labeled pareve, nondairy creamers, and oils may be used with meats. Fruits, vegetables, plain grains, pastas, plain legumes, and eggs are considered kosher and can be eaten with either dairy or meat products.

Pareve
dairy-free.

Kosher foods are labeled with a logo of the kosher-certifying agency, of which there are well over 100 in the United States alone. Of the estimated 12 million American kosher consumers, only 8% are religious Jews who eat only kosher food. The majority of kosher food users choose it for health, food safety, taste, lactose intolerance, or to satisfy halal requirements which have some common restrictions, such as prohibiting the intake of pork and blood (Lytton, 2014).

Food preparation is prohibited on the Sabbath. Religious holidays are celebrated with certain foods. For example, only unleavened bread is eaten during Passover, and a 24-hour fast is observed on Yom Kippur.

Islam

Halal
Islamic dietary laws.

Haram
foods that are prohibited.

Muslims eat as a matter of faith and for good health. Basic guidance concerning food laws is revealed in the Quran (the divine book) from Allah (the Creator) to Muhammad (the Prophet). For Muslims, health and food are considered acts of worship for which Allah must be thanked (Minority Nurse Staff, 2013a). There are 11 generally accepted rules pertaining to **halal** (permitted) and **haram** (prohibited) foods. The five major areas addressed by the halal are as follows:

- Kosher and halal animals are allowed. Not allowed are pork, carnivorous animals with fangs (lions, wolves, dogs, etc.), birds with sharp claws (falcons, eagles, owls, etc.), land animals without ears (frog, snakes, etc.), shark, and products containing gelatin made from the horns or hooves of cattle.
- Blood is not allowed.
- Proper methods must be used for slaughtering.
- Carrion (decaying carcass) is not allowed.
- Intoxicants are forbidden, including pure vanilla containing alcohol and wine vinegar.

As previously noted, many halal laws are similar to the food laws of Judaism; halal foods are also identified with symbols. Islam also stresses certain hygienic practices, such as washing hands before and after eating and frequent teeth cleaning.

Hinduism

A love of nature and desire to live a simple natural life are the basis of Hinduism (Minority Nurse Staff, 2013b). A number of health beliefs and dietary practices stem from the idea of living in harmony with nature and having mercy and respect for all of God's creations. Generally, Hindus avoid all foods that are believed to inhibit physical and spiritual development. Eating

Ahimsa
nonviolence as applicable to foods.

meat is not explicitly prohibited, but many Hindus are vegetarian because they adhere to the concept of **ahimsa**.

Another influential concept is that of purity. Some foods, such as dairy products (e.g., milk, yogurt, ghee [clarified butter]), are considered to enhance spiritual purity. When prepared together, pure foods can improve the purity of impure foods. Some foods, such as beef or alcohol, are innately polluted and can never be made pure.

Jainism, a branch of Hinduism, also promotes the nonviolent doctrine of ahimsa. Devout Jains are complete vegetarians and may avoid blood-colored foods (e.g., tomatoes) and root vegetables (because harvesting them may cause the death of insects).

Buddhism

The Buddhist code of morality is set forth in the Five Moral Precepts, which are to not (1) kill or harm living things; (2) steal; (3) engage in sexual misconduct; (4) lie; and (5) consume intoxicants, such as alcohol, tobacco, or mind-altering drugs. Believing that thoughtful food decisions can contribute to spiritual enlightenment, a Buddhist asks himself these questions (ElGindy, 2013):

- What food is this? This question evaluates the origin of the food and how it reached the individual.
- Where does it come from? This question considers the amount of work necessary to grow the food, prepare it, cook it, and bring it to the table.
- Why am I eating it? This question reflects on whether the individual deserves or is worthy of the food.
- When should I eat and benefit from this food? This question is based on the idea that food is a necessity and a healing agent and people are subjected to illness without food.
- How should I eat it? This question considers the premise that food is only received and eaten for the purpose of realizing the proper way to reach enlightenment.

In the Buddhist faith, life revolves around nature with its two opposing energy systems of yin and yang (ElGindy, 2013). Examples of these opposing energy systems are heat/cold, light/darkness, good/evil, and sickness/health. Illnesses may result from an imbalance of yin and yang. Most Buddhists subscribe to the concept of ahimsa (not killing or harming), so many are lacto-ovo vegetarians. Some eat fish; some avoid only beef. Buddhist dietary practices vary widely depending on the sect and country. Buddhist monks avoid eating solid food after the noon hour.

How Do You Respond?

Is all fast food bad? No, not all fast foods are "bad." "Bad" is a relative term that depends on how often and how much. But even when "healthy" selections are made, such as a grilled chicken sandwich or a plain baked potato, fast-food meals tend to be low in fiber, fruit, vegetables, and milk/dairy products. Although an occasional fast-food meal will not jeopardize someone's nutritional status, a steady diet of it can be detrimental for what it provides (too much fat, calories, and sodium) and for what it lacks.

REVIEW CASE STUDY

Elizabet moved to the Midwest at the age of 26 years from her native country, Iceland, where she ate seafood almost every evening for dinner. She ate fruit and vegetables daily, but the variety was limited. In her new home, she complains that good seafood is hard to find—that it is not as fresh as it is at home, it tastes different, and it is more expensive. She also misses the dark brown and black breads she is accustomed to; she is willing to try American breads but is unsure what variety is "good." American fast food is well known to her, but she does not want to rely on that to satisfy her need for

familiar foods. She wants to eat foods that are healthy, tasty, and affordable.

- What questions would you ask Elizabet before coming up with suggestions about foods she could try?
- What would you say to her about her frustration with the seafood available locally? What suggestions would you make to her?
- What would you tell her about healthy breads? What fruits would you recommend as healthy, tasty, and affordable? What vegetables?

STUDY QUESTIONS

1 Which of the following items would be the healthiest choice from a Mexican restaurant?
   a. Cheese quesadillas
   b. Arroz con pollo
   c. Taco salad
   d. Guacamole with taco chips

2 A descriptive word that indicates a low-fat cooking technique is
   a. Au gratin
   b. Breaded
   c. Roasted
   d. Battered

3 A first-generation Chinese American has been advised to consume less sodium. What native food would the nurse ask about to get an idea of how much sodium he consumes?
   a. Soybeans
   b. Soy sauce
   c. Wonton
   d. Bok choy

4 A negative impact of acculturation on Mexican American food choices is often a decrease in fiber intake related to a decrease in the intake of (select all that apply)
   a. Legumes
   b. Whole-grain cereals
   c. Nuts
   d. Vegetables
   e. Fruit

5 What are the nutritional characteristics of a traditional soul food diet? Select all that apply.
   a. High in fat
   b. High in sodium
   c. High in potassium
   d. High in cholesterol
   e. Low in calcium

6 Which of the following is a healthy traditional food practice of Chinese Americans that should be encouraged?
   a. None; an American diet is healthier
   b. High intake of milk and dairy products
   c. Frequent use of fresh fruit
   d. Extensive use of vegetables in mixed dishes

7 When developing a teaching plan for an overweight woman from Mexico, which approach would be best?
   a. Tell the client she will feel better if she loses some of the extra weight she is carrying around.
   b. Encourage more "nutritious" food choices.
   c. Advise the client that "healthy eating" will help her shed inches.
   d. Provide a low-calorie diet and encourage her to eat low-calorie American foods, such as artificially sweetened soda and low-fat ice cream.

8 Muslims are prohibited from consuming
   a. Alcohol
   b. Eggs
   c. Beef
   d. Shellfish

KEY CONCEPTS

- American cuisine has evolved from a melting pot of food, flavors, and cooking techniques contributed by immigrants over the course of U.S. history. It continues to undergo change.
- Convenience foods range from pre-prepared ingredients to use to make a home-cooked meal (e.g., fresh cut vegetables and bagged salad) to complete, heat-and-serve meals. Convenience "meals" tend to be high in sodium and low in fiber, fruit, vegetables, and whole grains. Portion sizes are smaller than most people normally consume.
- The average American eats dinner at home 5.7 times per week. Convenience products are frequently used to speed preparation time and range from precut vegetables to complete heat-and-eat meals. Generally, the more convenient the item, the higher the cost and greater the impact on nutrition.
- Suggestions to help control portion sizes while eating out include ordering two appetizers as a meal, splitting an entrée with a companion, ordering a "child"-sized meal, or creating a doggie bag before beginning to eat.

- Culture defines what is edible; how food is handled, prepared, and consumed; what foods are appropriate for particular groups within the culture; the meaning of food and eating; attitudes toward body size; and the relationship between food and health. Yet, food habits vary considerably among individuals and families within a cultural group based on personal factors, socioeconomic factors, and religious factors.
- Core foods are an indispensable part of the diet and consist of grains or starchy vegetables. Secondary foods are nutrient rich and add variety and ethnic identity to meals. Occasional or peripheral foods are used infrequently.
- Cultural values identify behavior that is desirable and define how people should interact within society. American values are often very different from values of other cultures. Understanding a client's cultural values facilitates communication.
- Culture defines body image and desirable weight. In the United States, thinness is valued, particularly for women.

In some other cultures, thinness is equated with poverty; heavier weight is considered desirable and a sign of prosperity.

- Dietary acculturation occurs as people who move to a new area change their food habits to some degree. New foods are added to their diet or substituted for traditional foods, and some traditional foods are rejected. Availability and cost influence food choices.

- Acculturation can have a negative or positive effect on nutrition and health. Generally, as immigrants adopt the "typical American diet," their intake of fat, sugar, and calories goes up, and their intake of fiber, fruits, vegetables, and vegetable protein goes down. New Americans should be encouraged to retain the healthy eating practices of their native diet.

- Generalizations can be made about traditional eating practices of subcultures within the United States. However, an individual's food choices deviate from these based on personal preferences, socioeconomic status, and degree of acculturation.

- Traditional soul food is high in fat, cholesterol, and sodium and low in fiber, fruit, vegetables, and calcium. Socioeconomic factors, geographic area, and work schedules have a greater impact on the intake of African Americans than does the traditional soul food diet.

- African Americans have a higher prevalence of overweight/obesity and hypertension than whites. The percentage of African Americans whose health is fair or poor in greater than in any other ethnic group as is infant mortality.

- Weight loss counseling for African American women should stress the health benefits of weight loss and be respectful of cultural values regarding body size and image.

- Mexican Americans have a higher prevalence of overweight/obesity than whites and lower rates of hypertension. As acculturation increases, eating out, eating at fast-food outlets, and eating salty snacks increase.

- Asian women have the longest life expectancy of all ethnic groups in the United States. Asian Americans are the group with the lowest percentage of people in fair or poor health. The prevalence of overweight/obesity among Asian Americans is lower than in whites, but their risk of type 2 diabetes appears to begin at lower BMI than other ethnic groups.

- Religion tends to have a greater impact on food habits than nationality or culture. People are more likely to eat ethnic food from a different culture than they are to eat food that is prohibited by the mandates of their religion.

Check Your Knowledge Answer Key

1 **TRUE** Religion tends to have a greater impact on food choices than culture does.

2 **FALSE** Race, ethnicity, and geographic region are often inaccurately assumed to be synonymous with culture. This misconception leads to stereotyping.

3 **TRUE** Core foods tend to be complex carbohydrates, such as cereal grains, starchy tubers, and starchy vegetables. These core foods are the indispensable foundation of the diet and provide significant calories.

4 **TRUE** Both Hinduism and Buddhism promote vegetarianism.

5 **FALSE** The hot–cold theory of health and diet refers to Asian cultures' belief that health and illness are related to the balance between yin and yang forces in the body. Yin represents female, cold, and darkness; yang represents male, hot, and light.

6 **TRUE** Usually, first-generation Americans adhere more closely to cultural food patterns to preserve their ethnic identity compared with subsequent generations.

7 **TRUE** For many ethnic groups who move to the United States, breakfast and lunch are most likely to be composed of convenient American foods, whereas traditional foods are retained for the major dinner meal, which has greater emotional significance.

8 **TRUE** Eating food prepared away from home tends to increase a person's intake of calories, sodium, added sugar, and saturated and solid fat.

9 **FALSE** Dietary acculturation can lead to positive or negative changes in food choices. For instance, Mexican Americans dramatically reduce their intake of lard and Mexican cream through the process of acculturation, which is a positive change. However, substituting sweetened drinks (e.g., Kool-Aid and soft drinks) for the traditional beverage made from fruit has a negative impact on nutritional intake.

10 **FALSE** Although restaurant portions tend to be much larger than the standard serving size, the same is not true for convenience foods. The portion sizes listed on the label of convenience meals tend to be much smaller than what Americans typically consume in a meal.

Websites

Cultural/Ethnic Food Guide Pyramids, USDA National Agricultural Library at http://fnic.nal.usda.gov/dietary-guidance/myplatefood-pyramid-resources/ethniccultural-food-pyramids

Ethnic medicine information including nutrition information: Harborview Medical Center, University of Washington at www.ethnomed.org

Office of Minority Health at http://minorityhealth.hhs.gov/

Oldways Preservation & Exchange Trust at www.oldwayspt.org

Website for information on fast food and eating out: Center for Science in the Public Interest at www.cspinet.org

References

Ayala, G., Baquero, B., & Klinger, S. (2008). A systemic review of the relationship between acculturation and diet among Latinos in the United States: Implications for future research. *Journal of the American Dietetic Association, 108,* 1330–1344.

Batis, C., Hernandez-Barrera, L., Barquera, S., Rivera, J. A., & Popkin, B. M. (2011). Food acculturation drives dietary differences among Mexicans, Mexican Americans, and non-Hispanic whites. *The Journal of Nutrition, 141,* 1898–1906.

Boyington, J., Carter-Edwards, L., Piehl, M., Hutson, J., Langdon, D., & McManus, S. (2008). Cultural attitudes toward weight, diet, and physical activity among overweight African American girls. *Preventing Chronic Disease, 5,* A36.

Brown, D. (2005). Dietary challenges of new Americans. *Journal of the American Dietetic Association, 105,* 1704–1706.

Caprio, S., Daniels, S., Drewnowski, A., Kaufman, F. R., Palinkas, L. A., Rosenbloom, A. L., & Schwimmer, J. B. (2008). Influence of race, ethnicity, and culture on childhood obesity: Implications for prevention and treatment: A consensus statement of Shaping America's Health and the Obesity Society. *Diabetes Care, 31,* 2211–2221.

Carr, C. (2012). Minority ethnic groups with type 2 diabetes: The importance of effective dietary advice. *Journal of Diabetes Nursing, 16,* 88–96.

Deurenberg, P., Deurenberg-Yap, M., & Guricci, S. (2002). Asians are different from Caucasians and from each other in their body mass index/body fat percent relationship. *Obesity Reviews, 3,* 141–146.

Eggenberger, S., Grassley, J., & Restrepo, E. (2006). Culturally competent nursing care for families: Listening to the voices of Mexican-American women. *Online Journal of Issues in Nursing, 11,* 7. doi:10.3912/OJIN.Vol11No03PPT01

ElGindy, G. (2013). *Understanding Buddhist patient's dietary needs.* Available at http://minoritynurse.com/understanding-buddhist-patients-dietary-needs/. Accessed on 1/5/17.

Ervin, B. (2011). Healthy Eating Index—2005 total and component scores for adults aged 20 and over: National Health and Nutrition Examination Survey, 2003–2004. *National Health Statistics Reports, 44,* 1–10.

Fitzgerald, N. (2010). Acculturation, socioeconomic status, and health among Hispanics. *NAPA Bulletin, 34,* 28–46.

Goody, C., & Drago, L. (2009). Using cultural competence constructs to understand food practices and provide diabetes care and education. *Diabetes Spectrum, 22,* 43–47.

Hiza, H., Casavale, K., Guenther, P., & Davis, C. (2013). Diet quality of Americans differs by age, sex, race/ethnicity, income, and education level. *Journal of the Academy of Nutrition and Dietetics, 113,* 297–306.

Hobson, K. (2016). *Supermarket prepared meals: What to watch out for.* Available at http://www.consumerreports.org/food-shopping/supermarket-prepared-meals-what-to-watch-out-for/. Accessed on 3/31/16.

Hoeffel, E., Rastogi, S., Kim, M., & Shahid, H. (2012). *The Asian population: 2010. 2010 Census Brief.* Available at www.census.gov//rpod/cen2010/briefs/c2010br-11.pdf. Accessed on 10/30/12.

James, D., Pobee, J., Oxidine, D., Brown, L., & Joshi, G. (2012). Using the health belief model to develop culturally appropriate weight-management materials for African-American women. *Journal of the Academy of Nutrition and Dietetics, 112,* 663–670.

Kagawa-Singer, M., Dadia, A., Yu, M., & Surbone, A. (2010). Cancer, culture, and health disparities: Time to chart a new course? *CA: A Cancer Journal for Clinicians, 60,* 12–39.

Kittler, P., Sucher, K., & Nahikian-Nelms, M. (2012). *Food and culture* (6th ed.). Belmont, CA: Wadsworth Cengage Learning.

Kulkarni, K. (2004). Food, culture, and diabetes in the United States. *Clinical Diabetes, 22,* 190–192.

Langellier, B., Brookmeyer, R., Wang, M., & Glik, D. (2015). Language use affects food behaviours and food values among Mexican-origin adults in the USA. *Public Health Nutrition, 18,* 264–274.

Lv, N., & Carson, D. (2004). Dietary pattern change and acculturation of Chinese Americans in Pennsylvania. *Journal of the American Dietetic Association, 104,* 771–778.

Lytton, T. (2014). Jewish foodways and religious self-governance in American: The failure of communal kashrut regulation and the rise of private kosher certification. *Jewish Quarterly Review, 104,* 38–45.

Minority Nurse. (2013a). *Hindu dietary practices: Feeding the body, mind and soul.* Available at http://minorityhnurse.com/?s=Hindu+dietary=practices. Accessed on 1/5/17.

Minority Nurse. (2013b). *Meeting Jewish and Muslim patient's dietary needs.* Available at http://minoritynurse.com/?s=Jewish+dietary+practices. Accessed on 1/5/17.

Office of Management and Budget. (1997). *Revisions to the standards for the classification of federal data on race and ethnicity.* Available at www.whitehouse.gov/omb/fedreg_1997standards/. Accessed on 10/31/12.

Office of Minority Health. (2014a). *Profile: Asian Americans.* Available at http://minorityhealth.hhs.gov/omh/browse.aspx?lvl=3&lvlid=63. Accessed on 3/31/16.

Office of Minority Health. (2014b). *Profile: Black/African Americans.* Available at http://minorityhealth.hhs.gov/omh/browse.aspx?lvl=3&lvlid=61. Accessed on 3/31/16.

Office of Minority Health. (2015). *Profile: Hispanic/Latino Americans.* Available at http://minorityhealth.hhs.gov/omh/browse.aspx?lvl=3&lvlid=64. Accessed on 3/31/16.

Oza-Frank, R., & Cunningham, S. (2010). The weight of US residence among immigrants: A systematic review. *Obesity Reviews, 11,* 271–280.

Parade. (2014). *What American eats: Our exclusive survey on the nation's changing tastes.* Available at http://parade.com/334779/parade/what-america-eats-our-exclusive-survey-on-the-nations-changing-tastes/. Accessed on 4/1/16.

Pérez-Escamilla, R. (2011). Acculturation, nutrition, and health disparities. *The American Journal of Clinical Nutrition, 93*(5), 1163S–1167S.

Satia, J. (2009). Diet-related disparities: Understanding the problem and accelerating solutions. *Journal of the American Dietetic Association, 109,* 610–615.

Satia, J., Patterson, R., Kristal, A., Hislop, T. G., Yasui, Y., & Taylor, V. M. (2001). Development of scales to measure dietary acculturation among Chinese-Americans and Chinese-Canadians. *Journal of the American Dietetic Association, 101,* 548–553.

Shai, I., Jiang, R., Manson, J. E., Stampfer, M. J., Willett, W. C., Colditz, G. A., & Hu, F. B. (2006). Ethnicity, obesity, and risk of type 2 diabetes in women: A 20-year follow-up study. *Diabetes Care, 29,* 1585–1590.

Sloan, A. (2016). What, when, and where American eats. *Food Technology, 70,* 23–35.

Sofianou, A., Fung, T., & Tucker, K. (2011). Differences in diet pattern adherence by nativity and duration of US residence in the Mexican-American Population. *Journal of the American Dietetic Association, 111,* 1563–1569.

Todd, J., Mancino, L., & Lin, B. (2010). *The impact of food away from home on adult diet quality (Feb 1, 2010)* (USDA-ERS Economic Research Report Paper No. 90). Available at http://ssrn.com/abstract=1557129. Accessed on 10/30/12.

U.S. Census Bureau. (2014). *QuickFacts.* Available at https://www.census.gov/quickfacts/table/PST045215/00. Accessed on 3/31/16.

U.S. Census Bureau. (2015). *Projections of the size and composition of the US population: 2014-2060.* Available at https://www.census.gov/library/publications/2015/demo/p25-1143.html. Accessed on 3/31/16.

U.S. Department of Agriculture, Economic Research Service. (2014). *Food-away-from-home.* Available at http://www.ers.usda.gov/topics/food-choices-health/food-consumption-demand/food-away-from-home.aspx. Accessed on 3/30/16.

Virudachalam, S., Long, J., Harhay, M., Polsky, D., & Feudtner, C. (2014). Prevalence and patterns of cooking dinner at home in the USA: National Health and Nutrition Examination Survey (NHANES) 2007-2008. *Public Health Nutrition, 17,* 1022–1030.

Wen, C. P., David Cheng, T. Y., Tsai, S. P., Chan, H. T., Hsu, H. L., Hsu, C. C., & Eriksen, M. P. (2009). Are Asians at greater mortality risks for being overweight than Caucasians? Redefining obesity for Asians. *Public Health Nutrition, 12,* 497–506.

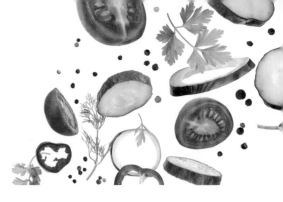

Chapter 11

Healthy Eating for Healthy Babies

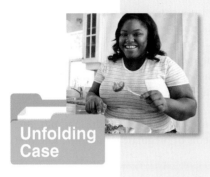

Unfolding Case

Rachel Stevens

Rachel is 27 years old and was diagnosed with polycystic ovary syndrome (PCOS) at age 18 years. She and her husband want to start a family, but she has irregular periods and fears she will have a hard time getting pregnant. She is 5 ft 5 in and weighs 183 pounds, which gives her a body mass index (BMI) of 30.5. She has noticed that her PCOS symptoms get worse the more weight she gains. She would also like to lose some weight and "get healthy" before getting pregnant.

Check Your Knowledge

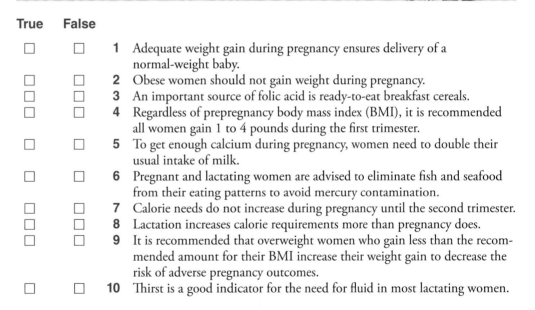

True	False		
☐	☐	**1**	Adequate weight gain during pregnancy ensures delivery of a normal-weight baby.
☐	☐	**2**	Obese women should not gain weight during pregnancy.
☐	☐	**3**	An important source of folic acid is ready-to-eat breakfast cereals.
☐	☐	**4**	Regardless of prepregnancy body mass index (BMI), it is recommended all women gain 1 to 4 pounds during the first trimester.
☐	☐	**5**	To get enough calcium during pregnancy, women need to double their usual intake of milk.
☐	☐	**6**	Pregnant and lactating women are advised to eliminate fish and seafood from their eating patterns to avoid mercury contamination.
☐	☐	**7**	Calorie needs do not increase during pregnancy until the second trimester.
☐	☐	**8**	Lactation increases calorie requirements more than pregnancy does.
☐	☐	**9**	It is recommended that overweight women who gain less than the recommended amount for their BMI increase their weight gain to decrease the risk of adverse pregnancy outcomes.
☐	☐	**10**	Thirst is a good indicator for the need for fluid in most lactating women.

Learning Objectives

Upon completion of this chapter, you will be able to

1 Evaluate a woman's pattern and amount of weight gain during pregnancy based on her prepregnancy body mass index (BMI).
2 Assess whether a woman may benefit from a multivitamin and mineral supplement during pregnancy.
3 Plan a day's intake for a pregnant woman based on her MyPlate food intake pattern.
4 Describe characteristics of a healthy eating pattern during pregnancy.

5 Give examples of nutrition interventions used for nausea, constipation, and heartburn during pregnancy.

6 Compare nutrition guidelines for healthy eating during pregnancy with the guidelines for lactation.

7 List benefits of breastfeeding for mother and infant.

Although an optimal eating pattern before and during pregnancy cannot *guarantee* a successful outcome of pregnancy, it can improve the chance of a healthy newborn baby, a healthy mom, and a healthy future for both. A woman who is well nourished and within her healthy weight range prior to conception provides an environment conducive to normal fetal growth and development during the critical first trimester of pregnancy. During pregnancy, the fetus cannot meet its genetic potential for development if the supply of energy and nutrients is inadequate. Conversely, excessive weight gain during pregnancy is strongly associated with maternal and fetal complications. An optimal eating pattern provides enough, but not too many, calories and nutrients to optimize maternal and fetal health.

This chapter discusses dietary guidelines for women before, during, and after pregnancy. Weight gain recommendations, common problems of pregnancy, and nutrition interventions for maternal health conditions are presented.

PREPREGNANCY NUTRITION

A mother's health and nutritional status at conception, and even before, can affect the infant's health, growth, and development over a life time. For instance,

Low Birth Weight (LBW)
a baby weighing less than 2500 g or 5.5 pounds.

- A low folate status prior to conception increases the risk of neural tube defects.
- An underweight mother has a higher risk of delivering a **low birth weight (LBW)** and small for gestational age (SGA) infant. Women who were LBW infants have a greater risk of having an LBW infant. LBW impairs infant growth and development.
- Prepregnancy overweight/obesity increases the risk of large for gestational age (LGA), high body weight, macrosomia, and childhood overweight and obesity (Yu et al., 2013).
- A preconception eating pattern containing fish, meat, chicken, fruit, and whole grains is associated with reduced risk for preterm delivery, whereas an eating pattern high in fat, refined grains, and added sugar is associated with preterm delivery and shorter birth length (Grieger, Grzeskowiak, & Clifton, 2014).

Ideally, when women enter pregnancy they are optimally nourished, at a healthy body weight, exercise regularly, and do not smoke, drink alcohol, or use street drugs. However, even among women planning to become pregnant, only a small proportion implement nutrition and lifestyle changes in the preconception period (Inskip, Crozier, Godfrey, Borland, & Robinson, 2009). Healthy eating patterns, body weight, folic acid supplementation, and other nutrition concerns are addressed in the following sections.

Healthy Eating Patterns

The basic principles of healthy eating that apply to healthy people are also appropriate before, during, and after pregnancy: Consume a calorie-appropriate eating pattern that includes plenty of fruits and vegetables of various kinds and colors; whole-grain bread and cereals; a variety of lean protein foods; low-fat or fat-free dairy products; and healthy oils in moderation. As with the general public, sodium, solid fats, added sugars, and refined grains should be limited. Nutrient needs should be met primarily through food, not supplements. Evidence suggests that healthy eating patterns prior to conception such as the Mediterranean-style eating pattern (Chapter 8) and the Dietary Approaches to Stop Hypertension (DASH) eating pattern (Chapter 20) are associated with a 24% to 48% lower risk of gestational diabetes (Tobias et al., 2012).

Common to both of these patterns are a high intake of fruit, vegetables, whole grains, and nuts and legumes, and a low intake of red and processed meats. It is likely that several potential mechanisms are responsible for the lower gestational diabetes mellitus (GDM) risk, including benefits related to weight, insulin resistance, and antioxidant content.

Healthy Weight

Healthy Weight
BMI of 18.5 to 24.9.

In the United States, more than half of pregnant women are overweight or obese (American College of Obstetricians and Gynecologists [ACOG], 2013b). Achieving a **healthy weight** prior to conception reduces the risk of neural tube defects, preterm delivery, diabetes, cesarean section, and hypertensive and thromboembolic diseases associated with obesity (Centers for Disease Control and Prevention [CDC], 2014c). All women with a BMI of 18.5 or lower or 25 or higher should be counseled about the risks of unhealthy weight to maternal health and future pregnancies, including the risk of infertility. Clinical care recommendations are based on BMI (CDC, 2014c).

- Women who are overweight (BMI 25–29.9) should be treated for overweight when two or more risk factors are present or when waist circumference is high. Treatment should focus on producing moderate weight loss through nutrition and physical activity.
- Women who are obese (BMI ≥30) should be treated to produce substantial weight loss over a prolonged period; comorbidities should be considered when determining treatment options. Prepregnancy obesity is associated with increased risk of gestational diabetes, pregnancy-induced hypertension, cesarean delivery, LGA, and macrosomia (Li et al., 2013).
- Women who are underweight (BMI ≤18.5) should be evaluated for eating disorders and distorted body image. Maternal prepregnancy underweight is associated with increased risks of SGA and LBW (Li et al., 2013).

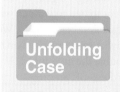

Unfolding Case

Recall Rachel. Weight loss and exercise can improve her PCOS symptoms, improve her chance of becoming pregnant, and lower her risk of adverse pregnancy outcomes. Counseling should include a healthy eating pattern, such as the DASH eating pattern or Mediterranean eating pattern. How is Rachel's BMI classified? What would be appropriate calorie and weight goals for Rachel? What tools would you recommend she use to help her eat healthy while working toward a healthier weight?

Folic Acid
synthetic form of folate found in multivitamins, fortified breakfast cereals, and enriched grain products.

Neural Tube Defect
a serious central nervous system birth defect, such as anencephaly (absence of a brain) and spina bifida (incomplete closure of the spinal cord and its bony encasement).

Folate
natural form of the B vitamin involved in the synthesis of DNA; only one-half is available to the body as synthetic folic acid.

Folic Acid

The World Health Organization (WHO, 2012), Institute of Medicine (IOM, 1998), CDC (2014c), U.S. Preventive Services Task Force (USPSTF, 2009), and *2015-2020 Dietary Guidelines for Americans* (U.S. Department of Health and Human Services [USDHHS] & U.S. Department of Agriculture [USDA], 2015) are among the many experts who recommend that synthetic **folic acid** be consumed prior to conception to prevent neural tube defects. Because **neural tube defects** originate in the first month of pregnancy before a woman may even know she is pregnant, all women of childbearing age who are capable of becoming pregnant are urged to consume 400 µg of synthetic folic acid every day from fortified food or supplements in addition to consuming natural **folate** in a varied eating pattern. Synthetic folic acid is recommended because it is better absorbed and has greater availability than natural folate in foods.

Quick Bite Sources of folic acid

100% fortified ready-to-eat breakfast cereals
White bread, rolls, pasta, and crackers (In the United States and Canada, enriched flour is required to be fortified with folic acid.)

Sources of naturally occurring folate

Leafy green vegetables, such as spinach
Citrus fruits
Dried peas and beans, such as lentils, soybeans, pinto beans

Other Nutrition Concerns

Because of the high prevalence of iron deficiency anemia among menstruating women, screening for anemia is recommended prior to conception. Counseling should include dietary sources of heme iron and how certain foods promote nonheme iron absorption (e.g., orange juice, meat), whereas others impair nonheme iron absorption (e.g., tea, coffee). Screening should also identify all supplements used, including vitamins, minerals, herbs, weight loss products, and home remedies so that safety and efficacy can be discussed.

NUTRITION AND LIFESTYLE DURING PREGNANCY

Epidemiologic evidence suggests that intrauterine environment plays a significant role in the origins of adult disease, including in utero programming of obesity and diabetes (Barker, 1990; Oken & Gillman, 2003). Many women are motivated during pregnancy to adopt healthy lifestyle changes, which have the potential to make a long-lasting impact on the health of mother and infant. Counseling on healthy weight and lifestyle should ideally start before conception or as soon as pregnancy is confirmed, particularly to prevent excess fat development in the fetus, infant, and adult (Davenport, Ruchat, Giroux, Sopper, & Mottola, 2013). Best practices for nutrition care are outlined in the following sections.

Recommended Amount and Pattern of Weight Gain

Current weight gain recommendations for pregnancy are based on prepregnancy BMI (see Table 11.1). Recommended weight gain is 25 to 35 pounds in women of normal weight, 28 to 40 pounds for underweight women, 15 to 25 pounds for overweight women, and 11 to 20 pounds for women who are obese at the time of conception (IOM, 2009). Although record numbers of American women have BMI values ≥35, the IOM (2009) stated there was insufficient data available to issue specific weight gain recommendations for this population. Recent data suggest that women with a BMI ≥40 who lose weight during pregnancy have a decreased risk of adverse birth outcomes compared to women who gained within the IOM recommendations (Blomberg, 2011). Women pregnant with twins need to gain somewhat more weight than that recommended for single births but not double the amounts.

Regardless of prepregnancy BMI, it is recommended that all women gain 1 to 4 pounds in the first trimester; thereafter, weekly weight is based on prepregnancy BMI (see Table 11.1). Normal-weight women are urged to gain approximately 1 pound per week during the second and third trimesters; recommended amounts of weekly gain for underweight, overweight, and obese women are slightly different (see Table 11.1) (IOM, 2009). Although slightly higher or lower rates of weight gain can be considered normal, obvious or persistent deviations warrant further investigation.

Quick Bite Weight gain distribution in normal pregnancy (pounds)

Birth weight of baby	7.5
Placenta	1.5
Increase in maternal blood volume	4
Increase in maternal fluid volume	4
Increase in uterus	2
Increase in breast tissue	2
Amniotic fluid	2
Maternal fat tissue	7
Total	30

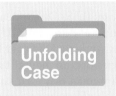

Consider Rachel. She was able to lose 10 pounds with exercise and healthy eating. After months of trying to conceive, her physician prescribed clomiphene (Clomid) to stimulate ovulation and she is now 4 weeks pregnant. How should she modify her eating pattern? What would you tell her about weight gain in the first trimester?

Unfolding Case

Table 11.1 — Recommended Weight Gain Ranges Based on Maternal Prepregnancy Body Mass Index (BMI)

BMI	Prepregnancy BMI Status	Total Weight Gain (pounds)	Rate of Weekly Weight Gain in Second and Third Trimester (mean range in pounds per week)*
Less than 18.5	Underweight	28–40	1 (1–1.3)
18.5–24.9	Normal weight	25–35	1 (0.8–1)
25–29.9	Overweight	15–25	0.6 (0.5–0.7)
30 or greater	Obese (all classes)	11–20	0.5 (0.4–0.6)

*Calculations assume 1.1- to 4.4-pound weight gain in the first trimester.
Source: National Research Council. (2009). *Weight gain during pregnancy: Reexamining the guidelines*. Washington, DC: The National Academies Press.

Calorie Requirements

According to Dietary Reference Intakes (DRIs), pregnant women do not need any additional calories until the second trimester. Even then, the increase is surprisingly small: An extra 340 cal/day is recommended during the second trimester and an additional 452 cal/day in the third (IOM, 2005). Most women of healthy prepregnancy weight need a total of 2200 to 2900 cal/day (Lessen & Kavanagh, 2015). Throughout pregnancy, adequacy of calorie intake is measured by adequacy of weight gain.

Healthy Eating Pattern

The foundation of a healthy eating pattern—as presented during preconception—is consistent throughout the lifespan, including during pregnancy. For pregnant women, choosing a variety of nutrient-dense foods within each food group is especially important so that the increase in nutrient needs can be met without exceeding the relatively small increase in calories recommended during the second and third trimesters.

A tool to help pregnant women choose a calorie-appropriate healthy eating pattern is MyPlate Daily Checklist for Moms (www.choosemyplate.gov/moms-daily-food-plan). For ease of use, patterns generated for pregnant women of healthy body weight increase by 400 cal/day beginning in the second trimester and lasting through the course of pregnancy. Figure 11.1 features eating patterns for a woman whose nonpregnant calorie requirements are 2000 cal/day. Notice the increase in food recommended during the second and third trimesters is relatively small, with a daily increase of

- ½ cup of vegetables
- 2 oz-equivalents of grains
- 1 oz-equivalent of protein

Additionally, although not part of the traditional food groups, oil allowance increases by 4 g/day, and an additional 80 calories are allotted for solid fat, added sugar, or more food from any of the food groups.

Figure 11.1 ▶

Sample MyPlate Daily. Checklists During Pregnancy and Lactation. *(Source: U.S. Department of Agriculture, Center for Nutrition Policy and Promotion. [2016]. Available at www.choosemyplate.gov. Accessed on 4/8/16.)*

		1st trimester 2000 cal	2nd & 3rd trimesters 2400 cal	Lactation 1st 6 mo exclusively breastfeeding 2400 cal
		Recommended servings per group		
Fruits	1 cup of fruits counts as • 1 cup raw or cooked fruit; or • 1/2 cup dried fruit; or • 1 cup 100% fruit juice	**2 c**	**2 c**	**2 c**
Vegetables	1 cup vegetables counts as • 1 cup raw or cooked vegetables; or • 2 cups leafy salad greens; or • 1 cup 100% vegetable juice	**2 1/2 c**	**3 c**	**3 c**
Grains	1 ounce of grains counts as • 1 slice bread; or • 1 ounce ready-to-eat cereal; or • 1/2 cup cooked rice, pasta, or cereal	**6 oz equivalents**	**8 oz equivalents**	**8 oz equivalents**
Protein	1 ounce of protein counts as • 1 ounce lean meat, poultry, or seafood; or • 1 egg; or • 1 Tbsp peanut butter; or • 1/4 cup cooked beans or peas; or • 1/2 ounce nuts or seeds	**5 1/2 oz equivalents**	**6 1/2 oz equivalents**	**6 1/2 oz equivalents**
Dairy	1 cup of dairy counts as • 1 cup milk; or • 1 cup yogurt; or • 1 cup fortified soy beverage; or • 1 1/2 ounces natural cheese or 2 ounces processed cheese	**3 c**	**3 c**	**3 c**

Nutrient Requirements

Although most nutrient requirements increase during pregnancy (Table 11.2),

- Nutrient needs are not constant throughout the course of pregnancy. Nutrient needs generally change little during the first trimester (folic acid is an exception) and are at their highest during the last trimester.
- Nutrient needs do not increase proportionately. For instance, the need for iron increases by 50% during pregnancy, yet the requirement for vitamin B_{12} increases by only about 10%.
- Actual requirements during pregnancy vary among individuals and are influenced by previous nutritional status and health history including chronic illnesses, multiple pregnancies, and closely spaced pregnancies.
- The requirement for one nutrient may be altered by the intake of another. For instance, women who do not meet their calorie requirements need higher amounts of protein.
- The intake of more food to meet increased calorie requirements and the increase in absorption and efficiency of nutrient use that occurs in pregnancy are generally enough to meet nutrient needs when healthy food choices are made (Lessen & Kavanagh, 2015). Exceptions are discussed in the following section.

Folic Acid

Dietary Folate Equivalents (DFE)
a measure of total folate available that accounts for the lower availability of natural folate in food compared to synthetic folic acid used in fortified foods and supplements. Total DFE = micrograms of food folate + 1.7 × micrograms of synthetic folic acid.

Folic acid has a vital role in DNA synthesis and thus is essential for the synthesis of new cells and transmission of inherited characteristics. Synthetic folic acid in fortified food and supplements is better absorbed than folate that occurs naturally in foods. It is recommended that before and during pregnancy, women consume a total of 600 μg of **dietary folate equivalents (DFE)** daily of which 400 μg is from a supplement or fortified food and the remaining amount is folate naturally present in food.

Table 11.2	Selected Nutritional Needs for Women (Aged 19–30 Years) During Pregnancy and Lactation		
Nutrient	**Nonpregnant Women**	**Pregnancy**	**Lactation**
Calories	Individualized	1st tri: +0	
		2nd tri: +340	1st 6 months: +330
		3rd tri: +450	2nd 6 months: +400
Protein (g)	46	71	71
Vitamin A (μg)	700	770	1300
Vitamin C (mg)	75	85	120
Vitamin D (IU)	600	600	600
Vitamin E (mg)	15	15	19
Vitamin K (μg)*	90*	90*	90*
Thiamin (mg)	1.1	1.4	1.4
Riboflavin (mg)	1.1	1.4	1.6
Niacin (mg)	14	18	17
Vitamin B₆ (mg)	1.3	1.9	2.0
Folate (μg)	400	600	500
Vitamin B₁₂ (μg)	2.4	2.6	2.8
Calcium (mg)	1000	1000	1000
Iron (mg)	18	27	9
Magnesium (mg)	310	350	310
Selenium (μg)	55	60	70
Zinc (mg)	8	11	12

Recommended Dietary Allowances are in **boldface;** Adequate Intakes (AIs) appear in roman type followed by an asterisk (*).
tri, trimester.

Quick Bite Good sources of iron

Heme iron
  Lean red meat, poultry, pork
Nonheme iron
  100% iron-fortified ready-to-eat cereals
  Dried peas and beans, such as soybeans,
    lentils, lim a beans
  Baked potato with skin
  Dried fruit

Iron

The Recommended Dietary Allowance (RDA) for iron increases from 18 to 27 mg/day during pregnancy to support the increase in maternal blood volume and to provide iron for fetal liver storage, which sustains the infant for the first 4 to 6 months of life. Even with careful selections, women are not likely to consume adequate amounts of iron during pregnancy from food alone. Most prenatal vitamins contain 30 mg of elemental iron. Prenatal supplementation with daily iron effectively lowers the risk of LBW and maternal anemia (Peña-Rosas, De-Regil, Dowswell, & Viteri, 2012); intermittent supplementation (one to two times a week) has also been shown effective in reducing maternal anemia or iron deficiency (Peña-Rosas & Viteri, 2009).

Nutrient Supplements

Vitamin and mineral supplements may be necessary for certain populations, such as women who (Kaiser & Campbell, 2014)

- Have anemia
- Have poor eating habits
- Are strict vegans
- Are dependent on tobacco, alcohol, or illicit drugs
- Have food insecurity

Specific vitamin and mineral supplements that may be needed based on individual circumstances are as follows:

- Pregnant women who consume little or no animal products should take a supplement of vitamin B_{12} if a reliable dietary source is not consumed. Reliable sources are vegan foods fortified with vitamin B_{12}, such as yeast extracts, vegetable stock, veggie burgers, textured vegetable protein, soymilk, vegetable and sunflower margarines, and ready-to-eat breakfast cereals.
- The RDA for calcium does not increase during pregnancy because the rate of absorption and maternal bone calcium mobilization increases (Procter & Campbell, 2014). However, women who consume less than 500 mg calcium per day may need supplements to meet maternal and fetal bone requirements (Procter & Campbell, 2014).
- Women who do not consume adequate vitamin D or have insufficient sunlight exposure are at risk of vitamin D deficiency. The ACOG (2011) maintains that supplements of 1000 to 2000 IU per day are probably safe for pregnant women who are vitamin D deficient.
- Zinc supplementation may be advisable in women who have impaired zinc absorption secondary to a plant-based eating pattern that is high in phytates, GI disorders, or use of high doses of supplemental iron.

Herbal Supplements

Because little is known about the safety and efficacy of herbal supplements during pregnancy, it is recommended that they not be used during pregnancy and lactation. Herbal products, including herbal teas, are technically unapproved drugs; most drugs cross the placental barrier to some degree, exposing the fetus to potentially teratogenic effects. Unlike approved drugs, little animal or human testing has been done to determine if herbs can cause birth defects or potentially harm mothers and infants.

Fetal Alcohol Syndrome
a condition characterized by varying degrees of physical and mental growth failure and birth defects caused by maternal intake of alcohol.

Teratogen
anything that causes abnormal fetal development and birth defects.

Alcohol

Alcohol use during pregnancy can cause physical and neurodevelopmental problems, such as mental retardation, learning disabilities, and **fetal alcohol syndrome**. Alcohol does its damage by dehydrating fetal cells, leaving them dead or functionless, or by causing secondary nutrient deficiencies. Because alcohol is a potent **teratogen** and a "safe" level of consumption is not known, women are advised to completely avoid alcohol before and during pregnancy.

Caffeine

The half-life of caffeine increases during pregnancy from 3 hours in the first trimester to 80 to 100 hours in late pregnancy (Procter & Campbell, 2014). Results of studies are mixed on the effect of caffeine on the risk of adverse pregnancy outcomes (Brent, Christian, & Diener, 2011; Hoyt, Browne, Richardson, Romitti, & Druschel, 2014). The ACOG (2010) recommends pregnant women limit their intake of caffeine to less than 200 mg/day, which is the approximate amount in 16 oz of coffee (Table 11.3).

Table 11.3 — Caffeine Content of Selected Beverages and Foods

Item	Serving Size	Average Caffeine Content (mg)
Coffee		
Brewed	8 oz	95
Instant	8 oz	64
Decaffeinated	8 oz	2
Starbucks brewed (grande)	16 oz	330
Tea		
Brewed, leaf or bag	8 oz	47
Brewed, green	8 oz	30
Instant	8 oz	26
Brewed, herbal	8 oz	0
Snapple iced tea (all flavors)	16 oz	42
Soft Drinks		
Mellow Yello	12 oz	51
Mountain Dew	12 oz	45
Dr. Pepper, Sunkist Orange	12 oz	36
Pepsi	12 oz	32
Coca-Cola	12 oz	30
Club soda, ginger ale, 7Up, Squirt, tonic water, Sprite	12 oz	0
Energy Drinks		
Sobe No Fear	16 oz	141
Aqua Blast	0.5 L	90
Red Bull	8.3 oz	67
Red Devil	8.4 oz	42
Other Beverages		
Chocolate milk or hot cocoa	8 oz	5
Yoo-hoo chocolate drink	9 oz	3
Candy		
Dark chocolate, semisweet	1 oz	18
Milk chocolate	1 oz	6

Sources: Adapted from U.S. Department of Agriculture, Agricultural Research Service. (2005). *USDA National Nutrient Database for Standard Reference*, Release 18. Available at https://www.ars.usda.gov/northeast-area/beltsville-md/beltsville -human-nutrition-research-center/nutrient-data-laboratory/docs/sr18-home-page/; Center for Science and the Public Interest. (2014). *Caffeine content of foods and drugs*. Available at http://www.cspinet.org/new/cafchart.htm. Accessed on 4/9/16; and McCusker, R. R., Goldberger, B. A., & Cone, E. J. (2006). Caffeine content of energy drinks, carbonated sodas, and other beverages. *Journal of Analytical Toxicology, 30,* 112–114.

Nonnutritive Sweeteners

The use of nonnutritive sweeteners during pregnancy has been studied extensively. The U.S. Food and Drug Administration (FDA) has approved advatame, acesulfame potassium (Sunette, Sweet One), aspartame (NutraSweet, Spoonful, Equal), neotame (Newtame), saccharin (Sweet'N Low), and sucralose (Splenda) as food additives appropriate for general use, which includes pregnancy. The exception is that women with phenylketonuria should not use aspartame because it is made from phenylalanine. However, the research that addresses the safety of nonnutritive sweeteners during healthy pregnancy or in gestational diabetes is limited (Procter & Campbell, 2014). Although occasional use may not be harmful, the question remains as to whether they are beneficial.

Fish and Shellfish

The intake of omega-3 fatty acids from at least 8 oz of fish/week during pregnancy, especially docosahexaenoic acid (DHA), is associated with improved infant visual and cognitive development (Mulder, King, & Innis, 2014). However, nearly all fish contain trace amounts of mercury because it occurs naturally in the environment, including waterways. Bacteria in the water convert mercury to methylmercury, which is absorbed by fish low on the food chain and becomes concentrated in larger, longer living predatory fish at the top of the food chain. Mercury accumulates in humans primarily by eating fish.

Mercury can be toxic, particularly to developing brains in fetuses and young children. Mercury poisoning in a fetus can result in learning delays in walking or talking to more severe problems such as cerebral palsy, seizures, and mental retardation. However, observational studies indicate that at relatively low levels of methylmercury exposure, cognitive ability improves as both fish intake and maternal methylmercury increase, perhaps due to protective benefits provided by omega-3 fatty acids and selenium in the fish (Strain et al., 2012).

The FDA and Environmental Protection Agency (EPA) are in the process of revising their advice on fish intake during pregnancy. The key message of the draft is to eat 8 to 12 oz of a variety of fish each week from choices that are lower in mercury (FDA & EPA, 2014). To obtain the benefits of seafood while reducing exposure to methylmercury, women who are pregnant or lactating are advised to (FDA & EPA, 2014).

- Eat 8 to 12 oz of seafood per week from a variety of fish and shellfish that are lower in mercury, such as shrimp, salmon, pollock, catfish, tilapia, cod, and canned light tuna.
- Avoid four types of fish: tilefish from the Gulf of Mexico, shark, swordfish, and king mackerel.
- Limit albacore ("white") tuna to 6 oz per week.
- Check local advisories about the safety of fish from local waters. If no advice is available, eat up to 6 oz per week of fish from local waters but don't consume any other fish that week.
- While increasing fish intake, stay within calorie needs.

Avoiding Foodborne Illness

Due to hormonal changes that decrease cell-mediated immune function, pregnant women and their fetuses are at increased risk of developing foodborne illness. *Listeria monocytogenes* is an unusual bacterium because it can grow in refrigerated temperatures, unlike most other foodborne pathogens. Many animals carry this bacterium without outward symptoms. During pregnancy, listeriosis, caused by this bacterium, may cause only mild, flu-like illness in the mother, although in serious cases, it can be fatal. Listeriosis can lead to miscarriage, stillbirth, or premature delivery. Infants may be born with cognitive impairments, paralysis, seizures, blindness, or other impairments (FDA, 2016a). Pregnant women are 10 times more likely to get listeriosis than other healthy adults and an estimated one-seventh of all listeria cases occur during pregnancy (CDC, 2013). To reduce the risk of listeriosis, pregnant women should *not* consume the following foods:

- Unpasteurized milk or products made with it
- Raw or undercooked meat, poultry, eggs, fish, or shellfish
- Refrigerated smoked seafood

- Refrigerated pâtés or meat spreads
- Certain unpasteurized soft cheeses such as feta, Brie, bleu, and Camembert
- Hot dogs and deli meats, unless heated until steaming hot just before serving

Healthy people infected by the parasite *Toxoplasma gondii* may be asymptomatic or may have flu-like symptoms. During pregnancy, the consequences are more serious: Toxoplasmosis passed to the fetus can cause mental retardation, blindness, and hearing loss, which may not develop until later in life. Pregnant women should be instructed on how to prevent transmission of the parasite, including

- Cook meat thoroughly.
- Peel or wash fresh fruits and vegetables before eating.
- Avoid cross-contamination in the kitchen by cleaning surfaces and utensils exposed to raw food.
- Avoid changing cat litter (cats pass an environmentally resistant form of the organism in their feces). If no one else can change the litter, women should be advised to wear disposable gloves and to thoroughly wash their hands in warm soapy water afterward. Litter should be changed daily because the parasite does not become infectious until 1 to 5 days after it is shed in the feces (FDA, 2016b).

Physical Activity

Physical activity in all stages of life promotes health and reduces the risk of chronic disease, such as cardiovascular disease, diabetes, and obesity. During pregnancy, studies show an inverse relationship between increased activity and excessive gestational weight gain and that exercise alone may be enough to lower weight gain in pregnancy (Streuling, Beyerlein, Rosenfeld, Schukat, & von Kries, 2011). Exercise also reduces the risk of gestational diabetes in obese women (ACOG, 2015). However, many women decrease their level of activity during pregnancy (Pereira et al., 2007).

According to the ACOG (2015) Committee Opinion, physical activity during pregnancy has minimal risks and benefits most women. Healthy women with uncomplicated pregnancies are urged to engage in aerobic and strength-training exercises before, during, and after pregnancy. A goal of 20 to 30 minutes of moderate exercise on most days of the week is recommended and adjusted as necessary (ACOG, 2015). Safe exercise should be encouraged, with attention paid to fall risk and avoiding supine positions during the second and third trimesters.

Maternal Health

Common complaints associated with pregnancy, such as nausea, heartburn, and constipation, may be prevented or alleviated by nutrition interventions (Table 11.4). Excessive weight gain, inadequate weight gain, pica, diabetes mellitus, hypertension and preeclampsia, and maternal phenylketonuria are discussed in the following sections.

Excessive Gestational Weight Gain

Excessive gestational weight gain (GWG) is associated with increased risk of pregnancy-induced hypertension, gestational diabetes, cesarean delivery, LGA infants, and complications during delivery (Guelinckx, Devlieger, Beckers, & Vansant, 2008). Excessive GWG is the strongest predictor of maternal overweight or obesity following pregnancy (Herring, Rose, Skouteris, & Oken, 2012) and is more common in women who are overweight or obese prior to pregnancy (Fraser et al., 2011). For the infant, excessive maternal weight gain is associated with childhood overweight and obesity (Tie et al., 2014) and abdominal adiposity (Ensenauer et al., 2013). Unfortunately, there are no evidence-based recommendations on the most appropriate dietary and/or physical activity interventions to use to control excessive maternal weight gain (Crozier et al., 2010).

The timing of excessive weight gain is also important. A study by Davenport et al. (2013) found that excessive weight gain the first half of pregnancy is a strong predictor of excessive infant body fat at birth and that timing of the excess weight is more important than the total excessive weight gain in predicting excessive infant adiposity.

A recent U.S. study found that 73% of pregnant women had excessive GWG based on the 2009 IOM guidelines (Johnson et al., 2013). Data suggest that actual GWG is strongly correlated with health-care provider advice (Stotland et al., 2005). Women who are given weight gain advice from their health-care provider are more likely to stay within the recommended range of weight

Table 11.4 Common Complaints Associated with Pregnancy

Complaint	Possible Causes	Nutrition Interventions
Nausea and vomiting (common during the first trimester)	Hypoglycemia, decreased gastric motility, relaxation of the cardiac sphincter, anxiety	Eat easily digested carbohydrate foods (e.g., dry crackers, melba toast, dry cereal, hard candy) before getting out of bed in the morning. Eat frequent, small snacks of dry carbohydrates (e.g., crackers, hard candy) to prevent drop in glucose. Eat small frequent meals. Avoid liquids with meals. Limit high-fat foods because they delay gastric emptying. Eliminate individual intolerances and foods with a strong odor.
Constipation	Relaxation of gastrointestinal (GI) muscle tone and motility related to increased progesterone levels Increasing pressure on the GI tract by the fetus Decrease in physical activity Inadequate fiber and fluid intake Use of iron supplements	Increase fiber intake, especially intake of whole-grain breads and cereals. Look for breads that provide at least 2 g fiber/slice and cereals with at least 5 g fiber/serving. Drink at least eight 8-oz glasses of liquid daily. Try hot water with lemon or prune juice upon waking to help stimulate peristalsis. Participate in regular exercise.
Heartburn	Decrease in GI motility Relaxation of the cardiac sphincter Pressure of the uterus on the stomach	Eat small, frequent meals and eliminate liquids immediately before and after meals to avoid gastric distention. Avoid coffee, high-fat foods, and spices. Eliminate individual intolerances. Avoid lying down or bending over after eating.

gain than women who do not receive advice. Strategies that may help avoid excess GWG include the following (Lessen & Kavanagh, 2015):

- Early and ongoing motivational counseling about healthy eating patterns and the recommended amount and pattern of gain based on their BMI
- Personalized one-on-one nutrition counseling
- Supervised group and/or home exercise programs
- Showing women their actual weight gain compared to target ranges

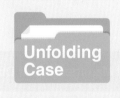

Unfolding Case

Consider Rachel. To help her avoid excessive weight gain, her weight is plotted against her target range at every prenatal visit. At her fourth month of pregnancy appointment, she showed a 1 month weight gain of almost double the recommended amount. What would you ask Rachel? What would you advise her to do?

Inadequate Weight Gain

In contrast, inadequate weight gain during pregnancy is associated with increased risk of preterm delivery and LBW (Li et al., 2013). A study by Davis, Hofferth, and Shenassa (2014) found a significant association between inadequate GWG and infant death that weakens with increasing prepregnancy BMI—that is, the risk of infant death was highest among underweight women who had inadequate weight gain and lowest among obese women.

Evidence is conflicting regarding the risk of less than recommended weight gain in overweight and obese women (Beyerlein, Lack, & von Kries, 2010; Siega-Riz et al., 2009). According to the ACOG, no evidence exists that encouraging more weight gain to conform to the IOM recommendations will improve maternal or fetal outcomes in overweight pregnant women who gain less than the recommended amount but have an appropriately growing fetus (ACOG, 2013a). Clearly, the relationships between maternal obesity, GWG, and maternal and newborn outcomes are complex (ACOG, 2013a).

Pica

Pica was first described by Hippocrates in 400 BCE (Miao, Young, & Golden, 2015). People who engage in pica may eat clay or dirt (geophagy); raw starch (amylophagy); ice and freezer frost (pagophagy); or other items including laundry starch, soap, ashes, chalk, paint, and burnt matches (Lessen & Kavanagh, 2015). Geophagy occurs most often. The reported mean prevalence among pregnant women in North/South America is 23% (Fawcett, Fawcett, & Mazmanian, 2016).

Pica has long been associated with micronutrient deficiencies, but the strength of this relationship is inconsistent (Miao et al., 2015). Possible mechanisms by which pica may cause deficiencies are that pica substances may prevent the absorption of micronutrients. It is also possible that micronutrient deficiencies cause humans to crave and eat minerals from nonfood substances. Miao et al. (2015) found that pica is associated with a 2.4 times higher risk of anemia, a lower hemoglobin concentration, lower hematocrit, and lower plasma zinc—whether the women practiced geophagy, pagophagy, or amylophagy. Screening pregnant women for pica could be a proxy for identifying risk of anemia or zinc deficiency. However, women may be reluctant to report the intake of nonfood substances.

Diabetes Mellitus

Gestational diabetes, defined as glucose intolerance diagnosed during the second or third trimester of pregnancy, is associated with increased risk of delivering an LGA infant, which in turn increases the risk of prolonged labor, cesarean delivery, shoulder dystocia, birth trauma, fetal hypoxia, and intrauterine death (Kim, Sharma, Sappenfield, Wilson, & Salihu, 2014). An LGA infant is more likely to develop diabetes, obesity, metabolic syndrome, asthma, and cancer later in life (Walsh & McAuliffe, 2012).

For the mother, GDM increases the risk of type 2 diabetes. Shortly after pregnancy, 5% to 10% of women with GDM are diagnosed with diabetes, usually type 2; women who have GDM have a 35% to 60% chance of developing diabetes in the next 10 to 20 years (CDC, 2014b).

The risk factors for GDM are similar to those for type 2 diabetes, namely, obesity, family history of diabetes, physical inactivity, and being of a certain race or ethnicity such as African American, Hispanics/Latinos, American Indians, some Asians, and Native Hawaiians or other Pacific Islanders (CDC, 2014b).

A systematic review and meta-analysis showed that treating GDM results in less preeclampsia, shoulder dystocia, and macrosomia, but there is little and inconsistent evidence that it helps neonatal hypoglycemia or future poor metabolic outcomes (Hartling et al., 2013). Nutrition recommendations for managing diabetes during pregnancy appear in Box 11.1.

BOX 11.1   Nutritional Management of Diabetes During Pregnancy

- The goals of diet are to achieve appropriate weight gain, keep blood glucose levels within the goal range, and avoid ketosis.
- Calorie intake for normal or underweight women should be based on DRIs for pregnant women. For overweight or obese women, a modest calorie restriction of the DRI for pregnant women is appropriate to slow weight gain. Weight loss in pregnancy is not recommended.
- Provide a minimum of 175 g carbohydrates daily for fetal brain and to prevent ketosis.
- Total carbohydrate intake should be less than 45% of total calorie intake to prevent hyperglycemia. Clinical measures such as blood glucose levels and ketones determine how carbohydrates are distributed during the day.
- Glucose control may be improved by allowing fewer carbohydrates at breakfast and more at other meals.
- Exercise is encouraged if there are no medical or obstetrical complications.

Source: Academy of Nutrition and Dietetics Evidence Analysis Library. (2008). *Gestational diabetes mellitus evidence-based nutrition practice guidelines.* Chicago, IL: American Dietetic Association. Available at http://www.andeal.org/topic.cfm?menu=3719&cat=3731. Accessed on 4/25/16.

Excessive GWG may present a greater risk for LGA than GDM in women who are not overweight or obese (Black et al., 2013). Interventions to effectively help overweight or obese women lose weight before pregnancy and prevent excessive GWG during pregnancy, regardless of GDM status, have the greatest potential to reduce the risk of LGA (Kim et al., 2014).

Hypertension and Preeclampsia

The prevalence of chronic hypertension is approximately 10% among women of reproductive age, primarily due to the increased prevalence of obesity (Robbins et al., 2014). Women who have hypertension before becoming pregnant are at increased risk maternal–fetal complications, including preeclampsia, placental abruption, gestational diabetes, preterm delivery, SGA delivery, and fetal mortality (Lo, Mission, & Caughey, 2013).

Gestational Hypertension
systolic blood pressure of 140 mmHg or greater or diastolic blood pressure of 90 mmHg or greater that develops in the second half of pregnancy and ends with childbirth.

Gestational hypertension is defined as a systolic blood pressure of greater than or equal to 140 mmHg or a diastolic reading of greater than or equal to 90 mmHg with onset after 20 weeks of gestation and without proteinuria. Often, gestational hypertension does not occur until 30 weeks or later. Studies suggest that the chance of developing gestational hypertension is more than 6 times higher among women who begin pregnancy obese compared to women who are at their ideal weight at conception (Stang & Huffman, 2016).

Preeclampsia
a toxemia of pregnancy characterized by hypertension accompanied by proteinuria or edema, or both.

The risk of developing **preeclampsia**, a potentially serious syndrome involving gestational hypertension plus proteinuria, is also correlated to BMI prior to conception, affecting an estimated 3.4% of women with a normal BMI, 10% of women with BMI ≥30, 12.8% of women with BMI ≥35, and 16.3% of women with BMI ≥40 (Schummers, Hutcheon, Bodnar, Lieberman, & Himes, 2015). Other risk factors include chronic hypertension or preeclampsia in a prior pregnancy; primiparity; multiple pregnancy; maternal age of 40 years or older; in vitro fertilization; and a history of diabetes, thrombophilia, or lupus (ACOG, 2014). Gestational hypertension and preeclampsia have been shown to double the risk of developing type 2 diabetes within 17 years postpartum, even when gestational diabetes was not diagnosed during pregnancy (Feig et al., 2013). Prevention of preeclampsia focuses on managing risk factors, such as controlling chronic hypertension and diabetes and losing weight if overweight.

Maternal intake is one of many factors suggested to play a role in the etiology of preeclampsia, but the hypotheses are varied and results are inconsistent. Endeshaw, Ambaw, Aragaw, and Ayalew (2014) found fruit and vegetables and folate to be protective against preeclampsia. A Cochrane review of randomized controlled trials concluded that calcium supplements (at least 1000 mg/day) lower blood pressure and the risk of preeclampsia but had no significant effect on reducing maternal and infant morbidity and mortality (Hofmeyr, Lawrie, Atallah, & Duley, 2010). Furthermore, only high-risk women with very low calcium intakes may benefit from calcium supplementation. Studies on the effects of supplemental omega-3 fatty acids, vitamin C, and vitamin E have not shown improved perinatal outcomes (Rossi, 2011; Zhou et al., 2012).

Maternal Phenylketonuria

Phenylketonuria (PKU)
an inborn error of phenylalanine (an essential amino acid) metabolism that results in retardation and physical handicaps in newborns if they are not treated with a low-phenylalanine diet beginning shortly after birth.

Microcephaly
abnormally small head.

Women who have **phenylketonuria (PKU)** and who consume a normal diet before and during pregnancy have very high blood levels of phenylalanine, which are devastating to the developing fetus. As a teratogen, excess serum phenylalanine can cause **microcephaly**, mental retardation, growth retardation, and/or congenital heart abnormalities in any offspring born to a woman with PKU. The primary determinants of infant outcome are the degree of elevated phenylalanine and the gestational age when phenylalanine control is achieved (van Calcar & Ney, 2012). Most of these infants do not inherit PKU and cannot benefit from a low-phenylalanine diet after birth.

Nutrition plays a key role in the outcome of maternal PKU pregnancies. To prevent mental retardation and other problems associated with maternal PKU, a low-phenylalanine diet is necessary at least 3 months before conception and throughout the duration of the pregnancy to strictly control blood phenylalanine levels and eliminate risks to the developing fetus. However, because phenylalanine is an essential amino acid, it must be provided in the diet in limited amounts to support growth and protein synthesis. Low-phenylalanine diets are very low in total protein, so a

BOX 11.2   Diet Guidelines for Pregnant Women with Phenylketonuria (PKU)

Pregnant women with PKU should be advised that

- Complete understanding and strict adherence to the diet are vital.
- Protein foods such as meat, fish, poultry, eggs, dairy products, and nuts are high in phenylalanine and must be eliminated.
- Diet drinks and foods sweetened with aspartame (NutraSweet) are strictly forbidden.
- PKU-appropriate medical foods (e.g., special PKU formula) may be expensive and offensive to adult palates but must be consumed in adequate amounts to support fetal growth and prevent maternal tissue breakdown that would have results similar to those caused by cheating on the diet.
- An adequate calorie intake is necessary for normal protein metabolism.
- Close monitoring of blood phenylalanine levels is essential.

Medical Foods
a food formulated to be consumed orally or administered enterally under the supervision of a physician for the specific dietary management of a disease or condition.

PKU medical food must be consumed as a source of protein. An excessive intake of phenylalanine is common without an adequate intake of calories provided by most **medical foods** (van Calcar & Ney, 2012). Deficiencies of vitamin B_6, vitamin B_{12}, calcium, folate, iron, and omega-3 fatty acids may develop from the restriction of protein foods. General diet guidelines are listed in Box 11.2.

NUTRITION FOR LACTATION

With rare exceptions, breastfeeding is the optimal method of feeding and nurturing infants. WHO recommends that infants be exclusively breastfed for the first 6 months of life with the introduction of complementary foods thereafter as breastfeeding continues up to the age of 2 years or beyond (WHO, 2016). In the United States, both the American Academy of Pediatrics (AAP) and the Academy of Nutrition and Dietetics recommend that infants be exclusively breastfed for the first 6 months of life and that breastfeeding continue with complementary foods until 1 year of age or longer (AAP, 2012; Lessen & Kavanagh, 2015). Breastfeeding is an important public health strategy for improving infant and child morbidity and mortality and improving maternal morbidity (Lessen & Kavanagh, 2015). The benefits of breastfeeding for both mother and infant are well recognized (Box 11.3).

Promoting Breastfeeding

The United States has seen a steady increase in breastfeeding rates since the late 1970s. Of infants born in 2011, 79% of newborns were breastfed, 49% were breastfeeding at 6 months, and 27% at 12 months (CDC, 2014a). Although these figures are improved, they still fall below the Healthy People 2020 objective to increase the proportion of infants who are breastfed to (CDC, 2014a)

- 81.9% ever breastfed
- 60.6% at 6 months
- 34.1% at 1 year
- 46.2% exclusively through 3 months
- 25.5% exclusively through 6 months

Despite the abundance of reasons to breastfeed, many women choose not to initiate breastfeeding, only partially breastfeed, or breastfeed for only a short duration. Factors influencing a mother's decision not to breastfeed or to breastfeed for a short duration include unsupportive hospital practices, lack of knowledge, personal beliefs, and family attitudes. A variety of factors may interfere with a woman's ability to successfully establish or continue breastfeeding (Box 11.4). Even a short period of breastfeeding is better than not breastfeeding at all. Women should be encouraged to breastfeed for as long as they are able and not be made to feel guilty if they fall short of the recommendations.

BOX 11.3   Benefits of Breastfeeding

For the Mother

- Promotes optimal maternal–infant bonding
- Simulates uterine contractions to help control postpartum bleeding and regain prepregnant uterus size
- Is readily available and requires no mixing or dilution
- Is less expensive than purchasing bottles, nipples, and formula
- Decreases risk of breast and ovarian cancer
- Delays resumption of menstruation, although not reliable for birth control
- Conserves iron stores by prolonging amenorrhea
- May hasten return to prepregnancy weight
- May lower the risk of breast cancer, rheumatoid arthritis, cardiovascular disease, hypertension, and diabetes
- Improves bone density and reduces risk for hip fracture
- Reduces risk of postpartum depression
- Enhances self-esteem as a competent mother

For the Infant

- Increases bonding with mother
- Is an optimal "natural" nutrition that contains no artificial colorings, flavorings, preservatives, or additives
- Is safe and fresh
- Reduces risk of acute otitis media, pneumonia, and severe lower respiratory tract infections
- Reduces the risk of nonspecific gastrointestinal tract infections and necrotizing enterocolitis
- Reduces the risk of sudden infant death syndrome and infant mortality
- Enhances immune system
- Reduces the risk of asthma, atopic dermatitis, and eczema
- Promotes better tooth and jaw development than bottle feeding because the infant has to suck harder
- Associated with higher IQ and school performance
- Reduces the risk of chronic diseases, such as obesity, type 1 and 2 diabetes, celiac disease, inflammatory bowel disease, and childhood leukemia and lymphoma
- Reduces risk for infant morbidity and mortality

Social support and support from health-care professional influence success with breast-feeding. As a learned behavior, not a physiologic response, the ability to successfully breastfeed and the duration of lactation can be positively affected by counseling. Preparation for breastfeeding should begin prenatally with counseling, guidance, and support for both the woman and her partner and continue throughout the gestational period. Hospital practices that promote breastfeeding appear in Box 11.5. Contraindications to breastfeeding are listed in Box 11.6.

BOX 11.4   Factors that May Interfere with Successful Breastfeeding

Impaired Letdown, Related to

Embarrassment or stress
Fatigue
Negative attitude, lack of desire, lack of family support
Excessive intake of caffeine or alcohol
Smoking
Drugs

Failure to Establish Lactation, Related to

Delayed or infrequent feedings
Weak infant sucking because of anesthesia during labor and delivery
Nipple discomfort or engorgement
Lack of support especially from baby's father

Decreased Demand, Related to

Supplemental bottles of formula or water
Introduction of solid food
Infant's lack of interest

BOX 11.5   Hospital Practices that Promote Breastfeeding

- Help mothers initiate breastfeeding within 1 hour of birth. Hospital procedures should allow for immediate maternal–infant contact after delivery.
- Infant rooming-in
- Encourage breastfeeding on demand.
- Inform all pregnant women about the benefits and management of breastfeeding.
- Show mothers how to breastfeed and maintain lactation even if they are separated from their infants.
- Feed only breast milk in the hospital.
- Give no artificial teats or pacifiers (e.g., dummies, soothers) to breastfeeding infants.
- Provide a phone number for breastfeeding help after discharge.

Eating Pattern

Nutritional needs during lactation are based on the nutritional content of breast milk and the "cost" of producing milk. Compared with pregnancy, the need for some nutrients increases, whereas the need for other nutrients falls (see Table 11.2). In general, an inadequate nutrient intake affects the quantity of milk produced but not the quality: The content of macronutrients and most minerals in breast milk is maintained at the expense of maternal stores if maternal intake is inadequate. Maternal intake does influence the quantity of some vitamins, such as vitamins B_6, B_{12}, A, and D, and also the fatty acid profile (Ballard & Morrow, 2013). The healthy eating pattern consumed during pregnancy should continue during lactation.

Calories

Well-nourished women who exclusively breastfeed need 450 to 500 more cal/day than normal, which can easily be met with modest increases to a balanced eating pattern. The recommendation is calorie intake increase by 330 for the first 6 months and 400 calories for the second 6 months. These figures are based on the idea that approximately 100 to 150 of the remaining required calories will be mobilized from fat stored during pregnancy, thereby helping women regain their prepregnancy weight. Breastfeeding supplemented with formula requires a smaller increase in calorie intake.

For the sample woman used for the MyPlate Daily Checklist in Figure 11.1, the eating pattern recommended while she exclusively breastfeeds for the first 6 months is 2400 calories, which is a recommended estimate using food groups, not an exact calorie prescription. This calorie level

BOX 11.6   Contraindications to Breastfeeding

- An infant diagnosed with galactosemia, a rare genetic metabolic disorder
- The infant whose mother
  - Uses illegal drugs
  - Is infected with HIV
  - Is taking antiretroviral medications
  - Has untreated active tuberculosis
  - Is infected with human T-cell lymphotropic virus type I or type II
  - Is undergoing radiation therapy (requires only a temporary interruption in breastfeeding)
  - Is taking prescribed cancer chemotherapy medications that interfere with DNA replication and cell division

Source: Centers for Disease Control and Prevention. (2015). *When should a mother avoid breastfeeding?* Available at http://www.cdc.gov/breastfeeding/disease/. Accessed on 4/10/16.

would allow her to mobilize fat accumulated during pregnancy to provide the additional calories needed to produce enough breast milk.

Adequacy of calorie intake is evaluated by changes in a woman's weight. Women who failed to gain enough weight during pregnancy, who have inadequate fat reserves, or who lose too much weight while breastfeeding may need to increase their calorie intake. Conversely, women who are not losing weight while lactating can reduce their calorie intake after lactation is established. Women should not restrict their calorie intakes below 1500 to 1800 per day because milk production may be decreased (Academy of Nutrition and Dietetics Nutrition Care Manual at https://www.nutritioncaremanual.org/).

Fluid

Another nutritional consideration during lactation is fluid intake. A rule-of-thumb suggestion is that breastfeeding mothers drink a glass of fluid every time the baby nurses and with all meals or approximately twelve 8-oz glasses of caffeine-free fluids per day. Thirst is a good indicator of need except among women who live in a dry climate or who exercise in hot weather. Fluids consumed in excess of thirst quenching do not increase milk volume.

Vitamins and Minerals

For many vitamins and minerals, requirements are higher during lactation than during pregnancy, but the increase in calories from nutrient-dense foods can generally meet increased needs. One exception is iron. Iron supplements may be needed to replace depleted iron stores, not to increase the iron content of breast milk. Although there is no routine recommendation for maternal supplements during lactation, many clinicians recommend continued use of prenatal vitamins (AAP, 2012).

Other Considerations

Other considerations concerning maternal intake and breast milk are as follows:

- Highly flavored or spicy foods may have an impact on the flavor of breast milk but need only be avoided if infant feeding is affected.
- The intake of alcohol should be minimized and limited to occasional use of moderate intake, ideally not until after 3 months postpartum. Nursing should not take place under 2 hours after alcohol intake to minimize its concentration in breast milk (AAP, 2012).
- Caffeine enters breast milk. Maternal intake should not exceed 2 to 5 cups of coffee, tea, or caffeinated soft drinks per day. Newborns are especially sensitive to caffeine (Academy of Nutrition and Dietetics Nutrition Care Manual at https://www.nutritioncaremanual.org/).
- Lactating women are urged to follow the same guidelines for seafood consumption as pregnant women: Eat 8 to 12 oz/week of a variety of seafood that is low in mercury because its omega-3 fatty acid content is important for neurologic development. Because they are high in mercury, lactating women should avoid shark, swordfish, king mackerel, and tilefish from the Gulf of Mexico; limit white albacore tuna to 6 oz/week; and check with authorities for advisories about fish from local waters.
- Herbal teas and supplements should be avoided unless approved by the physician.

Postpartum Weight Retention

Excessive GWG increases the risk of postpartum weight retention and long-term maternal weight gain (Nehring, Schmoll, Beyerlein, Hauner, & von Kries, 2011) and may be a significant contributor to the obesity epidemic in childbearing women (Rasmussen et al., 2010). Weight retention has been shown to occur in 68% of women at 12 months postpartum and may be as much as 20 pounds or more (Martin, Hure, Macdonald-Wicks, Smith, & Collins, 2014). A study by Kirkegaard et al. (2014) found that postpartum weight retention at 6 months and weight gain from 6 to 18 months postpartum had a major effect on maternal weight, BMI, and waist circumference 7 years later—independent of GWG and prepregnancy BMI.

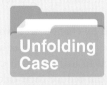

Unfolding Case

Think of Rachel. She gained 28 pounds during pregnancy— more than the 11 to 20 pounds her doctor recommended. She understands the importance of managing her weight for her own health and for future pregnancies. She has been successfully breastfeeding for 2½ months yet has not lost any weight, so she will lower her calorie intake to help promote weight loss. What would you recommend as an appropriate calorie level and goal weight? What kind of eating pattern may be healthiest for her given her high risk for type 2 diabetes and hypertension?

Although postpartum weight loss is critical to preventing and managing obesity in women, lifestyle interventions to achieve adequate postpartum weight loss have not been clearly identified (Lim et al., 2015). Findings from a meta-analysis of randomized controlled studies indicate that interventions that combine diet with exercise and include self-monitoring result in significantly greater postpartum weight loss (Lim et al., 2015). The most crucial time to intervene to prevent obesity later in life may be during the early postpartum period (Kirkegaard et al., 2014).

NURSING PROCESS

Normal Pregnancy

Jana is a 33-year-old professional who is 20 weeks pregnant with her first baby. Her prepregnancy BMI was 19.2. She has gained 7 pounds and complains of constipation. She plans on returning to work 6 weeks after delivery and wants to limit her weight gain so that she can fit into her clothes by the time she returns to work. She has asked you what she should eat that will be good for the baby but not cause her to get fat.

Assessment

Medical–Psychosocial History	Medical history such as diabetes, hypertension, lactose intolerance, PKU, or other chronic disease • Use of medications and over-the-counter drugs • Adequacy of sunlight exposure • Symptoms of constipation, including frequency, interventions attempted, and results • Other complaints related to pregnancy, such as heartburn • Usual frequency and intensity of physical activity • Attitude about pregnancy; knowledge about normal amount and pattern of weight gain during pregnancy • Attitude/plan regarding breastfeeding • Level of family/social support
Anthropometric Assessment	Height, prepregnancy weight, pattern of 7-pound weight gain during pregnancy
Biochemical and Physical Assessment	• Hemoglobin to screen for iron deficiency anemia (Many laboratory values change during pregnancy related to normal changes in maternal physiology and so cannot be validly compared with nonpregnancy standards.) • Glucose, other laboratory values as available • Blood pressure
Dietary Assessment	• How does the client describe her appetite? • Does the client follow a balanced and varied eating pattern that includes all food groups from MyPlate in reasonable amounts? • Does the client eat at regular intervals? • How has the client modified her intake since becoming pregnant? • Does the client eat nonfoods or have unusual eating habits? • Does the client take a vitamin and/or mineral supplement? • Does the client use alcohol, tobacco, caffeine, or herbal supplements? • Is the client knowledgeable about nutrient needs during pregnancy? • What cultural, religious, and ethnic influences affect the client's food choices?

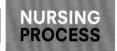

Normal Pregnancy

Diagnosis

Possible Nursing Diagnoses
- Constipation related to pregnancy
- Deficient knowledge of appropriate eating pattern for pregnancy
- Imbalanced nutrition: eating less than the body needs related to voluntary food restriction to limit weight gain

---

Planning

Client Outcomes

The client will
- Avoid constipation
- Identify measures that prevent constipation
- Explain the importance of nutrition for her health and for fetal growth and development
- Consume an adequate, varied, and balanced eating pattern based on MyPlate
- Explain the amount and pattern of recommended weight gain
- Gain approximately 1 pound of weight per week

Nursing Interventions

Nutrition Therapy

Increase fiber intake gradually to prevent constipation
- Provide an eating plan that includes all food groups and emphasizes ample fruits and vegetables, whole grains, lean protein, fat-free dairy, and healthy fats with total amounts per day based on her calorie needs
- Encourage adequate fluid intake due to increased fiber intake

Client Teaching

Instruct the client on
- The role of nutrition and weight gain in the outcome of pregnancy
- The role of fiber and fluids in preventing and alleviating constipation

Eating plan essentials, including
- Choosing a variety of foods within each major food group
- Selecting the appropriate number of servings from each major food group
- Consuming sources of fiber such as bran and whole-grain breads and cereals, dried peas and beans, fresh fruits, and vegetables

Behavioral matters including
- Abandoning the idea of limiting weight gain to fit into clothes after pregnancy
- Eating small, frequent meals
- The importance of maintaining physical activity

Where to find more information (see "Websites" at the end of this chapter)

Evaluation

Evaluate and Monitor
- Monitor for complaints of constipation
- Monitor amount and pattern of weight gain
- Suggest changes in the food plan as needed
- Provide periodic feedback and support

How Do You Respond?

Why don't pregnant women need to increase their calcium intake during pregnancy? The RDA for women age 19 to 50 years—whether pregnant or not—is 1000 mg. The reason why the RDA for calcium does not increase during pregnancy is that the body compensates for the increased need by more than doubling the rate of calcium absorption. If calcium intake was adequate before pregnancy, the amount consumed does not need to increase.

Should pregnant women avoid eating peanuts during pregnancy to reduce the risk of peanut allergy in their children? The advice to avoid peanuts and other allergens during pregnancy has been overturned. In fact, the opposite of that advice is now recommended: do not avoid peanuts during pregnancy and introduce them into the diets of high risk for allergy infants at an early age. Studies show that the early introduction of peanuts significantly decreases the frequency of developing a peanut allergy among children at high risk for this allergy (Toit et al., 2015). Similarly, a recent study found that higher maternal intake of three common allergens during early pregnancy, namely, peanut, milk, and wheat, is associated with a lower risk of mid-childhood allergy and asthma (Bunyavanich et al., 2014).

REVIEW CASE STUDY

Sarah is 28 years old and 7 months pregnant with her third child. Her other children are aged 2½ years and 1½ years. She had uncomplicated pregnancies and deliveries. Sarah is 5 ft 6 in tall; she weighed 142 pounds at the beginning of this pregnancy, which made her prepregnancy BMI 23. She has gained 24 pounds so far. Prior to her first pregnancy, her BMI was 20 (124 pounds). She is unhappy about her weight gain, but the stress of having two young children and being a stay-at-home mom made losing weight impossible.

She went online for her MyPlate plan, which recommends she consume 2400 cal/day. She doesn't think she eats that much because she seems to have constant heartburn. She takes a prenatal supplement, so she feels pretty confident that even if her intake is not perfect, she is getting all the nutrients she needs through her supplement. A typical day's intake for her is shown on the right:

- Does she have any risk factors for a high-risk pregnancy?
- Evaluate her prepregnancy weight and weight gain thus far. How much total weight should she gain?
- Based on the 2400-calorie meal pattern in Figure 11.1, what does Sarah need to eat more of? What is she eating in more

than the recommended amounts? How would you suggest she modify her intake to minimize heartburn?
- What would you tell her about weight gain during pregnancy? What strategies would you suggest to her after her baby is born that would help her regain her healthy weight?
- Is her attitude about supplements appropriate? What would you tell her about supplements?

Devise a 1-day menu for her that would provide all the food she needs in the recommended amounts and alleviate her heartburn.

Breakfast: Cornflakes with whole milk (because the children drink whole milk), Orange juice
Snack: Bran muffin and whole milk
Lunch: Either a peanut butter and jelly sandwich or tuna fish sandwich with mayonnaise, Snack crackers, Whole milk, Pudding or cookies
Snack: Ice cream
Dinner: Macaroni and cheese, Green beans, Roll and butter, Whole milk, Cake or ice cream for dessert
Evening: Chips and salsa

STUDY QUESTIONS

1 A woman trying to become pregnant was told by her physician to take a daily supplement containing 400 µg of folic acid. She asks why a supplement is better than eating folic acid through food. Which statement is the nurses' best response?
   a. "There are few natural sources of folate in food."
   b. "Synthetic folic acid in supplements and fortified foods is better absorbed, more available, and a more reliable source than the folate found naturally in food."
   c. "Folate in food is equally as good as folic acid in supplements. It is just easier to take it in pill form and then you don't have to worry about how much you're getting in food."
   d. "If you are sure that you eat at least five servings of fruits and vegetables every day, you don't really need to take a supplement of folic acid."

2 A woman who was at her healthy weight when she got pregnant is distraught by her 4-pound weight gain between 20 and 24 weeks of gestation. At this point in her pregnancy, her total weight gain is right on target. What is the nurse's best response?
   a. "A 4-pound-per-month weight gain at this point in your pregnancy is normal."
   b. "Although it is considerably less than the recommended amount, it is not a cause for concern. Just be sure to follow your meal plan next month so you get enough calories and nutrients."
   c. "I recommend you write down everything you eat for a few days so we can identify where the problem lies."
   d. "A 4-pound weight gain in 1 month at this point in your pregnancy may be a sign that you are at risk of preeclampsia. You should cut back on the 'extras' in your eating pattern to limit your weight gain for next month."

3 The nurse knows her instructions on healthy eating during pregnancy have been effective when the woman verbalizes she should
   a. Avoid seafood because of its mercury content
   b. Eliminate coffee and other sources of caffeine
   c. Increase her intake of milk to 4 cups/day
   d. Eliminate hot dogs and deli meats unless heated to steaming hot immediately before eating

4 At her first prenatal visit, an overweight woman asks how much weight she should gain during the course of her pregnancy. What is the nurse's best response?
   a. "You should not gain any weight during your pregnancy. You have adequate calorie reserves to meet all the energy demands of pregnancy without gaining additional weight."
   b. "You should try to gain less than 15 pounds."
   c. "Aim for a 15- to 25-pound weight gain."
   d. "The recommended weight gain for your weight is 25 to 35 pounds."

5 Which of the following statements indicates that the pregnant woman understands the recommendations about caffeine intake during pregnancy?
   a. "I have to give up drinking coffee and cola."
   b. "I will limit my intake of coffee to about 12 oz a day and avoid other sources of caffeine."
   c. "As long as I don't drink coffee, I can eat other sources of caffeine because they don't contain enough to cause any problems."
   d. "Caffeine is harmless during pregnancy, so I am allowed to consume as much as I want."

6 What nutrient is not likely to be consumed in adequate amounts during pregnancy so a supplement may be needed?
   a. Iron
   b. Calcium
   c. Vitamin B_{12}
   d. Vitamin C

7 A woman at 5 weeks of gestation is complaining of nausea throughout the day. What should the nurse recommend?
   a. Small, frequent meals of easily digested carbohydrates
   b. Small, frequent meals that are high in protein
   c. A liquid diet until the nausea subsides
   d. A low-fiber intake

8 Which of the following statements is true?
   a. "Women who breastfeed almost always achieve their pre-pregnancy weight at 6 weeks postpartum."
   b. "Weight loss during lactation is not recommended because it lowers the quantity and quality of breast milk produced."
   c. "Breastfeeding women do not have to increase their intake by the full amount of calories it 'costs' to produce milk because they can mobilize fat stored during pregnancy for some of the extra energy required."
   d. "Women do not need to increase their calorie intake at all for the first 6 months of breastfeeding because they can use calories stored in fat to produce milk."

KEY CONCEPTS

- Although proper nutrition before and during pregnancy cannot guarantee a successful pregnancy outcome, it does profoundly affect fetal development and birth.
- A screening performed at the first prenatal visit can identify women at potential nutritional risk during pregnancy and provides baseline data for ongoing monitoring. Nutrition counseling should be initiated early in prenatal care and continue throughout the pregnancy. It should stress the importance of appropriate weight gain, ways to improve overall intake, and the benefits of breastfeeding.
- A healthy eating pattern based on MyPlate food patterns is appropriate before, during, and after pregnancy, with few modifications.
- All women of childbearing age who are capable of becoming pregnant are urged to consume 400 μg of synthetic folic acid daily—through fortified foods or supplements—and consume foods that provide naturally occurring folate to reduce the risk of neural tube defects. The most critical period for the development of neural tube defects is the first month after conception when a woman may not even know she is pregnant.
- Screening for iron deficiency anemia should occur prior to conception. Women should be encouraged to consume rich sources of heme iron. Supplemental iron may be recommended.
- Ideally, women should attain a healthy weight prior to conception.
- Weight gain recommendations during pregnancy are based on a woman's BMI: 25 to 35 pounds for women of normal weight, 28 to 40 pounds for underweight women, 15 to 25 pounds for overweight women, and 11 to 20 pounds for obese women.
- The recommended pattern of weight gain for normal-weight women is 1.1 to 4.4 pounds in the first trimester and approximately 1 pound/week for the rest of pregnancy. This pattern is adjusted up or down for women who are not within their healthy weight range at the time of conception.
- Calorie requirements do not increase during the first trimester. In the second trimester, calorie needs increase by 340 cal/day and in the third trimester by 452 cal/day.
- A woman who eats a varied eating pattern with adequate calories should be able to meet her increased need for most vitamins and minerals through food alone. Iron supplements may be recommended. Folic acid requirements increase to 600 μg during pregnancy; supplements and/or fortified foods can provide this amount. Multivitamin and minerals are recommended for specific situations, such as during iron deficiency, for women carrying two or more fetuses, and when intake is poor.
- Women are urged to avoid alcohol before and during pregnancy because a safe level is not known.
- Herbal supplements should not be used during pregnancy because their safety has not been tested during pregnancy or lactation.
- Pregnant women are advised to limit their caffeine intake to 200 mg/day or less—the equivalent of approximately 12 oz of coffee. Findings on the impact of caffeine on pregnancy outcomes are mixed.
- Nonnutritive sweeteners are considered safe to use during pregnancy with the amounts specified by the FDA. However, not many studies have tested the effects of their use during pregnancy or lactation.
- Pregnant women should not eat shark, swordfish, king mackerel, and tilefish from the Gulf of Mexico and should limit albacore tuna to 6 oz/week. They should strive to eat 8 to 12 oz/week of a variety fish and shellfish.
- Pregnant women are at increased risk of foodborne illness due to changes in immune function from altered levels of hormones. The consequences of foodborne illness can be devastating for a developing fetus. Pregnant women are urged to take precautions to avoid foodborne illness.
- Pregnant woman should engage in moderate physical activity for at least 30 min/day on most days of the week. Safe activities include those that do not have a risk of fall or require lying down in the supine position after the second trimester of pregnancy.
- Excessive GWG is associated with increased risk of pregnancy-induced hypertension, gestational diabetes, cesarean delivery, LGA infants, and complications during delivery and is the strongest predictor of maternal overweight or obesity following pregnancy. Infants born to mothers who had excessive GWG have an increased risk of childhood overweight and obesity.
- Inadequate weight gain during pregnancy is associated with increased infant mortality. The risk is highest among underweight women with inadequate weight gain and is lowest in obese women.
- Diabetes, gestational hypertension, and maternal PKU are maternal health conditions that can greatly affect fetal development and the course of pregnancy. Nutrition therapy is vital. Women with these conditions must be closely monitored.
- Breastfeeding is recommended for the first 12 months of life. In addition to being uniquely suited to infant growth and development, it imparts other significant benefits to both infant and mother.
- Almost all women are capable of breastfeeding.
- The healthy eating pattern recommended during pregnancy should be continued during lactation. Although more calories are needed during lactation than pregnancy once lactation is well established, women can eat less than the total calories needed and mobilize calories stored as fat to help regain prepregnancy weight.
- Thirst is a reliable indicator of fluid need for most women during lactation.
- In the postpartum period, attaining a healthy BMI is important for avoiding obesity and its health risks later in life.

Check Your Knowledge Answer Key

1 **FALSE** The amount of weight a woman gains during pregnancy is an important indicator of fetal growth. However, adequate weight gain during pregnancy cannot by itself ensure the delivery of a normal-birth-weight infant.

2 **FALSE** Obese women should gain 11 to 20 pounds during pregnancy. It is not known how much weight severely obese women should gain during pregnancy.

3 **TRUE** Fortified cereals are a significant source of folic acid. In fact, the recommended amount of folic acid could easily be exceeded with large portions of fortified cereal.

4 **TRUE** Regardless of prepregnancy BMI, it is recommended all women gain 1 to 4 pounds during the first trimester.

5 **FALSE** The RDA for calcium does not increase during pregnancy because calcium absorption greatly increases. Calcium needs can be met with the equivalent of 3 cups of milk daily.

6 **FALSE** Pregnant and lactating women as well as women who may become pregnant are advised to eliminate only shark, swordfish, king mackerel, and tilefish from their eating patterns; white albacore tuna should be limited to 6 oz/week, and other fish and shellfish can be consumed in amounts up to 12 oz/week as long as any one particular type of fish is not eaten more than once a week. Local advisories about fish caught in local waters should also be heeded.

7 **TRUE** Calorie requirements do not increase until the second trimester, and even then, the increase is small: an additional 340 calories for the second trimester and an additional 452 calories in the third trimester.

8 **TRUE** Lactation increases calorie recommendations by 500 for the first 6 months of breastfeeding and by 400 for the second 6 months. Women may eat fewer calories than this and still produce enough milk by mobilizing calories stored as fat.

9 **FALSE** Evidence is lacking that pregnancy outcomes improve when overweight women who gain less than the recommended amount for their BMI increase their weight gain when the fetus is growing appropriately.

10 **TRUE** Thirst is a good indicator of the need for fluids except among women who live in a dry climate or exercise in hot weather.

Student Resources on thePoint®
For additional learning materials, activate the code in the front of this book at
http://thePoint.lww.com/activate

Websites

Academy of Nutrition and Dietetics at www.eatright.org

American Academy of Pediatrics at www.aap.org

American College of Obstetricians and Gynecologists at www.acog.org

La Lèche League International at www.lalecheleague.org

March of Dimes at www.marchofdimes.com

MyPlate for Pregnancy and Breastfeeding at www.choosemyplate.gov

Nutrition.gov at www.nutrition.gov

Supplemental Nutrition Program for Women, Infants, and Children (WIC) at http://www.fns.usda.gov/wic/women-infants-and-children-wic

References

American Academy of Pediatrics. (2012). *Breastfeeding and the use of human milk: Policy statement.* Available at http://pediatrics.aap publications.org/content/pediatrics/129/3/e827.full.pdf. Accessed on 4/5/16.

American College of Obstetricians and Gynecologists. (2010). ACOG Committee Opinion No. 462: Moderate caffeine consumption during pregnancy. *Obstetrics and Gynecology, 116,* 467–468.

American College of Obstetricians and Gynecologists. (2011). ACOG Committee Opinion No. 495: Vitamin D: Screening and supplementation during pregnancy. *Obstetrics and Gynecology, 118,* 197–198.

American College of Obstetricians and Gynecologists. (2013a). ACOG Committee Opinion No. 548: Weight gain during pregnancy. *Obstetrics and Gynecology, 121,* 210–212. doi:10.1097/01.AOG .0000425668.87506.4c

American College of Obstetricians and Gynecologists. (2013b). ACOG Committee Opinion No. 549: Obesity in pregnancy. *Obstetrics and Gynecology, 121,* 213–217. doi:10.1097/01.AOG.0000425667 .10377.60

American College of Obstetricians and Gynecologists. (2014). *Preeclampsia and high blood pressure during pregnancy.* Available at http://www .acog.org/Patients/FAQs/Preeclampsia-and-High-Blood-Pressure -During-Pregnancy. Accessed on 4/5/16.

American College of Obstetricians and Gynecologists. (2015). ACOG Committee Opinion No. 650: Physical activity and exercise during pregnancy and the postpartum period. *Obstetrics and Gynecology, 126,* e135–e142.

Ballard, O., & Morrow, A. (2013). Human milk composition: Nutrients and bioactive factors. *Pediatric Clinics of North America, 60,* 49–74.

Barker, D. J. (1990). The fetal and infant origins of adult disease. *BMJ, 301,* 1111.

Beyerlein, A., Lack, N., & von Kries, R. (2010). Within-populations average ranges compared with Institute of Medicine recommendations for gestational weight gain. *Obstetrics and Gynecology, 116,* 1111–1118.

Black, M., Sacks, D., Xiang, A., & Lawrence, J. (2013). The relative contribution of prepregnancy overweight and obesity, gestational weight gain, and IADPSG-defined gestational diabetes mellitus to fetal overgrowth. *Diabetes Care, 36*, 56–62.

Blomberg, M. (2011). Maternal and neonatal outcomes among obese women with weight gain below the new Institute of Medicine recommendations. *Obstetrics and Gynecology, 117*, 1065–1070.

Brent, R., Christian, M., & Diener, R. (2011). Evaluation of the reproductive and developmental risks of caffeine. *Birth Defects Research. Part B, Developmental and Reproductive Toxicology, 92*, 152–187.

Bunyavanich, S., Rifas-Shiman, S., Platts-Mills, T., Workman, L., Sordillo, J. E., Camargo, C. A., . . . Litonjua, A. A. (2014). Peanut, milk, and wheat intake during pregnancy is associated with reduced allergy and asthma in children. *The Journal of Allergy and Clinical Immunology, 133*, 1373–1382.

Centers for Disease Control and Prevention. (2013). *Listeria (Listeriosis).* Available at http://www.cdc.gov/listeria/risk.html. Accessed on 4/4/16.

Centers for Disease Control and Prevention. (2014a). *Breastfeeding report card—United States, 2014.* Available at http://www.cdc.gov/breastfeeding/pdf/2014breastfeedingreportcard.pdf. Accessed 4/5/16.

Centers for Disease Control and Prevention. (2014b). *National Diabetes Statistics Report: Estimates of diabetes and its burden in the United States.* Available at http://www.cdc.gov/diabetes/pubs/statsreport14/national-diabetes-report-web.pdf. Accessed on 4/4/16.

Centers for Disease Control and Prevention. (2014c). *Preconception care and health care. Health promotion.* Available at http://www.cdc.gov/preconception/careforwomen/promotion.html. Accessed on 4/2/16.

Chiang, J., Kirkman, M., Laffel, L., & Peters, A. L. (2014). Type 1 diabetes through the life span: A position statement of the American Diabetes Association. *Diabetes Care, 37*, 2034–2054.

Crozier, S., Inskip, H., Godfrey, K., Cooper, C., Harvey, N. C., Cole, Z. A., & Robinson, S. M. (2010). Weight gain in pregnancy and childhood body composition: Findings from the Southampton Women's Survey. *American Journal of Clinical Nutrition, 91*, 1745–1751.

Davenport, M., Ruchat, S., Giroux, I., Sopper, M., & Mottola, F. (2013). Timing of excessive pregnancy-related weight gain and offspring adiposity at birth. *Obstetrics and Gynecology, 122*, 255–261.

Davis, R., Hofferth, S., & Shenassa, E. (2014). Gestational weight gain and risk of infant death in the United States. *American Journal of Public Health, 104*, S90–S95.

Endeshaw, M., Ambaw, F., Aragaw, A., & Ayalew, A. (2014). Effect of maternal nutrition and dietary habits on preeclampsia: A case-control study. *International Journal of Clinical Medicine, 5*, 1405–1416. doi:10.4236/ijcm.2014.521179

Ensenauer, R., Chmitorz, A., Riedel, C., Fenske, N., Hauner, H., Nennstiel-Ratzel, U., & von Kries, R. (2013). Effects of suboptimal or excessive gestational weight gain on childhood overweight and abdominal adiposity: Results for a retrospective cohort study. *International Journal of Obesity, 37*, 505–512. doi:10.1038/ijo.2012.226

Fawcett, E., Fawcett, J., & Mazmanian, D. (2016). A meta-analysis of the worldwide prevalence of pica during pregnancy and the postpartum period. *International Journal of Gynecology and Obstetrics, 133*, 277–283.

Feig, D., Shah, B., Lipscombe, L., Wu, C. F., Ray, J. G., Lowe, J., . . . Booth, G. L. (2013). Preeclampsia as a risk factor for diabetes: A population-based cohort study. *PLoS Medicine, 10*, e1001425.

Fraser, A., Tilling, K., Macdonald-Wallis, C., Hughes, R., Sattar, N., Nelson, S. M., & Lawlor, D. A. (2011). Associations of gestational weight gain with maternal body mass index, waist circumference, and blood pressure measured 16 y after pregnancy: The Avon Longitudinal Study of Parents and Children (ALSPAC). *The American Journal of Clinical Nutrition, 93*, 1285–1291.

Grieger, J., Grzeskowiak, L., & Clifton, V. (2014). Preconception dietary patterns in human pregnancies are associated with preterm delivery. *The Journal of Nutrition*, 1075–1080.

Guelinckx, I., Devlieger, R., Beckers, K., & Vansant, G. (2008). Maternal obesity: Pregnancy complications, gestational weight gain and nutrition. *Obesity Reviews, 9*, 140–150.

Hartling, L., Dryden, D., Guthrie, A., Muise, M., Vandermeer, B., & Donovan, L. (2013). Benefits and harms of treating gestational diabetes mellitus: A systematic review and meta-analysis for the U.S. Preventive Services Task Force and the National Institutes of Health Office of Medical Applications of Research. *Annals of Internal Medicine, 159*(2), 123–129.

Herring, S., Rose, M., Skouteris, H., & Oken, E. (2012). Optimizing weight gain in pregnancy to prevent obesity in women and children. *Diabetes, Obesity, & Metabolism, 14*, 195–203.

Hofmeyr, G., Lawrie, T., Atallah, A., & Duley, L. (2010). Calcium supplementation during pregnancy for preventing hypertensive disorders and related problems. *Cochrane Database of Systematic Reviews, (8)*, CD001059.

Hoyt, A., Browne, M., Richardson, S., Romitti, P., & Druschel, C. (2014). Maternal caffeine consumption and small for gestational age births: Results from a population-based case-control study. *Maternal and Child Health Journal, 18*, 1540–1551.

Inskip, H., Crozier, S., Godfrey, K., Borland, S., & Robinson, S. (2009). Women's compliance with nutrition and lifestyle recommendations before pregnancy: General population cohort study. *BMJ, 338*, b481. doi:10.1136/bmj.b481

Institute of Medicine. (1998). *Dietary reference intakes for thiamin, riboflavin, niacin, vitamin B_6, folate, vitamin B_{12}, pantothenic acid, biotin, and choline.* Washington, DC: The National Academies Press.

Institute of Medicine. (2005). *Dietary reference intakes for energy, carbohydrates, fiber, fat, fatty acids, cholesterol, protein, and amino acids (macronutrients).* Washington, DC: The National Academies Press.

Institute of Medicine. (2009). *Weight gain during pregnancy: Reexamining the guidelines.* Washington, DC: The National Academies Press.

Johnson, J., Clifton, R. G., Roberts, J. M., Myatt, L., Hauth, J. C., Spong, C. Y., . . . Sorokin, Y. (2013). Pregnancy outcomes with weight gain above or below the 2009 Institute of Medicine guidelines. *Obstetrics and Gynecology, 121*, 969–975. doi:10.1097/aog.0b013e31828aea03

Kaiser, L., & Campbell, C. (2014). *Practice paper of the Academy of Nutrition and Dietetics: Nutrition and lifestyle for a healthy pregnancy outcome.* Available at http://www.eatrightpro.org/resource/practice/position-and-practice-papers/practice-papers/practice-paper-nutrition-and-lifestyle-for-a-healthy-pregnancy-outcome. Accessed on 9/20/16.

Kim, S., Sharma, A., Sappenfield, W., Wilson, H., & Salihu, H. (2014). Association of maternal body mass index, excessive weight gain, and gestation diabetes mellitus with large-for-gestational-age births. *Obstetrics and Gynecology, 12*, 737–744.

Kirkegaard, H., Stovring, H., Rasmussen, K., Abrams, B., Sørensen, T. I., & Nohr, E. A. (2014). How do pregnancy-related weight changes and breastfeeding relate to maternal weight and BMI-adjusted waist circumference 7 y after deliver? Results from a path analysis. *The American Journal of Clinical Nutrition, 99*, 312–319.

Lessen, R., & Kavanagh, K. (2015). Position of the Academy of Nutrition and Dietetics: Promoting and supporting breastfeeding. *Journal of the Academy of Nutrition and Dietetics, 115*, 444–449.

Li, N., Liu, E., Guo, J., Pan, L., Li, B., Wang, P., . . . Hu, G. (2013). Maternal prepregnancy body mass index and gestation weight gain on pregnancy outcomes. *PLos One, 8*(12), e82310. doi:10.1371/journal.pone.0082310

Lim, S., O'Reilly, S., Behrens, H., Skinner, T., Ellis, I., & Dunbar, J. (2015). Effective strategies for weight loss in post-partum women: A systematic review and meta-analysis. *Obesity Reviews, 16*, 972–987.

Lo, J., Mission, J., & Caughey, A. (2013). Hypertensive disease of pregnancy and maternal mortality. *Current Opinion in Obstetrics & Gynecology, 25*, 124–132.

Martin, J., Hure, A., Macdonald-Wicks, L., Smith, R., & Collins, C. (2014). Predictors of post-partum weight retention in a prospective longitudinal study. *Maternal & Child Nutrition, 10*, 496–509.

Miao, D., Young, S., & Golden, C. (2015). A meta-analysis of pica and micronutrient status. *American Journal of Human Biology, 27*, 84–93.

Mulder, K., King, J., & Innis, S. M. (2014). Omega-3 fatty acid deficiency in infants before birth identified using a randomized trial of maternal DHA supplementation in pregnancy. *PloS One, 9*(1), e83764.

Nehring, I., Schmoll, S., Beyerlein, A., Hauner, H., & von Kries, R. (2011). Gestational weight gain and long-term postpartum weight retention: A meta-analysis. *The American Journal of Clinical Nutrition, 94*, 1225–1231.

Oken, E., & Gillman, M. W. (2003). Fetal origins of obesity. *Obesity Research, 1*, 496–506.

Peña-Rosas, J., De-Regil, L., Dowswell, T., & Viteri, F. (2012). Daily oral iron supplementation during pregnancy. *Cochrane Database of Systematic Reviews*, (11), CD009997. doi:10.1002/14651858.CD009997.pub4

Peña-Rosas, J., & Viteri, F. (2009). Effects and safety of preventive oral iron or iron+folic acid supplementation for women during pregnancy. *Cochrane Database of Systematic Reviews*, (4), CD004736.

Pereira, M., Rifas-Shiman, S., Kleinman, K., Rich-Edwards, J. W., Peterson, K. E., & Gillman, M. W. (2007). Predictors of change in physical activity during and after pregnancy: Project Viva. *American Journal of Preventive Medicine, 32*, 312–319.

Procter, S., & Campbell, C. (2014). Position of the Academy of Nutrition and Dietetics: Nutrition and lifestyle for a healthy pregnancy outcome. *Journal of the Academy of Nutrition and Dietetics, 114*, 1099–1103.

Rasmussen, K., Abrams, B., Bodnar, L., Butte, N., Catalano, P., & Siega-Riz, M. (2010). Recommendations for weight gain during pregnancy in the context of the obesity epidemic. *Obstetrics and Gynecology, 116*, 1191–1195.

Robbins, C., Zapata, L., Farr, S., Kroelinger, C. D., Morrow, B., & Ahluwalia, I. (2014). Core state preconception health indicators—pregnancy risk assessment monitoring system and behavioral risk factor surveillance system, 2009. *MMWR Surveillance Summaries, 63*, 1–62.

Rossi, A. (2011). Prevention of preeclampsia with low-dose aspirin or vitamins A and C in women at high or low risk: A systematic review with meta-analysis. *European Journal of Obstetrics, Gynecology, and Reproductive Biology, 158*, 9–16.

Schummers, L., Hutcheon, J., Bodnar, L., Lieberman, E., & Himes, K. (2015). Risk of adverse pregnancy outcomes by prepregnancy body mass index: A population-based study to inform prepregnancy weight low counseling. *Obstetrics and Gynecology, 125*, 133–143.

Siega-Riz, A., Viswanathan, M., Moos, J., Dierlein, A., Mumford, S., Knaack, J., . . . Lohr, K. N. (2009). A systematic review of outcomes of maternal weight gain according to the Institute of Medicine recommendations: birthweight, fetal growth, and postpartum weight retention. *American Journal of Obstetrics and Gynecology, 201*, 339, e1–e14.

Stang, J., & Huffman, L. (2016). Position of the Academy of Nutrition and Dietetics: Obesity, reproduction, and pregnancy outcomes. *Journal of the Academy of Nutrition and Dietetics, 116*, 677–691.

Stotland, N., Haas, J., Brawarsky, P., Jackson, R., Fuentes-Afflick, E., & Escobar, G. J. (2005). Body mass index, provider advice, and target gestational weight gain. *Obstetrics and Gynecology, 105*, 633–638.

Strain, J., Davidson, P., Thurston, W., Harrington, D., Mulhern, M., McAfee, A., . . . Myers, G. (2012). Maternal PUFA status but not prenatal methylmercury exposure is associated with children's language functions at age 5 years in the Seychelles. *The Journal of Nutrition, 142*, 1943–1949.

Streuling, I., Beyerlein, A., Rosenfeld, E., Schukat, B., & von Kries, R. (2011). Weight gain and dietary intake during pregnancy in industrialized countries—a systematic review of observational studies. *Journal of Perinatal Medicine, 39*, 123–129.

Tie, H. T., Xia, Y. Y., Zeng, Y. S., Zhang, Y., Dai, C. L., Guo, J. J., & Zhao, Y. (2014). Risk of childhood overweight or obesity associated with excessive weight gain during pregnancy: A meta-analysis. *Archives of Gynecology and Obstetrics, 289*, 247–257. doi:10.1007/s00404-013-3053-z

Tobias, D., Zhang, C., Chavarro, J., Bowers, K., Rich-Edwards, J., Rosner, B. J., . . . Hu, F. B. (2012). Prepregnancy adherence to dietary patterns and lower risk of gestational diabetes. *The American Journal of Clinical Nutrition, 96*, 289–295.

Toit, G., Robers, G., Sayre, P., Bahnson, H., Radulovic, S., Santos, A. F., . . . Lack, G. (2015). Randomized trial of peanut consumption in infants at risk for peanut allergy. *The New England Journal of Medicine, 26*, 803–813.

U.S. Department of Health and Human Services & U.S. Department of Agriculture. (2015). *2015-2020 Dietary guidelines for Americans* (8th ed.). Available at http://health.gov/dietaryguidelines/2015/guidelines/. Accessed on 4/5/16.

U.S. Food and Drug Administration. (2016a). *Food safety for moms-to-be: While you're pregnant—Listeria.* Available at http://www.fda.gov/Food/FoodborneIllnessContaminants/PeopleAtRisk/ucm083320.htm. Accessed on 4/4/16.

U.S. Food and Drug Administration. (2016b). *Food safety for moms-to-be: While you're pregnant—toxoplasma.* Available at http://www.fda.gov/Food/FoodborneIllnessContaminants/PeopleAtRisk/ucm083327.htm. Accessed on 4/4/16.

U.S. Food and Drug Administration & Environmental Protection Agency. (2014). *Fish: What pregnant women and parents should know.* Available at http://www.fda.gov/downloads/Food/FoodborneIllness-Contaminants/Metals/UCM400358.pdf. Accessed on 4/10/16.

U.S. Preventive Services Task Force. (2009). *Final recommendation statement: Folic acid to prevent neural tube defects.* Available at http://www.uspreventiveservicestaskforce.org/Page/Document/RecommendationStatementFinal/folic-acid-to-prevent-neural-tube-defects-preventive-medication. Accessed on 4/3/16.

van Calcar, S., & Ney, D. (2012). Food products made with glycomacropeptide, a low-phenylalanine whey protein, provide a new alternative to amino acid-based medical foods for nutrition management of phenylketonuria. *Journal of the Academy of Nutrition and Dietetics, 112*, 1201–1210.

Walsh, J., & McAuliffe, F. (2012). Prediction and prevention of the macrosomic fetus. *European Journal of Obstetrics, Gynecology, and Reproductive Biology, 162*, 125–130.

World Health Organization. (2012). *Guideline: Daily iron and folic acid supplementation in pregnant women.* Geneva, Switzerland: World Health Organization. Available at http://apps.who.int/iris/bitstream/10665/77770/1/9789241501996_eng.pdf. Accessed on 4/3/16.

World Health Organization. (2016). *Infant and young child feeding.* Available at http://www.who.int/mediacentre/factsheets/fs342/en/. Accessed on 4/5/16.

Yu, Z., Han, S., Zhu, J., Sun, X., Ji, C., & Gio, X. (2013). Pre-pregnancy body mass index in relation to infant birth weight and offspring overweight/obesity: A systematic review and meta-analysis. *PLoS One, 8*, e61627. doi:10.137l/journal.pone.0061627

Zhou, S., Yelland, L., McPhee, A., Quinlivan, J., Gibson, R., & Makrides, M. (2012). Fish-oil supplementation in pregnancy does not reduce the risk of gestational diabetes or preeclampsia. *American Journal of Clinical Nutrition, 95*, 1378–1384.

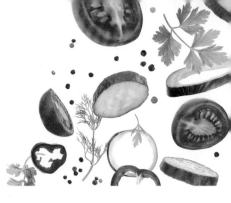

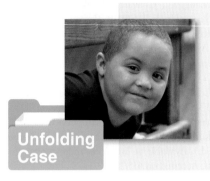

Luis Guzman

Luis is a 7-year-old boy who is 48 in tall and weighs 90 pounds. He is the only child of a single mother who worries that his weight is out of control. She admits she lets him eat whatever he wants, even though she knows he is eating inappropriately. His grandmother is his primary caregiver before school starts, and when school is not in session, and she also gives him whatever he wants, including fast food twice a week.

Check Your Knowledge

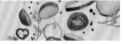

True	False		
☐	☐	**1**	Infants have higher requirements per kilogram of body weight for calories and most nutrients than adults do.
☐	☐	**2**	If breastfeeding is discontinued before the infant's first birthday, iron-fortified infant formula should be given until 12 months of age.
☐	☐	**3**	Protein is the nutrient most needed when solids are introduced into the diet.
☐	☐	**4**	Iron-fortified infant cereal should be the first solid introduced.
☐	☐	**5**	Peanut products should not be introduced in the diet until after the age of 12 months to reduce the risk of allergy.
☐	☐	**6**	The *2015-2020 Dietary Guidelines for Americans* do not apply to children, only adolescents and adults.
☐	☐	**7**	Iron deficiency in young children may be related to drinking too much milk.
☐	☐	**8**	Children who regularly skip breakfast have lower intakes of vitamins and minerals than children who normally eat breakfast.
☐	☐	**9**	Overweight and obese youth are at risk for the same complications from overweight that afflict adults—namely, type 2 diabetes, high blood pressure, and metabolic syndrome.
☐	☐	**10**	Like adults, children and adolescents underconsume potassium, vitamin D, calcium, and fiber because they do not eat enough fruits, vegetables, dairy, and whole grains.

Learning Objectives

Upon completion of this chapter, you will be able to

1 Compare breastfeeding to formula feeding.
2 Describe the process of introducing solid foods into the diet.
3 List eating behaviors of young children that may indicate nutrition risk.

4 Identify nutrients most likely to be under consumed by children and adolescents and the food groups that supply those nutrients.
5 Explain potential health risks of a poor quality eating pattern during childhood and adolescence.
6 Give examples of obesity prevention strategies for children and adolescents aimed at improving eating patterns, decreasing sedentary behaviors, increasing physical activity, and ensuring adequate sleep.
7 Evaluate an eating pattern based on MyPlate food intake recommendations.

The goals of nutrition and physical activity for children are to promote optimal physical and cognitive development, a healthy weight, an enjoyment of food, and a decreased risk of chronic disease (Ogata & Hayes, 2014). Actual nutrient requirements vary according to health status, activity pattern, and growth rate. The greater the rate of growth, the more intense the nutritional needs. Meeting needs is essential; also important is avoiding nutrient and calorie excesses.

The health trends of American children are mixed. Although deficiency diseases are rare and infant mortality has declined over recent decades, the prevalence of overweight and obesity are a public health concern. Today, nearly 1 out of 3 American children are overweight or obese, placing them at risk for chronic diseases that were once only diagnosed in adults, such as coronary artery disease, type 2 diabetes, hypertension, metabolic syndrome, and sleep apnea. Today's children may experience shorter life expectancies related to young onset obesity.

This chapter presents nutrition from birth through adolescence, including calorie and nutrient needs and eating practices. Nutrition concerns during childhood—namely, poor diet quality and overweight and obesity—are discussed.

INFANCY (BIRTH TO 1 YEAR)

Excluding fetal growth, growth in the first year of life is more rapid than at any other time in the life cycle. Birth weight doubles by 4 to 6 months of age and triples by the first birthday. Length increases by approximately 10 in during the first year. From birth through 23 months of age, size and growth rate are monitored by tracking weight-for-length and weight-for-age on World Health Organization growth charts (www.cdc.gov/growthcharts/who_charts.htm#). Adequate calories and nutrients are needed to support the unprecedented rate of growth.

Human milk has been the gold standard for estimating the nutritional needs of an infant even though the content is variable and the volume breastfed infants consume is impossible to measure (Stam, Sauer, & Boehm, 2013). Still, recommendations for the amount of calories, macronutrients, vitamins, and minerals infants should consume are based on the estimated average intakes of healthy full-term newborns who are exclusively breastfed by well-nourished mothers. Although the total amount of calories and nutrients are generally far less than what adults need, the infant's needs are much higher per kilogram of body weight. Proportionately, infants use large amounts of energy and nutrients to fuel their body processes and growth.

Because infants are born with low amounts of vitamin K stored in the body and a decreased ability to utilize vitamin K, infants are given a single intramuscular dose of vitamin K at birth to protect them from hemorrhagic disease of the newborn.

Breast Milk

Breast milk is specifically designed to support optimal growth and development in the newborn, and its composition makes it uniquely superior for infant feeding (Box 12.1) (American Academy of Pediatrics [AAP], 2012a). Breastfeeding is credited with numerous potential health benefits for the infant, including lower risks of otitis media, upper respiratory tract infection, lower respiratory tract infection, asthma, atopic dermatitis, gastroenteritis, obesity, celiac disease, type 1 and type 2 diabetes, certain types of leukemia, and sudden infant death syndrome (AAP, 2012a). Although many of these benefits are linked to breastfeeding for 3 months or more, some benefits occur with any duration of breastfeeding, such as the reduced risk of obesity and type 2 diabetes.

BOX 12.1   Composition of Breast Milk

- The protein content of breast milk is adequate to support growth and development without contributing to an excessive renal solute load.
- The majority of the protein is easy-to-digest whey.
- Breast milk contains small amounts of amino acids that may be harmful in large amounts (e.g., phenylalanine) and high levels of amino acids that infants cannot synthesize well (e.g., taurine).
- The fat in breast milk is easily digested because of fat-digesting enzymes contained in the milk.
- The content of linoleic acid (an essential fatty acid) is high.
- The high level of cholesterol is believed to help infants develop enzyme systems capable of handling cholesterol later in life.
- Breast milk contains amylase (a starch-digesting enzyme), which may promote starch digestion in early infancy when pancreatic amylase is low or absent.

- Breast milk contains enough minerals to support adequate growth and development but not excessive amounts that would burden immature kidneys with a high renal solute load.
- The minerals are mostly protein bound and balanced to enhance bioavailability. For instance, the rate of iron absorption from breast milk is approximately 50% compared with about 4% for iron-fortified formulas. Zinc absorption is better from breast milk than from either cow's milk or formula.
- All vitamins needed for growth and health are supplied in breast milk, but the vitamin content of breast milk varies with the mother's diet.
- The renal solute load of breast milk is suited to the immature kidneys' inability to concentrate urine.
- Although they are more abundant in colostrum, antibodies and anti-infective factors are present in mature breast milk. Bifidus factor promotes the growth of normal gastrointestinal (GI) flora (e.g., *Lactobacillus bifidus*) that protect the infant against harmful GI bacteria.

The AAP contends that because of the short- and long-term medical and neurodevelopmental benefits of breastfeeding, infant nutrition should be considered a public health issue and not simply a lifestyle choice (AAP, 2012a).

The AAP (2014) recommends exclusive breastfeeding for the first 6 months of life, which, with one exception, is considered a complete source of nutrition adequate to meet the needs of healthy, full-term infants. The exception is vitamin D, which is given in supplemental form until the age of 1 year or until the infant consumes 1 quart of vitamin D–fortified formula per day. Even after solid foods are introduced, breastfeeding should continue for at least the first 12 months of age. What the breastfeeding mother needs to know appears in Box 12.2.

The AAP (2014) also recommends breastfeeding for preterm infants, with the stipulation that infants who weigh less than 1500 g at birth receive human milk that is fortified with protein, minerals, and vitamins to ensure optimal nutrient intake.

BOX 12.2   Teaching Points for Breastfeeding

- The infant should be allowed to nurse for 5 minutes on each breast on the first day to achieve letdown and milk ejection. By the end of the first week, the infant should be nursing up to 15 minutes per breast.
- In the first few weeks of breastfeeding, the infant may nurse 8 to 12 times every 24 hours. Mothers should offer the breast whenever the infant shows early signs of hunger, such as increased alertness, physical activity, mouthing, or rooting. After breastfeeding is well established, eight feedings every 24 hours may be appropriate.
- The first breast offered should be alternated with every feeding so both breasts receive equal stimulation and draining.
- Even though the infant will be able to virtually empty the breast within 5 to 10 minutes once the milk supply is established, the infant needs to nurse beyond that point to satisfy the need to suck and to receive emotional and physical comfort.

- The supply of milk is equal to the demand—the more the infant sucks, the more milk is produced. Infants age 6 weeks or 12 weeks who suck more are probably experiencing a growth spurt and so need more milk.
- Water and juice are unnecessary for breastfed infants in the first 6 months of life, even in hot climates.
- Early substitution of formula or introduction of solid foods may decrease the chance of maintaining lactation.
- Infants weaned before 12 months of age should be given iron-fortified formula, not cow's milk.
- Both feeding the infant more frequently and manually expressing milk will help to increase the milk supply.
- Breast milk can be pumped, placed in a sanitary bottle, and immediately refrigerated or frozen for later use. Milk should be used within 24 hours if refrigerated or within 3 months if stored in the freezer compartment of the refrigerator.

Infant Formula

Infant formulas may be used in place of breastfeeding, as an occasional supplement to breastfeeding, or when exclusively breastfed infants are weaned before 12 months of age. The Infant Formula Act regulates the levels of nutrients in formulas, specifying both minimum and maximum amounts of each essential nutrient. Almost all formula used in the United States is iron fortified, a practice that has greatly reduced the risk of iron deficiency in older infants. Because the minimum recommended amount of each nutrient is more than the amount provided in breast milk, nutrient supplements are unnecessary for the first 6 months of life.

Categories of Formula

Box 12.3 features the categories of formulas for full-term and preterm infants. Full-term infant categories include "routine" cow's milk protein based, soy protein based, hydrolyzed formulas for infants with cow's milk protein allergy, and specialized formulas for infants with metabolic disorders. Within each of those categories there are a variety of formulas to choose. Currently, infant formula companies in the United States market directly to consumers and regularly release new formulas with or without slightly different compositions on a regular basis (Abrams, 2015). For instance, lutein (a phytonutrient) is not an essential nutrient and is therefore not required in

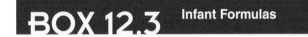

BOX 12.3 Infant Formulas

Full-Term Formulas

Milk based (e.g., Similac Advance or Enfamil Infant)

- For routine use; account for 80% of formula sold in the United States

Soy based (e.g., Isomil, ProSobee)

- For infants with galactosemia; lactase deficiency; allergy to cow's milk protein but not soy; vegan parents

Hydrolyzed

- Vary from partially hydrolyzed (e.g., Carnation Good Start) to extensively hydrolyzed (e.g., Alimentum or Nutramigen) depending on the how small the protein molecules are broken down
- Only extensively hydrolyzed formulas are hypoallergenic and suitable for infants with or at high risk of cow's milk protein allergy

Specialized

- For infants with inborn errors of metabolism, such as phenylketonuria (e.g., Phenyl-Free) or maple syrup urine disease (e.g., BCAD 1)
- Are intentionally lacking or deficient in one or more nutrients, so they do not supply adequate nutrition for normal infants
- Must be supplemented with small amounts of regular formula

For Infants Born Before Term

Preterm formulas (e.g., Enfamil Premature High Protein 24)

- For infants born before 34 weeks of gestation
- Designed to promote "catch-up" growth so are higher in calories, protein, calcium, magnesium, and phosphorus than routine formulas

Enriched formula (e.g., Enfamil EnfaCare, Similac NeoSure)

- For infants 34 to 36 weeks of gestation
- Provide more calories than term formula but less than preterm formula

Table 12.1   General Parameters for Formula Feeding

Age	Number of Feedings in 24 Hours	Amount per Feeding (oz)
1 month	6–8	2–4
2 months	5–6	5–6
3–5 months	4–5	6–7

formula, but a manufacturer is adding it to "support eye health." Other optional but increasingly common formula features include the following:

- The addition of docosahexaenoic acid (DHA) and arachidonic acid (ARA) to most formulas. Studies show these fatty acids promote eye and brain development.
- The addition of prebiotics and probiotics. Several studies suggest probiotics may benefit infants with diarrhea.
- Organic options
- Non-genetically modified organism (GMO) options

Surprisingly, the U.S. Food and Drug Administration (FDA) does not "approve" new formulas but rather reviews the proposed formula composition and background information provided by the formula manufacturer. The FDA is more empowered to evaluate safety than efficacy of infant formulas (Abrams, 2015).

Formula Feeding

The amount of formula provided per feeding and the frequency of feeding depend on the infant's age and individual needs. General parameters are provided in Table 12.1. Overfeeding is one of the biggest hazards of formula feeding. Caregivers should recognize that infants cry for reasons other than hunger and should not be fed every time they cry, nor should an infant be forced to finish his or her bottle. Feedings should always be supervised; bottles should never be propped for independent feeding. Nor should infant cereals be added to a bottle. To avoid nursing bottle caries, infants and children should not be put to bed with a bottle of formula, milk, juice, or other sweetened liquid (Fig. 12.1). Teaching points for formula feeding are summarized in Box 12.4.

Complementary Foods: Introducing Solids

The introduction of solids is dependent on the infant's developmental readiness and nutrient needs.

Developmental Readiness

Developmentally, most infants exhibit readiness to spoon-feed around 4 to 6 months of age as reflexes disappear, head control develops, and the infant is able to sit. Over time, control of the

Figure 12.1 ▶

Nursing bottle caries. Notice the extensive decay in the upper teeth. *(© K. L. Boyd, DDS/Custom Medical Stock Photo.)*

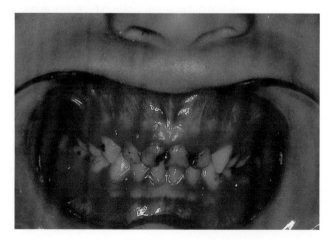

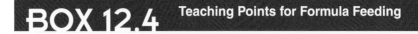

BOX 12.4 Teaching Points for Formula Feeding

- Never force the infant to finish a bottle or to take more than he or she wants.
- Signs that an infant is finished include biting the nipple, puckering the face, and turning away from the bottle.
- Discourage the misconception that "a fat baby = a healthy baby = good parents."
- Each feeding should last 20 to 30 minutes.
- Formula may be given at room temperature, slightly warmed, or directly from the refrigerator; however, always give formula at approximately the same temperature.
- Spitting up of a small amount of formula during or after a feeding is normal. Feed the infant more slowly and burp more frequently to help alleviate spitting up.
- Hold the infant closely and securely. Position the infant so that the head is higher than the rest of the body.
- Avoid jiggling the bottle and making extra movements that could distract the infant from feeding.
- Check the flow of formula by holding the bottle upside down. A steady drip from the nipple should be observed. If the flow is too rapid because of a too large nipple opening, the infant may overfeed and develop indigestion. If the flow rate is too slow because of a too small nipple opening, the infant may tire and fall asleep without taking enough formula. Discard any nipples with holes that are too large, and enlarge holes that are too small with a sterilized needle.
- Reassure caregivers that there is no danger of "spoiling" an infant by feeding him or her when the infant cries for a feeding.
- Burp the infant halfway through the feeding, at the end of the feeding, and more often if necessary to help get rid of air swallowed during feeding. Burping can be accomplished by gently rubbing or patting the infant's back as he or she is held on the shoulder, lies on his or her stomach over the caregiver's lap, or sits in an upright position.
- After the teeth erupt, the baby should be given only plain water for a bedtime bottle-feeding. Never prop the bottle or put the infant to bed with a bottle.

head, neck, jaw, and tongue; hand–eye coordination; and the ability to sit, grasp, chew, drink, and self-feed evolve. The eruption of teeth indicates readiness to progress from strained to mashed to chopped fine to regular consistency foods. Guidelines for introducing solids on the basis of developmental readiness appear in Table 12.2.

Nutrient Needs

Around 4 to 6 months of age, breast milk or formulas are not adequate as the sole source of nutrition and complementary foods become necessary, particularly for iron. Some experts recommend baby food meat as one of the first complementary foods because it provides iron and zinc, another important nutrient (AAP, 2012b). Traditionally, iron-fortified single-grain infant cereal has been the first solid food introduced, but there is no evidence to support any particular order for introducing solids. Formula-fed infants continue to need iron-fortified formula. The other nutrient of concern is fluoride. At 6 months of age, exclusively breastfed infants and infants who receive ready-to-use infant formula need supplemental fluoride. Infants who receive formula that has been prepared with local water need supplemental fluoride only if the water contains less than 0.3 ppm of fluoride.

Initiating Feeding

To increase the likelihood of acceptance, parents are urged to give a small amount of formula or breast milk to take the edge off hunger before introducing the first solid. After the infant learns to accept the first solid food, new foods are introduced in plain and simple form one at a time for a period of at least 2 to 3 days so that allergic reactions, such as rashes, vomiting, or diarrhea, can be identified. After tolerance is established, another new food is added. Within a few months, the infant is eating texture-appropriate meats, cereal, fruits, and vegetables in addition to breast milk and/or formula. The notion that infants who are fed fruits before vegetables will develop a preference for sweets and reject vegetables is not supported by evidence.

Table 12.2	Sequence of Infant Development and Feeding Skills in Normal, Healthy, Full-Term Infants*		
Developmental Skills			
Baby's Approximate Age	**Mouth Patterns**	**Hand and Body Skills**	**Feeding Skills or Abilities**
Birth through 5 months	• Suck/swallow reflex • Tongue thrust reflex • Rooting reflex • Gag reflex	• Poor control of head, neck, trunk • Brings hands to mouth around 3 months	• Swallows liquids but pushes most solid objects from the mouth
4 months through 6 months	• Draws in upper or lower lip as spoon is removed from mouth • Up-and-down munching movement • Can transfer food from front to back of tongue to swallow • Tongue thrust and rooting reflexes begin to disappear • Gag reflex diminishes • Opens mouth when sees spoon approaching	• Sits with support • Good head control • Uses whole hand to grasp objects (palmar grasp)	• Takes in a spoonful of pureed or strained food and swallows it without choking • Drinks small amounts from cup when held by another person, with spilling
5 months through 9 months	• Begins to control the position of food in the mouth • Up-and-down munching movement • Positions food between jaws for chewing	• Begins to sit alone unsupported • Follows food with eyes • Begins to use thumb and index finger to pick up objects (pincer grasp)	• Begins to eat mashed foods • Eats from a spoon easily • Drinks from a cup with some spilling • Begins to feed self with hands
8 months through 11 months	• Moves food from side-to-side in mouth • Begins to curve lips around rim of cup • Begins to chew in rotary pattern (diagonal movement of the jaw as food is moved to the side or center of the mouth)	• Sits alone easily • Transfers objects from hand to mouth	• Begins to eat ground or finely chopped food and small pieces of soft food • Begins to experiment with spoon but prefers to feed self with hands • Drinks from a cup with less spilling
10 months through 12 months	• Rotary chewing (diagonal movement of the jaw as food is moved to the side or center of the mouth)	• Begins to put spoon in mouth • Begins to hold cup • Good eye-hand-mouth coordination	• Eats chopped food and small pieces of soft, cooked table food • Begins self-spoon feeding with help

*Developmental stages may vary with individual babies.
Source: U.S. Department of Agriculture, Food and Nutrition Service. (2016). *Feeding infants: A guide for use in the child nutrition programs.* Available at http://www.fns .usda.gov/sites/default/files/feeding_infants.pdf. Accessed 4/18/16.

Choice of Foods

Like a healthy eating pattern for adults, infants should consume foods that provide variety, balance, and moderation with the following considerations:

- Fat intake should not be restricted because infants and young children need proportionately more fat than older children and adults.
- Fruit juice can contribute to excessive calorie intake and displace the intake of more nutrient-dense foods. The AAP recommends fruit juice not be given to infants younger than 6 months of (AAP, 2015a). If it is given to infants between 6 and 12 months, the juice should be served in a cup, not a bottle.
- Foods should be cooked without added salt or seasonings.
- Foods that may cause choking in infants and small children are avoided (Box 12.5).
- Empty calorie foods should not be given. The high nutritional requirements for healthy growth and development leave little room for foods with low nutritional value (May & Dietz, 2010).
- Because honey may contain botulism spores, infants under the age of 1 year should not have honey in any form, cooked or raw.

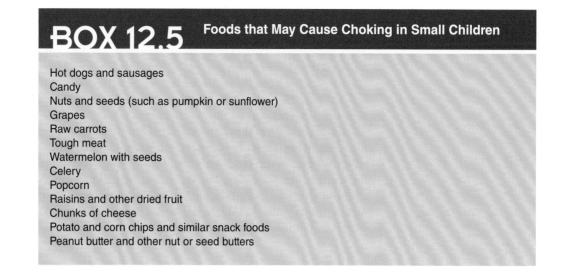

BOX 12.5   Foods that May Cause Choking in Small Children

Hot dogs and sausages
Candy
Nuts and seeds (such as pumpkin or sunflower)
Grapes
Raw carrots
Tough meat
Watermelon with seeds
Celery
Popcorn
Raisins and other dried fruit
Chunks of cheese
Potato and corn chips and similar snack foods
Peanut butter and other nut or seed butters

Food Allergies

Many pediatricians recommend against introducing eggs and fish before the age of 12 months, but there is no evidence that introducing these foods after 4 to 6 months affects the risk of allergy (AAP, 2012b). Similarly, the AAP advises health-care providers to recommend introducing peanut-containing products into the diets of high-risk infants between 4 and 11 months of age based on evidence that shows early introduction of peanuts into the diet of infants at high risk of peanut allergy can play a role in preventing peanut allergies (AAP, 2015b).

Food Amounts

Infants differ in the amount of food they want or need at each feeding. The amount of solid food taken at a feeding may vary from 1 to 2 tsp initially to ¼ to ½ cup as the infant gets older. To avoid overfeeding, infants and children should be allowed to self-regulate the amount of food consumed.

Tips for creating a positive eating environment are listed in Box 12.6.

BOX 12.6   Tips to Create a Positive Eating Environment

- Eat with the child. Be a role model.
- Eat at regular times. Offer three meals and up to three snacks at regular times each day.
- Prepare one meal for the whole family.
- Keep in mind that it is not important if a child refuses to eat a particular food (e.g., spinach), so long as the child has a reasonable intake from each major food group.
- Offer a variety of foods, not just the ones you like. Repeated exposures—up to 15 to 20 times—may be needed before a child accepts a new food.
- Fat and cholesterol should not be limited in the diets of very young children, who need fat and cholesterol for their developing brains and nervous systems.
- Never force a child to eat; if a healthy child is hungry, he or she will eat.
- Do not use food to reward, punish, bribe, or convey love.
- Let toddlers explore and enjoy food, even if it means eating with their fingers.
- Space meals further apart and limit snacking so the child will be hungry at mealtimes.
- Keep mealtime relaxed, pleasant, and unhurried, allowing 20 to 30 minutes per meal. After 30 minutes, put the food away and let the child leave the table.
- Children may refuse to eat because they are (1) too excited or distracted, (2) seeking attention, (3) expressing independence, (4) too tired, or (5) simply not hungry. When any of these instances occur, remove the child's plate without comment. If the child wants a snack later, make it nutritious.

NUTRITION FOR TODDLERS AND PRESCHOOLERS

Typically, every year from age 1 year until puberty, children typically grow 2 to 3 in taller and 5 to 6 pounds heavier. Beginning at age 2 years, Centers for Disease Control and Prevention (CDC) growth charts are used to monitor size and growth patterns by plotting body mass index (BMI) for age (Figs. 12.2 and 12.3). Non-healthy weight status (Table 12.3) and deviations in a child's percentile channel warrant further attention.

Early parental influence is associated with the development of a child's relationship with food later in life (Ogata & Hayes, 2014). Young children are especially dependent on parents and caregivers as to which foods are available, the portion sizes offered, how often eating occurs, and the social context of eating. For instance, eating all food on the plate, dessert used as a reward, and eating regularly scheduled meals are behaviors young adults report their parents instilled in them during childhood (Vauthier, Lluch, Lecomte, Artur, & Herbeth, 1996). Parents who offer large food portions (especially of calorie-dense, sweet, or salty foods), pressure their child to eat or

Figure 12.2 ▶

Body mass index-for-age percentiles for boys.

(Source: Adapted from the Centers for Disease Control and Prevention [CDC] Growth Chart, New York State Department of Health.)

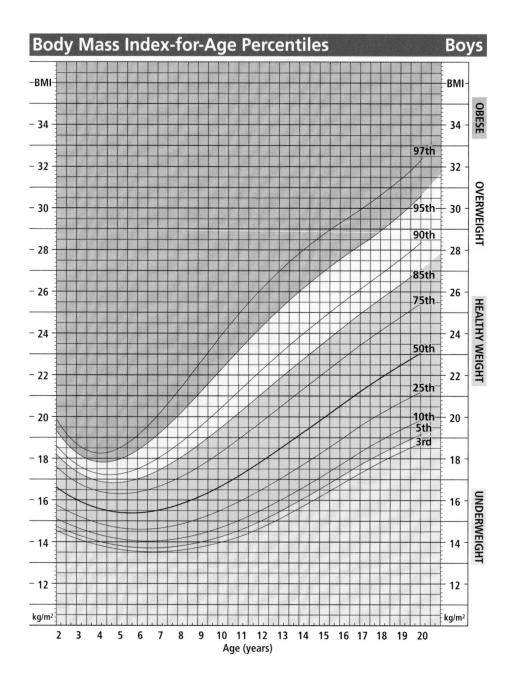

Figure 12.3 ▶

Body mass index-for-age percentiles for girls. *(Source: Adapted from the Centers for Disease Control and Prevention [CDC] Growth Chart, New York State Department of Health.)*

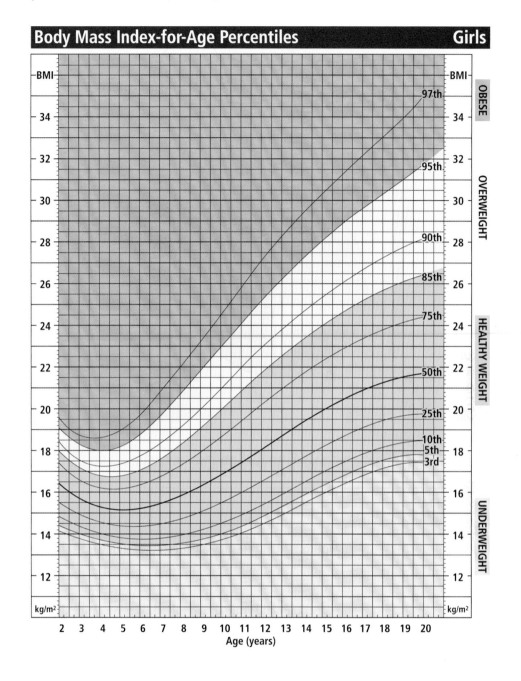

Table 12.3	Weight Status Based on Body Mass Index for Age Centers for Disease Control and Prevention Growth Charts

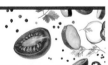

Weight Status Category	Percentile Range
Underweight	<5th percentile
Normal or healthy weight	5th percentile to <85th percentile
Overweight	85th percentile to <95th percentile
Obese	≥95th percentile

Source: Centers for Disease Control and Prevention. (2015). *BMI for children and teens*. Available at http://www.cdc.gov /obesity/childhood/defining.html. Accessed on 4/18/16.

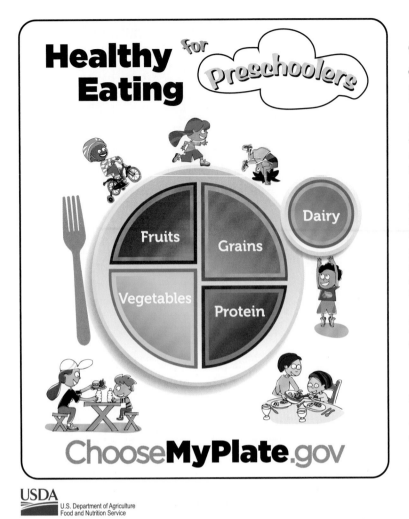

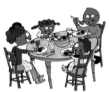

Get your child on the path to healthy eating.

Focus on the meal and each other.
Your child learns by watching you. Children are likely to copy your table manners, your likes and dislikes, and your willingness to try new foods.

Offer a variety of healthy foods.
Let your child choose how much to eat. Children are more likely to enjoy a food when eating it is their own choice.

Be patient with your child.
Sometimes new foods take time. Give children a taste at first and be patient with them. Offer new foods many times.

Let your children serve themselves.
Teach your children to take small amounts at first. Let them know they can get more if they are still hungry.

Cook together.
Eat together.
Talk together.
Make meal time family time.

USDA
U.S. Department of Agriculture
Food and Nutrition Service

FNS-451
October 2012
USDA is an equal opportunity provider and employer.

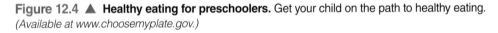

Figure 12.4 ▲ **Healthy eating for preschoolers.** Get your child on the path to healthy eating. *(Available at www.choosemyplate.gov.)*

restrict the child's eating, and model excessive eating undermine the child's ability to self-regulate food intake (Ogata & Hayes, 2014). Tips for getting children on the path to healthy eating appear in Figure 12.4.

Calories and Nutrients

There is very little research on the best ways to achieve optimal nutritional intakes from 1 to 2 years of age, the transition period between infancy and childhood. The dramatic decrease in growth rate is reflected in a disinterest in food, a "physiologic anorexia" due to lower calorie needs per kilogram of body weight.

At age 2 years, three meals a day with two to three snacks providing a total of 1000 calories is appropriate. Estimated calorie needs per day for males and females ages 3 to 18 years are illustrated in Figure 12.5.

The *Dietary Guidelines for Americans* are intended for all healthy Americans age 2 years and older; thus, the key recommendations for healthy eating remain consistent from early childhood throughout the lifespan (Box 12.7) (U.S. Department of Health and Human Services [USDHHS] & U.S. Department of Agriculture [USDA], 2015). By focusing on variety, nutrient density, and appropriate amounts recommended within the appropriate calorie level eating pattern, it is assumed nutrient needs will be met within calorie limits. Figure 12.6 also illustrates eating pattern recommendations for 2- to 5-year-olds, with ranges reflecting gender and activity variations. Figure 12.7 features sample 1000-calorie and 1600-calorie meal patterns.

Figure 12.5 ▶

Estimated calorie needs per day for males and females ages 3 to 18 years.

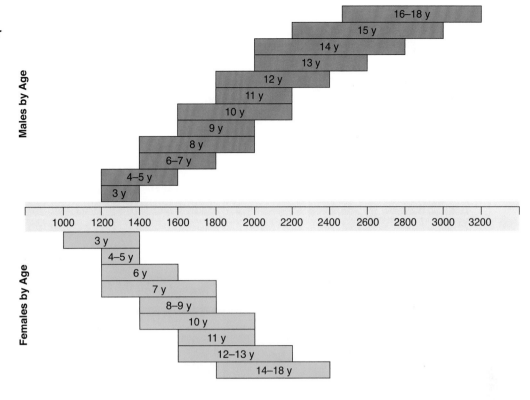

BOX 12.7

2015-2020 *Dietary Guidelines for Americans* Key Recommendations for Ages 2 Years and Older

Consume a healthy eating pattern that accounts for all foods and beverages within an appropriate calorie level.

A healthy eating pattern includes:

- A variety of vegetables from all of the subgroups—dark green, red and orange, legumes (beans and peas), starchy, and other
- Fruits, especially whole fruits
- Grains, at least half of which are whole grains
- Fat-free or low-fat dairy, including milk, yogurt, cheese, and/or fortified soy beverages
- A variety of protein foods, including seafood, lean meats and poultry, eggs, legumes (beans and peas), and nuts, seeds, and soy products
- Oils

A healthy eating pattern limits:

- Saturated fats and trans fats, added sugars, and sodium

Key recommendations that are quantitative are provided for several components of the diet that should be limited. These components are of particular public health concern in the United States, and the specified limits can help individuals achieve healthy eating patterns within calorie limits:

- Consume less than 10% of calories per day from added sugars
- Consume less than 10% of calories per day from saturated fats
- Consume less than 2300 mg/day of sodium

Source: U.S. Department of Health and Human Services & U.S. Department of Agriculture. *2015-2020 Dietary guidelines for Americans* (8th ed.). Available at http://health.gov/dietaryguidelines/2015/guidelines/. Accessed on 4/18/16.

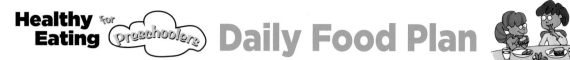

Healthy Eating for Preschoolers Daily Food Plan

Use this Plan as a general guide.

- These food plans are based on average needs. Do not be concerned if your child does not eat the exact amounts suggested. Your child may need more or less than average. For example, food needs increase during growth spurts.

- Children's appetites vary from day to day. Some days they may eat less than these amounts; other days they may want more. Offer these amounts and let your child decide how much to eat.

Food group	2 year olds	3 year olds	4 and 5 year olds	What counts as:
Fruits	1 cup	1 - 1½ cups	1 - 1½ cups	**½ cup of fruit?** ½ cup mashed, sliced, or chopped fruit ½ cup 100% fruit juice ½ medium banana 4-5 large strawberries
Vegetables	1 cup	1½ cups	1½ - 2 cups	**½ cup of veggies?** ½ cup mashed, sliced, or chopped vegetables 1 cup raw leafy greens ½ cup vegetable juice 1 small ear of corn
Grains Make half your grains whole	3 ounces	4 - 5 ounces	4 - 5 ounces	**1 ounce of grains?** 1 slice bread 1 cup ready-to-eat cereal flakes ½ cup cooked rice or pasta 1 tortilla (6" across)
Protein Foods	2 ounces	3 - 4 ounces	3 - 5 ounces	**1 ounce of protein foods?** 1 ounce cooked meat, poultry, or seafood 1 egg 1 Tablespoon peanut butter ¼ cup cooked beans or peas (kidney, pinto, lentils)
Dairy Choose low-fat or fat-free	2 cups	2 cups	2½ cups	**½ cup of dairy?** ½ cup milk 4 ounces yogurt ¾ ounce cheese 1 string cheese

Some foods are easy for your child to choke on while eating. Skip hard, small, whole foods, such as popcorn, nuts, seeds, and hard candy. Cut up foods such as hot dogs, grapes, and raw carrots into pieces smaller than the size of your child's throat—about the size of a nickel.

There are many ways to divide the Daily Food Plan into meals and snacks. View the "Meal and Snack Patterns and Ideas" to see how these amounts might look on your preschooler's plate at www.choosemyplate.gov/preschoolers.html.

Figure 12.6 ▲ **Healthy eating for preschoolers daily food plan.** *(Available at www .choosemyplate.gov.)*

Eating Practices

Parents and caregivers determine what food is served, when food is served, and where it is served. Children should be allowed to decide whether they eat and how much they eat. Although the food children need is the same as adults, the portion sizes are not. A rule-of-thumb guideline to determine age-appropriate serving sizes is to provide 1 tbsp of food per year of age (e.g., the serving size for a 3-year-old is 3 tbsp). By ages 4 to 6 years, recommended serving sizes are similar to those for adults. Eating behaviors in young children that warrant further investigation are listed in Box 12.8.

At age 1 year, the child should be drinking from a cup and eating many of the same foods as the rest of the family. Whole milk becomes a major source of nutrients, including fat; children between the ages of 1 and 2 years have a relatively higher need for fat to support rapid growth and development. However, milk intake should not exceed 2 to 3 cups per day because, in greater amounts, it may displace the intake of iron-rich foods from the diet and promote **milk anemia**. Gradual introduction of 2% milk occurs after age 2 years and eventually progresses to nonfat milk. However, when there is concern about the risk of obesity based on family history, low-fat milk beginning at 12 months of age may be appropriate (Daniels & Hassink, 2015).

New foods may take 15 to 20 exposures before they are accepted (Birch, 1999). Beginning around 15 months of age, a child may develop food jags as a normal expression of autonomy as the child develops a sense of independence. By the end of the second year, children can completely self-feed and can seek food independently.

Milk Anemia
an iron deficiency anemia related to excessive milk intake, which displaces the intake of iron-rich foods from the diet.

Meal and Snack Pattern

These patterns show one way a 1000 and 1600 calorie Daily Food Plan can be divided into meals and snacks for a preschooler. Sample food choices are shown for each meal or snack.

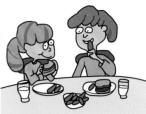

1000 Calorie Plan

Breakfast	
1 ounce grains 1/2 cup fruit 1/2 cup dairy*	Cereal and banana *1 cup crispy rice cereal* *1/2 cup sliced banana* *1/2 cup milk**

Morning Snack	
1/2 ounce grains 1/2 cup fruit	1/2 slice cinnamon bread 1/2 large orange

Lunch	
1 ounce grains 1/4 cup vegetables 1/2 cup dairy* 1 ounce protein foods	Open-faced chicken sandwich and salad *1 slice whole wheat bread* *1 slice American cheese** *1 ounce sliced chicken* *1/4 cup baby spinach (raw)* *2 Tbsp. grated carrots*

Afternoon Snack	
1/4 cup vegetables 1/2 cup dairy*	1/4 cup sugar snap peas 1/2 cup yogurt*

Dinner	
1/2 ounce grains 1/2 cup vegetables 1/2 cup dairy* 1 ounce protein foods	Chicken & potatoes *1 ounce chicken breast* *1/4 cup mashed potato* 1/4 cup green peas 1/2 small whole wheat roll 1/2 cup milk*

1600 Calorie Plan

Breakfast	
1 ounce grains 1/2 cup fruit 1/2 cup dairy*	Cereal and banana *1 cup crispy rice cereal* *1/2 cup sliced banana* 1/2 cup milk*

Morning Snack	
1 ounce grains 1/2 cup fruit 1 ounce protein foods	Egg sandwich *1 slice bread* *1 hard cooked egg* 1/2 large orange

Lunch	
1 ounce grains 1/2 cup vegetables 1/2 cup fruit 1/2 cup dairy* 1 ounce protein foods	Open-faced chicken sandwich and salad *1 slice whole wheat bread* *1 slice American cheese** *1 ounce sliced chicken* *1/2 cup baby spinach (raw)* *1/4 cup grated carrots* *1 small frozen banana*

Afternoon Snack	
1/2 cup vegetables 1/2 cup dairy*	1/2 cup sugar snap peas 1/2 cup yogurt*

Dinner	
2 ounce grains 1 cup vegetables 1 cup dairy* 3 ounces protein foods	Chicken & potatoes *3 ounces chicken breast* *1/2 cup mashed potato* 1/2 cup green peas 2 small whole wheat rolls 1 cup milk*

*Offer your child fat-free or low-fat milk, yogurt, and cheese.
Source: choosemyplate.gov

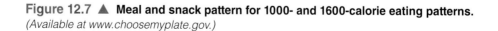

Figure 12.7 ▲ **Meal and snack pattern for 1000- and 1600-calorie eating patterns.**
(Available at www.choosemyplate.gov.)

Until the age of 4 years, young children are at risk for choking. To decrease the risk of choking, foods that are difficult to chew and swallow should be avoided (see Box 12.5); meals and snacks should be supervised; foods should be prepared in forms that are easy to chew and swallow (e.g., cut grapes into small pieces and spread peanut butter thinly); and infants should not be allowed to eat or drink from a cup while lying down, playing, or strapped in a car seat.

NUTRITION FOR CHILDREN AND ADOLESCENTS

Childhood represents a more latent period of growth compared to infancy and adolescence. Although there are individual differences, usually a larger child eats more than a smaller one; an active child eats more than a quiet one; and a happy, content child eats more than an anxious one. School-age children maintain a relatively constant intake in relation to their age group; children who are considered big eaters in second grade are also big eaters in sixth grade.

The slow growth of childhood abruptly and dramatically increases with pubescence until the rate is nearly as rapid as that of early infancy. Adolescence is a period of physical, emotional, social, and sexual maturation. Approximately 15% to 20% of adult height and 50% of adult weight are gained during adolescence. Fat distribution shifts and sexual maturation occurs. Subsequently, calorie and nutrient needs increase, as does appetite, but exactly when those increases occur depends on the timing and duration of the growth spurt. Because there are wide variations in the timing of the growth spurt among individuals, chronological age is a poor indicator of physiologic maturity and nutritional needs.

Gender differences are obvious. For instance, girls generally experience increases in growth between 10 and 11 years of age and peak at 12 years. Because peak weight occurs before peak height, many girls and parents become concerned about what appears to be excess weight. In contrast, boys usually begin the growth spurt at about 12 years of age and peak at 14 years. Stature growth ceases at a median age of approximately 21 years. Nutritional needs increase later for boys than for girls.

Calories and Nutrients

Calorie range recommendations for males and females appear in Figure 12.5. The lowest number within each range represents calorie estimates for a sedentary level of activity; for moderate activity, the number increases by 200 calories, and for an active individual, the increase is generally another 200 calories. Total calorie needs steadily increase during childhood, although calorie needs per kilogram of body weight progressively fall. The challenge in childhood is to meet nutrient requirements without exceeding calorie needs. Table 12.4 lists healthy U.S.-style eating patterns recommendations for calorie levels appropriate from childhood through adolescence. Generally, nutrient requirements are higher during adolescence than at any other time in the life cycles, with the exception of pregnancy and lactation.

The number of calories suggested for moderately active females aged 12 to 18 years is 2000, whereas for males, the need ranges from 2200 to 2800 calories. Females require fewer calories than males because they have proportionally more fat tissue and less muscle mass from the effects of estrogen. Girls also experience less bone growth than boys.

Table 12.4	Healthy U.S.-Style Eating Pattern: Recommended Amounts of Food from Each Food Group from 1400 Calories to 3200 Calories Levels									
	Amounts Recommended/Day per Calorie Level									
Food Groups	**1400**	**1600**	**1800**	**2000**	**2200**	**2400**	**2600**	**2800**	**3000**	**3200**
Vegetables (cup-eq)	1.5	2	2.5	2.5	3	3	3.5	3.5	4	4
Fruits (cup-eq)	1.5	1.5	1.5	2	2	2	2	2.5	2.5	2.5
Grains (oz-eq)	5	5	6	6	7	8	9	10	10	10
Dairy (cup-eq)	2.5	3	3	3	3	3	3	3	3	3
Protein Foods (oz-eq)	4	5	5	5.5	6	6.5	6.5	7	7	7
Oils (g)	17	22	24	27	29	31	34	36	44	51
Limit on calories of other uses	110	130	170	270	280	350	380	400	470	610

Source: U.S. Department of Health and Human Services & U.S. Department of Agriculture. (2015). *Healthy U.S.-style eating pattern: Recommended amounts of food from each food group.* Available at http://health.gov/dietaryguidelines/2015/guidelines/appendix-3/. Accessed on 4/20/16.

Quick Bite Sources of calcium

Milk
Yogurt
Hard cheeses, such as cheddar
Calcium-fortified orange juice
Calcium-fortified breakfast cereals
Canned fish with bones, such as salmon
"Greens," such as bok choy, collard greens, turnip greens, kale
Broccoli
Chinese/napa cabbage
Okra
Tofu, soymilk
Tortillas made from lime-processed corn

Quick Bite Sources of nonheme iron

Iron-fortified, ready-to-eat cereals
Whole wheat, enriched, or fortified bread
Noodles, rice, or barley
Canned plums
Cooked dried apricots
Raisins
Bean dip
Peanut butter

The Dietary Reference Intakes (DRIs) for children are divided into two age groups: 1- to 3-year-olds and 4- to 8-year-olds. Thereafter, age groups are further divided by gender: For males and females, the age groups through adolescence are 9- to 13-year-olds and 14- to 18-year-olds, respectively. Generally, nutrient needs increase with each age grouping, and most nutrient requirements reach their adult levels at the 14- to 18-year age group.

Calcium

For males and females from age 9 to 18 years, the Recommended Dietary Allowance (RDA) for calcium is 1300 mg—higher than at any other time in the life cycle. Approximately half of adult bone mass is accrued during adolescence; optimizing calcium intake during adolescence increases bone mineralization and may decrease the risk of fracture and osteoporosis later in life.

Iron

Iron is a concern because adolescents have increased needs for iron related to an expanding blood volume, the rise in hemoglobin concentration, and the growth of muscle mass. In boys, peak iron requirement occurs between 14 and 18 years of age as muscle mass expands. The requirement for iron in adolescent girls increases from 8 to 15 mg/day at the age of 14 years to account for menstrual losses. For girls who are not menstruating at 14 years old, the requirement for iron is 10.5 mg/day, not 15 mg/day. Girls tend to develop an iron deficiency slowly after puberty, particularly if menstrual losses are compounded by poor eating habits or chronic fad dieting. Heme iron, found in meats, is better absorbed than nonheme iron. Nonheme iron absorption increases when a source of vitamin C, such as orange juice or tomatoes, is consumed at the same time.

Eating Practices

As children get older, they consume more foods from outside the home and have more outside influences on their food choices. School, friends' houses, childcare centers, and social events present opportunities for children to make their own choices beyond parental supervision. Children who are home alone after school prepare their own snacks and, possibly, meals. In adolescence, peer pressure assumes a greater influence on food choices. As the adolescent becomes increasingly independent, more self-selected meals and snacks are purchased and eaten outside the home. A natural increase in appetite and a decrease in physical activity increase the risk of overeating.

Family Meals

Children and adolescents who have a high frequency of eating family meals tend to have better quality eating patterns as evidenced by higher intakes of fruits, vegetables, grains, fiber, and calcium-rich foods and lower intakes of carbonated beverages (Golden, Schneider, & Wood, 2016). Family meals promote social interaction and allow children to learn food-related behaviors. Food served at family meals may also be healthier than what teenagers would choose on their own.

Parents should provide and consume nutrient-dense meals and snacks (Box 12.9) and avoid or limit calorie-dense foods, such as fried foods, fatty meats, and high-fat sauces. The MyPlate graphic (see Fig. 12.4) that shows ½ the plate occupied by fruits and vegetables, ¼ by grains, and ¼ by protein with dairy on the side illustrates the concept of balance and proportion and is appropriate for all people over the age of 2 years.

Fast Food

Fast food represents the largest contributor to foods prepared away from home, surpassing the contribution of foods eaten at school (Ogata & Hayes, 2014). Compared to foods made at home, fast-food meals are low in fruit, vegetables, whole grains, and dairy and provide higher amounts of calories, fat, saturated fat, and sugar, contributing to poorer overall eating patterns compared to children who do not eat fast food (Powell & Nguyen, 2013).

Meal Skipping

The Dietary Guidelines Advisory Committee Report (2015) states that in the U.S. population, consumption of a three-meal-a-day pattern follows a U-shaped curve when plotted against age. Skipping meals is most likely to occur in children ages 2 to 5 years and then decline, reaching its lowest point during adolescence and young adulthood, after which it rises again. Breakfast is the meal most likely to be skipped by young people (Pearson, Biddle, & Gorely, 2009). Eating breakfast is associated with healthier eating patterns; a study among children aged 5 to 16 years found that children who ate breakfast had lower intakes of fat and healthier levels of serum vitamin C and folate than those who did not (Bhattacharya, Currie, & Haider, 2006). Although data are mixed, there seems to be a positive effect of breakfast eating on school performance (Adolphus, Lawton, & Dye, 2013). Whereas a high-fiber, nutrient-fortified, ready-to-eat cereal with nonfat milk and fruit may be a healthy traditional option for breakfast, nontraditional breakfasts may be more appealing to people who "don't like breakfast."

Quick Bite **Nontraditional breakfast ideas**

Pizza
Peanut butter sandwich
Soup with crackers
Yogurt parfait
Smoothies
Baked potato with cottage cheese
Dinner leftovers

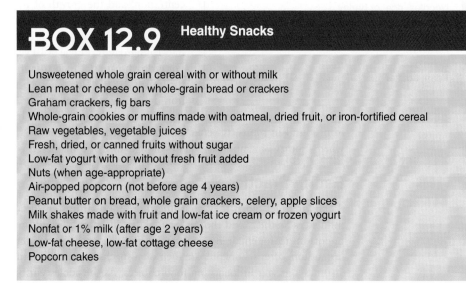

BOX 12.9   Healthy Snacks

Unsweetened whole grain cereal with or without milk
Lean meat or cheese on whole-grain bread or crackers
Graham crackers, fig bars
Whole-grain cookies or muffins made with oatmeal, dried fruit, or iron-fortified cereal
Raw vegetables, vegetable juices
Fresh, dried, or canned fruits without sugar
Low-fat yogurt with or without fresh fruit added
Nuts (when age-appropriate)
Air-popped popcorn (not before age 4 years)
Peanut butter on bread, whole grain crackers, celery, apple slices
Milk shakes made with fruit and low-fat ice cream or frozen yogurt
Nonfat or 1% milk (after age 2 years)
Low-fat cheese, low-fat cottage cheese
Popcorn cakes

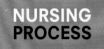

Well Child

Amanda is a 24-month-old girl who is seen regularly in the well-baby clinic for her checkups and immunizations. At this visit, you discover that her height and weight are in the 25th percentile for her age. Records indicate that previously, she had consistently ranked in the 75th percentile for weight and 50th percentile for height. The change has occurred over the last 6 months. Her mother complains that Amanda is "fussy" and has lost interest in eating.

Assessment

Medical–Psychosocial History
- Medical history including prenatal, perinatal, and birth history; specifically assess for gastrointestinal (GI) problems such as slow gastric emptying, constipation, diarrhea, and allergies
- Use of medications that can cause side effects such as delayed gastric emptying, diarrhea, constipation, or decreased appetite
- Level of development for age
- Elimination and reflux patterns, if applicable
- Caregiver's ability to understand; attitude toward health and nutrition and readiness to learn
- Psychosocial and economic issues such as the living situation, who does the shopping and cooking, adequacy of food budget, need for food assistance, and level of family and social support
- Use of vitamins, minerals, and nutritional supplements: what, how much, and why they are given

Anthropometric Assessment
- Obtain height and weight to calculate BMI; determine BMI-for-age percentile.
- Head circumference for age
- Pattern of weight gain and growth

Biochemical and Physical Assessment
- Laboratory values, including hemoglobin and hematocrit, and the significance of any other values that are abnormal

Dietary Assessment
- Food records, if available
- Interview the primary caregiver to assess the following:
  - What does Amanda usually eat in a 24-hour period, including types and amounts of food, frequency and pattern of eating, and texture of foods eaten?
  - How does her intake compare to a 1000-calorie (the calorie level appropriate for 2-year-olds) MyPlate intake pattern?
  - What food groups is she consuming less than recommended amounts of?
  - Are self-feeding skills appropriate for Amanda's age?
  - Is the mealtime environment positive?
  - What is the caregiver's attitude about Amanda's current weight, recent weight loss, and eating behaviors?
  - Are the caregiver's expectations about how much Amanda should eat reasonable and appropriate? What is the problem according to the caregiver?
  - Are there cultural, religious, and ethnic influences on the family's eating habits?

Diagnosis

Possible Nursing Diagnoses

Imbalanced nutrition: less than body requirements as evidenced by a decrease of two percentile channels in growth charts

Planning

Client Outcomes

The client will
- Experience appropriate growth in height and weight
- Consume, on average, an intake consistent with MyPlate recommendations for a 1000-calorie diet by eating a variety of foods within each food group
- Achieve or progress toward age-appropriate feeding skills

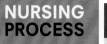

Well Child

Nursing Interventions

Nutrition Therapy	Promote MyPlate food plan of 1000 calories, which is appropriate for her age.
Client Teaching	Instruct the caregiver

- On the role of nutrition in maintaining health and promoting adequate growth and development, including the importance of adequate calories and protein
- On eating-plan essentials, including the importance of
  - Choosing a varied diet to help ensure an adequate intake
  - Providing foods of appropriate texture for age
  - Providing three meals plus three or more planned snacks to maximize intake
  - Providing liquids after meals, instead of with meals, to avoid displacing food intake
  - Limiting low-nutrient-dense foods (e.g., fruit drinks, carbonated beverages, sweetened cereals) because they displace the intake of more nutritious foods
  - The need to modify the diet, as appropriate, to improve elimination patterns

Address behavioral matters, such as

- Providing a positive mealtime environment (e.g., limiting distractions, having the child well rested before mealtime)
- Not using food to punish, reward, or bribe the child
- Promoting eating behaviors and skills appropriate for the age
- Keeping accurate food records
- Modifying foods to increase their nutrient density, such as by fortifying milk with skim milk powder; using milk in place of water in recipes; melting cheese on potatoes, rice, or noodles; and so on

Evaluation

Evaluate and Monitor	• Monitor growth in height and weight.
	• Evaluate food records to assess adequacy of intake according to a 1000-calorie MyPlate plan.
	• Progress toward age-appropriate feeding skills.

NUTRITION CONCERNS DURING CHILDHOOD AND ADOLESCENCE

Poor Diet Quality

Healthy Eating Index-2010
a tool to measure diet quality. Twelve component food groups are scored on how closely an individual adheres to the *2010 Dietary Guidelines for Americans*. Total possible score is 100; 80 is the minimum federal guideline for good health and disease prevention. The higher the score, the greater the adherence to the *Dietary Guidelines for Americans*.

A recent study in American youth using the **Healthy Eating Index-2010** found that although dairy and whole fruit intake are high in early childhood, overall diet quality was poor among all age and ethnic groups and worsened from early childhood to adolescence (Banfield, Liu, Davis, Chang, & Frazier-Wood, 2016). For Americans age 2 years throughout the lifespan, nutrition concerns are consistent: excessive intakes of calories, saturated fats, added sugars, and sodium and inadequate intakes of foods rich in calcium, potassium, vitamin D, and dietary fiber related to low intakes of dairy, vegetables, fruits, and whole grains (USDHHS & USDA, 2015). Iron is also underconsumed by adolescent females (USDA, Agricultural Research Service [ARS], 2014). In addition, a previous study among children and adolescents revealed 40% of calories consumed were from solid fats and added sugars, namely, empty calories (Reedy & Krebs-Smith, 2010). Empty calorie intake far exceeded empty calorie allowance in all age-sex groups.

Poor diet quality across childhood and adolescence is associated with adverse health outcomes, including early puberty (a risk factor for hormone-related cancers), high diastolic blood pressure, and possibly central obesity, although the link between diet quality and childhood obesity is controversial (Biro & Wien, 2010; Cheng et al., 2010; Marrodán et al., 2013).

Emerging evidence that eating habits developed during childhood often persist into adulthood raises concern because poor diet quality increases the risk of chronic diseases in adults, including type 2 diabetes, cardiovascular disease, and cancer (Banfield et al., 2016). Characteristics of a healthy eating pattern are those described in the *Dietary Guidelines for Americans* Key Recommendations (see Box 12.8).

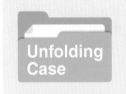

Think of Luis. His calorie intake is excessive as evidenced by his weight, and his essentially self-selected diet is of poor quality. Luis's doctor has warned his mother that his diastolic blood pressure is high and that he is overweight. His mother evades answering questions about Luis's typical eating pattern. How do you proceed with helping them achieve a healthier intake without knowing what his usual intake is?

OVERWEIGHT AND OBESITY

In less than one generation, the worldwide prevalence of childhood overweight and obesity has risen substantially (Lobstein et al., 2015). In 2011 to 2012, 8.1% of infants and toddlers from birth to 2 years had a weight-for-length greater than the 95th percentile, classifying them as obese (Ogden, Carroll, Kit, & Flegal, 2014). During that same period, approximately 15% of American children ages 2 to 19 years old were overweight and approximately 17% were obese (CDC, 2015a). By age grouping, obesity rates are

- 8.4% among children aged 2 to 5 years
- 17.7% among 6- to 11-year-olds
- 20.5% among 12- to 19-year-olds

Over the last three decades, the rate of childhood obesity has more than doubled and the rate of adolescent obesity has quadrupled (Golden et al., 2016). Although the rise in obesity prevalence may be reaching a plateau, current overall obesity rates remain too high and not significantly different from 2003 to 2004 (Ogden et al., 2014). In addition, the fastest growing subcategory of obesity in children and adolescents is severe obesity (Claire Wang, Gortmaker, & Taveras, 2011). Although the definition of severe pediatric obesity has not been unanimously agreed on, it is proposed that class II obesity ($\geq$120% of the 95th percentile or a BMI $\geq$35 kg/m^2, whichever is lower) and class III obesity ($\geq$140% of the 95th percentile or BMI $\geq$40, whichever is lower) be labeled severe pediatric obesity (Kelly et al., 2013).

Contributing Factors

Overweight and obesity are multifactorial in origin. Prenatal environment, such as smoking, and excessive gestational weight gain increase the risk for later obesity (Dattilo et al., 2012). A genetic predisposition toward obesity may account for 40% to 70% of observed obesity (Maes, Neale, & Eaves, 1997), but genetic factors alone do not explain the rapid increase in obesity prevalence. Parental weight status—especially maternal weight status—is a strong predictor of childhood obesity, which is not surprising given parents provide genes, environment, and food. In the majority of children, obesity is attributed to the interaction between multiple genetic factors and an obesogenic environment (Dattilo et al., 2012), which encourages calorie intake and discourages calorie expenditure. Home food environment is a key influence on childhood obesity (Rosenkranz & Dzewaltowski, 2008).

Within the last 30 years, the average weight of an American child has increased by more than 11 pounds (Lobstein et al., 2015). During that time period, the average calorie intake of American children has increased, a bigger proportion of the food budget is spent on food away from home, and portion sizes have grown. On the other side of the energy equation, a decrease in physical activity and increase in sedentary leisure activities, such as watching television, playing video games, and electronic social networking, are seen as major contributors to weight gain in children.

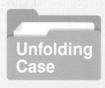

Unfolding Case

Recall Luis. At 48 in tall and 90 pounds, his BMI is approximately 27.5. His mother is obese and claims she gained 40 pounds during pregnancy, which is excessive. Although his mom says they rarely eat red meat or fried food, she admits he eats at will, often asking for sugar-sweetened and low-fiber cereal within 15 minutes of eating dinner. His favorite dinner is breaded chicken fingers, baked French fries, and a sweetened beverage. What recommendations would you make for improving the quality of his favorite dinner? How would you advise Luis's mother to respond to his request for more food so soon after eating dinner?

Risks Associated with Obesity

The risks of childhood overweight and obesity are significant:

- Obese infants and those with rapid weight gain during the first year of life are at increased risk of obesity later in life (Baird et al., 2005).
- Childhood overweight/obesity is a strong predictor of adult obesity (Brisbios, Farmer, & McGarga, 2012): Children obese at age 6 years have more than a 50% chance of being obese as adults regardless of parental weight status.
- A high adolescent BMI increases adult diabetes risk by almost threefold and coronary artery disease risk by almost fivefold (Tirosh et al., 2011).
- Risks of other comorbid conditions, such as hypertension, dyslipidemia, nonalcoholic fatty liver disease, gallstones, gastroesophageal reflux, polycystic ovary syndrome, obstructive sleep apnea, asthma, and bone and joint problems, are significantly increased in obese adolescents and in adults who were obese as adolescents (Freedman et al., 2005; Golden et al., 2016; Inge et al., 2013; C. Li, Ford, Zhao, & Mokdad, 2009).
- Children who are overweight and obese have significantly lower mean scores of quality of life (Keating, Moodie, & Swinburn, 2011).
- A study that followed almost 11,000 American adolescents found that obese girls were half as likely to attend college, were more likely to consider committing suicide and use alcohol and marijuana, and had a more negative self-image than normal-weight girls (Crosnoe, 2007).
- Teasing and psychological abuse by peers and adults can lead to social isolation, depression, low self-esteem, lower academic achievement, and lower economic productivity. Because they are social outcasts, a perpetuating cycle of weight gain, inactivity, and further weight gain makes weight control difficult.
- Evidence shows the medical and psychological consequences of childhood obesity continue into adulthood (Pulgarón, 2013).

Obesity Prevention and Treatment

The low success in treating obesity makes prevention crucial. Although most obesity intervention trials in youth focus on school-age children, attention is increasingly shifting toward younger ages (Lumeng, Taveras, Birch, & Yanovski, 2015). Obesity prevention strategies begin by monitoring growth from birth through every health-care visit to identify children at risk for becoming obese. Interventions should be implemented when a child's BMI percentile begins to increase instead of waiting until the child reaches the 85th or 95th percentile (Daniels & Hassink, 2015).

Intake patterns, eating habits, and food preferences begin to be established in in infancy and, although inconsistent, may be set as early as 2 years of age (Skinner, Carruth, Wendy, & Ziegler, 2002). Early life may be a critical period when appetite regulation and energy balance are programmed, with lifelong consequences for obesity risk (Robinson et al., 2015).

Early Life Obesity Prevention Strategies

Breastfeeding as a strategy to prevent obesity in infancy and childhood has received a lot of attention and a great deal of study in the last decade (Lumeng et al., 2015). Almost all observational studies suggest a lower risk of obesity in children who have been breastfed compared to those who were formula fed (Daniels & Hassink, 2015). However, in a large cluster of randomized controlled trials, breastfeeding had no effect on BMI in later childhood (R. Martin et al., 2013). Still, because breastfeeding imparts so many other benefits to mothers and infants, its promotion is strongly encouraged and should be part of any obesity prevention program (Daniels & Hassink, 2015).

Although evidence that breastfeeding effectively prevents obesity is inconsistent (Gillman, 2011), formula-fed infants are larger than breastfed infants by the age of 12 months (Kramer et al., 2004). Behavioral feeding practices and differences in the composition of formula compared to breast milk are cited as possible explanations. For instance,

- Formula-fed infants receive ~0.5 g/kg/day more protein than do breastfed infants (Michaelsen & Greer, 2014). The European Childhood Obesity Program (CHOP) study found that infants fed a lower protein formula similar to the amount of protein in breast milk had a growth pattern that did not significantly differ from the breastfed control group. In comparison, infants fed formula with the highest protein content had significantly higher weight gain and at ages 12 and 24 months and their BMIs were significantly higher even though the study stopped at 12 months (Koletzko et al., 2009). A follow-up study of that trial found that the children who had been given the higher protein formula had a significantly higher BMI at 6 years of age and that their risk of becoming obese was 2.43 times that of the lower protein formula group (Weber et al., 2014).

> *Concept Mastery Alert*
>
> Formula-fed infants consume more protein per kilogram of body weight than do breastfed infants. This may predispose the formula-fed infant to obesity later in life.

Although more data are needed before changes in formula content can be recommended, there has been a recent trend by formula manufacturers to lower the protein content in formula to approximate the protein intake of breastfed infants (Michaelsen & Greer, 2014). The U.S. Infant Formula Act allows for protein content to range from 1.8 to 4.5 g/100 calories (21 CFR Sect 106, 1996). By comparison, breast milk provides <1.4 g/100 calories.

- Bottle feeding is associated with emptying the bottle and greater weight gains (R. Li, Magalia, Fein, & Grummer-Strawn, 2012) whether the content is formula or expressed breast milk. The presumed mechanism is that the infant's satiety signals are not heeded.
- Other parental feeding and activity patterns that may increase the infant's risk of later obesity include putting the infant to bed with a bottle, propping a bottle, always feeding when the infant cries, early exposure to television viewing, and not meeting "tummy time" recommendations, which is considered physical activity for an infant (Perrin et al., 2014).
- Early introduction of solids is also speculated to increase the risk of obesity, but findings provide inconsistent evidence regarding the link to obesity in the short or long term (Grote et al., 2011). More research is needed on how the timing and composition of complementary feeding affects growth (Lumeng et al., 2015).

The AAP contends that the prevention of childhood obesity should start before 2 years of age by promoting (Daniels & Hassink, 2015)

- Healthy maternal weight
- Appropriate gestational weight gain
- No smoking during pregnancy
- Breastfeeding
- Appropriate weight gain during infancy
- A transition to healthy foods with weaning
- Eliminating sedentary entertainment
- Active play for physical activity
- Parental role modeling of healthy eating and physical activity behaviors

	Population	Strategies	Correspondence to staged approach for treatment of pediatric obesity	Example
Primary prevention	Population-wide interventions that include youth of all body sizes or weight	Eating and physical-activity messages or programs intended to prevent incidence of overweight/obesity and/or provide a supportive environment for weight maintenance	NA[a]	School-based health promotion programs for healthy eating and physical activity
Secondary prevention	Overweight or obese youth with no weight-related comorbidities	More structured and involved eating and physical-activity programs intended to help overweight and obese youth obtain a healthy weight; may require medical approval or limited supervision	Stage 1: Prevention Plus Stage 2: Structured Weight Management Stage 3: Comprehensive Multidisciplinary Intervention	Brief motivational interviewing on selected behaviors (e.g., decreased consumption of sugar-sweetened beverages), with progression to other stages if warranted
Tertiary prevention	Overweight or obese youth with comorbidities Severely obese youth	Intensive and comprehensive treatments for overweight and obese youth conducted under medical supervision with a focus on resolving weight-related comorbidities or at least decreasing their severity	Stage 1: Prevention Plus Stage 2: Structured Weight Management Stage 3: Comprehensive Multidisciplinary Intervention Stage 4: Tertiary Care Intervention	Multidisciplinary program offered at a pediatric weight-management center, which may include pharmacologic treatment or bariatric surgery

[a]NA = not applicable.

Figure 12.8 ▲ Continuum of pediatric obesity interventions from prevention to high-intensity medical treatment. (Source: Hoelscher, D., Kirk, S., Ritchie, L., & Cunningham-Sabo, L. [2013]. Position of the Academy of Nutrition and Dietetics: Interventions for the prevention and treatment of pediatric overweight and obesity. Journal of the Academy of Nutrition and Dietetics, 113, 1375–1394.)

Childhood and Adolescent Obesity Prevention Strategies

The American Academy of Nutrition and Dietetics position on the prevention and treatment of childhood and adolescent overweight and obesity combines a public health perspective with treatment approaches of the American Medical Association to create an intervention model along a continuum according to weight status (Fig. 12.8) (Hoelscher, Kirk, Ritchie, & Cunningham-Sabo, 2013). For all levels of prevention or treatment, strategies must be tailored to the child's developmental stage and family characteristics (Daniels & Hassink, 2015). Primary, secondary, and tertiary interventions are described in the following sections.

Primary Prevention

Primary prevention is recommended for all youth regardless of weight status with the goal of improving long-term health. Primary prevention is synonymous with lifestyle modification aimed at adopting permanent changes to eat healthy, become less sedentary, increase physical activity, and ensure adequate sleep (Box 12.10).

Parental role modeling of a healthy lifestyle is vital to initiating and sustaining changes in eating and physical activity behaviors. Parents often recognize that they need to set an example for their children but lack the time to do so. Still, other parents who are overweight may feel they cannot set a good example because they do not practice what they preach. Other barriers to parents taking action are (1) a belief that children will outgrow their excess weight, (2) a lack of knowledge about how to help children control their weight, and (3) a fear they will cause eating disorders in their children. Parents should be encouraged to not talk about weight but rather about healthy eating and healthy physical activity (Golden et al., 2016).

Secondary Prevention

Secondary obesity prevention interventions target overweight or obese youth with no weight-related comorbidities; in effect, secondary prevention is low level treatment (Hoelscher et al., 2013). Treating pediatric obesity is an ever-increasing challenge. Treatment is frequently unsuccessful, and evidence shows significant long-term weight loss maintenance is particularly difficult (Romirowsky, Kushner, Elliot, Nadler, & Mackey, 2015). Most intervention trials report small BMI benefits at most, despite considerable intervention efforts (Wake et al., 2015).

| BOX 12.10 | Lifestyle Modification Obesity Prevention Strategies |

Healthier Nutrition

- Eat family meals as often as possible.
- Promote a healthy eating pattern that emphasizes nutrient-dense foods such as fruits, vegetables, whole grains, low-fat or nonfat dairy, lean meats, legumes, and seafood.
- Consume age-appropriate daily calorie intake.
- Eat age-appropriate food portions.
- Eat foods low in calorie density, such as those high in fiber and/or water and modest in fat.
- Keep healthy foods and beverages available and in plain sight, such as water pitchers, fruits, vegetables, and other low calorie snacks.
- Limit sugar-sweetened beverages and high-calorie snacks and sweets. If purchased for a special occasion, buy them immediately before the event and remove them immediately afterward. Aim to eliminate all sugar-sweetened beverages.
- Limit the intake of 100% juice to 4 oz to 6 oz/day for children 1 to 6 years of age and 8 to 12 oz/day for children 7 to 18 years old.
- If high-calorie foods are in the home, they should be stored out of sight and made less visible by wrapping in foil.
- Decrease the size of serving spoons, plates, bowls, and glasses.
- Discourage eating directly from the package; repackage high-calorie snacks into smaller containers.
- Eat healthy snacks that are prepackaged in an age-appropriate size.
- Limit calorie-dense foods, such as fried foods, cheeses, and oil-based sauces.
- Eliminate artificially sweetened beverages and beverages containing caffeine.
- Eat breakfast daily.
- Choose healthy kids' meal side items and beverages when eating out, such as apple slices, water, and unflavored low-fat milk.

Reduce Sedentary Behaviors

- Reduce the number of televisions in the home and remove the television and other media from the child's bedroom and where meals are eaten.
- Limit sedentary entertainment (e.g., television and electronic entertainment or communication) to 2 hours or less per day for children 2 years and older. Eliminate sedentary entertainment for children under the age of 2 years.

Increase Physical Activity

- Meet national physical activity guideline of at least 60 minutes of moderate to vigorous physical activity daily.

Adequate Sleep

- Counsel parents on age-appropriate sleep durations. Children who sleep less than 9 hours a night have 1.5 times the risk of being obese compared to those who receive >11 hours of sleep a night (Pileggi, Lotito, Bianco, Nobile, & Pavia, 2013).

Source: Daniels, S., & Hassink, S. (2015). The role of the pediatrician in primary prevention of obesity. *Pediatrics, 136,* e275. doi:10.1542/peds2015-1558

Secondary prevention begins with lifestyle modification strategies similar to those in primary prevention. In overweight and obese youth without comorbidities, weight loss is usually not recommended due to the potential negative impact on growth and development. Depending on the age of the child and the degree overweight, the initial goal of intervention may be for children to maintain weight while the growing taller, leading to a lower BMI over time or actual weight loss. If BMI does not improve after 3 to 6 months, treatment progresses to stage 2, a more structured and intense level of intervention, which includes a low-calorie energy-dense eating pattern, structured meals, supervised physical activity of at least 60 minutes/day, 1 hour or less of screen time daily, and more intense behavior modification strategies, such as self-monitoring, goal setting, and cognitive restructuring (Barlow, 2007). If no improvement in BMI is seen after 3 to 6 months, intervention progresses to stage 3, a comprehensive multidisciplinary intervention involving obesity experts.

Parental involvement in treatment is crucial; family-based intervention programs are more successful than individual-centered programs (Epstein, Paluch, Roemmich, & Beecher, 2007).

Motivational Interviewing
a goal-oriented, client-centered counseling style that facilitates and engages intrinsic motivation to change behavior.

Motivational interviewing may be applied to inspire parents to serve as role models by providing healthy meals, eating with their children, avoiding talk about weight, engaging in regular physical activity, and limiting their own sedentary behaviors. Even in adolescence, parents are still the primary role models for eating and physical activity behaviors and have a direct impact on the adolescent's food and activity environment (Daniels & Hassink, 2015). Parents and other family members should be encouraged to implement the same changes as the child. Dieting is a risk factor for both obesity and eating disorders, so emphasis should be on healthy lifestyle, not restrictive eating.

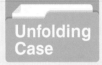
Unfolding Case

Consider Luis. He and his mother enroll in a 12-week-long weight management program at their community center. The program began by stressing healthy behaviors, including types of food to eat. What eating strategies would you encourage them to adopt? How much sedentary time per day is appropriate for Luis? What recommendations would you make about exercise, physical activity, and sedentary activity?

Tertiary Prevention

Tertiary prevention (highest level treatment) is intended for overweight or obese youth with comorbidities or for severely obese youth. This stage 4 of interventions includes comprehensive multidisciplinary interventions conducted under medical supervision with a focus on resolving or improving comorbidities (Hoelscher et al., 2013). For instance, very-low-calorie diets (<1000 cal/day) and/or meal replacements may be used as the dietary strategy and pharmacotherapy or bariatric surgery may be used.

Pharmacotherapy. Pharmacotherapy may be considered in obese children only after a formal program of intensive lifestyle modification fails or in overweight children only if severe comorbidities persist despite intensive lifestyle modification, especially in children with a strong family history of type 2 diabetes or premature cardiovascular disease (August et al., 2008). Drug therapy should only be prescribed by clinicians experienced in anti-obesity medications and their side effects.

Orlistat (Xenical) is the only medication currently approved by the FDA to treat obesity in adolescents and only in those ages 12 years and older (Kelly et al., 2013). It works by blocking the absorption of fat from the intestine. A large randomized trial in investigating the use of orlistat with lifestyle invention in adolescents found a significant decrease in BMI after 1 year (Chanoine, Hampl, Jensen, Boldrin, & Hauptman, 2005). Although it is generally considered safe, side effects are common (e.g., oily spotting, oily bowel movements, fecal urgency, and abdominal pain) and long-term effects on growth and developments are not known (Kelly et al., 2013).

Weight Loss Surgery

Bariatric surgery is the obesity treatment with the most weight loss success in adults (Romirowsky et al., 2015) and is increasingly accepted as an option for a select group of adolescents who have failed more conservative medically supervised treatment over a period of at least 6 months (Hoelscher et al., 2013). The American Society of Metabolic and Bariatric Surgery endorses bariatric surgery for adolescents with a BMI >35 with serious comorbidity or a BMI >40 with less severe comorbidities (Michalsky, Reichard, Inge, Pratt, & Lenders, 2012) based on evidence that bariatric surgery has been shown effective in producing sustained and significant weight loss in treatment-resistant severely obese adolescents (Hsia, Fallon, & Brandt, 2012). Other criteria such as developmental status, psychological status, and demonstrated ability to adhere to diet and physical activity recommendations are evaluated. Although bariatric surgery is effective at lowering BMI and improving cardiovascular and metabolic risk factors, the long-term effectiveness is not known and access is limited by insurance coverage (Kelly et al., 2013).

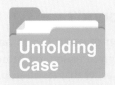

Recall Luis. He has not lost weight but has grown taller so there has been some improvement in his BMI. His mom continues counseling to improve her parenting skills, which she now admits influenced her son's overeating. She has had a hard time eating vegetables herself and tends to graze, although they are eating family dinners almost every day. How would you respond to her question of how long this "diet thing" needs to continue?

Adolescent Pregnancy

Adolescent pregnancy is associated with physiologic, socioeconomic, and behavioral factors that increase health risks to both infant and mother. Infants born to adolescent mothers are more likely to become teen mothers; adolescent pregnancy typically limits the mother's education and subsequent occupational opportunities. Infants born to adolescent mothers are at higher risk of low birth weight (LBW) and preterm delivery, which are precursors of infant morbidity and mortality (Mathews & MacDorman, 2013). Studies show that adolescent mothers are more likely to gain an excessive amount of weight (e.g., more than 40 pounds) during pregnancy compared to pregnant women who are at least 20 years old, placing both mother and infant at increased risk for becoming overweight or obese (Davis et al., 2013). Common complications among adolescent mothers include iron deficiency anemia and prolonged labor. The risks are highest for infants born to the youngest mothers (J. Martin et al., 2013). Compared with adult women, pregnant adolescents

- Are more likely to be physically, emotionally, financially, and socially immature. Low socioeconomic status may be a major reason for the high incidence of LBW infants and other complications of adolescent pregnancy.
- May not have adequate nutrient stores because they need large amounts of nutrients for their own growth and development. Although female adolescent growth is usually complete by the age of 15 years, physical maturity is not reached until 4 years after menarche, which usually occurs by age 17 years.
- May give low priority to healthy eating. Dieting, erratic eating patterns, reliance on fast foods, and meal skipping (especially breakfast) are common adolescent practices.
- May have poor intake and status of certain micronutrients, such as folate, iron, and vitamin D, which increases the risk of small-for-gestational-age births in pregnant adolescents (Baker et al., 2009).
- Often need to gain more weight for their BMI than older women to improve birth outcomes (Rasmussen & Yaktine, 2009).
- Are more concerned with body image and confused about weight gain recommendations. Many do not understand why they should gain more than 7 pounds, the weight of the average baby at birth.
- Are more likely to smoke during pregnancy. Smoking increases the risk of premature birth and its associated problems including death (CDC, 2015b).
- Seek prenatal care later and have fewer total visits during pregnancy.

Appropriate weight gain and adequate nutrition are among the most important modifiable factors that contribute to a healthful outcome of pregnancy for both mother and infant (Nielsen, Gittelsohn, Anliker, & O'Brien, 2006). Good nutrition has the potential to decrease the incidence of LBW infants and to improve the health of infants born to adolescents. Adolescents within the healthy BMI range should gain approximately 35 pounds to reduce the risk of delivering an LBW infant.

The MyPlate recommendations in Table 12.4 can also be used by pregnant teens. MyPlate is useful both in assessing dietary strengths and weaknesses and in providing a framework for implementing dietary changes in a way the adolescent can understand. Because adolescents living with one or more adults may have little control over what food is available to them, parents and significant others should also be encouraged to attend counseling sessions. Women, Infants, and Children (WIC) helps pregnant women obtain adequate and nutritious food for themselves and their infants.

How Do You Respond?

Does early introduction of solid foods help infants sleep through the night? A frequently given reason for introducing solids before 4 months of age is the unsupported belief that it will help infants to sleep through the night. A major objection to the early introduction of solids is that it may interfere with establishing sound eating habits and may contribute to overfeeding because infants less than 4 months old are unable to communicate satiety by turning away and leaning back.

What foods are most likely to cause allergies? Ninety percent of food allergy reactions are caused by proteins in these eight foods: milk, eggs, soy, peanuts, nuts (cashews, almonds), wheat, fish, and shellfish. Most people who have a food allergy are allergic to only one food.

Does diet contribute to acne prevalence? Diet may exacerbate acne. In a study based on self-reported acne among young adults, participants with moderate to severe acne reported a higher dietary glycemic index and higher intakes of total sugar, added sugar, fruit/ fruit juice, number of milk servings/day, saturated fat, and trans fats than participants with no or mild acne (Burris, Rietkerk, & Woolf, 2014). Also of interest was that fish intake was lower among participants with moderate to severe intake. Further research is needed to clarify the link between diet and acne and determine if nutrition therapy can play a role in acne treatment.

REVIEW CASE STUDY

Andrew is 16 years old and sedentary. He is 5 ft 8 in tall, weighs 218 pounds, and has a BMI of 33. He has been overweight for most of his life, as is most of his extended paternal family. His mother has tried "everything" over the years to get him to lose weight, from putting him on her own weight loss diet to hiding foods he shouldn't have, such as soft drinks and chips, to limit his access. He has a part-time job in a fast-food restaurant and is able to leave the school property at lunchtime to have lunch where he works. He is not good at sports but loves to play video games and watch movies. He hates that he's so big but feels hopeless about changing. His normal day's intake is shown on the right:

- Using the BMI-for-age percentile for boys, what is Andrew's weight status? Is it an appropriate approach to limit Andrew's calories to outgrow his current weight status?
- How many calories should Andrew consume daily? Based on the MyPlate intake levels, which food groups is he consuming the appropriate amounts of? Which groups is he overeating? Which groups is he not eating enough of? What are the sources of empty calories in his diet?
- What specific goals would you encourage Andrew to set regarding his intake, activity, and weight?
- What would you suggest his mother do to support better eating habits and a healthier weight?

Breakfast: Two doughnuts and a large glass of apple juice

Lunch: A double cheeseburger, large fries, and a large shake

Snacks: Frozen mini pizzas, a large soft drink, and a handful of cookies

Dinner: The same as lunch on nights he works; if he's home, he eats whatever is available, often pizza or sandwiches and chips, ice cream, and a soft drink

Snacks: Chips and salsa and a soft drink

STUDY QUESTIONS

1 Which statement indicates the mother understands the nurse's instructions about breastfeeding?
   a. "Breastfeeding should only last 5 minutes on each breast."
   b. "Sometimes, babies cry just because they are thirsty, so a bottle of water should be offered before breastfeeding begins to see if the infant is just thirsty."
   c. "The longer the baby sucks, the less milk I will have for the next feeding."
   d. "The first breast offered should be alternated with each feeding."

2 A mother asks why toddlers shouldn't drink all the milk they want. Which of the following is the nurse's best response?
   a. "Consuming more than the recommended amount of milk can displace the intake of iron-rich foods from the diet and increase the toddler's risk of iron deficiency anemia."
   b. "Consuming more than the recommended amount of milk increases the risk of milk allergy."
   c. "Too much milk can lead to overhydration."
   d. "Consuming more than the recommended amount of milk will provide too much protein."

3 The nurse knows her instructions about introducing solids into the infant's diet have been effective when the mother states
   a. "Babies should be introduced to solid foods at 1 to 3 months of age."
   b. "New foods should be given for at least 2 to 3 days so that allergic responses can be easily identified."
   c. "Infants are more likely to accept infant cereal for the first time if it is mixed with breast milk or formula and given from a bottle."
   d. "The appropriate initial serving size for solids is 1 to 2 tbsp."

4 Which of the following would be the best snack for a 2-year-old?
   a. Popcorn
   b. Banana slices
   c. Fresh cherries
   d. Raw celery

5 Which groups are adolescents most likely to eat in inadequate amounts? Select all that apply.
   a. Whole grains
   b. Vegetables
   c. Fruits
   d. Meat

6 The client asks if her 10-year-old daughter needs a weight loss diet. Which of the following would be the nurse's best response?
   a. "Rather than a diet at this age, you should just forbid her to eat sweets and empty calories."
   b. "Because prevention of overweight is more effective than treatment, you should start to limit her calorie intake by only serving low-fat and artificially sweetened foods."
   c. "Ten-year-old girls are about to enter the growth spurt of puberty, and it is natural for her to gain weight before she grows taller. Diets are not recommended for children, although healthy eating and moderation are always appropriate."
   d. "She needs extra calories for the upcoming growth spurt, so you should be encouraging her to eat more than she normally does."

7 Calorie requirements during adolescence
   a. Are higher than during adulthood because of growth and developmental changes
   b. Peak early and then fall until adulthood is reached
   c. Are lower than during childhood
   d. Cannot be generalized because individual variations exist

8 Nutrients most likely to be deficient in a female adolescent's diet are
   a. Vitamin A and folate
   b. Protein and vitamin C
   c. Zinc and phosphorus
   d. Iron and calcium

KEY CONCEPTS

- An optimal diet supports normal growth and development within calorie and nutrient guidelines.
- Because of varying rates of growth and activity, nutritional requirements are less precise for children and adolescents than they are for adults.
- Exclusive breastfeeding is recommended for the first 6 months of life. Breastfeeding should continue up to the age of 1 year.
- Iron-fortified infant formula is an acceptable alternative or supplement to breastfeeding. The biggest hazard of formula feeding is overfeeding.

- Adequacy of growth (height and weight) is the best indicator of whether or not an infant's intake is nutritionally adequate.
- Complementary foods should not be introduced before the infant is developmentally ready, usually around 6 months of age. The first food introduced should be a source of iron, such as baby food meat or iron-fortified infant cereal. New foods should be introduced one at a time for a period of at least 2 to 3 days so that any allergic reaction can be easily identified.
- Nutritional guidelines on how to achieve optimal nutritional intakes for toddlers do not exist. Infants and toddlers

are at low risk of nutrient deficiencies, yet their diets may already be beginning to be high in added sugars and fats and low in vegetables.

- The *2015-2020 Dietary Guidelines for Americans* are intended for all Americans age 2 years and older.
- Parents are the primary gatekeepers of their children's nutritional intake. They should make healthy foods available and not introduce foods into their children's diet that have no value other than calories.
- Children and adolescents who regularly eat family meals tend to have better quality eating patterns and eat more fruits and vegetables compared to youth who do not often eat family meals.
- Compared to food prepared at home, fast-food meals are lower in fruits, vegetables, whole grains, and dairy and provide more calories, fat, saturated fat, and sugar.
- The meal most likely to be skipped by youth is breakfast. Typically, breakfast eaters have lower intakes of fat and healthier levels of serum vitamin C and folate.
- In early childhood, the intake of dairy and fruit is high. However, among all age and ethnic groups, youth have poor overall diet quality that worsens as the child gets older.
- The food groups most likely to be consumed in inadequate amounts by children and adolescents are fruits, vegetables, whole grains, and dairy products, increasing their risk of inadequate intakes of calcium, potassium, vitamin D, and fiber.
- Poor diet quality—namely, low in nutrients and excessive in calories, saturated fat, sodium, and added sugar—increases the risk of early puberty, higher diastolic blood pressure, and maybe central obesity. Poor diet quality that begins in childhood often persists into adulthood.
- Overweight and obesity among youth are a major public health concern. Physical health risks include type 2 diabetes, coronary artery disease, dyslipidemia, hypertension, nonalcoholic fatty liver disease, gastroesophageal reflux disease, asthma, and obstructive sleep apnea. Psychological complications may also occur.

- Physical and psychological comorbidities in childhood and adolescence may continue into adulthood.
- The AAP recommends obesity prevention strategies begin before the age of 2 years. Recommendations include healthy maternal weight prior to conception, appropriate gestational weight gain, not smoking during pregnancy, breastfeeding, weaning to healthy foods, eliminating sedentary entertainment, active play, and parental role modeling.
- Lifestyle modification, namely, healthy eating, an increase in physical activity, a decrease in sedentary activity, and adequate sleep, is recommended to prevent and treat obesity in children and adolescents. Parents are urged to make the same changes to model healthy behaviors.
- Generally, the goal for overweight and obese children is to maintain weight while growing taller to improve BMI over time. Children and adolescents with comorbidities may require weight loss. The emphasis should be on healthy eating and increased activity, not weight.
- If lifestyle modification fails to improve BMI, a more structured approach including a low-calorie diet, supervised physical activity, less than 1 hour of screen time daily, and greater self-monitoring may be implemented.
- Even more intense treatment, such as pharmacotherapy and bariatric surgery may be considered when structured lifestyle modifications fail to produce improvements. Pharmacotherapy is generally reserved for obese adolescents or overweight adolescents with comorbidities. Bariatric surgery is considered only for severely obese adolescents who meet several other criteria. Long-term safety of these interventions is not known.
- Adolescents may have unhealthy eating habits, such as a high intake of sugar and inadequate intakes of iron and folate that increase their risk of poor pregnancy outcome.
- Pregnant adolescents should strive to gain 35 pounds during pregnancy.

Check Your Knowledge Answer Key

1 **TRUE** The amount of calories and protein needed per unit of body weight is greater for infants than for adults because growth in the first year of life is more rapid than at any other time in the life cycle (excluding the fetal period).

2 **TRUE** If breastfeeding is discontinued before the infant's first birthday, it should be replaced with iron-fortified infant formula. Cow's milk is not recommended before the age of 1 year.

3 **FALSE** Iron is the nutrient most needed when solids are introduced into the diet.

4 **TRUE** Overfeeding is a potential problem with early introduction of solid foods because young infants are unable to communicate satiety, the feeling of fullness.

5 **FALSE** To reduce the risk of allergy, it is recommended peanut products be introduced in the diet between 4 and 11 months of age in infants at high risk for allergy.

6 **FALSE** The *2015-2020 Dietary Guidelines for Americans* are intended for all healthy Americans over the age of 2 years.

7 **TRUE** Milk can displace the intake of iron-rich foods, increasing the risk of iron deficiency.

8 **TRUE** Children who regularly skip breakfast have lower intakes of vitamins and minerals than children who normally eat breakfast.

9 **TRUE** An overweight child is more likely to develop complications of adult overweight, such as diabetes, hypertension, and metabolic syndrome.

10 **TRUE** Like adults, children and adolescents underconsume potassium, vitamin D, calcium, and fiber because they do not eat enough fruits, vegetables, dairy, and whole grains.

Websites

American Academy of Pediatrics Institute for Healthy Childhood Weight at http://ihcw.aap.org provides obesity prevention and management and treatment resources Children's Nutrition Research Center at Baylor College of Medicine at www.bcm.edu/cnrc/

Choose MyPlate for food and nutrition recommendations based on the *Dietary Guidelines for Americans* at www.choosemyplate.gov

Healthychildren.org for dietary recommendations, parenting skills advice, etc. available at https://www.healthychildren.org

KidsHealth at www.kidshealth.org

Kids Eat Right at www.eatright.org/kids provides science-based resources for families

Let's Move at www.letsmove.gov provides links to many government and private efforts to raise a healthier generation of children

MyPlate Kid's Place at www.choosemyplate.gov/kids provides a variety of activities and resources

Nutri-eSTEP nutrition screen designed to screen toddlers 18 to 35 months and preschoolers 3 to 5 years available at www.nutritionscreen.ca

We Can! at http://www.nhlbi.nih.gov/health/educational/wecan/ contains dietary recommendations, physical activity recommendations, and monitoring tools

References

Abrams, S. (2015). Is it time to put a moratorium on new infant formulas that are not adequately investigated? *The Journal of Pediatrics, 166,* 756–760.

Adolphus, K., Lawton, C., & Dye, L. (2013). The effects of breakfast on behavior and academic performance in children and adolescents. *Frontiers in Human Neuroscience, 7,* 425.

American Academy of Pediatrics. (2012a). Policy statement: Breastfeeding and the use of human milk. *Pediatrics, 129,* e827–e841.

American Academy of Pediatrics. (2012b). Starting solid foods. Available at https://www.healthychildren.org/English/ages-stages/baby/feeding-nutrition/Pages/Switching-To-Solid-Foods.aspx. Accessed on 4/14/16.

American Academy of Pediatrics. (2014). Nutritional needs of the preterm infant. In R. Kleinman & F. Greer (Eds.), *Pediatric nutrition handbook* (pp. 79–112). Elk Grove Village, IL: Author.

American Academy of Pediatrics. (2015a). Fruit juice and your child's diet. Available at https://www.healthychildren.org/English/healthy-living/nutrition/Pages/Fruit-Juice-and-Your-Childs-Diet.aspx. Accessed on 4/16/16.

American Academy of Pediatrics. (2015b). Peanut allergies: What you should know about the latest research. Available at https://healthychildren.org/English/health-issues/conditions/allergies-asthma/Pages/Peanut-Allergies-What-You-Should-Know-About-the-Latest-Research.aspx. Accessed on 4/23/16.

August, G., Caprio, S., Fennoy, I., Freemark, M., Kaufman, F. R., Lustig, R. H., . . . Montori, V. M. (2008). Prevention and treatment of pediatric obesity: an endocrine society clinical practice guideline based on expert opinion. *The Journal of Clinical Endocrinology and Metabolism, 93,* 4576–4599. doi:10.1210/jc.2007-2458

Baird, J., Fisher, D., Lucas, P., Kleijnen, J., Roberts, H., & Law, C. (2005). Being big or growing fast: Systematic review of size and growth in infancy and later obesity. *BMJ, 331,* 929. doi:10.1136/bmj.38586.411273.EO

Baker, P., Wheeler, S., Sanders, T., Thomas, J. E., Hutchinson, C. J., Clarke, K., . . . Poston, L. (2009). A prospective study of micronutrient status in adolescent pregnancy. *The American Journal of Clinical Nutrition, 89,* 1114–1124.

Banfield, E., Liu, Y., Davis, J., Chang, S., & Frazier-Wood, A. (2016). Poor adherence to US dietary guidelines for children and adolescents in the National Health and Nutrition Examination Survey population. *Journal of the Academy of Nutrition and Dietetics, 116,* 21–27.

Barlow, S. (2007). Expert committee recommendations regarding the prevention, assessment, and treatment of child and adolescent overweight and obesity: Summary report. *Pediatrics, 120*(Suppl. 4), S164–S192.

Bhattacharya, J., Currie, J., & Haider, S. (2006). Breakfast of champions? The school breakfast program and the nutrition of children and families. *Journal of Human Resources, 41,* 445–466.

Birch, L. (1999). Development of food preferences. *Annual Review of Nutrition, 19,* 41–62.

Biro, F., & Wien, M. (2010). Childhood obesity and adult morbidities. *The American Journal of Clinical Nutrition, 91,* 1499S–1505S.

Brisbios, R., Farmer, A., & McGarga, L. (2012). Early markers of adult obesity: A review. *Obesity Reviews, 13,* 347–367.

Burris, J., Rietkerk, W., & Woolf, K. (2014). Relationships of self-reported dietary factors and perceived acne severity in a cohort of New York young adults. *Journal of the Academy of Nutrition and Dietetics, 114,* 384–392.

Centers for Disease Control and Prevention. (2015a). Prevalence of childhood obesity in the United States, 2011-2012. Available at http://www.cdc.gov/obesity/data/childhood.html. Accessed on 4/11/16.

Centers for Disease Control and Prevention. (2015b). Smoking, pregnancy, and babies. Available at http://www.cdc.gov/tobacco/campaign/tips/diseases/pregnancy.html. Accessed on 4/18/16.

Chanoine, J., Hampl, S., Jensen, C., Boldrin, M., & Hauptman, J. (2005). Effect of orlistat on weight and body composition in obese adolescents: A randomized controlled trial. *JAMA, 293,* 2873–2883.

Cheng, G., Gerlach, S., Libuda, L., Kranz, S., Günther, A. L., Karaolis-Danckert, N., . . . Buyken, A. E. (2010). Diet quality in childhood is prospectively associated with the timing of puberty but not with body composition at puberty onset. *The Journal of Nutrition, 140,* 95–102.

Claire Wang, Y., Gortmaker, S., & Taveras, E. (2011). Trends and racial/ethnic disparities in severe obesity among US children and adolescents, 1976-2006. *International Journal of Pediatric Obesity, 6,* 12–20.

Crosnoe, R. (2007). Gender, obesity, and education. *Sociology of Education, 80,* 241–260.

Daniels, S., & Hassink, S. (2015). The role of the pediatrician in primary prevention of obesity. *Pediatrics, 136,* e275. doi:10.1542/peds.2015.1558

Dattilo, A., Birch, L., Krebs, N., Lake, A., Taveras, E. M., & Saavedra, J. M. (2012). Need for early interventions in the prevention of pediatric overweight: A review and upcoming directions. *Journal of Obesity, 2012,* 123023. doi:10.1155/2012/123023

Davis, A., Gallagher, K., Taylor, M., Canter, K., Gillette, M. D., Wambach, K., & Nelson, E. L. (2013). An in-home intervention to improve nutrition, physical activity and knowledge among low-income teen mothers and their children: Results from a pilot study. *Journal of Developmental and Behavioral Pediatrics, 34*(8), 609–615. doi:10.1097/DBP.Ob013e3182a509df

Dietary Guidelines Advisory Committee. (2015). Scientific report of the 2015 Dietary Guidelines Advisory Committee. Part A. Executive summary. Available at http://health.gov/dietaryguidelines/2015-scientific-report/02-executive-summary.asp. Accessed on 9/22/16.

Epstein, J., Paluch, R., Roemmich, J., & Beecher, M. (2007). Family-based obesity treatment, then and now: Twenty-five years of pediatric obesity treatment. *Health Psychology, 26*, 381–391.

Freedman, D., Khan, L., Serdula, M., Dietz, W. H., Srinivasan, S. R., & Berenson, G. S. (2005). The relation of childhood BMI to adult adiposity: The Bogalusa Heart Study. *Pediatrics, 115*, 22–27.

Gillman, M. (2011). Commentary: Breastfeeding and obesity—the 2011 scorecard. *International Journal of Epidemiology, 40*, 681–684.

Golden, N., Schneider, M., & Wood, C. (2016). Preventing obesity and eating disorders in adolescents. *Pediatrics, 138*(3), e20161649.

Grote, V., Schiess, S., Closa-Monasterolo, R., Escribano, J., Giovannini, M., Scaglioni, S., . . . Koletzko, B. (2011). The introduction of solid food and growth in the first 2 y of life in formula-fed children: Analysis of data from a European cohort study. *The American Journal of Clinical Nutrition, 94*(6 Suppl.), 1785S–1793S.

Hoelscher, D., Kirk, S., Ritchie, L., & Cunningham-Sabo, L. (2013). Position of the Academy of Nutrition and Dietetics: Interventions for the prevention and treatment of pediatric overweight and obesity. *Journal of the Academy of Nutrition and Dietetics, 113*, 1375–1394.

Hsia, D., Fallon, S., & Brandt, M. (2012). Adolescent bariatric surgery. *Archives of Pediatrics & Adolescent Medicine, 166*, 757–766.

Inge, T., King, W., Jenkins, T., Courcoulas, A. P., Mitsnefes, M., Flum, D. R., . . . Daniels, S. R. (2013). The effect of obesity in adolescence on adult health status. *Pediatrics, 132*, 1098–1104.

Keating, C., Moodie, M., & Swinburn, B. (2011). The health-related quality of life of overweight and obese adolescents—a study measuring body mass index and adolescent-reported perceptions. *International Journal of Pediatric Obesity, 6*, 434–441.

Kelly, A., Barlow, S., Rao, G., Inge, T., Hayman, L. L., Steinberger, J., . . . Daniels, S. R. (2013). Severe obesity in children and adolescents: Identification, associated health risks, and treatment approaches: A scientific statement from the American Heart Association. *Circulation, 128*, 1689–1712.

Koletzko, B., von Kries, R., Closa, R., Escribano, J., Scaglioni S, Giovannini M., . . . Grote, V. (2009). Lower protein in infant formula is associated with lower weight up to age 2 y: A randomized clinical trial. *The American Journal of Clinical Nutrition, 89*, 1836–1845.

Kramer, M., Guo, T., Platt, R., Vanilovich, I., Sevkovskaya Z., Dzikovich, I., . . . Dewey, K. (2004). Feeding effects on growth during infancy. *The Journal of Pediatrics, 145*, 600–605.

Li, C., Ford, E., Zhao, G., & Mokdad, A. (2009). Prevalence of pre-diabetes and its association with clustering of cardiometabolic risk factors and hyperinsulinemia among U.S. adolescents: National Health and Nutrition Examination Survey 2005-2006. *Diabetes Care, 32*, 342–347.

Li, R., Magalia, J., Fein, S., & Grummer-Strawn, L. (2012). Risk of bottle-feeding for rapid weight gain during the first year of life. *Archives of Pediatrics & Adolescent Medicine, 166*, 421–436.

Lobstein, T., Jackson-Leach, R., Moodie, M., Hall, K., Gortmaker, S. L., Swinburn, B. A., . . . McPherson, K. (2015). Child and adolescent obesity: Part of a bigger picture. *Lancet, 385*, 2510–2520.

Lumeng, J., Taveras, E., Birch, L., & Yanovski, S. (2015). Prevention of obesity in infancy and early childhood: A National Institutes of Health workshop. *JAMA Pediatrics, 169*, 484–490.

Maes, H., Neale, M., & Eaves, L. (1997). Genetic and environmental factors in relative body weight and human adiposity. *Behavior Genetics, 27*, 325–351.

Marrodán, M., López-Ejeda, N., González-Montero de Espinosa, M., Martínez-Alvarez, J., Carmenate, M., Cabañas, M., . . . Romero-Collazos, J. F. (2013). High blood pressure and diet quality in the Spanish childhood populations. *Journal of Hypertension, 2*(2). doi:10.4172/2167-1095.1000115

Martin, J. A., Hamilton, B. E., Osterman, J. K., Curtin, S. C., & Mathews, T. J. (2013). Births: Final data for 2012. *National Vital Statistics Reports, 62*(9). Hyattsville, MD: National Center for Health Statistics. Available at http://www.cdc.gov/nchs/data/nvsr/nvsr62/nvsr62_09.pdf. Accessed on 4/18/16.

Martin, R., Patel, R., Kramer, M., Guthrie, L., Vilchuck, K., Bogdanovich, N., . . . Oken, E. (2013). Effects of promoting longer-term and exclusive breastfeeding on adiposity and insulin-like growth factor-I at age 11.5 years: A randomized trial. *JAMA, 309*, 1005–1013.

Mathews, T. J., & MacDorman, M. F. (2013). Infant mortality statistics from the 2010 period linked birth/infant death data set. *National Vital Statistics Reports, 62*(8). Hyattsville, MD: National Center for Health Statistics. Available at http://www.cdc.gov/nchs/data/nvsr/nvsr62/nvsr62_08.pdf. Accessed on 4/18/16.

May, A., & Dietz, W. (2010). The Feeding Infants and Toddlers Study 2008: Opportunities to assess parental, cultural, and environmental influences on dietary behaviors and obesity prevention among young children. *Journal of the American Dietetic Association, 110*, S11–S15.

Michaelsen, K., & Greer, F. (2014). Protein needs early in life and long-term health. *The American Journal of Clinical Nutrition, 99*(3), 718S–722S.

Michalsky, M., Reichard, K., Inge, T., Pratt, J., & Lenders, C. (2012). ASMBS pediatric committee best practice guidelines. *Surgery for Obesity and Related Diseases, 8*, 1–7.

Nielsen, J. N., Gittelsohn, J., Anliker, J., & O'Brien, K. (2006). Interventions to improve diet and weight gain among pregnant adolescents and recommendations for future research. *Journal of the American Dietetic Association, 106*, 1825–1840.

Ogata, B., & Hayes, D. (2014). Position of the Academy of Nutrition and Dietetics: Nutrition guidance for healthy children ages 2 to 11 years. *Journal of the Academy of Nutrition and Dietetics, 114*, 1257–1276,

Ogden, C., Carroll, M., Kit, B., & Flegal, K. (2014). Prevalence of childhood and adult obesity in the United States, 2011-2012. *JAMA, 311*, 806–814.

Pearson, N., Biddle, S., & Gorely, T. (2009). Family correlates of breakfast consumption among children and adolescents. A systematic review. *Appetite, 52*, 1–7.

Perrin, E., Rothman, R., Sanders, L., Skinner, A., Eden, S. K., Shintani, A., . . . Yin, H. S. (2014). Racial and ethnic differences associated with feeding-and activity-related behaviors in infants. *Pediatrics, 133*, e857–e867.

Pileggi, C., Lotito, F., Bianco, A., Nobile, C., & Pavia, M. (2013). Relationship between chronic short sleep duration and childhood body mass index: A school-based cross-sectional study. *PLoS One, 3*, e66680.

Powell, L., & Nguyen, B. (2013). Fast-food and full-service restaurant consumption among children and adolescents: Effect on energy, beverage, and nutrient intake. *JAMA Pediatrics, 167*, 14–20.

Pulgarón, E. (2013). Childhood obesity: A review of increased risk for physical and psychological comorbidities. *Clinical Therapeutics, 35*, A18–A32. doi:10.1016/j.clinthera.2012.12.014

Rasmussen, K. M., & Yaktine, A. L. (2009). *Weight gain during pregnancy: Reexamining the guidelines*. Washington, DC: The National Academies Press.

Reedy, J., & Krebs-Smith, S. (2010). Dietary sources of energy, solid fats, and added sugars among children and adolescents in the United States. *Journal of the American Dietetic Association, 110*, 1477–1484.

Robinson, S., Crozier, S., Harvey, N., Barton, B., Law, C. M., Godfrey, K. M., . . . Inskip, H. M. (2015). Modifiable early-life risk factors for childhood adiposity and overweight: An analysis of their combined impact and potential for prevention. *The American Journal of Clinical Nutrition, 101*, 368–375.

Romirowsky, A., Kushner, M., Elliot, C., Nadler, E., & Mackey, E. (2015). Evidence-based psychological interventions to support an adolescent undergoing bariatric surgery: A case report. *Clinical Practice in Pediatric Psychology, 3*, 71–79.

Rosenkranz, R., & Dzewaltowski, D. (2008). Model of the home food environment pertaining to childhood obesity. *Nutrition Reviews, 66*, 123–140.

Skinner, J., Carruth, B., Wendy, B., & Ziegler, P. (2002). Children's food preferences: A longitudinal analysis. *Journal of the American Dietetic Association, 102*, 1638–1647.

Stam, J., Sauer, P., & Boehm, G. (2013). Can we define an infant's need from the composition of human milk? *The American Journal of Clinical Nutrition, 98*(2), 521S–528S.

Tirosh, A., Shai, I., Afek, A., Dubnov-Raz, G., Ayalon, N., Gordon, B., . . . Rudich, A. (2011). Adolescent BMI trajectory and risk of diabetes versus coronary disease. *The New England Journal of Medicine, 364*, 1315–1325.

U.S. Department of Agriculture, Agricultural Research Service. (2014). Nutrient intakes from food and beverages: Mean amounts consumed per individual, by gender and age. What We Eat in America, NHANES 2011–2012. Available at www.ars.usda.gov/ba/bhnrc/fsrg. Accessed on 1/22/16.

U.S. Department of Health and Human Services & U.S. Department of Agriculture. (2015). 2015-2020 Dietary guidelines for Americans (8th ed.). Available at http://health.gov/dietaryguidelines/2015/guidelines/ Accessed on 4/14/16.

Vauthier, J., Lluch, A., Lecomte, E., Artur, Y., & Herbeth, B. (1996). Family resemblance in energy and macronutrient intakes: The Stanislas Family Study. *International Journal of Epidemiology, 25*, 1030–1037.

Wake, M., Clifford, S., Lycett, K., Jachno, K., Sabin, M. A., Baldwin, S., & Carlin, J. (2015). Natural BMI reductions and overestimation of obesity trial effectiveness. *Pediatrics, 135*, e292–e295. doi:10.1542/peds.2014-1832

Weber, M., Grote, V., Closa-Monasterolo, R., Escribano, J., Langhendries, J. P., Dain, E., . . . Koletzko, B. (2014). Lower protein content in infant formula reduces BMI and obesity risk at school age: Follow-up of a randomized trial. *The American Journal of Clinical Nutrition, 99*, 1041–1051.

Chapter 13

Nutrition for Older Adults

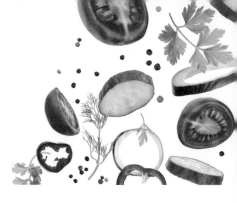

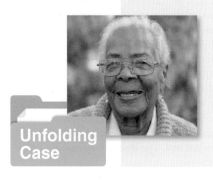

Unfolding Case

Clara Wellington

Clara, 74 years old, lives alone in her own home. A home health aide visits 2 hours per week to help Clara with light housekeeping. Clara is relatively healthy. Her only medication is an occasional antacid for gastroesophageal reflux disease. She is 5 ft 5 in, and for all of her adult life, she has weighed 135 pounds, giving her a body mass index (BMI) of 22.5. At her most recent doctor visit, she was down 7 pounds from the previous visit 6 months ago.

Check Your Knowledge

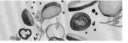

True	False		
☐	☐	1	It is too late to reap health benefits of a healthy eating pattern when it is not adopted until midlife.
☐	☐	2	In general, calorie needs in older adults decrease while the need for other nutrients stays the same or increases.
☐	☐	3	Older adults may not feel thirsty even when they are becoming dehydrated.
☐	☐	4	Older adults should get vitamin B_{12} from supplements or fortified foods.
☐	☐	5	Older adults generally do not consume enough iron.
☐	☐	6	Sarcopenia is inevitable and irreversible.
☐	☐	7	Obesity in older adults is not a health risk.
☐	☐	8	Older adults may need more protein than the current RDA for protein.
☐	☐	9	Calorie and protein supplements may help reverse frailty.
☐	☐	10	A key risk factor for malnutrition in older adults is loss of appetite.

Learning Objectives

Upon completion of this chapter, you will be able to

1 Give examples of physiologic changes that occur with aging and that have an impact on nutrition.
2 Compare calorie and nutrient needs of older adults to those of younger adults.
3 Compare modified MyPlate for Older Adults with MyPlate for younger adults.
4 Explain why older adults may need supplements of calcium, vitamin D, and vitamin B_{12}.
5 Discuss risk factors for malnutrition in older adults.
6 Debate the benefits of using a liberal diet in long-term care facilities.
7 Propose strategies for enhancing food intake in long-term care residents.

The population of adults age 65 years and older is increasing at a faster rate than the under 65 years population of adults (U.S. Department of Health and Human Services [USDHHS], Administration on Aging [AOA], 2014). Not only is the older population increasing, it is also getting increasingly older. In 2013, an estimated 44.7 million people, or 14.1% of the population, were age 65 years and over; more than 67,000 of this group were over the age of 100 years (USDHHS, AOA, 2014). Despite the misconceptions and stereotypes people have of older adults, they are a heterogeneous group that varies in age, marital status, social background, financial status, health status, and living arrangements.

With the exception of Chapter 11 (pregnancy and lactation) and Chapter 12, (infants, children, and adolescents), this book implicitly addresses nutrition as it pertains to adults. Yet, adulthood represents a wide age range, from young adults at 18 years to the "oldest old." Adults over 50 years, and especially those over 70 years, have different nutritional needs and concerns than do younger adults. This chapter focuses on how aging affects nutrition for older adults.

AGING AND OLDER ADULTS

Aging is a gradual, inevitable, complex process of progressive physiologic, cellular, cultural, and psychosocial changes that begin at conception and end at death. As cells age, they undergo degenerative changes in structure and function that eventually lead to impairment of organs, tissues, and body functioning. Changes that may occur with aging are listed in Box 13.1; selected changes are presented in the following sections.

Changes in Body Composition

In general, aging causes a loss of bone and muscle and an increase in body fat due in part to hormonal changes that regulate metabolism. For instance, a decrease in growth hormone and

---

BOX 13.1 Changes that May Occur with Aging

Composition and Energy Expenditure Changes

- Decrease in lean body mass
- Decrease in basal metabolic rate
- Increase in fat tissue
- Decrease in physical activity

Oral and Gastrointestinal Changes

- Difficulty in chewing related to loss of teeth and periodontal disease
- Constipation is more common and may be related to decreased peristalsis from loss of abdominal muscle tone, inadequate fluid and fiber intake, secondary reaction to drug therapy, or a decrease in physical activity.
- Digestive disorders may occur from a decreased secretion of hydrochloric acid (HCl) in the stomach and digestive enzymes, decreased GI motility, and decreased organ function.
- Prevalence of atrophic gastritis increases
- Nutrient absorption may decrease because of decreased mucosal mass and decreased blood flow to and from the mucosal villi.

Metabolic Changes

- Altered glucose tolerance; the underlying reason may be a decrease in insulin secretion or a decrease in tissue sensitivity to insulin.
- Synthesis of vitamin D in the skin decreases with age.

Central Nervous System Changes

- Tremors, slowed reaction time, short-term memory deficits, personality changes, and depression may occur secondary to a decrease in the number of brain cells or the decrease in blood flow to the brain.

Renal Changes

- Ability to concentrate urine decreases

Sensory Losses

- Hearing loss, loss of visual acuity, decreased sense of smell, decreased number of taste buds, and decreased sensation of thirst

Other Changes

- Change in income related to retirement
- Reliance on medications
- Social isolation related to death of spouse, living alone, impaired mobility
- Poor self-esteem related to change in body image, lack of productivity, feelings of aimlessness

androgens contributes to the loss of lean body mass and insulin resistance reduces the ability to use protein. Prolactin, a hormone that helps maintain body fat, increases with age. These changes in body composition are one of the reasons why calorie needs decrease with aging.

Progressive loss of muscle mass is a common feature of aging (Paddon-Jones et al., 2015). Physiologic and behavioral changes account for the 1% to 2% annual loss of muscle mass that begins around the age of 50 years. Because the reserve of muscle mass is large, function is not impaired. In the early 60s, a person's loss of muscle becomes evident as muscle strength declines an average of 3% per year. An estimated 20% to 40% of muscle strength may be lost by the time a person reaches the 70s. Acute or chronic illness and inactivity—alone or in combination with malnutrition or inadequate protein intake—hastens the loss of lean body mass and functionality (English & Paddon-Jones, 2010).

Sarcopenia
the loss of skeletal muscle mass, strength, and function that occurs with aging.

Sarcopenia occurs when age-related loss of skeletal muscle mass is accompanied by loss of muscle strength and function; it is a main determinant of disability and mortality (Manini & Clark, 2012). Advanced sarcopenia is characterized by physical frailty, increased likelihood of falls, impaired ability to perform activities of daily living, and diminished quality of life (Paddon-Jones, Short, Campbell, Volpi, & Wolfe, 2008). Sarcopenia is estimated to affect 8% to 40% of adults over the age of 60 years and approximately 50% of those over the age of 75 years (Berger & Doherty, 2010). Sarcopenia should be considered in all older adults with observed declines in physical function, strength, or overall health and especially in older adults who are bedridden, who cannot rise independently from a chair, or who have a slow gait (Evans, 2010).

Decreased Appetite

Older adults exhibit less hunger and earlier satiety than younger adults (Bernstein & Munoz, 2012). Among the possible causes of diminished appetite are a decrease in physical activity, decrease in metabolic rate, a decrease in gastrointestinal (GI) hormone secretions, delayed gastric emptying, social isolation, cognitive impairments, medication side effects, and impaired chewing or swallowing. Diminished appetite contributes to undernutrition in both community and institutional settings and can lead to unintentional weight loss, which is often associated with poor health outcomes and is a marker for deteriorating well-being in older adults (Bernstein & Munoz, 2012).

Functional Limitations

Activities of Daily Living (ADLs)
bathing, dressing, eating, and getting around the house, and using the toilet.

Instrumental Activities of Daily Living (IADLs)
using the telephone, doing housework, preparing meals, shopping, managing money, and taking medication.

A decrease in muscle mass and strength can lead to a progressive decline in physical function. Among community-resident Medicare beneficiaries 65 years and older in 2013, 33% had difficulty performing one or more **activities of daily living (ADLs)** and an additional 12% reported difficulty with one or more **instrumental activities of daily living (IADLs)** (USDHHS, AOA, 2014). Functional limitations may impair the ability to eat or prepare or shop for food. Chronic diseases that increase the risk of functional limitations include cerebrovascular accident, diabetes, ischemic heart disease, and arthritis (Bernstein & Munoz, 2012).

Immune System Changes

With aging, levels of inflammatory mediators typically increase, even in the absence of acute infection or other physiologic stress (Szarc vel Szic, Declerck, Vidaković, & Vanden Berghe, 2015). "Inflammaging" is the term used to describe the phenomenon of chronic, systemic low-grade inflammation that is characteristic of aging (Franceschi & Campisi, 2014). Many age-related chronic diseases are low-lying inflammatory states, such as cardiovascular disease, chronic obstructive pulmonary disease, congestive heart failure, diabetes, metabolic syndrome, and obesity (Malone & Hamilton, 2013). Inflammaging is a significant risk factor for morbidity and mortality in older people (Franceschi, 2007). Among the potential strategies that may prevent or cure inflammaging and its pathologies are a healthy lifestyle, namely, age-appropriate exercise and a healthy eating pattern that includes pro- and prebiotics (Franceschi & Campisi, 2014).

Psychosocial Changes

Loss of a spouse, difficulty ambulating, and sensory impairments such as loss of vision or hearing are factors that contribute to social isolation. Eating alone is a risk factor for poor nutritional status among older adults, especially among men. Food choices are not necessarily poor; rather, it is the quantity of food consumed that is often inadequate.

Depression is not a normal consequence of aging but occurs in many older adults. As many as 5% of community-dwelling older adults meet the diagnostic criteria for major depression and up to 15% have clinically significant symptoms of depression that interfere with functioning (Hybels & Blazer, 2003). The prevalence of depression is even higher among older adults with medical illnesses. Weight loss or gain is among the many symptoms of depression.

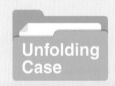

Recall Clara. A history, physical exam, and lab tests fail to find an underlying pathology for her weight loss. When questioned about her usual food intake, Clara admits that she has lost interest in cooking and shopping and that her appetite isn't what it used to be. Her family reveals that her intake has decreased, as evidenced by the spoiled food they find in her refrigerator and out of date items in her pantry. What percentage of weight has Clara lost over the last 6 months? What is an appropriate intervention to recommend at this point?

Polypharmacy

A study of community-dwelling older adults found that 51% reported using five or more medications daily (Heuberger & Caudell, 2011). Medications can cause side effects that interfere with intake, such as changes in taste and smell, dry mouth, early satiety, anorexia, and GI upset. Polypharmacy in older adults is associated with a decrease in walking speed, disability, mortality, cognitive decline, and delirium (Husson et al., 2014). Nutritionally, an inverse relationship has been observed between the number of medications used and the intakes of fiber, fat-soluble vitamins, B vitamins, and minerals; a positive relationship was noted for the intake of cholesterol, carbohydrate, and sodium (Heuberger & Caudell, 2011).

HEALTHY AGING

Genetic and environmental "life advantages"—such as genetic potential for longevity, intelligence, motivation, curiosity, good socialization, religious affiliation, marriage and family, avoidance of substance abuse, availability of health care, adequate sleep, and sufficient rest and relaxation—have positive effects on both length and quality of life. Although there is no universally agreed upon definition of healthy or successful aging, a major study used the following as its criteria: no major chronic diseases, no cognitive impairment, no physical disabilities, and no mental health limitations (Sun et al., 2009). Healthy lifestyle behaviors—being physically active, eating healthy, maintaining healthy weight, and not smoking—may help prevent or delay physical and mental deteriorations associated with aging (Bernstein & Munoz, 2012).

Physical Activity

Older adults are urged to follow the adult guidelines for physical activity or as their abilities allow (Box 13.2). Strong evidence shows that for adults and older adults, physical activity lowers the risk of heart disease, stroke, type 2 diabetes, hypertension, dyslipidemia, metabolic syndrome,

BOX 13.2   Physical Activity Guidelines for Americans Age 65 Years and Older

For important health benefits, adults need at least

- Two hours and 30 minutes a week of moderate intensity or 1 hour and 15 minutes (75 minutes) a week of vigorous-intensity aerobic physical activity, or an equivalent combination of moderate- and vigorous-intensity aerobic physical activity and
- Muscle strengthening activities that work all major muscle groups (legs, hips, back, abdomen, chest, shoulders, arms) performed on 2 or more days per week

For even greater health benefits, older adults should increase their activity to

- Five hours (300 minutes) a week of moderate-intensity aerobic physical activity, or 2 hours and 30 minutes a week of vigorous-intensity physical activity, or an equivalent combination of both and
- Muscle-strengthening activities that work all major muscle groups (legs, hips, back, abdomen, chest, shoulders, arms) performed on 2 or more days per week

Additional points:

- Physical activity is safe for almost everyone and the health benefits of physical activity far outweigh the risks.
- People without diagnosed chronic conditions (e.g., diabetes, heart disease, or osteoarthritis) and who do not have symptoms (e.g., chest pain or pressure, dizziness, or joint pain) do not need to consult with a health-care provider about physical activity. If the given recommendations are not possible due to limiting chronic conditions, older adults should be as physically active as their abilities allow. For all individuals, some activity is better than none.
- Older adults should do exercises that maintain or improve balance if they are at risk of falling.

Sources: Centers for Disease Control and Prevention. (2015). *How much physical activity do older adults need?* Available at http://www.cdc.gov/physicalactivity/basics/older_adults/index.htm. Accessed on 4/25/16; U.S. Department of Health and Human Services. (2008). *Physical activity guidelines for Americans. At-a-glance: A fact sheet for professionals.* Available at http://health.gov/paguidelines/factsheetprof.aspx. Accessed on 4/25/16.

and weight gain in addition to improving cardiovascular and muscular fitness, preventing falls, reducing depression, and improving cognitive function (USDHHS, 2008).

Healthy Eating

Healthy eating can enhance wellness, improve nutritional status, reduce the risk of chronic disease, help manage chronic disease, and help maintain energy levels. Although a lifetime of healthy eating is optimal, adopting a healthy eating pattern even in later life has health benefits. A study among women who began a Mediterranean-style eating pattern in their 50s and 60s found they had a 40% greater chance of living beyond 70 years with greater health and well-being (Samieri et al., 2013).

Dietary Guidelines for Americans

The *Dietary Guidelines for Americans* are intended to help all people age 2 years and older, including older adults, choose healthier eating plans to support a healthy body weight and help prevent and reduce the risk of chronic disease throughout the life span (USDHHS & U.S. Department of Agriculture [USDA], 2015a) (see Chapter 8). The key recommendations are to

- Consume a calorie-appropriate healthy eating pattern
- Eat more vegetables, fruits, whole grains, lean protein foods, and low-fat or fat-free dairy
- Choose foods low in added sugars and saturated fats
- Limit sodium to 2300 mg
- Drink alcohol only in moderation

Older adults, like the general population, consume too much added sugar, saturated fat, and sodium. Also consistent with the U.S. population as a whole, adults aged 50 years and older underconsume vegetables, fruits, whole grains, seafood, dairy, and oils (USDHHS & USDA, 2015b). Low intakes of these groups are to blame for the overall low intakes of potassium, fiber,

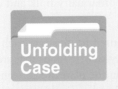

Unfolding Case

Consider Clara. She lives alone, has lost weight, and has lost interest in preparing food. She tried going to the senior center for noon time meals but told her family she "quit" because they give her food she doesn't like—too much meat, milk, and vegetables and not enough sweets. She also got lost driving there one day and fears she may be developing dementia. She agrees to more extensive help in the home. What criteria should the in-home health aide be monitoring regarding Clara's intake? What suggestions would you give the aide to promote Clara's intake?

calcium, and vitamin D—the nutrients of public health concern. Women age 50 years and older and men age 71 years and older may also underconsume the protein group.

MyPlate

MyPlate for Older Adults, produced by Tufts University, is designed to help healthy, older adults who are living independently choose an eating pattern that reflects the *2015-2020 Dietary Guidelines for Americans* (Fig. 13.1). The graphic features a variety of colorful fruits and vegetables,

MyPlate for Older Adults

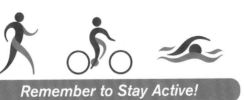

Fruits & Vegetables

Whole fruits and vegetables are rich in important nutrients and fiber. Choose fruits and vegetables with deeply colored flesh. Choose canned varieties that are packed in their own juices or low-sodium.

Healthy Oils

Liquid vegetable oils and soft margarines provide important fatty acids and some fat-soluble vitamins.

Herbs & Spices

Use a variety of herbs and spices to enhance flavor of foods and reduce the need to add salt.

Fluids

Drink plenty of fluids. Fluids can come from water, tea, coffee, soups, and fruits and vegetables.

Grains

Whole grain and fortified foods are good sources of fiber and B vitamins.

Dairy

Fat-free and low-fat milk, cheeses and yogurts provide protein, calcium and other important nutrients.

Protein

Protein rich foods provide many important nutrients. Choose a variety including nuts, beans, fish, lean meat and poultry.

Remember to Stay Active!

 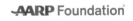

Figure 13.1 ▲ **MyPlate for Older Adults.** (*Source: Copyright © 2016 Tufts University. For details about the MyPlate for Older Adults, please see http://hnrca.tufts.edu/myplate/files/MPFOA2015.pdf.*)

whole and fortified grains, low-fat and nonfat dairy milk and dairy products, lean proteins, and oils. Noteworthy features are as follows:

- Nutrient-dense food choices are used to illustrate each food group. As calorie needs decrease, there is less room for empty-calorie foods that are high in solid fats or added sugar.
- The examples of foods featured on the plate are convenient, affordable, and readily available. For instance, frozen broccoli and canned legumes are shown because they are easy to prepare and have a long shelf life.
- Low-sodium canned vegetables appear as an option to help lower sodium intake.
- A variety of beverages are featured next to the plate to highlight the importance of adequate fluid intake.
- The use of herbs and spices is recommended to enhance flavors and reduce the use of salt.
- Older adults engaged in common activities appear in an icon on the bottom of the placemat as a reminder that there are a variety of options for engaging in physical activity.

Frequently, food choices of older adults are based on considerations other than food preferences, such as income; the individual's physical ability to shop, prepare, chew, and swallow food; and the occurrence of food intolerances related to chronic disease or side effects of medication. Box 13.3 features tips for eating well for the older adult.

NUTRITIONAL NEEDS OF OLDER ADULTS

Although the healthy eating patterns recommended by the *Dietary Guidelines* and illustrated in MyPlate are appropriate for older Americans, actual nutrient needs among older adults may differ from those of younger people due to changes in metabolic processes, physical functioning, body composition, and nutrient absorption and other factors such as frailty, comorbidities, and polypharmacy (Bolzetta et al., 2015). Health status, physiologic functioning, physical activity, and nutritional status vary more among older adults (especially people older than 70 years) than among individuals in any other age group, so nutrient recommendations may not be appropriate for all older adults at all times.

Calories

Calorie recommendations decrease with aging related to the typical decrease in physical activity and the changes in body composition that lower metabolic rate (Fig. 13.2). As with other age groups, individual variations in activity exist. Compared to younger adults, older adults need fewer calories yet generally have the same or higher requirements for vitamins and minerals, making the concept of nutrient density even more important.

Protein

The Recommended Dietary Allowance (RDA) for protein remains constant at 0.8 g/kg for both sedentary and physically active men and women from the age of 19 years on (Institute of Medicine, 2005a). This level represents the minimum protein intake necessary to avoid progressive loss of **lean body mass** as determined by nitrogen balance studies (Wolfe, Miller, & Miller, 2008). However, the data were gathered almost entirely in college-aged men who can maintain nitrogen balance on less protein than can older adults (Wolfe et al., 2008). This one-size-fits-all protein recommendation does not consider age-related changes in metabolism, immunity, hormone levels, or progressing frailty (Bauer et al., 2013).

Lean Body Mass
all body components except stored fat; the fat-free mass of the body.

A protein intake greater than the RDA has been shown to improve muscle mass, strength, and function in older adults and may also improve immune status, wound healing, blood pressure, and bone health (Wolfe et al., 2008). One reason why older adults need more protein than younger adults is that they have a declining anabolic response to protein intake; that is, their threshold for the amount of protein needed to stimulate protein synthesis is higher. Protein need may be higher in response to the inflammatory and catabolic impact of chronic and acute diseases that commonly occur with aging (Walrand, Guillet, Salles, Cano, & Boirie, 2011). Paradoxically, although older adults

BOX 13.3   Tips for Eating Well As You Get Older

Enjoy Your Meals

Eating is one of life's pleasures, but some people lose interest in eating and cooking as they get older. They may find that food no longer tastes good. They may find it harder to shop for food or cook, or they don't enjoy meals because they often eat alone. Others may have problems chewing or digesting the food they eat.

Why Not Eating Can Be Harmful

If you don't feel like eating because of problems with chewing, digestion, or gas, talk with your doctor or a registered dietitian. Avoiding some foods could mean you miss out on needed vitamins, minerals, fiber, or protein. Not eating enough could mean that you don't consume enough nutrients and calories.

Problems with Taste or Smell?

One reason people lose interest in eating is that their senses of taste and smell change with age. Foods you once enjoyed might seem to have less flavor when you get older. Some medicines can change your sense of taste or make you feel less hungry. Talk with your health-care provider if you have no appetite, or if you find that food tastes bad or has no flavor.

If you don't feel like eating because food no longer tastes good, you can enhance the flavor of food by cooking meals in new ways or adding different herbs and spices.

Problems Chewing?

If you have trouble chewing, you might have a problem with your teeth or gums. If you wear dentures, not being able to chew well could also mean that your dentures need to be adjusted. Talk to your health-care provider or dentist if you're finding it hard to chew food.

Chewing problems can sometimes be resolved by eating softer foods. For instance, you could replace raw vegetables and fresh fruits with cooked vegetables or juices. Also, choose foods like applesauce and canned peaches or other fruits.

Meat can also be hard to chew. Instead, try eating ground or shredded meat, eggs, or dairy products like fat-free or low-fat milk, cheese, and yogurt. You could also replace meat with soft foods like cooked beans and peas, eggs, tofu, tuna fish, etc.

Problems with Digestion?

If you experience a lot of digestive problems, such as gas or bloating, try to avoid foods that cause gas or other digestive problems. If you have stomach problems that don't go away, talk with your health-care provider. If you do not have an appetite or seem to be losing weight without trying, talk to your health-care provider or ask to see a registered dietitian.

Try New Dishes

Making small changes in the way you prepare your food can often help overcome challenges to eating well. These changes can help you to enjoy meals more. They can also help make sure that you get the nutrients and energy you need for healthy, active living.

- Look for ways to combine foods from the different food groups in creative ways. You can do this while continuing to eat familiar foods that reflect your cultural, ethnic, or family traditions.
- Experiment with ethnic foods, regional dishes, or vegetarian recipes.
- Try out different kinds of fruits, vegetables, and grains that add color to your meals.
- Try new recipes from friends, newspapers, magazines, television cooking shows, or cooking websites.
- Take a cooking class to learn new ways to prepare meals and snacks that are good for you. Grocery stores, culinary schools, community centers, and adult education programs offer these classes.

Eat with Others

Eating with others is another way to enjoy meals more. For instance, you could share meals with neighbors at home or dine out with friends or family members. You could also join or start a breakfast, lunch, or dinner club.

Many senior centers and places of worship host group meals. You might also arrange to have meals brought to your home.

When Eating Out

When you eat out, you can still eat well if you choose carefully, know how your food is prepared, and watch portion sizes. Here are some tips:

- Eat reasonable amounts of food and stay within your calorie needs for the day.
- Select main dishes that include vegetables, such as salads, vegetable stir fries, or kebabs.
- Order your food baked, broiled, or grilled instead of fried.
- Make sure it is thoroughly cooked, especially dishes with meat, poultry, seafood, or eggs.
- Choose dishes without gravies or creamy sauces.
- Ask for salad dressing on the side so you can control the amount you eat.
- Ordering half portions or splitting a dish with a friend can help keep calorie intake down.

Ask for Substitutions

Also, don't be afraid to ask for substitutions. Many restaurants and eating establishments not only offer healthful choices but let you substitute healthier foods. For example, you might substitute fat-free yogurt for sour cream on your baked potato. Instead of a side order of onion rings or French fries, you could have the mixed vegetables. Ask for brown rice instead of white rice. Try having fruit for dessert.

Meals are an important part of our lives. They give us nourishment and a chance to spend time with friends, family members, and others. If physical problems keep you from eating well or enjoying meals, talk with a health-care professional. If you need help shopping or preparing meals or want to find ways to share meals with others, look for services in your community. Your area Agency on Aging can tell you about these services. To contact your area Agency on Aging, call the Eldercare Locator toll-free at 1-800-677-1116.

Source: National Institute on Aging, National Institutes of Health, U.S. Department of Health and Human Services. (n.d.). *Eating well as you get older enjoy your meals.* Available at http://nihseniorhealth.gov/eatingwellasyougetolder/enjoyyourmeals/01.html. Accessed on 2/10/17.

Figure 13.2 ▶
Estimated calorie needs per day for males and females ages 51 to 76 years and older.

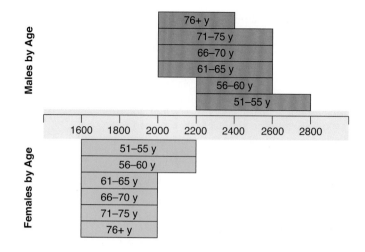

need more protein, their intake is less than that of younger adults. Approximately one-third of adults over the age of 50 years do not even meet the RDA for protein (Houston et al., 2008). Factors that may contribute to a decrease in protein intake include the cost of high-protein foods, the decreased ability to chew meats, lower overall calorie intake, and changes in digestion and gastric emptying.

The PROT-AGE Study Group, composed of an international panel of experts, met for the first time in 2012 for the purpose of developing updated evidence-based recommendations for optimal protein intake for older adults (Bauer et al., 2013). A summary of PROT-AGE recommendations is listed in Box 13.4. In addition to consuming more total protein, it is recommended that protein be evenly distributed throughout the day (e.g., 25–30 g protein per meal, the equivalent of 3–4 oz protein foods) to maximally stimulate muscle protein synthesis and thus slow or prevent the progression of sarcopenia in older adults (Paddon-Jones et al., 2015). Animal protein, but not vegetable protein, may be associated with less lean mass loss. Higher amounts of leucine, an essential amino acid that stimulates the majority of protein synthesis, are recommended (Bauer et al., 2013). Researchers are also considering whether increasing protein intake earlier in life, such as during middle-age, will promote long-term muscle health. More research is needed to determine protein and leucine thresholds, what causes anabolic resistance to low protein intakes in older adults, and who best benefits from protein interventions to prevent or manage sarcopenia (Rodriguez, 2015).

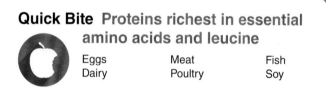

Quick Bite   **Proteins richest in essential amino acids and leucine**

Eggs	Meat	Fish
Dairy	Poultry	Soy

Water

The Adequate Intake (AI) for water, which includes total water from drinking water, other beverages, and water in solid foods, is constant from the age of 19 years on (Institute of Medicine, 2005b). However, older adults are at increased risk of dehydration for several reasons, including

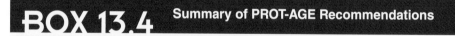

BOX 13.4   Summary of PROT-AGE Recommendations

Older adults

- Who are healthy should consume at least 1.0 to 1.2 g/kg/day. Because the per-meal anabolic threshold of dietary protein is higher for older adults than young adults, older adults should consume 25 to 30 g protein/meal, containing about 2.5 to 2.8 g leucine.
- Who have an acute or chronic disease should consume 1.2 to 1.5 g protein/kg/day.
- With severe illness or injury or with marked malnutrition may need as much as 2.0 g protein/kg/day
- With severe kidney disease who are not on dialysis should limit protein intake

Source: Bauer, J., Biolo, G., Cederholm, T., Cesari, M., Cruz-Jentoft, A. J., Morley, J. E., . . . Boirie, Y. (2013). Evidence-based recommendations for optimal dietary protein intake in older people: A position paper from the PROT-AGE Study Group. *Journal of the American Medical Directors Association, 14,* 542–559.

a diminished sense of thirst, alterations in mental status and cognition, adverse effects of medications, impaired mobility, and an age-related decrease in the ability to concentrate urine. Fear of incontinence and pain from arthritis may cause voluntary restriction in fluid intake. Dehydration can contribute to constipation, cognitive impairment, functional decline, and death (Bernstein & Munoz, 2012). Older adults should be encouraged to drink fluids at regular intervals throughout the day and not rely on thirst to indicate need.

Fiber

The recommendation for fiber decreases for adults age 50 years and older because the AI for fiber is based on total calorie intake: 14 g fiber/1000 calories of intake. This value is based on median intake levels observed to protect against coronary heart disease (CHD) (Institute of Medicine, 2005a). However, fiber also helps prevent constipation, a condition older adults are more prone to due to changes in decreased abdominal muscle tone, decrease in physical activity, or as a side effect of drug therapy. Older adults may benefit from increasing their fiber intake despite the lower AI for their age group. Fiber sources that promote laxation include wheat bran, whole grains, fruits, and vegetables.

Vitamin D

Low blood levels of vitamin D appear to be widespread in healthy adults and children in the United States and other countries. Older adults are particularly at risk for vitamin D deficiency because of various risk factors, including inadequate intake, limited sun exposure, reduced skin thickness, impaired GI absorption, and impaired activation by the liver and kidneys. Low levels of vitamin D may increase the risk of hip fracture. There are few dietary sources of vitamin D: fortified milk and other vitamin D fortified foods, egg yolks, fatty fish, and beef liver. Supplements of vitamin D may be necessary to achieve adequacy. The Endocrine Society recommends a daily supplement of 1000 to 2000 IU/day for adults as maintenance therapy; higher doses are needed to correct vitamin D deficiency (Holick et al., 2011).

Calcium

Consuming adequate amounts of calcium, vitamin D, and other nutrients is critical for optimum bone health. Low bone mineral density and osteoporosis are common in the United States, especially in older adults, and can lead to fractures and increased risk of morbidity and mortality (USDHHS & USDA, 2015b).

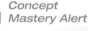 *Concept Mastery Alert*

The best option for a client concerned about an osteoporosis diagnosis after fracturing his or her hip is medication to treat osteoporosis. Once bone loss has occurred, medications are necessary.

Calcium recommendations are 1000 mg/day for men 50 to 70 years old and 1200 mg/day for women 51 years and over and men 71 and older—preferably obtained from food. Generally, three daily servings of milk, yogurt, or cheese plus nondairy sources of calcium are needed to ensure an adequate calcium intake. People who are unwilling or unable to consume adequate calcium through food sources need calcium supplements (Cosman et al., 2014).

Vitamin B$_{12}$

As many as 20% of older adults may have a mild atrophic gastritis that causes malabsorption of vitamin B$_{12}$ from food sources (Lewerin, Jacobsson, Lindstedt, & Nilsson-Ehle, 2008): Low gastric acid secretion impairs the freeing of protein-bound vitamin B$_{12}$ in foods. Medications that suppress gastric acid secretion also impair vitamin B$_{12}$ absorption. Vitamin B$_{12}$ deficiency has been associated with neurologic and psychiatric symptoms, including cognitive impairment (Morris, Selhub, & Jacques, 2012). As a preventive measure, the National Academy of Sciences Institute of Medicine recommends that people older than age 50 years obtain most of their requirement from fortified foods (e.g., fortified ready to eat cereal) or supplements (Institute of Medicine, 1998).

Iron

The recommendation for iron for men does not change with aging. In women, the requirement for iron decreases after menopause. However, iron deficiency may occur in older adults secondary

Table 13.1	Sources of Nutrients that May Be Lacking in the Diets of Older Adults
Food Component	**Sources**
Vitamin A	Green and orange vegetables, especially **green leafy vegetables**; orange fruits, liver, **milk**
Vitamin D	**Milk**, fortified soy milk, fatty fish, some fortified ready-to-eat cereals
Vitamin E	Vegetable oils, margarine, salad dressing made with vegetable oil, nuts, seeds, **whole grains**, **green leafy vegetables**, fortified cereals
Calcium	**Milk**, yogurt, cheese, fortified orange juice, **green leafy vegetables**, **legumes**
Magnesium	**Green leafy vegetables**, nuts, **legumes**, **whole grains**, seafood, chocolate, **milk**
Potassium	Fruit and **vegetables**, **legumes**, **whole grains**, **milk**, meats
Fiber	**Whole grains**; **legumes**; fruit and **vegetables**, especially the skin and seeds

Boldface type used to illustrate the commonality of sources among these nutrients.

to low stomach acid, the use of antacids, or chronic blood loss from diseases or medications. Iron intake may be low in adults who do not regularly eat red meat.

Vitamin and Mineral Supplements

In theory, older adults should be able to obtain adequate amounts of all essential nutrients through well-chosen foods. In practice, mean intakes of vitamin A, vitamin D, vitamin E, calcium, magnesium, and potassium fall below recommended amounts for adults age 50 years and older (Table 13.1) (USDA, Agricultural Research Service [ARS], 2014). As noted earlier, supplements of vitamin D, calcium, and vitamin B_{12} may be necessary for older adults. According to 2007–2010 data, 67% of adults over the age of 60 years reported taking at least one supplement in the previous 30 days, with multivitamins the most common supplement used (Baily, Gahche, Miller, Thomas, & Dwyer, 2013). Low-dose multivitamin and mineral supplements can be helpful to achieve adequate intake when food selection is limited (Bernstein & Munoz, 2012).

NUTRITION-RELATED CONCERNS IN OLDER ADULTS

Most adults age 65 years and older have at least one chronic health problem, such as arthritis, heart disease, cancer, diabetes, or hypertension; the number of chronic health conditions increases as older adults age (Fig. 13.3) (USDHHS, AOA, 2014). Common conditions that present unique challenges in the older population include obesity, Alzheimer disease, undernutrition/malnutrition, and frailty.

Obesity

Slightly more than one-third of adults age 60 years and older are obese (CDC, 2015). Obesity is a major cause of preventable disease and premature death. It increases the risk of hypertension, diabetes, cardiovascular disease, certain cancers, and osteoarthritis (OA)—disorders that become more prevalent with aging. Obesity impairs quality of life by exacerbating age-related declines in health and physical function, which lead to increased dependence, disability, and morbidity (Bernstein & Munoz, 2012). Sarcopenic obesity is obesity characterized by loss of muscle mass and strength combined with an increase in body fat mass, which causes greater declines in physical functioning than either sarcopenia or obesity alone (Houston, Nicklas, & Zizza, 2009).

Certainly, obesity is not unique to older adults; what is controversial is the question of what is appropriate obesity treatment for older adults. There is a lack of evidenced-based data showing that *long-term* weight loss is beneficial or harmful (Waters, Ward, & Villareal, 2013). Loss of

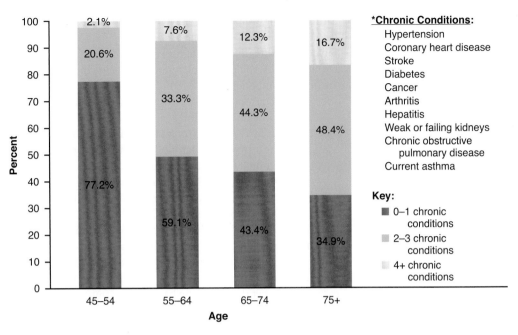

Figure 13.3 ▶
Percentage of respondent-reported chronic conditions from 10 selected conditions, 2013. *(Source: U.S. Department of Health and Human Services, Centers for Disease Control and Prevention, National Center for Health Statistics.* Health, United States, 2014. With special feature on adults aged 55–64. *Available at www.cdc.gov /nchs/hus/contents2015.html. Accessed on 4/28/16.)*

*Chronic Conditions:
Hypertension
Coronary heart disease
Stroke
Diabetes
Cancer
Arthritis
Hepatitis
Weak or failing kidneys
Chronic obstructive
   pulmonary disease
Current asthma

Key:
■ 0–1 chronic
   conditions
▨ 2–3 chronic
   conditions
▢ 4+ chronic
   conditions

weight is not synonymous with, or does it have the same benefit as, loss of fat. Intentional weight loss causes loss of muscle—even when the goal is fat loss—which can have a negative impact on functional capacity. In fact, loss of muscle and bone is a common outcome in weight loss trials and one of the primary reasons why recommending weight loss for older adults is controversial. Other challenges include the difficulty of changing behavior with advancing age: Many older people may not feel a need to make changes at this point in life. Active participation in physical activity may be difficult because of medical problems, financial limitations, or impaired hearing or vision. Diminished sense of taste, living alone, depression, and limited food budget may impede changes in intake.

There are relatively few randomized controlled trials on weight loss interventions in obese adults over the age of 65 years (Waters, Ward, et al., 2013). From the limited data available, Waters, Ward, et al. (2013) found that weight loss is attainable in this age group and that a combination of diet and exercise is able to achieve a 10% weight loss over 3 to 12 months. The short-term benefits of weight loss included positive changes in physical functioning, metabolic markers, and cardiovascular risks—benefits that occurred despite losses of muscle mass and bone mass density. Long-term maintenance of weight loss and long-term health implications are not known (Waters, Vawter, et al., 2013). Research is needed to examine the complex interaction between age-related changes, lifestyle modifications, and weight management.

Alzheimer Disease

Alzheimer disease (AD) is an irreversible, progressive brain disorder that gradually destroys memory and cognition. Although not a normal consequence of aging, the risk of AD increases with age and symptoms usually appear after the age of 60 years (National Institute on Aging [NIA], National Institutes of Health [NIH], 2015).

AD appears to result from a complex series of events in the brain that occur over decades. Disruptions in nerve cell communication, metabolism, and repair eventually cause many nerve cells to stop functioning, lose connections with other nerve cells, and die, resulting in gradual atrophy of the brain. The cause of early-onset AD is usually a genetic mutation. Suspected causes of late-onset AD include a combination of genetic, environmental, and lifestyle factors (NIA, NIH, 2015). Like CHD, AD is at least partially a vascular problem, but plaques and tau tangles that form with AD are filled with beta-amyloid, an indissoluble protein, not fat and cholesterol. Increased age and family history of AD are known risk factors for AD; cardiovascular disease, stroke, hypertension, and diabetes may also increase the risk (CDC, 2016). Interventions that lower serum cholesterol levels or other risk factors and improve cardiovascular health, such as healthy eating and physical activity, may also lower the risk of cognitive decline and AD. Although more research is needed, emerging evidence suggests that a Mediterranean diet supplemented with olive oil or nuts improves cognitive function in older adults (Valls-Pedret et al., 2015). A review by Huhn, Kharabian Masouleh, Stumvoll, Villringer, and Witte (2015) found evidence that two particular components of a Mediterranean diet, specifically omega-3 fatty acids and polyphenols such as resveratrol, have a positive effect on brain health in aging. Omega-3 fatty acids may provide protection against AD through their **antithrombosis** and anti-inflammatory activity because inflammation is part of the AD syndrome. At midlife, consuming a healthy eating pattern rich in fruits and vegetables, whole grains, and seafood and limited in sodium, added fats, added sugars, and alcohol is associated in older adults with better verbal memory, a cognitive domain particularly vulnerable to AD (Kesse-Guyot et al., 2011). Large-scale randomized controlled trials are needed to define the role of nutrition in the development of AD.

Antithrombosis
against the formation of a thrombosis or blood clot.

AD can have a devastating impact on an individual's nutritional status. Compared with healthy older adults, older adults diagnosed with cognitive impairment or AD may have lower intakes of all nutrients (Bernstein & Munoz, 2012). Early in the disease, impairments in memory and judgment may make shopping, storing, and cooking food difficult. The patient may forget to eat or may forget that he or she has already eaten and consequently may eat again. Changes in the sense of smell may develop, a preference for sweet and salty foods may occur, and unusual food choices are not uncommon. Agitation and fidgeting increases energy expenditure, and weight loss is common. Choking may occur if the patient forgets to chew food sufficiently before swallowing or hoards food in the mouth. Eating of nonfood items may occur, and eventually self-feeding ability is lost. Patients in the latter stage of AD no longer know what to do when food is placed in the mouth. When this occurs, a decision regarding the use of other means of nutritional support (e.g., nasogastric or percutaneous endoscopic gastrostomy tube feedings) must be made.

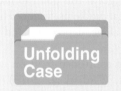

Unfolding Case

Recall Clara. In hindsight, her loss of interest in shopping and cooking were early signs of declining cognitive ability. Her symptoms are characteristic of the progressive decline in function seen in adults with Alzheimer disease. She is admitted to a memory care facility and diagnosed as frail. What interventions may help improve Clara's intake?

Malnutrition

Older adults represent the largest demographic group at disproportionate risk for inadequate intake and protein–calorie malnutrition (PCM) (Skates & Anthony, 2012). Cross-sectional and longitudinal studies indicate that the quantity of food and calorie intake decreases substantially with age (Bernstein & Munoz, 2012). As food and calorie intake decreases, so does protein and micronutrient intake; weight loss and nutrient deficiencies may result. Loss of appetite, which may arise from physiologic, psychosocial, and medical factors, is a key predictor of malnutrition in older adults.

The exact prevalence of malnutrition is unknown because there is currently no gold standard for diagnosis; studies vary in their methodologies and how they measure malnutrition. Malnutrition is reported to affect 12% to 70% of older adults in hospitals (Heersink, Brown, DiMaria-Ghalili, & Locher, 2010) and 1.5% to 67% in nursing homes (Bell, Lee, & Tamura, 2015). An estimated 56% of community-dwelling older adults are at risk of malnutrition and 6% are malnourished (DiMaria-Ghalili, Michael, & Rosso, 2013).

Common symptoms of malnutrition, such as confusion, fatigue, and weakness are often attributed to other conditions and are misdiagnosed or unrecognized as malnutrition (Marshall, Young, Bauer, & Isenring, 2016). Malnutrition among hospitalized adults is associated with many adverse outcomes, including increased risk of pressure ulcers, impaired wound healing, immune

BOX 13.5   Selected Risk Factors to Assess for Malnutrition in Older Adults

Physical and Medical Conditions

- Chronic diseases, which can affect intake by
  - Altering appetite
  - Impairing the ability to eat, prepare, or purchase food
  - Restricting food choices
  - Increasing nutrient needs through inflammation
- Geriatric syndromes, such as pressure ulcers, falls, functional decline, delirium, incontinence, sleeping problems, dizziness, and self-neglect

Physical Assessment

- Loss of subcutaneous fat
- Muscle loss
- Oral impairments, such as loss of teeth, ill-fitting dentures, or dry mouth
- Dysphagia
- Impaired sense of taste or smell
- Appetite changes
- Constipation or diarrhea

Nutrition Assessment

- Intentional or unintentional weight loss
- Diet history, although food recall may be inaccurate especially in adults with cognitive impairment
- Nutrition screening, such as the MNA-SF

- Medications, including prescriptions, over-the-counter medications, vitamins, and supplements
- Side effects that affect appetite or intake, such as dry mouth, slow GI motility, early satiety, etc.
- Number of medications used

Mental Health Status

- Cognition and dementia
- Mood and anxiety disorders
- Depression

Functioning

- Gait, strength, and balance
- Ability to perform ADLs and IADLs

Social Domain

- Social networks
- Financial constraints
- Living arrangements

Environment

- Housing, such as ability to use stairs to gain access to outside
- Adequacy of transportation to purchase food
- Accessibility to grocery stores

Source: DiMaria-Ghalili, R. (2014). Integrating nutrition in the comprehensive geriatric assessment. *Nutrition in Clinical Practice, 29*, 420–427.

suppression, increased risk of infection, muscle wasting, functional loss, increased risk of falls, longer hospitalizations, higher readmission rates, higher treatment costs, and increased mortality (Barker, Gout, & Crowe, 2011; Tappenden et al., 2013). Selected risk factors for malnutrition in older adults appear in Box 13.5.

Frailty

Frailty is a medical syndrome characterized by diminished strength, endurance, and physiologic function that increases an individual's vulnerability for developing increased dependency and/or death when exposed to a stressor (Morley et al., 2013). Frailty has multiple causes and is either physical or psychological or a combination of both. Frailty can improve or worsen over time. Although sarcopenia may be a component of frailty, frailty is more multidimensional than sarcopenia alone (Fielding et al., 2011).

The prevalence of physical frailty among adults age 65 years and older is estimated to be 4% to 17% (Collard, Boter, Schoevers, & Oude Voshaar, 2012). Women are almost twice as likely as men to be frail. Prevalence significantly increases in adults over the age of 80 years.

Simple validated screening tools are available to enable physicians to quickly identify adults with physical frailty syndrome who are in need of a more in-depth assessment. One example is the simple FRAIL questionnaire screening tool (Fig. 13.4). Frailty screening is recommended for all adults age 70 years and older and anyone with significant weight loss (≥5% over the last year) due to chronic illness (Morley et al., 2013).

Proposed interventions to potentially prevent or treat physical frailty include exercise, protein–calorie supplementation, vitamin D, and reducing polypharmacy (Morley et al., 2013). Weight loss is a major element of frailty (Landi, Laviano, & Cruz-Jentolf, 2010), although frailty

Figure 13.4 ▶

The "FRAIL" questionnaire.

(Source: Morley, J. E.,
Vellas, B., van Kan, G. A.,
Anker, S. D., Bauer, J. M.,
Bernabei, R., . . . Walston,
J. [2013]. Frailty consensus:
A call to action. Journal of the
American Medical Directors
Association, 14[6], 392–397.)

Fatigue:	Are you fatigued?	
Resistance:	Cannot walk up 1 flight of stairs?	
Aerobic:	Cannot walk 1 block?	
Illness:	Do you have more than 5 illnesses?	
Loss of weight:	Have you lost more than 5% of your weight in the past 6 months?	

3 or greater = frailty
1 or 2 = prefrail

can occur in people who are morbidly obese (Waters, Vawter, et al., 2013). Oral nutrition supplements can provide several benefits, including an increase in muscle mass, weight gain, and decreased risk of complications. Vitamin D supplements for older adults who are deficient in vitamin D may reduce the risk of falls, hip fractures, and mortality and may improve muscle function (Morley et al., 2013).

NUTRITION SCREENING OF OLDER ADULTS

Nutrition screening to identify presence or risk of malnutrition is appropriate in any setting where older adults receive services or care, such as in hospitals, long-term care facilities, community-based care, home health, and physician offices (Kamp, Wellman, & Russell, 2010). There are many screening tools that may be used in older adults; however, none take the place of an individualized nutrition assessment when a nutritional issue is suspected or confirmed. The Mini Nutritional Assessment-Short Form (MNA-SF) is a widely used, evidence-based screening tool for use in adults age 65 years and older (Skipper, Ferguson, Thompson, Castellanos, & Porcari, 2012). It has been validated in hundreds of international studies by a range of healthcare professionals and a variety of settings (Huhmann, Perez, Alexander, & Thomas, 2013). Decreased intake and weight loss are among the six criteria it uses to assess risk. The tool appears as Figure 1.1 in Chapter 1.

The Self-MNA is a tool derived from the MNA-SF to enable older adults to assess their own nutritional status (Fig. 13.5). The six criteria are the same but are worded more simply for non-health professionals. Ideally, the Self-MNA could be completed by individuals or their caregivers prior to or during an outpatient clinical appointment to allow for ongoing monitoring of nutritional status (Huhmann et al., 2013). The Self-MNA has been scientifically validated to have excellent sensitivity and specificity for identifying "normal nutritional status," "at risk of malnutrition," and "malnourished" in community-dwelling adults age 65 years and older. The screening tool is easy to use, efficient, and demonstrates sufficient inter-rater reliability among community-dwelling older adults.

Potential Intervention Strategies Appropriate for Older Adults

Regardless of living situation, ongoing screening that identifies actual or potential malnutrition should be followed by a nutrition assessment that leads to an individualized plan to improve overall intake. One option is to increase the nutrient density of foods eaten by adding ingredients that provide calories and/or protein. The effect is to increase the nutritional value while the volume of food served remains the same.

Homemade or commercial protein supplements are an effective option to increase overall nutrient intake for nursing home

Quick Bite Examples of foods made more nutrient/calorie dense

Mashed potatoes made with extra butter, whole milk, and/or cheese

Milk fortified with nonfat dry milk powder to make "double strength" milk that can be used in cereal, soups, milk based desserts, milk shakes

Casseroles, soups, rice, noodles, or sandwiches with added cheese or chopped fine hard-cooked eggs

Fruit, plain cake, or other desserts topped with vanilla Greek yogurt

Oatmeal made with added butter, nonfat dry milk, and sugar

Coffee with half and half, whole milk and/or honey

Scrambled eggs with added cheese

**Nestlé
Nutrition Institute**

Self-MNA®

Mini Nutritional Assessment

For Adults 65 years of Age and Older

Last name: _____   First name: _____

Date: _____   Age: _____

Complete the screen by filling in the boxes with the appropriate numbers. Total the numbers for the final screening score.

Screening		
A **Has your food intake declined over the past 3 months?** **[ENTER ONE NUMBER]** *Please enter the most appropriate number (0, 1, or 2) in the box to the right.*	0 = severe decrease in food intake 1 = moderate decrease in food intake 2 = no decrease in food intake	☐
B **How much weight have you lost in the past 3 months?** **[ENTER ONE NUMBER]** *Please enter the most appropriate number (0, 1, 2 or 3) in the box to the right.*	0 = weight loss greater than 7 pounds 1 = do not know the amount of weight lost 2 = weight loss between 2 and 7 pounds 3 = no weight loss or weight loss less than 2 pounds	☐
C **How would you describe your current mobility?** **[ENTER ONE NUMBER]** *Please enter the most appropriate number (0, 1, or 2) in the box to the right.*	0 = unable to get out of a bed, a chair, or a wheelchair without the assistance of another person 1 = able to get out of bed or a chair, but unable to go out of my home 2 = able to leave my home	☐
D **Have you been stressed or severely ill in the past 3 months?** **[ENTER ONE NUMBER]** *Please enter the most appropriate number (0 or 2) in the box to the right.*	0 = yes 2 = no	☐
E **Are you currently experiencing dementia and/or prolonged severe sadness?** **[ENTER ONE NUMBER]** *Please enter the most appropriate number (0, 1, or 2) in the box to the right.*	0 = yes, severe dementia and/or prolonged severe sadness 1 = yes, mild dementia, but no prolonged severe sadness 2 = neither dementia nor prolonged severe sadness	☐
Please total all of the numbers you entered in the boxes for questions A-E and write the numbers here:		☐☐

Figure 13.5 ▲ **Self-Mini Nutritional Assessment screening tool. *(continued)***

Now, please CHOOSE ONE of the following two questions – F1 or F2 – to answer.

Question F1

Height (feet & inches)   **Body Weight** (pounds)

Height	Group 0	Group 1	Group 2	Group 3
4'10"	Less than 91	91 – 99	100 – 109	110 or more
4'11"	Less than 94	94 – 103	104 – 113	114 or more
5'0"	Less than 97	97 – 106	107 – 117	118 or more
5'1"	Less than 100	100 – 110	111 – 121	122 or more
5'2"	Less than 104	104 – 114	115 – 125	126 or more
5'3"	Less than 107	107 – 117	118 – 129	130 or more
5'4"	Less than 110	110 – 121	122 – 133	134 or more
5'5"	Less than 114	114 – 125	126 – 137	138 or more
5'6"	Less than 118	118 – 129	130 – 141	142 or more
5'7"	Less than 121	121 – 133	134 – 145	146 or more
5'8"	Less than 125	125 – 137	138 – 150	151 or more
5'9"	Less than 128	128 – 141	142 – 154	155 or more
5'10"	Less than 132	132 – 145	146 – 159	160 or more
5'11"	Less than 136	136 – 149	150 – 164	165 or more
6'0"	Less than 140	140 – 153	154 – 168	169 or more
6'1"	Less than 144	144 – 158	159 – 173	174 or more
6'2"	Less than 148	148 – 162	163 – 178	179 or more
6'3"	Less than 152	152 – 167	168 – 183	184 or more
6'4"	Less than 156	156 –171	172 – 188	189 or more
Group	**0**	**1**	**2**	**3**

Please refer to the chart on the left and follow these instructions:

1. Find your height on the left-hand column of the chart.
2. Go across that row and circle the range that your weight falls into.
3. Look to the bottom of the chart to find out what group number (0, 1, 2, or 3) your circled weight range falls into.

Write the Group Number (0, 1, 2, or 3) here: ☐

Write sum of questions A-E (from page 1) ☐

Lastly, calculate the sum of these 2 numbers. This is your SCREENING SCORE: ☐

Question F2

Measure the circumference of your LEFT calf by following the instructions below:

1. Loop a tape measure all the way around your calf to measure its size.
2. Record the measurement in cm: _____
   - If less than 31cm, enter "0" in the box to the right.
   - If 31cm or greater, enter "3" in the box to the right.

© SIGVARIS

☐

Write the sum of questions A-E (from page 1) here: ☐ ☐

Lastly, calculate the sum of these 2 numbers. This is your SCREENING SCORE: ☐ ☐

Screening Score (14 points maximum)

12–14 points:	Normal nutritional status	
8–11 points:	At risk of malnutrition	
0–7 points:	Malnourished	**Copy your SCREENING SCORE:** ☐ ☐

If you score between 0-11, please take this form to a healthcare professional for consultation.

Figure 13.5 ▲ *(continued)*

residents as well as community-dwelling older adults. Smoothies, milk shakes, and protein powder–based milk drinks can be consumed between meals; liquids leave the stomach more quickly than solids and are less likely to interfere with the next meal. Commercial supplements offer convenience but are more expensive. Many people find that supplements are an easy way to boost intake; however, taste fatigue may occur over time. Consider altering the amount, timing, flavors, or types to maintain acceptance. Monitor overall intake to ensure that supplements are adding to instead of replacing food intake.

Potential Additional Interventions for Community-Dwelling Adults

Among community-dwelling adults, eating with others may help improve the intake and nutritional status of those who live alone. Efforts should be made to eat with friends and relatives whenever possible. Other potential options are the federally funded nutrition programs—congregate meals and Meals on Wheels. These programs are designed to provide low-cost, nutritious, hot meals; education about food and nutrition; opportunities for socialization and recreation; and information on other health and social assistance programs. The congregate meal program provides a hot, balanced, midday meal and the opportunity to socialize in senior citizen centers and other public or private facilities. Those who choose to pay may do so; otherwise, the meal is free. Meals on Wheels is a home-delivered meal program for elderly persons who are unable to get to congregate meal centers because they live in an isolated area or have a chronic illness or physical limitations. Usually, a hot meal is served at midday and a bagged lunch is included to be used as the evening meal. Modified diets, such as carbohydrate-controlled diets and low-sodium diets, are provided as needed.

Another option to improve intake may be to discontinue therapeutic diet restrictions. Restrictive diets have the potential to negatively affect quality of life by limiting food choices and dulling appetite; potential benefits should be weighed against the potential negative impact on intake and weight. Restrictive diets should be used only when a significant improvement in health can be expected, such as in cases of ascites or constipation.

Potential Additional Interventions for Long-Term Care Residents

Preventing malnutrition is a quality of life issue. Efforts should be made to optimize food and fluid intake at each meal and snack. Mealtime should be made as enjoyable experience as possible. Encourage independence in eating and supervise dining areas so that proper feeding techniques are used when residents are assisted or fed by certified nursing assistants. Food preferences should be honored whenever possible. Family involvement increases residents' intake. Additional strategies to promote food intake appear in Box 13.6.

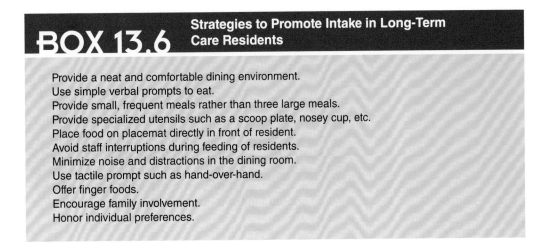

BOX 13.6 Strategies to Promote Intake in Long-Term Care Residents

Provide a neat and comfortable dining environment.
Use simple verbal prompts to eat.
Provide small, frequent meals rather than three large meals.
Provide specialized utensils such as a scoop plate, nosey cup, etc.
Place food on placemat directly in front of resident.
Avoid staff interruptions during feeding of residents.
Minimize noise and distractions in the dining room.
Use tactile prompt such as hand-over-hand.
Offer finger foods.
Encourage family involvement.
Honor individual preferences.

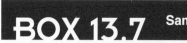

BOX 13.7 Sample Liberal Eating Pattern for Older Adults

Breakfast

Orange juice
Oatmeal
One soft-cooked egg
One slice buttered whole wheat toast
Low-fat milk
Coffee/tea

Lunch

Turkey sandwich made with two slices whole wheat bread, tomato, romaine lettuce, and low-fat
  salad dressing
Vegetable soup
Sliced strawberries over angel food cake
One cup low-fat milk
Coffee/tea

Dinner

Roast pork
Oven roasted potatoes
Baked acorn squash
Fresh fruit salad
Ice cream
Coffee/tea

Snack

One cup low-fat yogurt

To meet the needs of individual residents, a holistic approach is advocated that includes the individual's personal goals, overall prognosis, risk/benefit ratio, and quality of life. A liberalized eating pattern, which is a healthy diet of nutrient-dense foods that contains neither excessive nor restrictive amounts of cholesterol, sodium, and added sugar, may help improve intake and lower the risk of weight loss (Box 13.7).

A liberal eating pattern can be modified to meet the requirements of residents with increased needs, such as those who have pressure ulcers. A liberal diet with foods made more nutrient-dense or extra meat and/or milk will provide increased amounts of calories, protein, and fluid. Supplemental vitamin C and zinc may be ordered to promote healing.

As with any nutritional intervention, frequent and accurate monitoring of the resident's intake, weight, and hydration status is vital to prevent or treat nutrition-related problems. Intakes <75% and weight loss of 5% in 30 days warrant investigation.

Unfolding Case

Think of Clara. A nutrition screen revealed malnutrition. Clara is consuming <50% of her food at each meal. She pushes food around her plate and hides it under the plate. She also prefers wandering the halls to sitting. Clara has a health-care proxy who explicitly states she does not want artificial food or fluids should there be no hope of recovery. What strategies may help improve her intake?

<table>
<tr><td>**NURSING PROCESS**</td><td>**Older Adult**</td></tr>
</table>

Harold Hausman is a regular participant of the monthly congregational nursing program sponsored at his church. He is a sedentary 82-year-old widower who lives alone. You have noticed that he has lost weight over the last several months. He has asked you to answer a few questions he has about the low-sodium, low-cholesterol diet his doctor recommended.

Assessment

Medical–Psychosocial History
- Medical history including hyperlipidemia, hypertension, cardiovascular disease, or GI complaints
- Ability to understand, attitude toward health and nutrition, and readiness to learn
- Attitude about his present weight and recent weight loss
- Usual activity patterns
- Use of prescribed and over-the-counter drugs
- Functional limitations such as impaired ability to shop, cook, and eat
- Psychosocial and economic issues such as who does the shopping and cooking, adequacy of food budget, need for food assistance, and level of family and social support

Anthropometric Assessment
- Height, current and usual weight
- Percentage of weight change
- Determine BMI

Biochemical and Physical Assessment
- Cholesterol level, if available
- Blood pressure
- Dentition and ability to swallow

Dietary Assessment
- Why did your doctor give you this low-sodium, low-cholesterol eating plan?
- How many daily meals and snacks do you usually eat?
- What is a normal day's intake for you?
- What changes have you made in implementing this eating plan? For instance, did you stop using the saltshaker at the table or are you reading labels for sodium content? Did you change the type of butter/margarine you use? The type of salad dressing?
- Do you prepare food with added fat, or do you bake, broil, steam, or boil your food?
- How does your intake compare to a 2000-cal/day meal plan recommended by MyPlate for people your age?
- Do any cultural, religious, or ethnic considerations influence your eating habits?
- Do you use vitamins, minerals, or nutritional supplements? If so, which ones, how much, and why are they taken?
- Do you use alcohol, tobacco, and caffeine?
- How is your appetite?

Diagnosis

Possible Nursing Diagnoses

Imbalanced nutrition: eating less than the body needs related to restrictive diet and eating alone as evidenced by weight loss

Planning

Client Outcomes

The client will
- Attain/maintain a "healthy" weight
- Consume, on average, a varied and balanced eating pattern that meets the recommended number of servings from the 2000-calorie MyPlate meal plan
- Implement healthy low-sodium, low-cholesterol changes to his usual intake without compromising nutritional or caloric adequacy

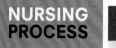

NURSING PROCESS

Older Adult

Nursing Interventions

Nutrition Therapy

Encourage a varied and balanced eating pattern that meets the recommended number of servings from each of the major MyPlate food groups for a 2000-calorie eating pattern.

Client Teaching

Instruct the client on
- The role of nutrition in maintaining health and quality of life, including the following:
  - A balanced eating pattern consisting of a variety of nutrient-dense foods helps maximize the quality of life
  - Avoiding excess salt is prudent for all people; recommendations on sodium intake should be made on an individual basis according to the client's cardiac and renal status, appetite, and use of medications.
  - Although it is wise to avoid high-fat, nutrient-poor foods such as most cakes, cookies, pastries, pies, chips, full-fat dairy products, and fried foods, observing too severe fat restriction compromises calorie intake and may result in undesirable weight loss.
- Eating plan essentials, including the importance of
  - Choosing a varied of foods to help ensure an average adequate intake; limiting food choices or skipping a food group increases the risk of both nutrient deficiencies and excesses
  - Eating enough food to avoid unfavorable weight loss
  - Eating enough high-fiber foods such as whole-grain breads and cereals, dried peas and beans, and fresh fruits and vegetables
  - Drinking adequate fluid regularly throughout the day
- Behavioral matters, including
  - The importance of discussing the rationale for the low-sodium, low-cholesterol diet with his physician, particularly because he has had an unfavorable weight loss
  - How to read labels to identify low-sodium foods
- Physical activity goals that may help improve appetite and intake

Evaluation

Evaluate and Monitor

- Monitor weight and blood pressure.
- Provide periodic feedback and reinforcement on food intake and questions about the eating plan.

How Do You Respond?

Do chondroitin sulfate and glucosamine hydrochloride (CS + GH) work for arthritis pain? These two products have been used for more than 40 years to prevent or treat OA based on the premise that the disease is caused by a deficiency of these components of cartilage. Although study results on the use of CS + GH in the treatment of OA have been conflicting, recent findings show that CS + GH have comparable efficacy to celecoxib in reducing pain, stiffness, functional limitation, and joint swelling/effusion after 6 months of use in patients with painful knee OA (Hochberg et al., 2016). Because it has a good safety profile, it may be beneficial to try, but it may take 4 months of use before improvement is evident.

REVIEW CASE STUDY

Annie is an 80-year-old widow who lives alone. She has a long history of hypertension and diabetes and suffers from the complications of CHD and neuropathy. She has diabetic retinopathy, which has left her legally blind. She has never been compliant with a diabetic diet but takes insulin as directed. She is 5 ft 5 in tall and weighs 170 pounds, down from her usual weight of 184 pounds 5 months ago.

Annie reluctantly agreed to receive Meals on Wheels so she does not have to prepare lunch and dinner except on weekends. Her daughter buys groceries for Annie every week, and her grocery list generally consists of milk, oatmeal, two cans of soup, two bananas, a bag of chocolate candy, a layer cake, two doughnuts, and mixed nuts. Her weekend meals consist of whatever she has available to eat.

- What is Annie's BMI? How would you assess her weight status?
- Is her recent weight loss significant? Is it better for her to lose weight, maintain her present weight, or try to regain what she has lost?
- What would you recommend Annie eat for breakfast? For snacks? For weekend meals? Would you discourage her from eating sweets?
- What arguments would you make for her to eat better?

STUDY QUESTIONS

1 A 68-year-old man who has steadily gained excess weight over the years complains that it is too late for him to make any changes in diet or exercise that would effectively improve his health, particularly the arthritis he has in his knees. Which of the following would be the nurse's best response?
   a. "You're right. You should have made changes long ago. You cannot benefit from a change in diet and exercise now."
   b. "It is too hard for older people to change their habits. You should just continue what you've been doing and know that it's a quality of life issue to enjoy your food."
   c. "It may not help to change your intake and exercise, but it certainly wouldn't hurt. Why don't you give it a try and see what happens?"
   d. "It is not too late to make changes, and losing weight through diet and exercising are more effective at relieving arthritis pain than either strategy is alone. And older people often are better at making lifestyle changes than are younger adults."

2 The nurse knows her instructions about vitamin B_{12} are effective when the client verbalizes he will
   a. Consume more meat.
   b. Consume more fruits and vegetables.
   c. Eat vitamin B_{12}–fortified cereal.
   d. Drink more milk.

3 A client complains that she is not eating any more than she did when she was 30 years old and yet she keeps gaining weight. Which of the following would be the nurse's best response?
   a. "As people get older, they lose muscle mass, which lowers their calorie requirements, and physical activity often decreases too. You can increase the number of calories you burn by building muscle with resistance exercises and increasing your activity."
   b. "You may not think you are eating more calories but you probably are because the only way to gain weight is to eat more calories than you burn."
   c. "Weight gain is an inevitable consequence of getting older related to changes in your body composition. Do not worry about it because older people are healthier when they are heavier."
   d. "Weight gain among older adults is inevitable and untreatable. Concentrate on eating a healthy eating pattern and forget about weight."

4 A mineral likely to be consumed in inadequate amounts by older adults is
   a. Iron
   b. Potassium
   c. Iodine
   d. Sodium

5 The best dietary advice for the possible prevention of AD is to
   a. Eat more fiber.
   b. Eat a heart healthy eating pattern rich in fruits, vegetables, whole grains, and seafood.
   c. Take a multivitamin every day.
   d. Avoid foods with a high glycemic index.

6 Risk factors for malnutrition in older adults include (select all that apply)
   a. A decrease in food intake in the last 3 months
   b. Weight loss
   c. Stress or severe illness in the last 3 months
   d. Dementia and/or prolonged severe sadness
   e. Impaired mobility

7 A source of leucine that may help stimulate protein synthesis is
   a. Milk
   b. Nuts
   c. Legumes
   d. Grains

8 Which of the following may help promote the intake of a resident in long-term care? Select all that apply.
   a. Use simple verbal prompts to eat.
   b. Provide three meals a day; avoid snacks.
   c. Minimize noise and distractions in the dining room.
   d. Offer finger foods.
   e. Honor individual preferences; solicit input from resident and family.

KEY CONCEPTS

- The population of older adults is increasing and is getting older. Older adults represent a heterogeneous group that varies in health, activity, and nutritional status.
- Aging begins at birth and ends in death. Exactly how and why aging occurs is not known.
- Numerous changes occur with aging that have an impact on nutritional needs or intake.
- Loss of bone and muscle mass and an increase in fat tissue in older adults leads to a lower metabolic rate and decrease in the number of calories needed.
- Sarcopenia occurs when loss of muscle leads to a decrease in strength and function. It is a risk factor for morbidity and mortality.
- Various factors may cause a decrease in appetite, including changes in energy expenditure and GI hormone secretions.
- Functional limitations may impair the ability to eat, procure, prepare, or consume food.
- Immune system changes leading to inflammaging increase the risk of morbidity and mortality. A healthy eating pattern and physical activity may prevent or reverse inflammaging.
- Psychosocial changes can lead to social isolation and a decrease in appetite and intake.
- Polypharmacy is associated with adverse side effects and a worsening of nutritional intake overall.
- Healthy aging may mean the absence of chronic disease, cognitive impairments, physical disabilities, and mental health limitations. Healthy lifestyle behaviors promote healthy aging.
- The *Dietary Guidelines for Americans* apply to older adults as well as younger people. Like the population as a whole, older adults tend to under consume fruits, vegetables, whole grains, dairy, seafood, and oils, which leads to low intakes of the nutrients of concern—vitamin D, calcium, potassium, and fiber.
- MyPlate for Older Adults illustrates the *Dietary Guidelines for Americans* with an emphasis on choosing nutrient-dense foods, foods lower in sodium, and ample fluid.
- Older adults need fewer calories than younger adults but generally have the same or higher nutrient needs, particularly calcium, vitamin D, and possibly protein.
- Older adults may not be able to effectively absorb vitamin B_{12} that occurs in protein foods and so are urged to consume vitamin B_{12} through fortified foods (e.g., cereal) or supplements.
- The requirement for iron decreases in women after menopause.
- Water needs do not change with aging but older adults have a diminished sense of thirst, which contributes to their greater risk of dehydration.

- Fiber recommendations decrease based on the decrease in calorie intake, but older adults may benefit from increasing their fiber intake because it helps prevent or treat constipation.
- Supplements of vitamin D, calcium, and vitamin B_{12} may be necessary. A large percentage of older adults take a multivitamin, which may help ensure an adequate intake.
- Most older adults have at least one chronic health problem. At least in part, eating patterns are involved in most chronic health problems.
- Long-term benefits of weight loss in obese older adults are not known. Short-term benefits of weight loss in obese older adults include improvements in physical functioning, metabolic markers, and cardiovascular risks.
- Many known risk factors for AD are similar to those for CHD. Although the role of diet has not clearly been established, a heart healthy diet may help reduce the risk of AD.
- The prevalence of malnutrition among older adults is unknown because there is not an agreed upon standard by which it is defined. Older adults are at risk for malnutrition for numerous reasons, including physical, medical, nutritional, social, mental, and environmental factors.
- Frailty may be prevented or reversed with calorie and protein supplements and vitamin D supplements.
- Nutrition screening to identify actual or potential malnutrition is appropriate in all settings. The MNA-SF is a widely used, validated tool designed for health professionals. The Self-MNA is designed to enable older adults to assess their nutritional status which can serve as a monitoring tool for physicians.
- Interventions to improve intake for either community-dwelling older adults or nursing home residents are to increase the nutrient density of foods consumed and use oral nutritional supplements with or between meals.
- Adults living in the community may benefit from food assistance programs such as congregate dining or Meals on Wheels. Forgoing a restrictive diet may also improve intake.
- For residents in long-term care, additional efforts to prevent malnutrition should focus on maintaining an adequate calorie and protein intake. Honor special requests, encourage food from home, and provide assistance with eating as needed. A liberal eating pattern may help prevent malnutrition and improve quality of life.

Check Your Knowledge Answer Key

1 **FALSE** Midlife is not too late to reap health benefits of adhering to a healthy eating pattern. People of all ages can benefit from improving their eating pattern.

2 **TRUE** In general, calorie needs in older adults decrease due to a decrease in lean body mass and physical activity while the need for other nutrients stays the same or increases.

3 **TRUE** Due to a diminished sense of thirst that occurs with aging, older adults may not feel thirsty even when they are becoming dehydrated.

4 **TRUE** Older adults do not need more vitamin B_{12} than younger adults, but their ability to absorb the natural form of vitamin B_{12} from food may be impaired. Adults over the age of 50 years are urged to consume the RDA for vitamin B_{12} from fortified foods or supplements to ensure adequacy.

5 **FALSE** Most older adults consume adequate amounts of iron. In fact, they are cautioned against consuming supplements that contain iron so as not to exceed the upper limit for iron.

6 **FALSE** Although loss of lean body mass is a normal consequence of aging, muscle mass can be increased with resistance exercises and a diet adequate in protein.

7 **FALSE** Obesity is a health risk at any age. Studies show obese older adults experience improvements in physical functioning, metabolic markers, and cardiovascular risks after losing weight. However, there is a lack of evidence on the long-term benefits or risks of weight loss in obese older adults.

8 **TRUE** Due to a reduced ability to use protein (e.g., from insulin resistance and protein anabolic resistance), studies support the need for a higher protein intake by older adults.

9 **TRUE** Calorie and protein supplements can promote weight gain and an increase in muscle mass and thus may help improve or reverse frailty in older adults.

10 **TRUE** Loss of appetite is a key risk factor for malnutrition in older adults.

Student Resources on the**Point®**
For additional learning materials, activate the code in the front of this book at
http://thePoint.lww.com/activate

Websites

Administration on Aging at www.aoa.gov
Alzheimer's Association at www.alz.org
American Association of Retired Persons at www.aarp.org
Arthritis Foundation at www.arthritis.org
National Institute of Aging Information Office at www.nia.nih.gov
The American Geriatrics Society at www.americangeriatrics.org

References

Baily, R., Gahche, J., Miller, P., Thomas, R., & Dwyer, J. (2013). Why US adults use dietary supplements. *JAMA Internal Medicine, 173,* 355–361.

Barker, L., Gout, B., & Crowe, T. (2011). Hospital malnutrition: Prevalence, identification and impact on patients and the healthcare system. *International Journal of Environmental Research and Public Health, 8,* 514–527.

Bauer, J., Biolo, G., Cederholm, T., Cesari, M., Cruz-Jentoft, A. J., Morley, J. E., . . . Boirie, Y. (2013). Evidence-based recommendations for optimal dietary protein intake in older people: A position paper from the PROT-AGE Study Group. *Journal of the American Medical Directors Association, 14,* 542–559.

Bell, C., Lee, A., & Tamura, B. (2015). Malnutrition in the nursing home. *Current Opinion in Clinical Nutrition and Metabolic Care, 18,* 17–23.

Berger, M., & Doherty, T. (2010). Sarcopenia: Prevalence, mechanisms, and functional consequences. *Interdisciplinary Topics in Gerontology, 37,* 94–114.

Bernstein, M., & Munoz, N. (2012). Position of the Academy of Nutrition and Dietetics: Food and nutrition for older adults: Promoting health and wellness. *Journal of the Academy of Nutrition and Dietetics, 112,* 1255–1277.

Bolzetta, F., Veronese, N., De Rui, M., Berton, L., Toffanello, E. D., Carraro, S., . . . Sergi, G. (2015). Are the Recommended Dietary Allowances for vitamins appropriate for elderly people? *Journal of the Academy of Nutrition and Dietetics, 115,* 1789–1797.

Centers for Disease Control and Prevention. (2015). *Adult obesity facts.* Available at http://www.cdc.gov/obesity/data/adult.html. Accessed on 5/4/16.

Centers for Disease Control and Prevention. (2016). *Arthritis quick stats.* Available at http://www.cdc.gov/arthritis/press/quickstats.html. Accessed on 5/2/16.

Collard, R., Boter, H., Schoevers, R., & Oude Voshaar, R. (2012). Prevalence of frailty in community-dwelling older persons: A systematic review. *Journal of the American Geriatrics Society, 60,* 1487–1492.

Cosman, F., de Beur, S., LeBoff, M., Lewiecki, E. M., Tanner, B., Randall, S., & Lindsay, R. (2014). Clinician's guide to prevention and treatment of osteoporosis. *Osteoporosis International, 25,* 2359–2381.

DiMaria-Ghalili, R., Michael, Y., & Rosso, A. (2013). Malnutrition in a sample of community-dwelling older Pennsylvanians. *The Journal of Aging Research & Clinical Practice, 2,* 39–45.

English, K., & Paddon-Jones, D. (2010). Protecting muscle mass and function in older adults during bed rest. *Current Opinion in Clinical Nutrition and Metabolic Care, 13,* 34–39.

Evans, W. (2010). Skeletal muscle loss: Cachexia, sarcopenia, and inactivity. *The American Journal of Clinical Nutrition, 91*(4), 1123S–1127S.

Fielding, R., Vellas, B., Evans, W., Bhasin, S., Morley, J. E., Newman, A. B., . . . Zamboni, M. (2011). Sarcopenia: An undiagnosed condition in older adults. Current consensus definition: Prevalence, etiology, and consequences. International Working Group on Sarcopenia. *Journal of the American Medical Directors Association, 12*, 249–256.

Franceschi, C. (2007). Inflammaging as a major characteristic of old people: Can it be prevented or cured? *Nutrition Reviews, 65*(12 Pt. 2), S173–S176. doi:10.1111/j.1753-4887.2007.tb00358.x

Franceschi, C., & Campisi, J. (2014). Chronic inflammation (inflammaging) and its potential contribution to age-associated diseases. *The Journals of Gerontology, Series A: Biological Sciences and Medical Sciences, 69*(Suppl. 1), S4–S9.

Heersink, J., Brown, C., DiMaria-Ghalili, R., & Locher, J. (2010). Undernutrition in hospitalized older adults: Patterns and correlates, outcomes, and opportunities for intervention with a focus on processes of care. *Journal of Nutrition for the Elderly, 29*, 4–41.

Heuberger, R., & Caudell, K. (2011). Polypharmacy and nutritional status in older adults: A cross-sectional study. *Drugs and Aging, 28*, 315–323.

Hochberg, M., Martel-Pelletier, J., Monfort, J., Möller, I., Castillo, J. R., Arden, N., . . . Pelletier, J. P. (2016). Combined chondroitin sulfate and glucosamine for painful knee osteoarthritis: A multicentre, randomised, double-blind, non-inferiority trial versus celecoxib. *Annals of the Rheumatic Diseases, 75*, 37–44. doi:10.1136/annrheumdis-2014-20672

Holick, M., Binkley, N., Bischoll-Ferrari, H., Gordon, C., Hanley, D. A., Heaney, R. P., . . . Weaver, C. M. (2011). Evaluation, treatment, and prevention of vitamin D deficiency: An Endocrine Society clinical practice guideline. *The Journal of Clinical Endocrinology and Metabolism, 96*, 1911–1930.

Houston, D. K., Nicklas, B., Ding, J., Harris, T. B., Tylavsky, F. A., Newman, A. B., . . . Kritchevsky, S. B. (2008). Dietary protein intake is associated with lean mass change in older, community-dwelling adults: The Health, Aging, and Body Composition (Health ABC) Study. *The American Journal of Clinical Nutrition, 87*, 150–155.

Houston, D. K., Nicklas, B., & Zizza, C. (2009). Weighty concerns: The growing prevalence of obesity among older adults. *Journal of the American Dietetic Association, 109*, 1886–1895.

Huhmann, M., Perez, V., Alexander, D., & Thomas, D. (2013). A self-completed nutrition screening tool for community-dwelling older adults with high reliability: A comparison study. *The Journal of Nutrition, Health & Aging, 17*, 339–344.

Huhn, S., Kharabian Masouleh, S., Stumvoll, M., Villringer, A., & Witte, A. V. (2015). Components of a Mediterranean diet and their impact on cognitive functions in aging. *Frontiers in Aging Neuroscience, 7*, 132. doi:10.3389/fnagi.2015.00132

Husson, N., Watfa, G., Laurain, M., Perret-Guillaume, C., Niemier, J. Y., Miget, P., & Benetos, A. (2014). Characteristics of polymedicated (≥4) elderly: A survey in a community-dwelling population aged 60 years and over. *The Journal of Nutrition, Health & Aging, 18*, 87–91.

Hybels, C., & Blazer, D. (2003). Epidemiology of late-life mental disorders. *Clinics in Geriatric Medicine, 19*, 663–696.

Institute of Medicine. (1998). *Dietary reference intakes for thiamin, riboflavin, niacin, vitamin B6, folate, vitamin B12, pantothenic acid, biotin, and choline.* Washington, DC: The National Academies Press.

Institute of Medicine. (2005a). *Dietary reference intakes for energy, carbohydrate, fiber, fat, fatty acids, cholesterol, protein, and amino acids* (macronutrients). Washington, DC: The National Academies Press.

Institute of Medicine. (2005b). *Dietary reference intakes for water, potassium, sodium, chloride, and sulfate.* Washington, DC: The National Academies Press.

Kamp, B., Wellman, N., & Russell, C. (2010). Position of the American Dietetic Association, American Society for Nutrition, and Society for Nutrition Education: Food and nutrition programs for community-residing older adults. *Journal of Nutrition Education and Behavior, 42*, 72–82.

Kesse-Guyot, E., Amieva, H., Castetbon, K., Henegar, A., Ferry, M., Jeandel, C., . . . Galan, P. (2011). Adherence to nutritional recommendations and subsequent cognitive performance: Findings from the prospective Supplementation with Antioxidant Vitamins and Minerals 2 (SU.VI.MAX 2) study. *The American Journal of Clinical Nutrition, 93*, 200–210.

Landi, F., Laviano, A., & Cruz-Jentolf, A. (2010). The anorexia of aging: Is it a geriatric syndrome? *Journal of the American Medical Directors Association, 11*, 153–156.

Lewerin, C., Jacobsson, S., Lindstedt, G., & Nilsson-Ehle, H. (2008). Serum biomarkers for atrophic gastritis and antibodies against Helicobacter pylori in the elderly: Implication for vitamin B12, folic acid and iron status and response to oral vitamin therapy. *Scandinavian Journal of Gastroenterology, 43*, 1050–1056.

Malone, A., & Hamilton, C. (2013). The Academy of Nutrition and Dietetics/the American Society for Parenteral and Enteral Nutrition consensus malnutrition characteristics: Application in practice. *Nutrition in Clinical Practice, 28*, 639–650.

Manini, T., & Clark, B. (2012). Dynapenia and aging: An update. *The Journals of Gerontology, Series A: Biological Sciences and Medical Sciences, 67*(1), 28–40.

Marshall, S., Young, A., Bauer, J., & Isenring, E. (2016). Malnutrition in geriatric rehabilitation: Prevalence, patient outcomes, and criterion validity of the Scored Patient-Generated Subjective Global Assessment and the Mini Nutritional Assessment. *Journal of the Academy of Nutrition and Dietetics, 116*, 785–794.

Morley, J., Vellas, B., van Kan, G., Anker, S. D., Bauer, J. M., Bernabei, R., . . . Walston, J. (2013). Frailty consensus: A call to action. *Journal of the American Medical Directors Association, 14*, 392–397.

Morris, M., Selhub, J., & Jacques, P. (2012). Vitamin B-12 and folate status in relation to decline in scores on the Mini-Mental State Examination in the Framingham Cohort study. *Journal of the American Geriatrics Society, 60*, 1457–1464.

National Institute on Aging, National Institutes of Health. (2015). *Alzheimer's disease fact sheet.* Available at https://d2cauhfh6h4x0p.cloudfront.net/s3fs-public/ad_fact_sheet-2015_update-final.pdf?yc_RAJLU3wLHTP0mQDmeO4le0OcwR8T9. Accessed on 5/2/16.

Paddon-Jones, D., Campbell, W., Jacques, P., Kritchevsky, S. B., Moore, L. L., Rodriguez, N. R., & van Loon, L. J. (2015). Protein and healthy aging. *The American Journal of Clinical Nutrition, 101*(Suppl), 1339S–1345S.

Paddon-Jones, D., Short, K., Campbell, W., Volpi, E., & Wolfe, R. R. (2008). Role of dietary protein in the sarcopenia of aging. *The American Journal of Clinical Nutrition, 87*(5), 1562S–1566S.

Rodriguez, N. (2015). Introduction of Protein Summit 2.0: Continued exploration of the impact of high-quality protein on optimal health. *The American Journal of Clinical Nutrition, 101*(6), 1317S–1319S. doi:10.39445/ajcn.114.083980

Samieri, C., Sun, Q., Townsend, M., Chiuve, S. E., Okereke, O. I., Willett, W. C., . . . Grodstein, F. (2013). The association between dietary patterns at midlife and health in aging: An observational study. *Annals of Internal Medicine, 159*, 584–591.

Skates, J., & Anthony, P. (2012). Identifying geriatric malnutrition in nursing practice: The Mini Nutritional Assessment (MNA®)—an evidence-based screening tool. *Journal of Gerontological Nursing, 38*, 18–27.

Skipper, A., Ferguson, M., Thompson, K., Castellanos, V. H., & Porcari, J. (2012). Nutrition screening tools: An analysis of the evidence. *Journal of Parenteral and Enteral Nutrition, 36*, 292–298.

Sun, Q., Townsend, M., Okereke, O., Franco, O. H., Hu, F. B., & Grodstein, F. (2009). Adiposity and weight change in mid-life in relation to healthy survival after age 70 in women: Prospective cohort study. *BMJ, 339*, b3796.

Szarc vel Szic, K., Declerck, K., Vidaković, M., & Vanden Berghe, W. (2015). From inflammaging to healthy aging by dietary lifestyle choices: Is epigenetics the key to personalized nutrition? *Clinical Epigenetics, 7*, 33. doi:10.1186/s13148-015-0068-2

Tappenden, K., Quatrara, B., Parkhurst, M., Malone, A. M., Fanjiang, G., & Ziegler, T. R. (2013). Critical role of nutrition in improving quality of care: An interdisciplinary call to action to address adult hospital malnutrition. *Journal of the Academy of Nutrition and Dietetics, 113*, 1219–1237.

U.S. Department of Agriculture, Agricultural Research Service. (2014). Nutrient intakes from food and beverages: Mean amounts consumed per individual, by gender and age. *What we eat in America, NHANES 2011-2012.* Available at https://www.ars.usda.gov/ARSUserFiles/80400530/pdf/1112/Table_1_NIN_GEN_11.pdf. Accessed on 1/22/16.

U.S. Department of Health and Human Services. (2008). *2008 Physical activity guidelines for Americans: At-a-glance: A fact sheet for professionals.* Available at www.health.gov/paguidelines/factsheetprof.aspx. Accessed on 11/20/12.

U.S. Department of Health and Human Services, Administration on Aging. (2014). *A profile of older Americans: 2014.* Available at https://aoa.acl.gov/aging_statistics/profile/2014/docs/2014-profile.pdf. Accessed on 4/26/16.

U.S. Department of Health and Human Services & U.S. Department of Agriculture. (2015a). *2015-2020 Dietary guidelines for Americans* (8th ed.). Available at http://health.gov/dietaryguidelines/2015/guidelines/. Accessed on 5/2/16.

U.S. Department of Health and Human Services & U.S. Department of Agriculture. (2015b). *Scientific report of the 2015 Dietary Guidelines Advisory Committee.* Available at http://health.gov/dietaryguidelines/2015-scientific-report/PDFs/Scientific-Report-of-the-2015-Dietary-Guidelines-Advisory-Committee.pdf. Accessed on 5/6/16.

Valls-Pedret, C., Sala-Vila, A., Serra-Mir, M., Corella, D., de la Torre, R., Martínez-González, M. Á., . . . Ros, E. (2015). Mediterranean diet and age-related cognitive decline: A randomized clinical trial. *JAMA Internal Medicine, 175*, 1094–1103.

Walrand, S., Guillet, C., Salles, J., Cano, N., & Boirie, Y. (2011). Physiopathological mechanism of sarcopenia. *Clinics in Geriatric Medicine, 27*, 365–385.

Waters, D., Vawter, R., Qualls, C., Chode, S., Armamento-Villareal, R., & Villareal, D. T. (2013). Long-term maintenance of weight loss after lifestyle intervention in frail, obese older adults. *The Journal of Nutrition, Health & Aging, 17*, 3–7.

Waters, D., Ward, A., & Villareal, D. (2013). Weight loss in obese adults 65 years and older: A review of the controversy. *Experimental Gerontology, 48*, 1054–1061.

Wolfe, R., Miller, S., & Miller, K. (2008). Optimal protein intake in the elderly. *Clinical Nutrition, 27*, 675–684.

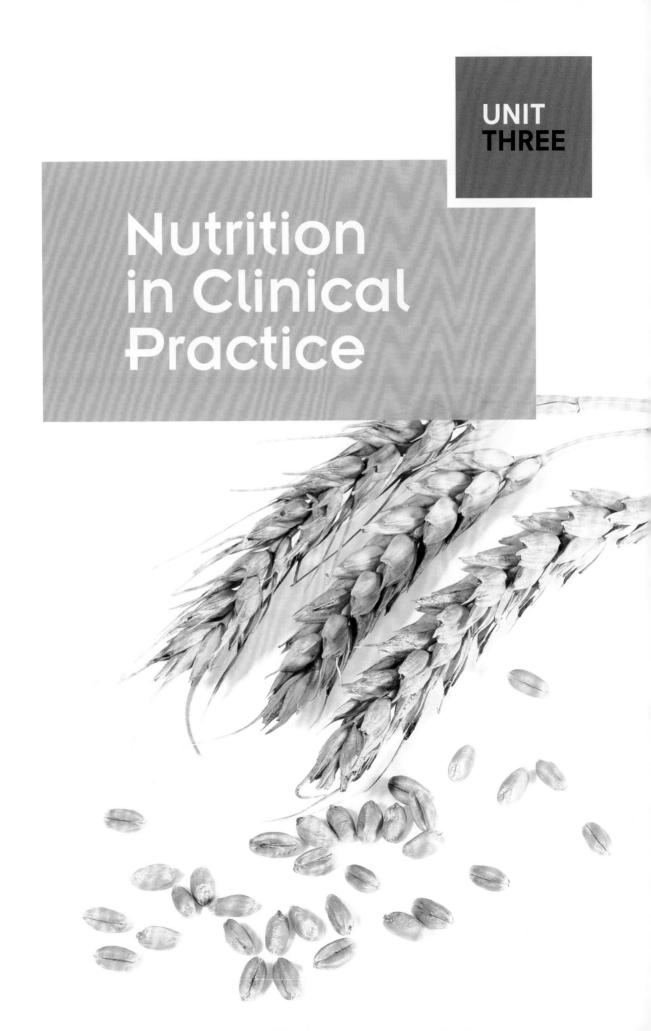

Nutrition
in Clinical
Practice

Chapter 14

Hospital Nutrition: Defining Nutrition Risk and Feeding Patients

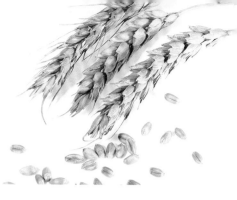

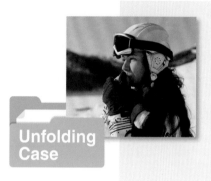

Unfolding Case

Sandy Arnold

Sandy is a 21-year-old downhill skier who is training for international competition. She has been hospitalized for the last 7 days after a skiing accident in which she sustained multiple fractures and internal injuries. She is intubated, a nasoduodenal (ND) feeding tube is placed, and the enteral nutrition order is written for 2200 mL/day of a standard formula that provides 1.0 cal/mL to be given over 18 hours. She has no medical history, is 5 ft 8 in, and weighed 130 pounds upon admission.

Check Your Knowledge

True	False		
☐	☐	1	Adult malnutrition may be related to starvation (e.g., social or environmental related), chronic disease, or acute illness or injury.
☐	☐	2	One of the criteria for the diagnosis of severe malnutrition in a patient with chronic illness is a weight loss of >5% in the previous 6 months.
☐	☐	3	Patient tolerance is improved when oral intake progresses slowly after surgery from a clear liquid diet to regular food.
☐	☐	4	Osmolality is a primary consideration in selecting an appropriate enteral formula.
☐	☐	5	The terms *fiber* and *residue* are synonymous.
☐	☐	6	The patient's ability to digest nutrients is a primary consideration when deciding the type of enteral formula to use.
☐	☐	7	A continuous drip delivered by a pump is recommended for administering tube feedings to patients who are critically ill.
☐	☐	8	Parenteral nutrition can be infused through a peripheral or central vein.
☐	☐	9	The biggest source of calories in parenteral nutrition infusions is protein.
☐	☐	10	Coloring tube-feeding formulas with food dye helps to prevent aspiration.

Learning Objectives

Upon completion of this chapter, you will be able to

1 Modify a menu to an altered consistency diet (e.g., clear liquid diet, pureed diet, mechanically altered diet).
2 Give examples of therapeutic diets and their uses.
3 Compare polymeric enteral formulas with hydrolyzed formulas.

4 Choose the most appropriate enteral formula for a given patient.

5 Discuss the advantages and disadvantages of various enteral nutrition delivery methods.

6 Propose interventions to combat various nutrition-related problems that may occur with enteral nutrition.

7 Explain the potential benefits of using enteral nutrition over parenteral nutrition when enteral nutrition is not contraindicated.

8 List indications for using parenteral nutrition.

9 Discuss the components of parenteral nutrition and the usual concentration of macronutrients provided.

The primary focus of clinical nutrition is to prevent or treat malnutrition. The first step in the process is to identify patients with, or at risk for, malnutrition via a nutrition screen (see Chapter 1). A nutrition assessment follows along with classification of the degree of malnutrition and implementation of a nutrition care plan. The nurse facilitates the nutrition care process by sharing assessment data; facilitating nutrition therapy interventions; reinforcing nutrition education; monitoring the patient's intake, weight, and function; and communicating findings so that the plan can be revised as needed. The nurse plays a critical role in combatting malnutrition.

This chapter begins with the etiology and characteristics of malnutrition and leads to options for "feeding" patients, including oral diets, nutritional supplements, enteral nutrition, and parenteral nutrition.

HOSPITAL MALNUTRITION

The prevalence of malnutrition among hospitalized adults is estimated at 30% to 50% (Jensen, Compher, Sullivan, & Mullin, 2013); however, only 3.2% of these patients are discharged with the diagnosis of malnutrition (Corkins et al., 2014). This discrepancy may be explained in part by the failure to identify patients with malnutrition and the lack of a universally agreed upon definition of malnutrition. It is well recognized that malnutrition is associated with numerous adverse outcomes, including an increased risk of pressure ulcers, impaired wound healing, immune suppression, increased rate of infection, muscle wasting, prolonged hospital stay, higher readmission rates, higher health-care costs, and increased mortality (Barker, Gout, & Crowe, 2011). The deleterious effect of malnutrition not only affects virtually all organ systems but it can also impair cognitive ability, leaving patients unable to make independent, informed consent when they are in a severely compromised nutritional state (Russo, Gupta, & Merriman, 2016). Timely identification and treatment of malnutrition is critical to improving patient outcomes (Field & Hand, 2015).

Diagnosis of Malnutrition

The International Classification of Diseases, 10th Revision, Clinical Modification (ICD-10-CM) includes diagnosis codes for adult protein calorie malnutrition for billing and research purposes. However, the lack of a universally accepted set of signs and symptoms for defining and classifying the severity of malnutrition results in widespread confusion and potential misdiagnosis (White, Guenter, Jensen, Malone, & Schofield, 2012).

Recognizing the need to standardize how malnutrition is defined and classified, the Academy of Nutrition and Dietetics and the American Society of Parenteral and Enteral Nutrition proposed a standardized approach for defining malnutrition in the adult hospitalized patient (White et al., 2012). The etiology-based approach involves assessing the patient for the presence of inflammation, which is a potent contributor to disease related malnutrition (Fig. 14.1) (Malone & Hamilton, 2013). Although there is not one single criteria to confirm the presence of inflammation, a variety of lab values and clinical symptoms may be used, such as low serum albumin, elevated C-reactive protein, high blood glucose, altered white blood

Figure 14.1 ▶
Etiology-based malnutrition definitions.

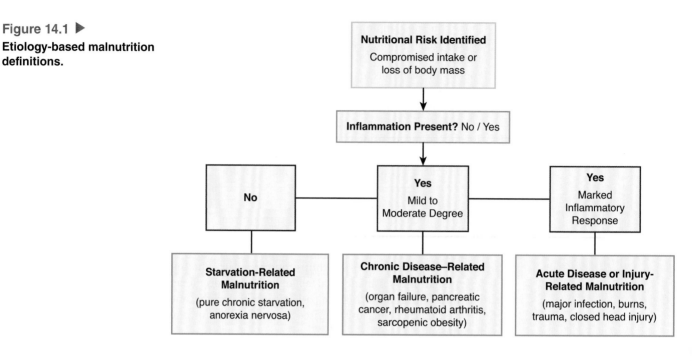

cell count, fever, and infection (Malone & Hamilton, 2013). The etiology-based definitions of malnutrition are

- **Starvation-related**, which occurs when food is not available due to environmental or social circumstances. It usually develops slowly and may be caused by abuse, neglect, famine, poverty, or disordered eating (Skipper, 2012).
- **Chronic disease–related**, which may occur in patients with diseases such as congestive heart failure or chronic obstructive pulmonary disease. A mild to moderate degree of inflammation impedes appetite, intake, or nutrient utilization.
- **Acute disease or injury-related**, which may occur in patients with critical illness, multitrauma, or major infection due to a marked inflammatory response. These patients may be adequately nourished upon admission but are at high risk for malnutrition due to the nature of their illness.

Six characteristics have been proposed for diagnosing and classifying the degree of malnutrition (Table 14.1). Malnutrition is diagnosed when a patient demonstrates two or more characteristics and is classified as severe or nonsevere (moderate) based on specific thresholds and/or descriptions for each etiology of malnutrition. Table 14.2 illustrates the interpretation of weight loss.

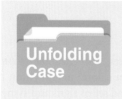

Unfolding Case

Recall Sandy. What was Sandy's body mass index (BMI) on admission? For her age and activity level, 2200 calories is appropriate to meet the needs of healthy females. Is 2200 calories adequate to meet Sandy's needs?

Nutrition Therapy for Malnutrition

Nutrition intervention is well documented to improve key clinical outcomes (Tappenden et al., 2013). Numerous studies, mostly in patients 65 years of age and older, show specific nutrition interventions have the potential to substantially lower complication rates, length of hospital stay, readmission rates, cost of care, and, in some cases, mortality (Cawood, Elia, & Stratton, 2012; Somanchi, Tao, & Mullin, 2011). Actual nutrient requirements are affected by the underlying etiology of malnutrition. For instance, the nutrition prescription for a patient whose malnutrition is caused by cirrhosis will differ from malnutrition caused by major burns.

Table 14.1   Characteristics to Assess for Malnutrition

Malnutrition Characteristics	How Obtained	Potential Problems
Weight loss over time	Actual or stated measurement upon admission Weight history	Fluid overload or dehydration will skew admission weights. Usual weight may be unknown or difficult for the patient or caregiver to recall.
Inadequate food and nutrition intake compared with requirements	History obtained from the patient or caregiver Meal consumption documentation	If indirect calorimetry is not available, calorie needs are estimated by using predictive equations which are less valid.
Loss of muscle mass	Physical assessment of various muscles, such as quadriceps, trapezius, deltoid	Requires experience and training
Loss of fat mass	Physical assessment of subcutaneous fat, such as the orbital region, upper arm, and thoracic regions	Requires experience and training
Fluid accumulation	Physical exam for the presence of local or generalized fluid retention, such as in the lower and upper extremities, face and eyes, and scrotal area	Fluid accumulation may be caused by other conditions such as congestive heart failure or chronic kidney disease.
Measurably diminished hand grip strength	Measured by a dynamometer	Requires experience and training Diseases such as rheumatoid arthritis, dementia, and neuromuscular diseases may limit validity of measure.

Source: Malone, A., & Hamilton, C. (2013). The Academy of Nutrition and Dietetics/The American Society for Parenteral and Enteral Nutrition consensus malnutrition characteristics: Application in practice. *Nutrition in Clinical Practice, 28,* 639–650.

Nutrition intervention strategies include oral diets, supplements, enteral nutrition, and/or parenteral nutrition. Often, a combination of nutrition therapies is needed to meet increased nutritional needs (Russo et al., 2016).

Although timely implementation of a nutrition care plan is clinically important, it is often delayed (Russo et al., 2016). For instance, patients may be nothing by mouth (NPO) for extended periods of time due to medical diagnostic tests or procedures. Patients with poor intake due to changes in mental status may be candidates for enteral nutrition, but it may not be implemented in the hope of quick improvement in mentation. These and other scenarios leave a gap between what is recommended and what is actually implemented. Efforts should be made to monitor "holds" on oral diets or enteral nutrition for procedures and to ensure that enteral or parenteral formulas are infused at the prescribed rate to maximize benefits (Tappenden et al., 2013).

Table 14.2   Interpretation of Weight Loss by Malnutrition Etiology

Etiology of Malnutrition	Moderate Malnutrition	Severe Malnutrition
Starvation or chronic disease	5%/1 month 7.5%/3 months 10%/6 months 20%/1 year	>5%/1 month >7.5%/3 months >10%/6 months >20%/1 year
Acute disease or injury	1–2%/1 week 5%/1 month 7.5%/3 months	>2%/1 week >5%/1 month >7.5%/3 months

Source: Malone, A., & Hamilton, C. (2013). The Academy of Nutrition and Dietetics/The American Society for Parenteral and Enteral Nutrition consensus malnutrition characteristics: Application in practice. *Nutrition in Clinical Practice, 28,* 639–650.

FEEDING HOSPITAL PATIENTS

The goal of nutrition intervention for all hospitalized patients, whether or not they have been diagnosed with malnutrition, is to provide sufficient calories and nutrients to meet the patient's estimated needs in a form the patient can tolerate and utilize. Feeding strategies are presented in the following text.

Oral Diets

Oral diets are the easiest and most preferred method of providing nutrition. In most facilities, patients choose what they want to eat from a menu representing the diet ordered by the physician. Oral diets may be categorized as "regular," modified consistency, or therapeutic. Often, combination diets are ordered, such as a pureed low-sodium diet or a high-protein, soft diet. The actual foods allowed on a diet vary among institutions and the diet manual used.

Private and government regulatory agencies stipulate meal timing, frequency, and nutritional content and require that hospital menus be supervised by a qualified dietitian. Many hospital food service departments offer a room service, cook-to-order menu. Compared to more traditional food service menus, a restaurant-style service gives patients greater control over what and when they eat, provides more menu choices, improves food quality and service temperatures, reduces food waste, and improves patient satisfaction (Fitzpatrick, 2010).

A study by van Bokhorst-de van der Schueren, Roosemalen, Weijs, and Languis (2012) found that although meals provided adequate amounts of calories and protein, most patients do not consume complete meals: 61% of patients consumed <90% of their calorie requirement and 75% consumed <90% of their protein requirement. Appetite may be impaired by fear, pain, or anxiety. Hospital food may be refused because it is unfamiliar, tasteless (e.g., cooked without salt), inappropriate in texture (e.g., pureed meat), religiously or culturally unacceptable, or served at times when the patient is unaccustomed to eating. Inadequate liquid diets may not be advanced to a solid food diet in a timely manner. Patients may underestimate the importance of nutrition in their recovery process. Giving the right food to the patient is one thing; getting the patient to eat (most of it) is another. See Box 14.1 for suggestions on how to promote an adequate intake.

BOX 14.1 Promoting an Adequate Intake

Attention to details can make a big difference in the patient's acceptance of hospital food.

- Let the patient select his or her own menu whenever possible. This gives the patient a greater sense of control, increases the likelihood that the food will be consumed, and may prompt the patient to ask questions about the particular diet or provide information about his or her personal food and nutrition history.
- Offer patients who do not like menu selections the daily "standby" or choices as alternatives. Be aware that "hospital food" is frequently used as a vehicle for patients to vent anger and frustration over their loss of control.
- Be aggressive about diet progressions. Keep in mind that advancing the diet as quickly as possible allows the patient to meet nutritional requirements sooner and increases patient satisfaction.
- Set the stage for a pleasant meal. Be sure trays are delivered promptly to ensure foods are at the proper temperatures. Adjust the lighting and make sure the patient is in an appropriate sitting position. Screen the patient from offensive sights and remove unpleasant odors from the room. Encourage family to visit at mealtime, if appropriate. Offer mouth care to improve appetite, if appropriate.

- Be positive. Refrain from negative comments about the food. Also be aware of what your body language is saying to the patient. A frown or raised eyebrows can speak volumes.
- Provide assistance when necessary. Encourage the patient to self-feed to the greatest extent possible. Some patients may benefit from minor help such as opening milk cartons or buttering bread; others may need to be completely fed. Monitor the patient's ability to self-feed and adjust the intensity of help accordingly.
- Gently motivate the patient to eat. Sometimes, encouragement is all that is needed to get the patient to eat. For other patients, motivation comes from being made aware of the importance of food in the recovery process. Thinking of food as part of treatment instead of a social function may improve intake even when appetite is compromised.
- Identify eating problems. Patients who feel full quickly should be encouraged to eat the most nutritious items first (meat, milk) and save the less dense items for last (juice, soup, coffee). Patients who have difficulty chewing benefit from a mechanical soft diet. Determine if the patient would accept between-meal supplements and a bedtime snack to help maximize intake.

Regular Diet

Regular diets are used to achieve or maintain optimal nutritional status in patients who do not have altered nutritional needs. No foods are excluded, and portion sizes are not limited on a normal diet. The nutritional value of the diet varies significantly with the actual foods chosen by the patient.

Regular diets are adjusted to meet age-specific needs throughout the life cycle. For instance, a regular diet for a child differs from that of an adult. Regular diets are also altered to meet specifications for vegetarian or kosher eating.

Sometimes, physicians order a *diet as tolerated* (*DAT*) on admission or after surgery. This order is interpreted according to the patient's appetite and ability to eat and tolerate food. The nurse has the authority to advance the DAT.

Modified Consistency Diets

Modified consistency diets include clear liquid and mechanically altered diets (Table 14.3). A clear liquid diet is the most frequently ordered postoperative meal, based on the rationale that a gradual progression from a clear liquid diet to a regular diet is important for maximizing tolerance when

Table 14.3   Characteristics of Modified Consistency Diets

Diet Characteristics	Foods Allowed	Indications
Clear liquid A short-term, highly restrictive diet composed only of fluids or foods that are transparent and liquid at body temperature (e.g., gelatin). It requires minimal digestion and leaves a minimum of residue. Inadequate in calories and all nutrients except vitamin C if vitamin C–fortified juices are used.	Clear broth or bouillon Coffee, tea, and carbonated beverages, as allowed and as tolerated Fruit juices; clear (apple, cranberry, grape) and strained (orange, lemonade, grapefruit) Fruit ice made from clear fruit juice Gelatin Popsicles Sugar, honey, hard candy Commercially prepared clear liquid supplements	In preparation for bowel surgery or colonoscopy; acute gastrointestinal disorders; transitional feeding after parenteral nutrition Practice of using clear liquids as initial feeding after surgery may not be warranted.
Pureed diet A diet composed of foods that are blended, whipped, or mashed to pudding-like consistency All foods should be smooth and free of lumps. Most foods can be liquefied by combining equal parts of solids and liquids; fruits and vegetables need less liquid. Broth, gravy, cream soups, cheese, tomato sauce, milk, and fruit juice are preferable to water for blenderizing due to their higher calorie and nutritional value. Liquids may be thickened to improve ease of swallowing.	All foods are allowed, but consistency is changed to liquid.	Used after oral or facial surgery; for wired jaws; chewing and swallowing problems
Mechanically altered diet A regular diet modified in texture only; excludes most raw fruits and vegetables and foods containing seeds, nuts, and dried fruit Gravies, sauces, milk, and water are used to soften foods that are chopped, ground, mashed, or cooked soft. Sticky foods such as peanut butter are avoided.	Chopped or ground diet: milk; yogurt; pudding; cottage cheese; mashed, soft ripened fruit (peaches, pears, bananas); cooked, mashed soft vegetables (peas, carrots, yams); ground meats; soft casseroles; smooth cooked cereals; soft bite-sized pasta; bread products made into a slurry with the addition of gravy or syrup	Used for patients who have limited chewing ability, such as patients who are edentulous, have ill-fitting dentures, or have undergone surgery to the head, neck, or mouth
Soft diet A regular diet that features soft-textured foods that are easy to chew and swallow. Hard, sticky, dry, or crunchy foods are excluded.	Soft cooked vegetables; shredded lettuce; canned fruit; soft, peeled fresh fruit; well-moistened, thin sliced, tender, or ground meats, poultry, or fish; eggs; milk; yogurt; mashed potatoes; white rice; well-cooked pasta; well-moistened cereals without dried fruits or nuts	Used to limit gastrointestinal irritation and minimize gut activity for healing purposes Not intended for long-term use because it can cause constipation

eating resumes. However, there is little scientific evidence to support this practice. In a randomized controlled trial of patients undergoing major gastrointestinal (GI) surgery, giving "normal food" on the first postoperative day did not increase morbidity or mortality; postop nausea occurs in approximately 20% of patients whether they are advanced first to clear liquids or to solid food (Lassen et al., 2008). A regular diet as the first meal has been shown to be well tolerated and provides more nutrition and greater patient satisfaction than a clear liquid diet (Warren, Bhalla, & Cresci, 2011).

Mechanically altered diets contain foods that are pureed, chopped/ground, or soft for patients who have difficulty chewing or swallowing. Dysphagia diets are another variation of modified consistency diets that are covered in Chapter 17.

Therapeutic Diets

Therapeutic diets differ from a regular diet in the amount of one or more nutrients or food components for the purpose of preventing or treating disease or illness. The number or timing of meals may also be altered. Table 14.4 outlines the characteristics and indications of selected therapeutic diets.

Table 14.4 Selected Therapeutic Diets: Characteristics and Indications

Type of Diet	Characteristics	Indications
Heart-healthy or Therapeutic Lifestyle Changes (TLC)	Limited in saturated fats, trans fats, and cholesterol; encourages intake of omega-3 fats; high in fiber, recommends 25%–35% of total calories come from fat; encourages more plant-based meals and attaining/maintaining healthy weight	High cholesterol; prevention or treatment of cardiovascular disease
Consistent carbohydrate	Total daily carbohydrate content is consistent with emphasis on general nutritional balance. Calories are based on attaining and maintaining healthy weight. A high-fiber intake is encouraged, sodium may be limited, and heart-healthy fats are encouraged over saturated fat.	Type 1 and type 2 diabetes, gestational diabetes; impaired glucose tolerance; impaired fasting glucose
Fat restricted	Limits total fat; limitations vary from <50 or <25 g fat/day to 25%–35% of total calories.	Malabsorption syndromes, liver disease, pancreatic disease, chronic cholecystitis, gastroesophageal reflux
High fiber	A general diet with low-fiber foods replaced by foods high in fiber with a goal of 25–35 g or more per day	To prevent or treat constipation, diabetes, irritable bowel syndrome, hypercholesterolemia, obesity
Low fiber	Limits fiber by eliminating skins, membranes, and seeds from fruits and vegetables; allows grains with <2 g fiber/serving; and excludes nuts, seeds, and dried fruits. Lactose may also be restricted.	Before surgery to minimize fecal residue; during acute phases of intestinal disorders, such as ulcerative colitis, Crohn disease, and diverticulitis; radiation therapy to the pelvis and lower bowel; recent intestinal surgery; new colostomy or ileostomy
High calorie, high protein	A diet rich in calorie-dense and/or protein-dense foods	To meet increased nutritional requirements; also used in patients with poor intakes
Renal	Slightly lower in protein, adequate in calories, with sodium, potassium, and phosphorus levels adjusted depending on the stage of chronic kidney disease	Stages 1–4 chronic kidney disease
Potassium modified	Potassium may be increased or restricted by manipulating potassium-rich foods, such as fruits, vegetables, whole grains, milk, and meats.	Low-potassium diets may be used in the treatment of certain renal diseases, in conjunction with certain medications, or in adrenal insufficiency; high-potassium diets may be used in conjunction with certain medications and with certain renal diseases.
Sodium restricted	Sodium limit may be set at 1500 mg/day or 2000 mg/day.	Hypertension, congestive heart failure, acute and chronic renal disease, liver disease
Gluten free	Sources of gluten (a protein in wheat, rye, and barley) are eliminated from the diet; gluten-free grains, such as corn, potato, rice, soy, and quinoa are encouraged as sources of complex carbohydrates.	Celiac disease (celiac sprue, nontropical sprue, gluten-sensitive enteropathy) and dermatitis herpetiformis rash
Lactose restricted	Limits foods with lactose ("milk sugar") to the amount tolerated by the individual.	Lactose intolerance or lactase insufficiency, which may occur secondary to certain inflammatory gastrointestinal disorders such as ulcerative colitis and Crohn disease

Table 14.5   Oral Nutrition Supplements

Type	Examples	Characteristics	Comments
Clear liquid	Ensure Active Ensure Clear Boost Breeze	Provide protein and carbohydrates with 0 g fat for patients on clear liquid diets	Although they come in flavors, they are not as well accepted as the other types of supplements.
Milk based	Carnation Breakfast Essentials Ready-to-Drink Carnation Instant Breakfast Essentials Powder Resource Milk Shake Mix	Contain nonfat milk; powdered forms are mixed with milk. Provide significant amounts of protein and calories; are relatively inexpensive and palatable	Not suitable for patients with lactose intolerance
Commercially prepared liquid	Ensure products: Regular, High Protein, Plus, and other varieties Boost products: Regular, High Protein, Plus, Glucose Control, and other varieties Carnation Instant Breakfast Lactose-Free	Regular varieties: 8 g protein, 250 cal/8 oz High protein: 12–15 g protein/8 oz Plus: 14 g protein, 360 cal/8 oz Are lactose free	Generally sweet and flavored Are quick, easy, varied in flavor, often available in grocery stores Most provide complete nutrition, so they can be used as sole source of nutrition.
Commercially prepared supplemental foods	Hormel Solutions Chocolate Chip Cookie Resource Broth Plus Mix Hormel Solutions High Protein Orange Gelatin Mix Ensure Original Pudding ZonePerfect Nutrition Bars	Specially designed to provide a concentrated source of protein and calories	Offer an alternative to sweetened drinks
Bariatric meal replacement	Bariatric Fusion Meal Replacement Bariatric Advantage High Protein Meal Replacement	Provides 27 g high-quality protein/160 calorie serving; low fat, low carbohydrate; provide fiber, vitamins, and minerals	Formulated for before and after weight loss surgery

Oral Nutrition Supplements

Some patients are unable or unwilling to eat enough food to meet their requirements, either because intake is poor or because their nutritional needs are so high that it is difficult to meet requirements in a normal volume of food. For these patients, oral nutrition supplements (ONS) play a key role in boosting calorie and nutrient intake.

Categories of supplements include clear liquid supplements, milk-based drinks, prepared liquid supplements, specially prepared foods, and bariatric meal replacements (Table 14.5). Liquid supplements are easy to consume, are generally well accepted, and tend to leave the stomach quickly, making them a good choice for between-meal snacks.

A systematic review of ONS therapy found an overall mean compliance rate of 78%, providing an average of 433 cal/day (Hubbard, Elia, Holdoway, & Stratton, 2012). Actions that help promote compliance include obtaining taste preferences, explaining the potential benefits, serving supplements cold, and rotating different types of supplements and various flavors to help forestall or prevent taste fatigue that tends to occur over time. Acceptance should be closely monitored and the percentage consumed documented.

ENTERAL NUTRITION

Enteral nutrition (EN) has long been considered the standard of care for providing nutrition support for patients who are unable to consume adequate calories and protein orally but have at least a partially functional GI tract that is accessible and safe to use. EN may augment an oral diet or may be the sole source of nutrition. Indications for EN include dysphagia, mechanical ventilation, chronic history of poor oral intake, critical illness, head and neck surgeries, and malnutrition with inadequate oral intake. EN is contraindicated when the GI tract is nonfunctional or inaccessible, in severe short bowel syndrome,

> **Enteral Nutrition (EN)**
> the delivery of nutrients by tube, catheter, or stoma into the GI tract beyond the oral cavity; commonly known as tube feeding.

FIGURE 14.2 ▶

**Selecting the appropriate
type and method of feeding.**

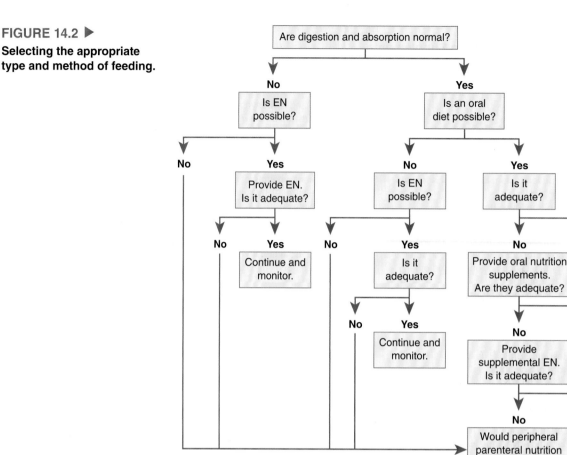

FIGURE 14.2 ▶

**Selecting the appropriate
type and method of feeding.**

intractable vomiting and/or diarrhea, GI ischemia, bowel obstruction, high-output fistula, perito-
nitis, and paralytic ileus. Figure 14.2 illustrates the process of selecting an appropriate method of
feeding based on GI function.

EN is significantly less costly than parenteral nutrition, helps maintain gut integrity and
gut-associated lymphoid tissue, and helps prevent translocation of bacteria (American Academy
of Nutrition and Dietetics, 2016a). Even in critically ill patients, it is practical and safe to use EN
instead of PN (McClave et al., 2016). However, EN has not been proven to affect mortality, and
there is little evidence that EN, when compared to PN, reduces length of hospital stay (Academy
of Nutrition and Dietetics Evidence Analysis Library, 2012).

Enteral Access

The choice of enteral access, or placement of the feeding tube, is highly dependent on the anticipated
length of time tube feeding will be used. Short-term access (<4 weeks) is most commonly obtained
through nasal passage of a feeding tube into the stomach (nasogastric or NG). Less commonly used **transnasal routes** are ND and nasojejunal (NJ). For permanent or long-
term enteral access, a surgical incision or needle puncture is used to create an opening
in the abdominal wall, either into the stomach (gastrostomy) or jejunum (jejunostomy).
The advantages of **ostomy routes** are that they can be hidden under clothing and eliminate irritation to the mucous membranes. The correct placement of any feeding tube
should be verified by radiographs before the first feeding is initiated. Table 14.6 summarizes the advantages and disadvantages of various feeding routes.

Transnasal Routes
feeding routes that extend from the nose to
either the stomach or the small intestine.

Ostomy Routes
a surgically created opening (stoma) made
to deliver feedings directly into the stomach
or intestines.

Table 14.6 Advantages and Disadvantages of Various Feeding Routes

Route	Indications	Advantages	Disadvantages
Nasogastric (NG)	Inability to safely and adequately consume oral intake Short-term feeding (<4 weeks) with functional gastrointestinal tract	Easy to place and remove tube Uses stomach as reservoir Can use intermittent feedings Dumping syndrome less likely than with NI feedings	Contraindicated for clients at high risk for aspiration Potentially irritating to the nose and esophagus May be removed by uncooperative or confused patients Not appropriate for long-term use Unaesthetic for patient
Nasointestinal (NI)	Short-term feeding for patients at high risk of aspiration, delayed gastric emptying, or gastroesophageal reflux disease (GERD)	Less risk of aspiration, especially important for patients who have impaired gag or cough reflex, decreased consciousness, ventilator dependence, or a history of aspiration pneumonia	Increased risk of dumping syndrome Not appropriate for intermittent or bolus feedings Not appropriate for long-term use Unaesthetic for patient
Gastrostomy	For long-term use in patients with a functional gastrointestinal tract Frequently used for patients with impaired ability to swallow	Same advantages as NG but more comfortable and aesthetic for patient Confirmation of tube placement easier Cannot be misplaced into the trachea	Percutaneous endoscopic gastrostomy insertion contraindicated for clients who cannot have an endoscopy Risk of aspiration pneumonia in clients with GERD Stoma care required Danger of peritonitis Potential for tube dislodgment
Jejunostomy	For long-term use in patients at high risk for aspiration pneumonia and in clients with altered gastrointestinal integrity above the jejunum For short-term use after gastrointestinal surgery	Low risk of aspiration No risk of misplacing tube into the trachea More comfortable and aesthetic for clients than transnasal tubes Because motility resumes more quickly in the intestines than in the stomach after gastrointestinal surgery, feedings can begin sooner than other feedings.	Small-diameter tubes easily become clogged Peritonitis can occur from tube dislodgment. Cannot be used for intermittent or bolus feedings Stoma care required

Formula Types

There are currently more than 110 EN formulas and modular products available in the United States for adult and pediatric patients (Academy of Nutrition and Dietetics, 2016a). Enteral formulas are considered medical foods, which the U.S. Food and Drug Administration (FDA) defines as "a food which is formulated to be consumed or administered enterally under the supervision of a physician and which is intended for the specific dietary management of a disease or condition for which distinctive nutritional requirements, based on recognized scientific principles, are established by medical evaluation" (FDA, 2016). Because formulas are food, not medications, their composition is determined by the manufacturer and does not require FDA approval. For instance, the amount of protein in a standard formula varies among brands from 40 to 48 g/L. Table 14.7 features characteristics of various types of enteral formulas. Most institutions have a formulary of specific enteral products available within major categories.

Standard Formulas

Standard formulas, also known as polymeric or intact formulas, are the most commonly used formulas and appropriate for most patients requiring EN. They are designed to mimic a regular diet in that they provide complex molecules of carbohydrate, protein, and fat. They contain whole proteins extracted from milk or soybeans, such as casein, caseinates, soy protein, whey protein, and milk protein or a combination of these proteins. Common sources of carbohydrate include corn maltodextrin, corn syrup solids, sucrose, and sugar alcohols. Sources of fat include canola, soybean, safflower oil, soy lecithin, and

Standard Formulas
tube-feeding formulas that contain whole molecules of protein; also known as intact or polymeric formulas.

Table 14.7   Enteral Formulas: Types, Characteristics, Recommended Uses, and Product Examples

Formula Type	Characteristics	Recommended for Use	Product Examples
Polymeric	Contain complex molecules of carbohydrate, protein, and fat Provide 1–2 cal/mL 1–1.5 L needed to meet RDA for vitamins and minerals Varieties include high protein and high calorie	Intended for patients with normal digestion and absorption	Standard: Osmolite High protein: Promote High calorie: Nutren 2.0
Fiber enriched	A subclass of polymeric formulas intended to improve GI health by regulating frequency and/or consistency of stool by promoting healthy GI microbiota Fiber content is usually well below total daily fiber recommendations. May contain prebiotics (e.g., oligofructose or inulin) May also contain probiotics	Intended for patients with diarrhea or to promote or maintain GI microbiota	Jevity 1.0 Nutren 1.0 Fiber
Blenderized	Includes made at home formulas made from blended whole foods and commercial formulas made from whole foods Appeal to consumers who want "natural" products Provides phytochemicals that are not in standard formulas	Only considered in medically stable patients with a healed feeding tube side and no signs of infection	Compleat (made with chicken, peas, carrots, tomatoes, and cranberry juice)
Diabetes/glucose intolerance	Composed of 40% carbohydrate, 20% protein, 40% fat Fat and soluble fiber content may slow gastric emptying time and prevent elevated glucose.	Not currently supported by strong evidence; instead effort should be made to avoid overfeeding	Glucerna Diabetisource AC Glytrol
Renal	Formulated to meet specific recommendations in acute and chronic renal failure Calorically dense for patients who require fluid restriction Low electrolyte content	For chronic renal disease on dialysis or acute kidney injury	Novasource Renal Nepro with Carb Steady
Hepatic	Low total protein, higher content of branched chain amino acids, lower in aromatic amino acids to decrease hepatic encephalopathy Restricted in fluid and sodium	For hepatic insufficiency or liver disease with encephalopathy refractory to standard treatment	NutriHep
Pulmonary	Low in carbohydrate, high in fat to help reduce CO_2 production and respiratory quotient Calorically dense	For chronic pulmonary disease, respiratory disorders, ventilator dependency Use with caution in septic, critically ill patients	Nutren Pulmonary Pulmocare
Hydrolyzed/ semihydrolyzed	Macronutrients in simple form to promote absorption	Intended for patients with malabsorption problems	Tolerex Peptamen
Immunonutrition	Contains immune-modulating ingredients such as arginine, glutamine, omega-3 fatty acids, and nucleotides	Potentially beneficial for patients undergoing elective surgery; evidence lacking to recommend for routine use among critically ill patients	Impact Peptide 1.5 Pivot 1.5 Cal

RDA, Recommended Daily Allowance; GI, gastrointestinal.
Source: Brown, B., Roehl, K., & Betz, M. (2015). Enteral nutrition formula selection: Current evidence and implications for practice. *Nutrition in Clinical Practice, 30,* 72–85.

medium chain triglycerides (MCT) from coconut and/or palm kernel oil. Variations of standard formulas include formulas that are high in protein, high in calories, and fiber enriched. Normal digestion and absorption are necessary for standard formulas.

Blenderized formulas are a type of standard formula made from a mixture of whole foods, such as chicken, vegetables, fruits, and oil and fortified with vitamins and minerals. They may be homemade or commercially available and appeal to people who want a more natural formula.

Hydrolyzed Formulas

Hydrolyzed
broken down.

Hydrolyzed, or elemental formulas, are intended for patients with impaired digestion or absorption, such as people with inflammatory bowel disease, short-gut syndrome, cystic fibrosis, and pancreatic disorders. They contain nutrients that are partially or completely broken down to their simplest form, such as predigested protein in the form of amino acids, dipeptides, and tripeptides; simple carbohydrates such as hydrolyzed cornstarch, maltodextrin, or fructose; and a small amount of fat in the form of fatty acid esters or MCT. Hydrolyzed formulas are more expensive than intact formulas.

Disease-Specific Formulas

A variety of disease-specific formulas are available to meet the altered nutrient needs of patients with certain illnesses, such as for diabetes/glucose intolerance, kidney disease, liver failure, acute respiratory distress syndrome, chronic obstructive pulmonary disease, immune compromised, and metabolic stress. Use of most disease-specific formulas is not well supported by scientific studies (Academy of Nutrition and Dietetics, 2016a). Expert consensus suggests avoiding the routine use of all specialty formulas in critically ill patients in a medical intensive care unit (ICU) and disease-specific formulas in the surgical ICU (McClave et al., 2016). However, immune-modulating formulas containing arginine should be considered in patients with severe trauma and postop patients in the surgical ICU.

Modular Formulas

An infrequently used option to improve intake is to use a modular formula. Modular formulas are incomplete liquid supplements usually of a single nutrient, such as either carbohydrate (e.g., hydrolyzed cornstarch), protein (e.g., whey protein), or fat (e.g., MCT oil). These products can be combined to make a customized tube feeding or added to existing formulas or foods to boost calorie or nutrient density. For instance, a patient with chronic kidney failure may receive carbohydrate-fortified mashed potatoes to increase calorie intake without increasing protein or altering taste. The disadvantages of using modular products are ineffective quality control (calculation errors), bacterial contamination, and higher costs than standard formulas. Modular products added to tube feedings increase the risk of nutrient imbalances and clogged tubes.

Nutrient Content

Formulas are designed to provide complete nutrition when consumed in sufficient volume. Formulas differ in their macronutrient content, micronutrient density, calorie density, water content, fiber content, and osmolality. Virtually all commercially available enteral formulas are gluten and lactose free.

Macronutrient Content

The amounts of carbohydrate, fat, and protein vary significantly among enteral products. Standard formulas generally provide 30% to 60% of calories from carbohydrate, 10% to 25% of calories from protein, and 10% to 45% of calories from fat. The concentrations of fat and carbohydrate are usually not a primary concern, unless they are important because of disease, such as diabetic formulas, high-fat formulas for patients with respiratory disease, and modified-fat formulas for patients with malabsorption.

Micronutrient Density

Micronutrient density, as indicated by the amount of formula needed to meet 100% of adult Dietary Reference Intakes (DRIs) for vitamins and minerals, varies among formulas. Generally, the amount of formula needed to meet nutrient DRIs ranges from 1000 to 1500 mL/day. When a tube feeding is the patient's sole source of nutrition, it is important to ensure nutritional adequacy within the volume of formula the patient receives.

Calorie Density

The calorie density of a product determines the volume of formula needed to meet the patient's estimated needs. Most routine formulas provide 1.0 to 1.2 cal/mL, which is adequate for most patients needing EN support. High-calorie formulas provide 1.5 to 2.0 cal/mL and are appropriate for patients who need a fluid restriction or those who are intolerant of higher volumes of formula.

Water Content

The water content of tube feedings varies with the caloric concentration. Generally, formulas that provide 1.0 cal/mL provide approximately 850 mL of water per liter. The water content of high-calorie formulas is lower at 690 to 720 mL/L. Adults generally need 30 to 40 mL/kg/day, so most patients who received EN need additional free water to meet fluid requirements. Free water is administered when water is used to flush the tube and as a bolus administration specifically for the purpose of meeting fluid requirements.

Fiber Content

Fiber
the group name for carbohydrates that are not digested in the human GI tract.

Residue
what remains in the GI tract after digestion, namely, fiber, undigested food, intestinal secretions, bacterial cell bodies, and cells shed from the intestinal lining.

Blenderized Formula
a type of standard formula made from blenderized whole foods.

Although they are not synonymous, the terms fiber and residue are frequently used interchangeably. Fiber stimulates peristalsis, increases stool bulk, and is degraded by GI bacteria to short-chain fatty acids that promote repair and maintenance of the intestinal lining. Fiber combines with undigested food, intestinal secretions, and other cells to make residue. Fiber is one component of residue, but residue encompasses other substances as well.

Hydrolyzed formulas are essentially residue free because they are completely absorbed. Standard formulas come in low residue or fiber-enriched varieties that provide 10 to 15 g fiber per liter in the form of oat, soy, pea, guar gum, or other fibers. Blenderized formulas are made from whole foods and thus contain natural sources of fiber, generally about 4 g fiber per liter.

EN formulas containing fiber may improve digestive health and normal bowel function (Brown, Roehl, & Betz, 2015). Research indicates diarrhea may be prevented or managed in critically ill adults when guar gum is included in the EN regimen (Academy of Nutrition and Dietetics Evidence Analysis Library, 2012). Results of a meta-analysis showed that formulas containing soluble fiber may be most beneficial in reducing diarrhea in patients with the higher occurrence of loose stools (Elia, Engfer, Green, & Silk, 2008). Only limited evidence supports the use of high-fiber formulas to improve glycemic control in patients with diabetes (Brown et al., 2015). Fiber-containing formulas should be avoided in patients with acute intestinal disorders and before or after some intestinal surgeries.

Osmolality

Osmolality
the measure of the number of particles in solution; expressed as milliosmoles per kilogram (mOsm/kg).

Isotonic
a formula that has approximately the same osmolality as blood, about 300 mOsm/kg.

Hypertonic
a formula with an osmolality greater than that of blood (>300 mOsm/kg).

In enteral formulas, osmolality is determined by the concentration of sugars, amino acids, and electrolytes. Isotonic formulas have approximately the same osmolality as blood (approximately 300 mOsm/kg). Most enteral formulas are hypertonic, with osmolalities between 300 to 700 mOsm/kg. Generally, the more digested the protein, the greater the osmolality; thus, hydrolyzed formulas are higher in osmolality than standard formulas.

For most people, osmolality does not affect tolerance. However, some patients develop diarrhea when a hypertonic formula is infused into the small intestine. Initiating the formula at a slow rate and advancing the rate gradually and slowly improves tolerance.

Equipment

Formulas come in cans or sealed containers to which the tubing is attached for administration. Tubing size and pump availability affect formula selection. Generally, high-fiber formulas have a high viscosity and require a large-bore tube (8 French or greater) to prevent clogging. Adding a modular product to a formula to increase the nutrient or calorie density may also necessitate the use of a larger tube. Hydrolyzed formulas have very low viscosity but should be delivered by pump to ensure controlled administration. The minimum tube size required for pump or gravity feeding should be verified from the EN product guide or manufacturer website (Academy of Nutrition and Dietetics, 2016a).

Delivery Methods

Formulas may be given intermittently or continuously over a period of 8 to 24 hours. The rates may be regulated either by a pump or by gravity drip. The type of delivery method to be used depends on the type and location of the feeding tube, the type of formula being administered, and the patient's tolerance.

Intermittent Tube Feedings

Intermittent feedings are administered four to six times daily in equal portions of 250 to 400 mL of formula infused over 30 to 45 minutes with or without a pump. The number of feedings given per day depends on the total volume of feeding needed. Feedings may be spaced throughout an entire 24-hour period or may be scheduled only during waking hours to give patients time for uninterrupted sleep. Intermittent feedings are generally used for noncritical patients, home tube feedings, and patients in rehabilitation. They offer the advantage of resembling a more normal pattern of intake, and they allow the client more freedom of movement between feedings. Tolerance of intermittent feedings is optimized by infusing the formula at room temperature. To decrease the risk of aspiration, **gastric residuals** are checked before each feeding until tolerance is clearly established. Water flushes should occur before and after each intermittent feeding.

Intermittent Feedings
tube feedings administered in equal portions at selected intervals.

Gastric Residuals
the volume of feeding that remains in the stomach from a previous feeding.

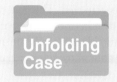

Unfolding Case

Think of Sandy. The doctor has ordered 2200 mL/day of a standard formula that provides 1.0 cal/mL which is to be given over 18 hours. What will the infusion rate be? Will she meet her fluid requirement without additional free water?

Bolus Feedings

Bolus Feedings
rapid administration of a large volume of formula.

Dumping Syndrome
a group of symptoms, such as nausea, vomiting, diarrhea, distention, and cramps, caused by the rapid emptying of an osmotic load from the stomach into the small intestine.

Bolus feedings are a variation of intermittent feedings. The formula is poured into the barrel of a large syringe attached to the feeding tube. A large volume of formula (500 mL maximum; usual volume is 250–400 mL) is delivered relatively quickly, usually in 5 to 15 minutes every 3 to 4 hours. They are used only for feedings into the stomach and allow greater independence for patients. Bolus feedings are usually tolerated when infused into the stomach; when infused into the intestine, they may cause **dumping syndrome**.

Continuous Drip Method

Continuous drip feedings are the most commonly used administration method in hospitalized patients, especially those who are critically ill or who receive intestinal feedings. They are given at a constant rate over a 24-hour period to maximize tolerance and nutrient absorption. Infusion pumps are used to ensure consistent flow rates. This method is associated with smaller residual volumes, lower risk for aspiration, and a decrease in the severity of diarrhea when compared to other delivery methods. Continuous feedings should be interrupted every 4 hours so that 20 to 30 mL of warm water can be infused into the line to clear the tubing and hydrate the client.

Cyclic Feedings

A variation of continuous drip feedings, cyclic feedings deliver a constant rate of formula over 8 to 20 hours, often during sleeping hours. Extra care must be taken to keep the head of the bed continuously elevated more than 30 degrees to avoid aspiration. Because there is "time off," the rate of infusion tends to be higher than for continuous feedings. Cyclic feedings are usually well tolerated and are often used to maintain a reliable source of nutrition while transitioning from total EN to an oral intake or in noncritical, undernourished patients unable to meet their nutritional needs orally.

Initiating and Advancing the Feeding

Before initiating a feeding, tube placement is verified, ideally by radiography, and the tube is marked with indelible ink or adhesive tape where it exits the nose (Simons & Abdallah, 2012). Other common verification methods, such as auscultation, aspirating gastric contents, and pH testing, are less

Quick Bite

Periodic flushing of the tube helps meet water requirements and ensures patency (openness). Although cranberry juice and cola have been used, water is the preferred flush (Bankhead et al., 2009). The often-cited standard for maintaining tube patency in adults is to flush with a minimum of 20 to 30 mL of warm water (Charney & Malone, 2013)

● Every 4 hours for continuous feedings
● Before and after bolus or intermittent feedings
● Before and after residual checks
● Before and after medication administration

If a tube becomes clogged, activated pancreatic enzyme solutions and products to mechanically eliminate clogs are commercially available but studies on the safety and efficacy of these methods are lacking (Charney & Malone, 2013).

reliable and not recommended. Elevate the patient's upper body to at least a 30-degree angle, preferably to 45 degrees, for all patients receiving EN, unless it is medically contraindicated to reduce the risk of aspiration.

Regardless of the access route, tube-feeding formulas are initiated at full strength. The previous practice of diluting hypertonic feedings has not been shown to improve tolerance, prolongs the period of inadequate nutrition support, and may increase the risk of bacterial contamination. Initiating feedings at full strength has not been found to cause tube-feeding intolerance or diarrhea.

To enhance tolerance in critically ill patients and those who have not eaten in a long time, conservative initiation and advancement rates are recommended. Regardless of the type of formula used, the initial rate may begin at 10 to 40 mL/hour and advance by 10 to 20 mL/hour every 8 to 12 hours as tolerated until the desired rate is achieved. The goal rate should be achieved within 24 to 36 hours. The sooner the goal rate is achieved, the sooner the patient's nutritional needs are met. Stable patients may tolerate beginning enteral feedings at the goal rate.

Tube-Feeding Complications

EN is generally considered safe, but GI, metabolic, and mechanical complications are possible. Monitoring ensures that the patient is tolerating the EN regimen and that it is adequately meeting the patient's needs (Box 14.2).

Aspiration is the most serious potential complication with EN. Patients with inhibited cough reflex related to debilitation, unconsciousness, or pulmonary complications are at high risk for aspiration as are those with delayed gastric emptying or gastroesophageal reflux. More common than large-volume aspirations is a series of clinically silent small aspirations. Aspiration increases the risk of aspiration-related pneumonia. Table 14.8 summarizes potential nutrition-related problems in tube-fed patients.

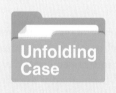

Unfolding Case

Recall Sandy. She develops diarrhea after 2 days on the tube feeding. What are the possible causes? What would you recommend to resolve her diarrhea?

BOX 14.2   Criteria to Monitor in Tube-Fed Hospitalized Patients

● Daily weight to detect fluid shifts
● Daily intake and output
● Gastric residual character and volume every 4 to 8 hours or before each intermittent feeding in patients fed via the stomach. Return all aspiration secretions to the stomach because they contain nutrients, electrolytes, and digestive enzymes.
● Character and frequency of bowel movements
● Signs and symptoms of intolerance: vomiting, nausea, distention, constipation
● Daily electrolyte levels, serum glucose, blood urea nitrogen (BUN), and creatinine until goal rate is achieved; thereafter, two to three times per week or as needed. Minerals and a weekly blood count may be ordered.
● External length of the tube, to check for displacement
● Tube site for infection

Table 14.8	Troubleshooting Nutrition-Related Problems in Tube-Fed Patients	

Potential Problem	Possible Cause	Nursing Interventions and Considerations
Aspiration	Feeding infused into the lung	Confirm proper placement of the feeding tube by radiograph prior to initiating a feeding.
	Gastroesophageal reflux	Elevate the bed's headboard 30–45 degrees during feeding and for approximately 1 hour afterward.
	Impaired cough reflex	Consider a nasointestinal or jejunostomy feeding.
	Delayed gastric emptying	Monitor gastric residuals. Switch to a continuous drip delivery method.
Diarrhea	Infusion of a formula that is too cold	Give canned formulas at room temperature. Warm refrigerated formulas to room temperature in a basin of warm water.
	Bacterially contaminated formula	Follow handwashing and sanitation protocol. Refrigerate unused formula promptly. Discard opened cans within 24 hours. Flush the tubing as per protocol. Hang formulas for less than 6 hours. Change extension tubing every 24 hours. Initiate and advance feedings as per protocol.
	Feeding rate too rapid	For existing feedings, decrease the rate to the level tolerated and then advance at half the original increment (e.g., 12 mL/hour instead of 25 mL/hour). Feed smaller volumes more frequently or switch to continuous drip method.
	Volume of formula too great Side effect of antibiotics or other medications	Consider a high-calorie formula if problem persists. Investigate drugs used for possible causes/possible alternatives. Administer antidiarrheals as ordered. Consider using intermittent feeding that are coordinated with antibiotic dosing
	Malplacement of feeding tube	Check the position of the tube.
	Feeding rate too rapid	Slow the rate of feeding; switch to a continuous drip method of delivery.
Nausea (Discontinue the feeding. Administer antiemetics if ordered by the physician.)	Volume of formula too great → delayed gastric emptying Feeding too soon after intubation	Check gastric residual and proceed as per facility protocol. If distention is contributing to nausea, encourage ambulation. Optimal time to initiate feeding varies with type of access (e.g., NG, open surgical gastrostomy); follow facility protocol.
	Anxiety Intolerance to a specific formula, especially high-fat formulas	Explain the procedures to the client and encourage questions. Allow client to verbalize his or her feelings; provide emotional support. Switch to a different formula.
Distention and bloating	High-fat content of formula	Switch to lower-fat formula.
	Decrease in gastrointestinal function, especially among critically ill clients	Check for active bowel sounds; switch to a hydrolyzed formula if bowel sounds are hypoactive.
Dehydration	Excessive protein intake → compensatory increase in urine output to excrete nitrogenous wastes	Switch to a formula with less protein; increase water intake, if possible.
	Inadequate fluid intake	Provide additional water.
	Glycosuria (glucose in urine)	Test for glucose in the urine; notify physician of glycosuria of 3+ or 4+. Administer insulin if ordered by physician. Switch to a continuous drip method to avoid giving a high-carbohydrate load with each feeding.
Fluid overload	Excessive use of water to flush tube	Use only 20–30 mL of water to rinse tubing after each feeding.

(continued)

Table 14.8	Troubleshooting Nutrition-Related Problems in Tube-Fed Patients (continued)

Potential Problem	Possible Cause	Nursing Interventions and Considerations
Constipation	Low residue content of formula	Increase fiber content if appropriate (i.e., change to a formula with added fiber or increase fruits and vegetables in a blenderized diet).
	Inactivity	Encourage ambulation as much as possible.
	Dehydration	Monitor intake and output; add free water if intake is not greater than output by 500–1000 mL.
	Obstruction	Stop feeding and notify physician.
Gastric rupture	Dangerous retention of feeding in the stomach related to gastric atony or obstruction	Observe for signs of impending gastric rupture: distention, epigastric and upper quadrant pain, nausea, a large residual; if observed, discontinue feeding immediately and notify the physician.
Clogged tube	Improper cleaning of tube	Regular flushing with appropriate volumes of warm water as per facility protocol Replace the feeding tube and bag every 12–24 hours. Flush the tube before and after each infusion (regardless of method) with 30–50 mL of water; if flushing fails to remove clog, the tube must be removed and replaced.
	Deprivation of food → lack of sensory, social, and cultural satisfaction from eating	Allow oral intake of food that the client requests, if possible; if oral intake is contraindicated, allow the client to chew his or her favorite food without swallowing. Encourage the client to leave the room when others are eating and find other enjoyable activities. Encourage client and family to view tube feeding as another way of eating rather than a form of treatment.
Anxiety	Altered body image	Encourage client to verbalize his or her feelings. Stress positive aspects of tube feeding.
	Loss of control; fear	Encourage client to become involved in preparation and administration of the formula, if possible. Inform client of problems that may occur and how to prevent or cope with them. Encourage socialization with other well-adapted tube-fed clients.
	Limited mobility	Encourage normal activity.
	Discomfort related to tube or formula intolerance	Control gastrointestinal symptoms, such as diarrhea, nausea, vomiting, and constipation, that interfere with normal activity. Observe for intolerances; alleviate with appropriate interventions. Be sure to inspect and properly care for the tube exit site to avoid potential complications.
Dry mouth	Irritation of mucous membranes related to lack of oral intake	Encourage good oral hygiene to alleviate soreness and dryness: mouthwash, warm water rinses, regular brushing. Apply petroleum jelly to the lips to prevent cracking. Allow ice chips, sugarless gum, and hard candies, if possible, to stimulate salivation.
	Breathing through the mouth	Encourage client to breathe through the nose as much as possible.

Giving Medications by Tube

Although many medications are frequently given through feeding tubes to patients who are unable to swallow, they should never be given while a feeding is being infused. Some drugs become ineffective if added directly to the enteral formula; also, adding acidic drugs to the formula may cause the protein to coagulate and clog the tube. It is important to stop the feeding before administering drugs and to make sure the tube is flushed with 10 to 30 mL of water before and after the drug is given. If more than one drug is given, flush the tube between doses with 5 mL of water. See Box 14.3 for other drug considerations.

BOX 14.3 — Considerations for Giving Medications Through a Feeding Tube

- Drugs absorbed from the stomach should never be given through a nasointestinal tube.
- The liquid form of a medication diluted with 30 mL of water should be used for feeding tube administration. If there is no alternative, a drug can be crushed to a fine powder and mixed with water before it is administered. Slow-release drugs should never be crushed.
- Dilute highly viscous and hyperosmolar liquid medications with 10 to 30 mL of water before administering.
- Drugs should be given orally whenever possible.
- Tube feeding may need to be temporarily stopped to permit drug administration on an empty stomach or to avoid drug–nutrient interaction. Some experts recommend stopping a continuous feeding for 15 minutes before and after the delivery of the medication.

Transition to an Oral Diet

The goal of diet intervention during the transition period between EN and an oral diet is to ensure an adequate nutritional intake while promoting an oral diet. To begin the transition process, the tube feeding should be stopped for 1 hour before each meal. Gradually increase meal frequency until six small oral feedings are accepted. Actual intake should be recorded and evaluated daily. When oral calorie intake consistently reaches 500 to 700 cal/day, tube feedings may be given only during the night. When the patient consistently consumes two-thirds of protein and calorie needs and 1000 mL fluid orally for 3 consecutive days, the tube feeding may be totally discontinued.

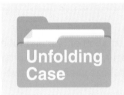

Unfolding Case

Consider Sandy. Her condition improves and she desperately wants to have the feeding tube removed but knows she has to demonstrate that she can orally consume at least a "fair" intake. What measures can you take to encourage and maximize her oral intake?

NURSING PROCESS

Enteral Nutrition Support

Vince is 48 years old, 6 ft tall, and has weighed 170 to 175 pounds throughout his adult life. Two weeks ago, he was admitted to the ICU after an industrial accident caused first- and second-degree burns over 20% of his body. He was initially fed via an NG tube and then started on an oral diet. Vince was only able to achieve 40% of the calorie goal set by the dietitian, so he has reluctantly agreed to be fed by tube for 8 hours during the night to supplement his daytime oral intake.

Assessment

Medical–Psychosocial History

- Medical history, such as diabetes or GI disorder
- Medications that may affect nutrition
- Current treatment plan
- Level of tube-feeding acceptance, including fears or apprehension about being tube fed during the night
- If Vince may need a tube feeding after discharge, assess living situation, such as availability of running water, electricity, refrigeration, cooking and storage facilities, employment, social support system, and financial status

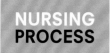

Enteral Nutrition Support

Anthropometric Assessment	Height, current weight, body mass index Percentage of usual body weight
Biochemical and Physical Assessment	• Check laboratory values—hemoglobin, hematocrit, glucose, electrolytes; other abnormal values for their nutritional significance • Check tube for proper positioning; check external length of tube every 4 hours to monitor tube placement. • Monitor hydration status. • Ask if the client has any physical complaints associated with oral food intake or tube feeding, such as nausea or bloating. • Observe abdomen for distention. • Measure gastric residual volumes. • Monitor stool frequency, volume, and consistency.
Dietary Assessment	• How many calories and how much protein are being provided via the tube feeding? • Do the nocturnal tube feedings affect the amount of food consumed orally during the day? • Is protocol being followed for administering the tube feeding and documenting administration and tolerance? • Is Vince able and willing to learn how to use tube feeding at home if necessary?

Diagnosis

Possible Nursing Diagnoses	Imbalanced nutrition: consuming fewer calories than the body requires related to hypermetabolism secondary to thermal injuries

Planning

Client Outcomes	The patient will • Meet calorie and protein goals via combination of oral and tube feeding • Be free of any signs or symptoms of aspiration and other complications • Discontinue tube feedings when oral intake is consistently two-thirds of calorie and protein goal

Nursing Interventions

Nutrition Therapy	• Administer tube feeding as ordered. • Encourage oral intake.
Client Teaching	Instruct the client • On the importance of tube feedings for supplemental nutrition until oral intake meets at least two-thirds of goal • On the signs and symptoms of intolerance of tube feeding and to alert the nurse if any problems arise • Not to adjust the flow rate unless otherwise instructed • On formula preparation, administration, and monitoring as well as the rationales and interventions for tube-feeding complications, if home enteral nutrition is indicated

Evaluation

Evaluate and Monitor	• Monitor weight. • Monitor calorie and protein intake. • Monitor flow rate and administration. • Monitor for signs and symptoms of intolerance: aspiration, complaints of nausea, bloating, high gastric residuals, and diarrhea.

PARENTERAL NUTRITION

Parenteral Nutrition (PN)
the delivery of nutrients by vein; parenteral literally means "outside the intestinal tract."

Parenteral nutrition (PN) was developed in the 1960s when researchers from the University of Pennsylvania discovered how to deliver nutrients into the bloodstream via central venous access, thereby bypassing the GI tract (Koretz, 2007). Using a large-diameter central vein allows for the infusion of a nutritionally complete, hypertonic formula because it is quickly diluted; smaller veins are not able to handle such concentrated solutions. PN is a lifesaving therapy in patients who have a nonfunctional GI tract, such as in the case of small bowel obstruction, mesenteric ischemia, severe short bowel syndrome, GI fistula (and not able to tube feed distal to the fistula), paralytic ileus, or in patients who are unable to meet their estimated calorie needs after 7 to 10 days of EN (Academy of Nutrition and Dietetics, 2016b). In practice, PN is used for other clinical conditions, such as critical illness, acute pancreatitis, liver transplantation, and AIDS, and in cancer patients receiving bone marrow transplants.

PN is invasive, costly, and associated with infectious, metabolic, and mechanical complications (Box 14.4). Although PN serves an important role in the nutrition management of specific diseases, it is losing favor as the treatment of choice in some conditions in which PN was previously considered required, such as acute pancreatitis (Martin et al., 2011). PN is never an emergency procedure, and it should be discontinued as soon as possible. PN is not indicated when the prognosis does not warrant aggressive nutrition support (Academy of Nutrition and Dietetics, 2016b).

When EN is not feasible, it is recommended that (McClave et al., 2016)

- Exclusive PN be withheld for the first 7 days in patients at low nutrition risk.
- Exclusive PN begin as soon as possible following ICU admission in patients who are severely malnourished or high risk of malnutrition. During the first week of hospitalization, a hypocaloric dose ($\leq$20 cal/kg/day or 80% of estimated needs) with adequate protein ($\leq$1.2 g/kg/day) should be considered.
- In patients who are receiving EN, supplemental PN should be considered after 7 to 10 days if the patient is unable to meet >60% of calorie and protein requirements by EN alone.

BOX 14.4 — Potential Complications of Parenteral Nutrition

Infection and Sepsis Related to

Catheter contamination during insertion
Long-term indwelling catheter
Catheter seeding from bloodborne or distant infection
Contaminated solution

Mechanical Complications

Dehydration; hypovolemia
Bone demineralization
Hyperglycemia
Rebound hypoglycemia
Hyperosmolar, hyperglycemic state
Azotemia
Electrolyte disturbances
    Hypocalcemia
    Hypophosphatemia, hyperphosphatemia
    Hypokalemia
    Hypomagnesemia
High serum ammonia levels
Deficiencies of
    Essential fatty acids
    Trace elements
    Vitamins and minerals

Altered acid–base balance
Elevated liver enzymes
Fluid overload

Mechanical Complications Related to Catheterization

Catheter misplacement
Hemothorax (blood in the chest)
Pneumothorax (air or gas in the chest)
Hydrothorax (fluid in the chest)
Hemomediastinum (blood in the mediastinal spaces)
Subcutaneous emphysema
Hematoma
Arterial puncture
Myocardial perforation
Catheter embolism
Cardiac dysrhythmia
Air embolism
Endocarditis
Nerve damage at the insertion site
Laceration of lymphatic duct
Chylothorax
Lymphatic fistula
Thrombosis

Catheter Placement

PN may be infused via peripheral or central veins. Peripheral parenteral nutrition (PPN) is not widely used because solutions infused into peripheral veins must have lower osmolarity (<900 mOsm/L) (i.e., they must have low concentrations of dextrose and amino acids) to prevent phlebitis and increased risk of thrombus formation (Boullata et al., 2014). Because the caloric and nutritional value of PPN is limited, it is best suited for patients who need short-term nutrition support (≤10–14 days) and do not require more than 2500 cal/day. PPN is contraindicated in patients who need a fluid restriction, such as in patients with renal failure, liver failure, or congestive heart failure.

Central PN
the infusion of nutrients into the bloodstream by way of a central vein. Central PN solutions are nutritionally complete.

Central PN is administered via central venous catheters (CVCs) that access large veins; their distal tip lies in the distal vena cava or right atrium. CVC, which may be single or multilumen, are most commonly placed in the jugular, subclavian, femoral, cephalic, or basilic veins (Academy of Nutrition and Dietetics, 2016b). CVC catheters may be nontunneled (percutaneous nontunneled central catheter, peripherally inserted central catheter [PICC]), tunneled, or implanted ports.

Composition of Parenteral Nutrition

PN solutions are a complex admixture of protein, carbohydrate, fat, electrolytes, vitamins, and trace elements in sterile water. PN solutions are commercially available as premade formulas in single container or multichamber bags, often referred to as "premixed" (although they require mixing in the pharmacy) or may be prepared in the hospital pharmacy using manual or automated compounding techniques, which allows individualization of the solution based on the patient's fluid and nutrient requirements (Boullata et al., 2014). PN may be compounded as a 2-in-1 solution with dextrose and amino acids with additional additives mixed in one bag. A fat emulsion is administered separately via intravenous (IV) piggyback. The other option is a 3-in-1 solution or total nutrient admixture that contains dextrose, amino acids, and lipids in one bag.

Protein

Protein is provided as a solution of crystalline essential and nonessential amino acids with the amounts of specific amino acids varying insignificantly among manufacturers. Amino acid solutions range in concentration from 3% to 20%, providing 30 to 200 g protein per liter, respectively. Specially modified amino acid solutions are available for renal failure (only essential amino acids), liver failure (high in branched-chain amino acids, low in aromatic amino acids), and high stress (high in branched-chain amino acids), but they are rarely used because there is little evidence of benefit (Academy of Nutrition and Dietetics, 2016b).

Dextrose

Dextrose Monohydrate
a molecule of glucose combined with a molecule of water.

Glucose, in the form of **dextrose monohydrate**, is the main source of calories in PN. It provides 3.4 cal/g and is available in concentrations ranging from 2.5% to 70% that provide 25 to 700 g/L, respectively. Only concentrations at 10% or less are used for PPN to avoid damage to the peripheral vein. In adults, 100 to 125 g of carbohydrate are needed daily to optimally suppress hepatic gluconeogenesis and to meet glucose requirements for the central nervous system. It is estimated that an adult is not able to oxidize glucose at rates higher than 5 to 7 mg/kg/min (≤4 mg/kg/min in critically ill patients) (Academy of Nutrition and Dietetics, 2016b). However, this rate is individualized and dependent on the patient's condition.

Although carbohydrate is an important energy source, giving a patient too much can have negative consequences. Hyperglycemia is associated with immune function impairments and increased risk of infectious complications. A high carbohydrate load may also lead to excessive carbon dioxide production, which may complicate weaning from mechanical ventilation. The trend toward less aggressive feeding has decreased the incidence of this complication.

Fat

Lipid emulsions provide essential fatty acids in an isotonic solution. They are made from 100% soybean oil or 50:50 mixes of safflower plus soybean oil. Lipid emulsions are available in

10%, 20%, and 30% concentrations, supplying 1.1, 2.0, and 3.0 cal/mL, respectively. Lipids are a significant source of calories and so are useful when volume must be restricted or when dextrose must be lowered because of persistent hyperglycemia. Patients with egg allergies may not tolerate lipid emulsions because they contain egg phospholipids as emulsifiers.

All lipid emulsions in the United States are composed of omega-6 fatty acids, which are implicated as contributing to the inflammatory response (Academy of Nutrition and Dietetics, 2016b). The minimum amount of lipid recommended is 10% (500 mL) or 20% (250 mL) given twice a week. However, they are often given daily and may provide 20% to 30% of total calories. IV lipid emulsions should not exceed 1 g/kg/day in critically ill and septic patients and are restricted in patients with hypertriglyceridemia. Due to a propensity for microbial growth, IV piggyback lipids should not hang longer than 12 hours.

Electrolytes, Vitamins, and Trace Elements

Standard electrolyte packages include sodium, potassium, chloride, calcium, magnesium, acetate, and phosphorus. The amounts of these nutrients infused parenterally are lower than DRI recommendations because DRI values take into account the efficiency of intestinal absorption when nutrients are consumed orally. Electrolyte content of PN is adjusted according to the patient's acid–base status and fluid–electrolyte status. Standard adult and pediatric preparations exist for vitamins and trace elements. The standard IV multivitamin for PN is multivitamin infusion (MVI)-13, which contains all fat and water soluble vitamins; although a preparation without vitamin K is available for patients on warfarin therapy. Multiple trace element (MTE) vials and single-entity vials are commercially available. MTE mixtures have four or five different trace elements, including zinc, copper, chromium, manganese, and selenium. Because iron destabilizes other ingredients in parenteral solutions, a special form of iron must be injected separately as needed.

Medications

Medications are sometimes added to IV solutions by the pharmacist or infused into them through a separate port. For instance, insulin may be given by piggyback to improve glucose tolerance. Heparin may be added to reduce fibrin buildup on the catheter tip. In general, medications should not be added to PN solutions because of the potential incompatibilities of the medication and nutrients in the solution.

Initiation and Administration

PN is initiated and administered according to patient characteristics and facility protocol. Generally, the goal rate for adult patients is achieved within 72 to 96 hours after PN is initiated (Academy of Nutrition and Dietetics, 2016b). Because protein has minimal metabolic consequences, up to 60 to 70 g/L may be provided on the first day. It is recommended that dextrose be limited to 100 to 150 g on the first day of PN in patients with hyperglycemia or diabetes; the limit for other patients is 150 to 200 g on the first day. Nursing management considerations appear in Box 14.5.

PN may be infused continuously over 24 hours or cyclically over 8- to 16-hour periods. Continuous infusions are given to patients who are malnourished or critically ill and are often used to begin PN. Rapid changes in the infusion rate are discouraged in some patients due to the potential for hyperglycemia or hypoglycemia.

Cyclical infusions offer patients periodic freedom from the equipment and allow serum glucose and insulin levels to drop during the periods when PN is not infused, which may reduce the risk of impaired liver function related to excessive glycogen and fat deposition. When it is given during the night, **cyclic PN** frees the patient to participate in normal activities during the day. Overall, studies support the use of cyclic PN instead of continuous PN for stable patients who require long-term or home PN (Stout & Cober, 2011). Cyclical PN is often used as a transition between PN and EN or an oral intake. During the switch from continuous to cyclic PN, the infusion time may be gradually decreased by several hours each day, as ordered, and assessment is ongoing for signs of glucose intolerance.

Cyclic PN
infusing PN at a constant rate for 8 to 16 hours/day.

BOX 14.5 Nursing Management Considerations for Parenteral Nutrition

- Once parenteral nutrition solutions are prepared, they must be used immediately or refrigerated. It is recommended that solutions be removed from the refrigerator 1 hour before infusion because they must reach approximately room temperature before they are hung. Once hung, the solution is infused or discarded within 24 hours.
- Inspect the solution for "cracking" (appearance of a layer of fat on top or oily globules in the solution), which may occur in 3-in-1 mixtures if the calcium or phosphorus content is relatively high or if salt-poor albumin has been added. A "cracked" solution cannot be infused; notify the pharmacy and the physician, who may need to adjust the original PN order to eliminate or reduce the offending component.
- Monitor the flow rate to avoid complications and ensure adequate intake.
- Observe for side effects of PN: weight gain greater than 1 kg/day (indicative of fluid overload), elevated temperature or sepsis, high blood glucose levels, shortness of breath, tightness of chest, anemia, nausea and vomiting, jaundice,

allergy to protein content of the solutions, pneumothorax, or cardiac arrhythmias.
- Monitor laboratory data and clinical signs to prevent the development of nutrient deficiencies or toxicities.
- Some patients may feel hungry while receiving PN and should be allowed to eat, if possible. If oral intake is contraindicated, give mouth care.
- Begin weaning the client from PN to EN or oral intake as soon as possible. Gradual weaning is necessary to prevent rebound hypoglycemia. PN can be discontinued when enteral intake (an oral diet, tube feeding, or combination of the two) provides at least 60% of estimated calorie requirements.
- Patients who have permanently nonfunctional gastrointestinal tracts require PN indefinitely. For home PN to be successful, clients and their families must be physically and emotionally prepared. Intensive counseling focuses on preparation and administration of the solution, catheter and equipment care, and assessment skills as well as the psychological impact of permanent PN.

PN, parenteral nutrition; EN, enteral nutrition.

Refeeding Syndrome

Refeeding Syndrome
a potentially fatal complication that occurs from an abrupt change from a catabolic state to an anabolic state and an increase in insulin caused by a dramatic increase in carbohydrate intake.

When PN was first introduced, it was widely and enthusiastically embraced as state-of-the-art therapy. The prevailing school of thought was that "if some is good, more is better" and overfeeding was common practice (Koretz, 2007). At that time, PN was called "hyperalimentation"—literally excessive nourishment. The practice of overfeeding has been replaced with a more conservative, lower-in-calories approach because it is now known that overfeeding, particularly overfeeding carbohydrates in nutritionally debilitated patients, can lead to a life-threatening complication known as the refeeding syndrome.

Giving aggressive PN to patients who are starved and/or malnourished, such as those with cancer, alcohol abuse, disordered eating, chronic malnutrition, or significant weight loss, may cause refeeding syndrome, which is characterized by hyperglycemia and fluid and electrolyte imbalances. The spike in insulin following the infusion of dextrose promotes anabolism; cells quickly draw potassium, phosphate, and magnesium out of the bloodstream. The resulting decrease in serum electrolyte levels can lead to fluid retention, heart failure, and respiratory failure. Symptoms include edema, cardiac arrhythmias, muscle weakness, and confusion. Thiamin deficiency occurs from the increased metabolism of carbohydrates and may cause acidosis, hyperventilation, and neurological impairments. The risk of refeeding syndrome can be minimized by ensuring normal electrolyte levels prior to initiating PN and beginning PN at a lower rate and advancing the infusion slowly. A higher protein, low carbohydrate regimen is recommended. Monitoring of glucose and electrolyte levels is essential.

Transitioning from Parenteral Nutrition

The transition from PN to EN and/or an oral intake begins only after GI function is adequate. PN is usually tapered as EN feedings or oral intake resumes; the transition rate is influenced by how long the patient has been dependent on PN and their overall health. Intake progresses from clear liquids to solid food, possibly a low-fat, lactose-free diet, as the patient's tolerance improves. When the patient is able to consume 60% of estimated calorie needs through EN and/or an oral intake, PN may be discontinued (McClave et al., 2016).

How Do You Respond?

Should I save my menus from the hospital to help me plan meals at home? This is not a bad idea if the in-house and discharge food plans are the same, but the menus should serve as a guide, not as a gospel. Just because shrimp was never on the menu doesn't mean it is taboo. Likewise, if the client hated the orange juice served every morning, he or she shouldn't feel compelled to continue drinking it. By necessity, hospital menus are more rigid than at-home eating plans.

Is it good practice to color tube feedings? The Academy of Nutrition and Dietetics Evidence Analysis Library (2012) states that blue dye should not be added to EN for the detection of aspiration. The potential risks of using blue dye, such as skin discoloration, contamination of dye, allergic reactions, and association with mortality (exact method unknown), far outweigh any perceived benefit. Furthermore, the presence of blue dye in tracheal secretions is not a sensitive indicator for aspiration.

My patient claims he can taste his tube feeding. Can he? Except for patients who experience gastric reflux, patients cannot truly taste a tube feeding. However, the appearance and aroma of the formula may influence the patient's acceptance and perception of palatability. If the formula's appearance is offensive, cover the feeding reservoir or remove it from the patient's field of vision, if possible.

REVIEW CASE STUDY

Eugene is a 73-year-old man who weighs 168 pounds and is 5 ft 10 in tall. He has had progressive difficulty swallowing related to supranuclear palsy. He has no other medical history other than hypertension, which is controlled by medication. He denies that the disease interferes with his ability to eat, even though he coughs frequently while eating and has lost 20 pounds over the last 6 months. He is currently hospitalized with pneumonia, and a swallowing evaluation concluded that he should have NPO. He has agreed to an NG tube because he believes the "problem" will be short term and he will be able to resume a normal oral diet after he is discharged from the hospital. Based on his age and activity, and considering his weight and health status, the dietitian has determined he needs 2000 calories/day and approximately 90 g protein per day to help maintain muscle mass.

- What type of formula would be most appropriate for him? How much formula would he need to meet his calorie requirements? How much formula would he need to meet his vitamin and mineral requirements?
- What type of delivery would you recommend? What would the goal rate be?
- If the doctor convinces him to agree to having a percutaneous endoscopic gastrostomy (PEG) tube placed, what formula and feeding schedule would you recommend for use at home? What does his family need to be taught about tube feedings?

STUDY QUESTIONS

1 Which of the following strategies may help promote an adequate oral intake in hospitalized patients? Select all that apply.
   a. Tell the patient that you wouldn't want to eat the food either but that it is important for the patient's recovery.
   b. Encourage the patient to select his or her own menu.
   c. Offer standby alternatives when the patient cannot find anything on the menu he or she wants to eat.
   d. Advance the diet as quickly as possible, as appropriate.

2 For which of the following situations is a pureed diet most appropriate?
   a. As an initial oral diet after surgery to establish tolerance
   b. As a transition between a full liquid diet and a regular diet
   c. For patients who need a low-fiber diet
   d. For patients who have had their jaw wired

3 Which type of enteral formula would be most appropriate for a patient experiencing malabsorption related to inflammatory bowel disease?
   a. A standard intact formula
   b. A fiber-enriched intact formula
   c. A hydrolyzed formula for malabsorption
   d. A patient with malabsorption cannot receive EN

4 Which type of formula may normalize either constipation or diarrhea in tube-fed patients?
   a. A fiber-enriched formula
   b. An isotonic formula
   c. A hydrolyzed formula
   d. A standard, intact formula

5 Which tube-feeding delivery method is most likely to cause dumping syndrome?
   a. Intermittent feedings
   b. Bolus feedings infused into the small intestine
   c. Bolus feedings infused into the stomach
   d. Continuous drip feedings

6 Nausea in a tube-fed patient may be caused by which of the following? Select all that apply.
   a. Malplacement of the feeding tube
   b. A feeding rate that is too rapid
   c. Providing an excessive volume of formula
   d. Feeding too soon after intubation
   e. Anxiety
   f. Using a formula that is low in residue

7 Which of the following are indications for using PN? Select all that apply.
   a. Paralytic ileus
   b. Severe short bowel syndrome
   c. Dysphagia
   d. Coma

8 When EN is not feasible, how long can initiation of PN be delayed after admission in patients who are at low risk of malnutrition?
   a. 2 to 3 days
   b. 5 days
   c. 7 days
   d. 10 days

KEY CONCEPTS

- The focus of clinical nutrition is to prevent or treat malnutrition. Nurses are instrumental in many aspects of the nutrition care process.
- Hospitalized patients are at risk of malnutrition. Malnutrition is associated with many adverse outcomes, including increased morbidity and mortality.
- Timely identification and treatment of malnutrition is vital; however, the definition of malnutrition is not universally agreed upon.
- The underlying causes of malnutrition may be due to starvation (social or environmental related), chronic disease, or acute disease/injury.
- Clinical characteristics to diagnose malnutrition and its severity include weight loss, inadequate intake, loss of muscle mass, loss of fat mass, fluid accumulation, and measurably diminished grip strength.
- Nutrition interventions for feeding patients are oral diets, ONS, EN, and PN. A combination of approaches may be used.
- Oral diets are classified as "regular," consistency modified, and therapeutic. Combination diets (e.g., a low-sodium, soft diet) are often ordered.
- ONS can boost calorie and protein intake in patients with impaired appetite or high nutrient needs. A variety of supplements are available (clear liquid, milk based, routine, modified routine, puddings, and bars); they vary in nutritional composition, cost, and taste.

- EN is defined as any feeding through the GI tract and is commonly referred to as a tube feeding. Tube feedings are preferred to PN whenever the GI tract is at least partially functional, accessible, and safe to use. Tube feedings may be delivered through transnasal tubes or through ostomy sites into the GI tract.
- The choice of tube-feeding method depends on the patient's digestive and absorptive capacities, where the feeding is to be infused, the size of the feeding tube, the patient's nutritional needs, present and past medical history, and tolerance.
- Standard tube-feeding formulas require normal digestion; they contain intact molecules of protein, carbohydrate, and fat. Intact formulas come in several varieties: high protein, high calorie, fiber added, and disease specific.
- Hydrolyzed formulas are made from partially or totally predigested nutrients; they are higher in cost and osmolality; and they are used when digestion is impaired. Specially defined formulas are available for specific metabolic disorders (e.g., renal failure, hepatic failure).
- Routine formulas provide 1.0 to 1.2 cal/mL; high-calorie or "plus" formulas range from 1.5 to 2.0 cal/mL.
- The volume of formula needed to meet Reference Daily Intakes (RDIs) for vitamins and minerals is available from the manufacturer.
- Most patients receiving EN need additional free water to meet their estimated requirements. Free water includes water used to flush the tube and bolus infusions of water.

- Most hydrolyzed formulas are low residue or residue free. Intact formulas range from low-residue to fiber-enriched formulas, which may help regulate bowel patterns, but study results are conflicting.
- Osmolality, the concentration of particles in solution, does usually not affect tolerance in most people.
- Policies for initiating and advancing tube feedings vary among facilities. Generally, enteral feedings are started at full strength. Stable patients may begin an enteral feeding at the goal rate; enteral feedings in critically ill patients may begin at a rate of 10 to 40 mL/hour and increase by 10 to 20 mL/hour every 8 to 12 hours as tolerated.
- Continuous drip infusion with a pump is the preferred method for delivering tube feedings to critically ill patients and should be used whenever feedings are infused into the jejunum. Intermittent feedings may be preferable for long-term tube feeding and home EN because they more closely resemble a normal intake and allow the client freedom between feedings. Bolus feedings into the intestine are not recommended.
- EN is safe but not without the risk of various GI, metabolic, and respiratory complications. Aspiration is one of the most serious complications of enteral feedings and may be related to inhibited cough reflex, delayed gastric emptying, or gastroesophageal reflux. Ensuring the tube is properly placed and that it remains in position and elevating the head of the bed at least 30 degrees help reduce the risk of aspiration.
- PN delivers nutrients directly into the bloodstream when the GI tract is nonfunctional or when oral or enteral intake is inadequate to meet the patient's needs.
- PN is usually infused into a central, large-diameter vein, which quickly dilutes the hypertonic solution. Less frequently used is peripheral PN; it must be near-isotonic to avoid collapsing small-diameter veins, so the amount of calories it supplies is limited.
- Various concentrations of amino acids, dextrose, lipid emulsions, electrolytes, multivitamins, and trace elements may be given by vein. Compounding is the process of combining the formula ingredients.
- Because PN has numerous potential metabolic, infectious, and mechanical complications, it should be used only when necessary and discontinued as soon as feasible. It is never an emergency procedure.

Check Your Knowledge Answer Key

1 **TRUE** Adult malnutrition may be related to starvation, chronic disease, or acute illness/injury. Some patients are admitted with malnutrition related to starvation or chronic illness; others develop malnutrition while hospitalized because intake is poor and needs are high, especially in patients with an intense inflammatory response to acute illness or injury.

2 **FALSE** One of the criteria for the diagnosis of severe malnutrition in patients with chronic illness is weight loss >5% in 1 month.

3 **FALSE** There is little evidence to support a slow diet progression after surgery. Most patients can tolerate a regular diet by the first or second postoperative meal. Dietary restrictions are not necessarily helpful in relieving flatulence, nausea, or vomiting that occurs secondary to anesthesia and decreased bowel motility.

4 **FALSE** For most people, osmolality does not affect tolerance.

5 **FALSE** Although the terms *fiber* and *residue* are often used interchangeably, they are not synonymous. Fiber refers to carbohydrates not digested in the GI tract. Residue is composed of fiber along with undigested food, intestinal secretions, bacterial cell bodies, and cells from the intestinal lining.

6 **TRUE** The individual's capability to digest food is a primary consideration when choosing a tube-feeding formula for a patient. Intact formulas are appropriate when digestion is normal; hydrolyzed formulas are necessary when digestion is altered.

7 **TRUE** Continuous drip feedings are recommended for critically ill patients because there is a lower risk for aspiration, a decreased risk of diarrhea, and a decrease in the hypermetabolic response to stress when compared to other delivery methods.

8 **TRUE** PN may be infused into a peripheral or central vein, but because smaller diameter veins cannot handle hypertonic formulas, they are limited in the amount of calories they can provide. Most PN is infused through a central vein.

9 **FALSE** The biggest source of calories in PN infusions is carbohydrate (dextrose).

10 **FALSE** Coloring tube formulas with food dye does not prevent aspiration and is associated with potential complications, such as contamination of the dye, allergy to the dye, and increased mortality from unknown cause.

Websites

American Society for Parenteral and Enteral Nutrition at www .nutritioncare.org

Enteral product information at www.abbottnutrition.com and www .nestle-nutrition.com

European Society for Parenteral and Enteral Nutrition at www.ESPEN.org

The Oley Foundation, a nonprofit organization to help patients, families, and clinicians involved with home parenteral or enteral nutrition, at www.oley.org

References

Academy of Nutrition and Dietetics. (2016a). *Nutrition care manual: Enteral nutrition.* Available at https://www.nutritioncaremanual.org/topic .cfm?ncm_category_id=11&ncm_toc_id=255696. Accessed on 5/9/16.

Academy of Nutrition and Dietetics. (2016b). *Nutrition care manual: Parenteral nutrition.* Available at https://www.nutritioncaremanual.org/topic .cfm?ncm_category_id=11&ncm_toc_id=255697. Accessed on 5/9/16.

Academy of Nutrition and Dietetics Evidence Analysis Library. (2012). *Critical illness evidence-based nutrition practice guidelines.* Available at http://www.andeal.org/topic.cfm?menu=5302&cat=4800. Accessed on 5/17/16.

Bankhead, R., Boullata, J., Brantley, S., Corkins, M., Guenter, P., Krenitsky, J., . . . Wessel, L. (2009). Enteral nutrition practice recommendations. *Journal of Parenteral and Enteral Nutrition, 33,* 122–167.

Barker, L., Gout, B., & Crowe, R. (2011). Hospital malnutrition: Prevalence, identification and impact on patients and the healthcare system. *International Journal of Environmental Research and Public Health, 8,* 514–527.

Boullata, J., Gilbert, K., Sacks, G., Labossiere, R., Crill, C., Goday, P., . . . Holcombe, B. (2014). A.S.P.E.N. clinical guidelines: Parenteral nutrition ordering, order review, compounding, labeling, and dispensing. *Journal of Parenteral and Enteral Nutrition, 38,* 334–377. doi:10.1177/0148607114521833

Brown, B., Roehl, K., & Betz, M. (2015). Enteral nutrition formula selection: Current evidence and implications for practice. *Nutrition in Clinical Practice, 30,* 72–85.

Cawood, A., Elia, M., & Stratton, R. (2012). Systematic review and meta-analysis of the effects of high protein oral nutritional supplements. *Ageing Research Reviews, 11,* 278–296.

Charney, P., & Malone, A. (2013). *Academy of Nutrition and Dietetics pocket guide to enteral nutrition* (2nd ed.). Chicago, IL: Academy of Nutrition and Dietetics.

Corkins, M., Guenter, P., DiMaria-Ghalili, R., Jensen, G. L., Malone, A., Miller, S., . . . Resnick, H. E. (2014). Malnutrition diagnoses in hospitalized patients: United States, 2010. *Journal of Parenteral and Enteral Nutrition, 38,* 186–195.

Elia, M., Engfer, M., Green, C., & Silk, D. (2008). Systematic review and meta-analysis: The clinical and physiological effects of fibre-containing enteral formulae. *Alimentary Pharmacology & Therapeutics, 27,* 120–145.

Field, L., & Hand, R. (2015). Differentiating malnutrition screening and assessment: A nutrition care process perspective. *Journal of the Academy of Nutrition and Dietetics, 115,* 824–828.

Fitzpatrick, T. (2010). Room service refined. *Food Management, 8,* 52–54.

Hubbard, G., Elia, M., Holdoway, A., & Stratton, R. (2012). A systematic review of compliance to oral nutritional supplements. *Clinical Nutrition, 31,* 293–312.

Jensen, G., Compher, C., Sullivan, D., & Mullin, G. (2013). Recognizing malnutrition in adults: Definitions and characteristics, screening,

assessment, and team approach. *Journal of Parenteral and Enteral Nutrition, 37,* 802–807.

Koretz, R. (2007). Do data support nutrition support? Part I: Intravenous nutrition. *Journal of the American Dietetic Association, 107,* 988–996.

Lassen, K., Kjaeve, J., Fetveit, T., Tranø, G., Sigurdsson, H. K., Horn, A., & Revhaug, A. (2008). Allowing normal food at will after major upper gastrointestinal surgery does not increase morbidity: A randomized multicenter trial. *Annals of Surgery, 247,* 721–729.

Malone, A., & Hamilton, C. (2013). The Academy of Nutrition and Dietetics/The American Society for Parenteral and Enteral Nutrition consensus malnutrition characteristics: Application in practice. *Nutrition in Clinical Practice, 28,* 639–650.

Martin, K., DeLegge, M., Nichols, M., Chapman, E., Sollid, R., & Grych, C. (2011). Assessing appropriate parenteral nutrition ordering practices in tertiary care medical centers. *Journal of Parenteral and Enteral Nutrition, 35,* 122–130.

McClave, S., Taylor, B., Martindale, R., Warren, M. Johnson, D. R., Braunschweig, C., . . . Compher, C. (2016). Guidelines for the provision and assessment of nutrition support therapy in the adult critically ill patient: Society of Critical Care Medicine (SCCM) and American Society for Parenteral and Enteral Nutrition (A.S.P.E.N.). *Journal of Parenteral and Enteral Nutrition, 40,* 159–211.

Russo, E., Gupta, R., & Merriman, L. (2016). Implementing the care plan for patients diagnosed with malnutrition—why do we wait? *Journal of the Academy of Nutrition and Dietetics, 116,* 865–867.

Simons, S., & Abdallah, L. (2012). Bedside assessment of enteral tube placement: Aligning practice with evidence. *The American Journal of Nursing, 112,* 40–46.

Skipper, A. (2012). Agreement on defining malnutrition. *Journal of Parenteral and Enteral Nutrition, 36,* 261–262.

Somanchi, M., Tao, X., & Mullin, G. (2011). The facilitated early enteral and dietary management effectiveness trial in hospitalized patients with malnutrition. *Journal of Parenteral and Enteral Nutrition, 35,* 209–216.

Stout, S., & Cober, M. (2011). Cyclic parenteral nutrition infusion: Considerations for the clinician. *Practical Gastroenterology, Nutrition Issues in Gastroenterology, 97,* 11–24.

Tappenden, K., Quatrara, B., Parkhurst, M., Malone, A. M., Fanjiang, G., & Ziegler, T. R. (2013). Critical role of nutrition in improving quality of care: An interdisciplinary call to action to address adult hospital malnutrition. *Journal of Parenteral and Enteral Nutrition, 113,* 1219–1237.

U.S. Food and Drug Administration. (2016). *Guidance for industry: Frequently asked questions about medical foods* (2nd ed.). Available at http://www.fda.gov/Food/GuidanceRegulation/GuidanceDocuments RegulatoryInformation/MedicalFoods/ucm054048.htm. Accessed on 12/2/16.

van Bokhorst-de van der Schueren, M., Roosemalen, M., Weijs, P., & Languis, J. (2012). High waste contributes to low food intake in hospitalized patients. *Nutrition in Clinical Practice, 27,* 274–280.

Warren, J., Bhalla, V., & Cresci, G. (2011). Postoperative diet advancement: Surgical dogma vs. evidence based medicine. *Nutrition in Clinical Practice, 26,* 115–125.

White, J., Guenter, P., Jensen, G., Malone, A., & Schofield, M. (2012). Consensus statement of the Academy of Nutrition and Dietetics/ American Society for Parenteral and Enteral Nutrition: Characteristics recommended for the identification and documentation of adult malnutrition (undernutrition). *Journal of the Academy of Nutrition and Dietetics, 112,* 730–738.

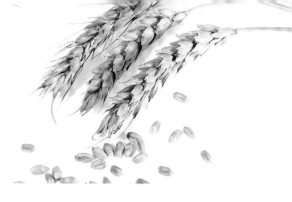

Chapter 15

Nutrition for Obesity and Eating Disorders

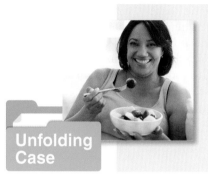

Emma Guido

Emma is 33 years old, measures 5 ft 1 in tall, and weighs 160 pounds. Since the age of 21 years, her weight has ranged from 100 to 160 pounds. Her goal is to weigh 110 pounds. She is a certified personal trainer but changed professions because it was "fueling bad behaviors." She does not have a medical history, although she admits to being hospitalized at one point because of very low potassium levels. She wants to achieve "more normal" eating behaviors.

Check Your Knowledge

True	False		
☐	☐	**1**	Comprehensive lifestyle treatment for obesity is appropriate only when body mass index (BMI) is ≤30.
☐	☐	**2**	People with a BMI >30 (obese) who are not ready to make lifestyle changes should be treated with medication to achieve weight loss.
☐	☐	**3**	Changes in metabolism that occur after weight loss make it more difficult to maintain weight loss, especially in the short term.
☐	☐	**4**	People who successfully lose weight are advised to participate in a long-term comprehensive weight loss maintenance program.
☐	☐	**5**	A weight loss of 10% of initial weight is needed to achieve improvements in cardiovascular disease risk factors.
☐	☐	**6**	If a person will try only one strategy, lowering calories is more effective at promoting short-term weight loss than increasing activity.
☐	☐	**7**	Micronutrient deficiencies are common after bariatric surgery.
☐	☐	**8**	A general calorie target to produce weight loss in men is 1200 to 1500 cal/day.
☐	☐	**9**	For weight loss, it is better to cut carbohydrates than to cut fat grams.
☐	☐	**10**	Bulimia poses fewer nutritional problems than anorexia does.

Learning Objectives

Upon completion of this chapter, you will be able to

1 Discuss the impact an obesogenic environment has on the prevalence of obesity.
2 Assess a person's need to lose weight based on body mass index (BMI), comorbidities, and readiness to change.
3 Describe general calorie targets for weight loss diets for men and women.
4 Give examples of evidence-based diets that are associated with weight loss if calorie intake is appropriately lowered.

5 Discuss characteristics of people who are successfully able to maintain weight loss.
6 Describe the risks and benefits of medication in promoting weight loss.
7 Describe a general diet progression after bariatric surgery.
8 Calculate excess body weight.
9 Summarize nutritional complications that may occur after bariatric surgery.
10 Contrast nutrition therapy for anorexia nervosa with that of bulimia nervosa.

Obesity is a chronic condition that typically develops over an individual's lifetime. At its most basic level, obesity is a problem of excessive calorie intake. A far less common weight issue is disordered eating manifested as anorexia nervosa or bulimia. Historically, the study of obesity and eating disorders has been separate: The former has been rooted in medicine, and the latter has been the focus of psychiatry and psychology. Yet, there are commonalities between them, such as questions of appetite regulation, concerns with body image, and similar etiologic risk factors.

    This chapter focuses on obesity—its causes, complications, and treatment approaches, including nutrition therapy, behavior change, physical activity, pharmacology, and surgery. Eating disorders and their nutrition therapy are described.

OBESITY

Obesity can be defined as an excessive amount of fat that increases the risk of illness and premature death (Fock & Khoo, 2013). The National Institutes of Health definitions of **overweight** and **obesity** are based on population studies that assess the relationship between obesity and rates of mortality and morbidity that are related to weight (Table 15.1).

Overweight
a body mass index (BMI) of 25 or greater.

Obesity
a BMI of 30 or greater.

    Obesity is a major health issue and a global public health challenge. In the United States, in 2011 to 2014, the prevalence of obesity among adults was just over 36% (Fig. 15.1) (Ogden, Carroll, Fryar, & Fiegal, 2015). Trends in overweight, obesity, and extreme obesity are depicted in Figure 15.2 (Fryar, Carroll, & Ogden, 2014). The dramatic increase in extreme obesity is particularly noteworthy. Obesity prevalence has increased in both men and women, in all age groups, and in all racial and ethnic groups.

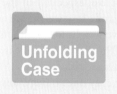

Unfolding Case

Consider Emma. What is her current BMI? Does it present a health risk? What was her BMI when she weighed 100 pounds? Was that a healthier weight?

Table 15.1   National Institutes of Health Definitions of Overweight and Obesity

	Body Mass Index	Risk of Developing Health Problems
Underweight	<18.5	Increased
Normal weight	18.5–24.9	Lowest
Overweight	25–29.9	Increased
Obesity*	≥30	
Class I	30–34.9	High
Class II	35–39.9	Very high
Class III (extreme obesity)	≥40	Extremely high

*Because evidence suggests health risks begin at lower BMIs in Asians, China uses a cutoff of 28 for obesity, Japan uses 25, and the World Health Organization recommends a cutoff for Asians of >27.5.
U.S. Department of Health & Human Services, National Institutes of Health, National Heart, Lung, and Blood Institute. (n.d.). *Classification of overweight and obesity by BMI, waist circumference, and associated disease risks.* Available at http://www.nhlbi.nih.gov/health/educational/lose_wt/BMI/bmi_dis.htm. Accessed on 6/9/16.

Figure 15.1 ▶

Prevalence of obesity in the United States, 2011–2014.

(Source: Ogden, C., Carroll, M., Fryar, C., and Fiegal, K. [2015]. Prevalence of obesity among adults and youth: United States, 2011–2014. NCHS Data Brief No. 219. Available at https://www.cdc.gov/nchs /data/databriefs/db219.pdf. Accessed on 1/17/17.)

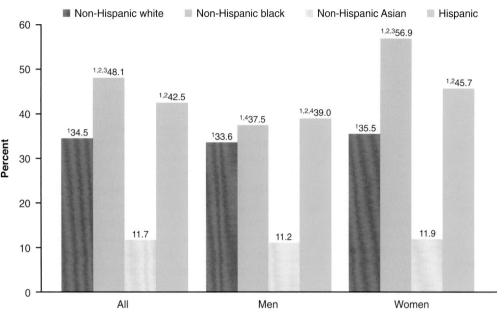

■ Non-Hispanic white   ■ Non-Hispanic black   ■ Non-Hispanic Asian   ■ Hispanic

[1,2,3]48.1   [1,2]42.5   [1]34.5   11.7   [1]33.6   [1,4]37.5   [1,2,4]39.0   11.2   [1]35.5   [1,2,3]56.9   [1,2]45.7   11.9

(All / Men / Women)

[1]Significantly different from non-Hispanic Asian persons.
[2]Significantly different from non-Hispanic white persons.
[3]Significantly different from Hispanic persons.
[4]Significantly different from women of the same race and Hispanic origin
  Note: All estimates are age-adjusted by the direct method to the 2000 U.S. census population using the age groups 20–39, 40–59, and 60 and over.

Complications of Obesity

Obesity significantly increases mortality. On average, class I obesity lowers life expectancy by 2 to 4 years. Much less information is available for BMI >35, but in those with a BMI of 40 to 50, life expectancy seems to be reduced by 8 to 10 years, comparable to the effects of smoking (Prospective Studies Collaboration, 2009). Studies suggest that overweight and obesity were likely responsible for approximately 18% of deaths in black and white adult Americans from 1986 to 2006 (Masters et al., 2013). Beginning at a BMI of 30, as BMI increases, so does the risk of all-cause mortality (Jensen et al., 2014).

Figure 15.2 ▶

Trends in adult overweight, obesity, and extreme obesity among men and women aged 20 to 74 years.

(Source: Fryar, Carroll, & Ogden, 2014.)

NOTES: Age-adjusted by the direct method to the year 2000 U.S. Census Bureau estimates using age groups 20–39, 40–59, and 60–74. Pregnant females were excluded. Overweight is body mass index (BMI) of 25 or greater but less 30; obesity is BMI greater than or equal to 30; and extreme obesity is BMI greater than or equal to 40.

Complications of obesity have far-reaching negative effects on health—either directly because of obesity or indirectly, such as a sedentary lifestyle or poor-quality eating pattern (Fock & Khoo, 2013). Obesity increases the risk of morbidity from hypertension, dyslipidemia, type 2 diabetes, coronary heart disease, stroke, gallbladder disease, osteoarthritis, sleep apnea, respiratory problems, and some cancers (Jensen et al., 2014). Other complications include gastroesophageal reflux disease, nonalcoholic fatty liver disease (NAFLD), and polycystic ovary syndrome. Obesity increases the risk of complications during and after surgery and the risk of complications during pregnancy, labor, and delivery. The biomedical, psychosocial, and economic consequences of obesity have significant impact on the health and well-being of the U.S. population (Jensen et al., 2014).

Central Obesity
waist circumference exceeding 35 in in women or 40 in in men.

Metabolic Syndrome
a cluster of interrelated symptoms, including obesity, insulin resistance, hypertension, and dyslipidemia, which together increase the risk of cardiovascular disease and diabetes.

Where excess body fat is stored also influences the risk of comorbidities. **Central obesity**, as part of the **metabolic syndrome**, increases the risk of coronary heart disease and type 2 diabetes (see Chapter 19). Central obesity also increases the risk of stroke, sleep apnea, hypertension, dyslipidemia, insulin resistance, inflammation, and some types of cancer (Tchernof & Després, 2013). This risk is usually confirmed at any degree of total body fatness. Evidence shows that as waist circumference increases, so do risk of obesity comorbidities (Jensen et al., 2014).

Causes of Obesity

The cause of obesity seems obvious: Obesity occurs when calorie intake exceeds calorie expenditure (i.e., people eat more calories than they expend over time). Although we know *how* obesity occurs, *why* it occurs is not fully understood despite intensive study. A recent literature review found that there is no consensus among previously published reviews regarding the primary cause of obesity; however, combined "physical activity and diet" was the most popular cause identified in adult studies (Ross, Flynn, & Pate, 2015). It is likely that obesity occurs from a dynamic interaction of variables, such as metabolic, genetic, environmental, cultural, behavioral, and socioeconomic factors.

Body Fat Metabolism

The body converts an excess of calories from any source to fat (triglycerides) and stores it in fat cells in adipose tissue. The number of fat cells a person has increases most rapidly during the growth periods of late childhood and early puberty. Thereafter, the number of fat cells increases only in response to an excess calorie intake; an excess of calories leads to triglyceride accumulation in fat cells, which, as they expand, stimulate the formation of more fat cells. Obesity is caused by an increase in the number and/or size of fat cells.

When calorie intake exceeds need and adipose tissue cells and subcutaneous fat cells are saturated and unable to further expand, excess fat accumulates in organs such as the heart, liver, and kidney. Fat stored in these organs promotes insulin resistance and increased cardiometabolic risk (Tchernof & Després, 2013). Excess fat may also accumulate in the pancreas, impairing insulin secretion and increasing the risk of type 2 diabetes.

When calorie intake is less than calorie expenditure, stored triglycerides are metabolized for energy and the size of fat cells decreases, but their number does not. When excess calories are later available, these fat cells readily expand in size. In part, this explains why people with extra fat cells tend to regain lost weight more quickly than people with an average number of fat cells. Preventing an excess accumulation of fat cells during childhood and adolescence may have a critical role in preventing obesity later in life.

Lipoprotein Lipase

Lipoprotein lipase (LPL) is an enzyme found in adipose tissue and muscle. It functions to remove triglycerides from the blood to store them in adipose and muscle tissue. In women, LPL is abundant in the fat cells of the breasts, hips, and thighs; in men, LPL is abundant in the fat cells of the abdomen. These different enzyme levels account for the difference in where women and men tend to gain excess weight.

Obese people have higher levels of LPL in their adipose tissue than do lean people. The result is an increased propensity to store fat, even when the excess calorie intake is relatively small.

Adipose LPL activity increases after weight loss to promote fat deposition—the body's attempt to maintain weight or composition through its own internal controls despite variations in calorie intake and energy expenditure. This phenomenon is known as the set-point theory.

Resetting Set-Point Theory

It appears that the body is more efficient in protecting against weight loss when calories are restricted than it is at preventing weight gain when calorie intake is excessive (Farias, Cuevas, & Rodriguez, 2011). Findings by Briggs et al. (2013) suggest that obesity caused by an excessive calorie intake changes the body's set point to a higher weight, making it difficult for obese people to lose weight. Researchers speculate that when subjected to a low-calorie intake, the body interprets the negative energy balance as a threat to the set point and secretes ghrelin to stimulate appetite and defend this higher body weight. These physiologic mechanisms appear to have been designed to enable our primitive ancestors to survive through long intervals without food (Demaria, 2013).

Genetics

Genetic factors are to blame for very rare, single-gene forms of obesity. For instance, massive obesity and excessive appetite are characteristics of Prader-Willi syndrome, a genetic disorder caused by a chromosomal abnormality. Among the other characteristics of this syndrome are mental retardation and reproductive problems.

Emerging research has begun to identify the genetic influence on "common" obesity, which is not controlled by a single gene but probably influenced by dozens if not hundreds of genes. Supporting the case for a genetic basis to weight status is the tendency of adopted children to have similar weights to their biological parents, not their adoptive parents (Silventoinen, Rokholm, Kaprio, & Sorensen, 2010). Similarly, studies on twins show that identical twins are twice as likely as fraternal twins to weigh the same (Wardle, Carnell, Haworth, & Plomin, 2008).

Study results suggest that genetics play a role in whether a person may be *predisposed* to obesity, not that genes *predestine* a person to obesity. Even when a genetic susceptibility exists, exposure to an **obesogenic environment** is necessary for obesity to develop (Herrera & Lindgren, 2010). Likewise, in people with a genetic predisposition to obesity, the severity of the disease is largely determined by lifestyle and environmental conditions (Loos & Rankinen, 2005). The rapid rise in obesity around the globe has occurred without changes in the gene pool, suggesting that the root cause is lifestyle and environment, not biology.

Obesogenic Environment
an environment that produces and supports overweight and obesity.

Leptin

The Ob gene is one of the main genes linked to the obesity phenotype in humans. It directs fat cells in adipose tissue to secrete the protein leptin, which acts in the hypothalamus and other areas of the brain to decrease appetite and increase energy expenditure. The circulating level of leptin varies with the proportion of fat mass (Nabi, Rafiq, & Qayoom, 2016). For instance, an increase in body fat leads to an increase in leptin, which leads to a decrease in appetite and an increase in metabolism and energy expenditure. Conversely, when body fat decreases, leptin levels decrease which stimulates appetite and lowers metabolism and energy expenditure.

Leptin deficiency is very rare in humans. It is characterized by rapid weight gain in the first few months of life leading to severe obesity (Farooqi & O'Rahilly, 2009). Appetite is intense, and satiety after eating is impaired. Leptin therapy that raises leptin levels from undetectable to detectable has profound effects on diminishing appetite and promoting weight and fat loss. Interestingly, leptin levels increase with increasing BMI, yet the high leptin levels in people who are obese seem ineffective in suppressing appetite or increasing energy expenditure, suggesting leptin resistance (Nabi et al., 2016). Studies with leptin demonstrate that appetite and eating behavior is in part determined by biology.

Ghrelin

Ghrelin
a protein produced by stomach cells that enhances appetite and decreases energy expenditure.

The hormone-like protein **ghrelin**, which is secreted mostly by the stomach cells, promotes weight gain by stimulating appetite and promoting efficient energy storage. Ghrelin levels fall after eating and whenever the body is in a positive calorie balance (e.g., when the body is gaining weight). Ghrelin levels are usually high before eating and when there is a negative energy balance or low-calorie intake, which may explain why maintaining weight loss is so difficult. Researchers have found that eventually—perhaps a year after weight loss—ghrelin levels adjust to a new lower weight and revert toward before-weight loss levels (Iepsen, Lundgren, Holst, Madsbad, & Torekov, 2016), which may then help maintain weight loss.

Obesogenic Environment

The increasing prevalence of obesity has been associated with changing culture, lifestyles, and economics (Demaria, 2013). The current environment, which encourages energy intake and discourages energy expenditure, has been labeled *obesogenic*. It, along with behavior, is believed to account for the increased prevalence of overweight and obesity in the world today (Corsica & Hood, 2011). Factors that contribute to an obesogenic environment include the following:

- An abundance of readily accessible, low-cost, palatable, high-calorie foods in large portions
- Increasing consumption of snacks
- A high intake of added sugars, including soft drinks
- A great proportion of the food budget spent on food away from home
- The increasing portion size of restaurant meals
- A decrease in energy expenditure related to labor-saving devices, such as remote control devices and motorized walkways
- An increase in sedentary leisure activities, such as watching television, playing video games, and sitting in front of a computer. Television watching may promote obesity by leaving less time for physical activity, lowering resting metabolic rate, and/or promoting greater meal frequency and food intake (Chaput, Klingenberg, Astrup, & Sjodin, 2011).

MANAGEMENT OF OVERWEIGHT AND OBESITY

An expert panel convened in 2008 to update the National Institutes of Health's 1998 Clinical Guidelines on the Identification, Evaluation, and Treatment of Overweight and Obesity in Adults—The Evidence Report (Jensen et al., 2014). Guided by critical questions, the panel evaluated new evidence related to key issues on overweight and obesity evaluation and treatment, particularly in people with diabetes and other risk factors for cardiovascular disease. The culmination of their work is the next generation evidence-based report entitled "2013 American Heart Association/American College of Cardiology/The Obesity Society Guidelines for the Management of Overweight and Obesity in Adults" (Jensen et al., 2014). The report includes a treatment management algorithm, identifies the best low-calorie diets, and summarizes the expected impact of comprehensive lifestyle and surgical interventions. The following sections include many of the expert panel's recommendations.

Identifying Patients Who Need to Lose Weight

The first step in managing overweight and obesity is to identify who should lose weight based on BMI, cardiovascular risk factors, and the patient's readiness for behavior change (Jensen et al., 2014).

- Weight loss is indicated for anyone with a BMI ≥30 (obese) or with a BMI of 25 to 29.9 (overweight) who have one risk for cardiovascular disease, such as diabetes, prediabetes, hypertension, dyslipidemia, high waist circumference, or other obesity-related comorbidities. Patients who are not ready or able to lose weight should be advised to avoid additional weight gain and are treated for cardiovascular and obesity-related conditions.
- People who are overweight but without any risk factors or who are of normal weight with a history of overweight or obesity should be advised to frequently monitor their weight and adjust their calorie intake if they start to gain weight. They should also be encouraged to engage in regular physical activity to help avoid weight gain.
- People who are at normal weight (BMI 18.5–24.9) should be advised to not gain weight.

Evaluating Readiness to Lose Weight

Objectively identifying who may benefit from weight loss is not the only criterion to be considered before beginning treatment; assessing the patient's level of readiness to make changes is crucial. Because patients at the two earliest stages of the transtheoretical stages of behavior change model are ambivalent about behavior change, patients in those stages are not likely to benefit from weight loss counseling (Fig. 15.3) (Wee, Davis, & Phillips, 2005). Even worse, counseling before readiness may preclude subsequent attempts at weight loss when the patient may be more likely to succeed.

To assess the patient's stage of readiness, ask (Rhee, McEachern, & Jelalian, 2014)

- If the patient intends to make changes to improve intake, physical activity level, and behavior, such as keeping a food diary, monitoring weight, and limiting sedentary time.
- If the patient has made any changes to eat healthier, be more physically active, or improve specific behaviors in the last month.
- How long the patient has been eating healthier, engaging in greater physical activity, and using behavior strategies.

Goals of Treatment

Ideally, treatment would "cure" overweight and obesity; that is, weight would gradually fall into the healthy BMI category and would be permanently maintained. In reality, this ideal is seldom achieved. The goal of losing large amounts of weight may be unrealistic and overwhelming and, from a health perspective, not necessary to achieve medically significant health benefits. A sustained weight loss of as little as 3% to 5% of body weight can cause clinically significant improvements in some cardiovascular risk factors, such as lower levels of triglycerides, blood glucose, hemoglobin A1c, and lowered risk of type 2 diabetes (Jensen et al., 2014). Greater weight loss leads to greater benefits, such as improved blood pressure and low-density lipoprotein (LDL) cholesterol

Figure 15.3 ▶
Stages of change graphic.

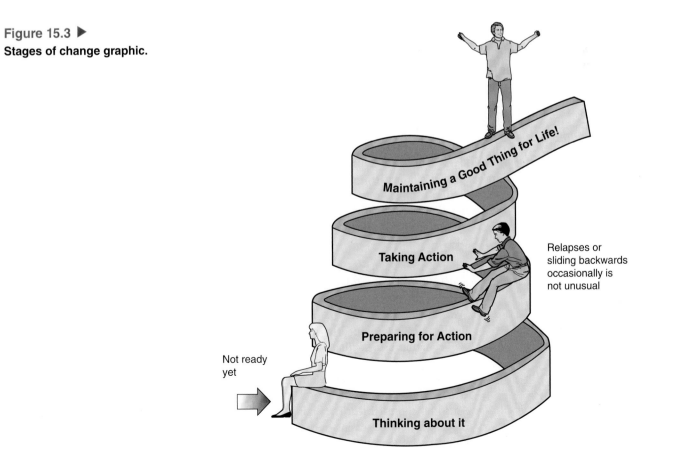

and reduced need for medications to control blood glucose, triglycerides, and cholesterol. A 5% to 10% weight loss within 6 months is recommended.

Setting a modest weight loss goal and sustaining that weight loss are far more realistic than striving for thinness. Yet, for some people, even modest weight loss may be unattainable. A more appropriate weight management goal for clients who are not ready or unable to lose weight is to prevent additional weight gain. Although this may sound like a passive approach, it requires active intervention, not simply maintenance of the status quo.

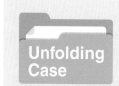

Unfolding Case   **Think of Emma.** Would you identify her as a candidate for weight loss? If so, what would a reasonable weight goal be?

WEIGHT LOSS INTERVENTIONS

Weight loss interventions include

- Comprehensive lifestyle treatment, which serves as the foundation of weight management for all people. It includes nutrition therapy, physical activity, and behavioral strategies to facilitate adherence to a low-calorie diet and increased physical activity. Comprehensive lifestyle treatment alone will cause a substantial proportion of patients to lose enough weight to improve health (Jensen et al., 2014).
- Medication may be considered as adjunct therapy for those who are not able to lose weight or maintain weight loss and have a BMI ≥30 or BMI ≥27 with comorbidity.
- Bariatric surgery may be considered as an adjunct therapy when BMI ≥40 or BMI ≥35 with comorbidity.

Nutrition Therapy for Weight Loss

Weight loss requires a negative calorie balance, which is achieved by eating fewer calories, increasing physical activity, or both. Based on the assumption that 1 pound of fat mass is approximately equivalent to 3500 calories, a deficit of 500 cal/day theoretically leads to a 1 pound weight loss in 7 days. However, metabolic adaptations occur during weight loss (e.g., fewer calories expended during daily activities because body weight is lower) that require a further decrease in calorie intake to achieve a negative calorie balance and continued weight loss (Finkler, Heymsfield, & St-Onge, 2012). This is one factor that contributes to the decreasing rate of weight loss that occurs as the duration of a diet increases (Finkler et al., 2012).

A hypocaloric eating pattern may be achieved by any of the following methods (Jensen et al., 2014).

- Choose a general target to create a calorie deficit, such as 1200 to 1500 cal/day for women and 1500 to 1800 cal/day for men. These levels are adjusted according to the individual's body weight and physical activity levels.
- Prescribe a calorie level that is 500 to 750 cal/day less than estimated need. Estimated need can be determined by indirect calorimeter if available. If it is not, the Mifflin-St. Jeor equation using actual body weight is used to estimate resting metabolic rate, which is then multiplied by an activity factor to estimate total calorie needs per day (Box 15.1). A hypocaloric plan is achieved by either subtracting 500 to 750 cal or 30% from the total estimated needs.
- An ad lib approach that does not necessarily prescribe a specific calorie level but achieves a calorie deficit by restricting or eliminating particular food groups, such as a low-carbohydrate or low-fat eating plan

BOX 15.1   Calculating Calorie Needs

1. Use Mifflin-St. Jeor equation to estimate resting metabolic rate.
   Men: RMR = (10W) + (6.25H) − (4.92A) + 5
   Women: RMR = (10W) + (6.25H) − (4.92A) − 161

2. Multiply RMR by a physical activity factor to estimate total calorie needs.
   Sedentary: 1.0 or more to < 1.4
   Low active: 1.4 to < 1.6
   Active: 1.6 to < 1.9
   Very active: 1.9 to < 2.5

RMR, resting metabolic rate in calories; W, actual weight in kilograms; H, height in centimeters; A, age in years.
Source: Raynor, H., & Champagne, C. (2016). Position of the Academy of Nutrition and Dietetics: Interventions for the treatment of overweight and obesity in adults. *Journal of the Academy of Nutrition and Dietetics, 116*, 129–147.

Quick Bite   One pound of body fat equals approximately 3500 calories

To lose 1 pound per week, 3500 fewer calories per week should be consumed
   3500 calories ÷ 7 days/week = 500 calorie deficit per day
To lose 2 pounds per week, 7000 fewer calories per week should be consumed
   7000 calories ÷ 7 days/week = 1000 calorie deficit per day

Concept Mastery Alert

To lose 2 pounds each week, a person should consume 1000 fewer calories each day. If a client consumes 2500 calories each day, the goal for weight loss is 1500 calories.

The "Best" Weight Loss Diet

The question of which diet is the "best" diet for weight loss has been debated for decades. Attention has focused on the relevance of the macronutrient composition of the diet—the proportion of carbohydrates, protein, and fat—in achieving and maintaining weight loss (Hooper et al., 2012; Johnston et al., 2014). Keep in mind that as the percentage of calories from one macronutrient changes, so do the proportion of calories provided by one or both other macronutrients. For instance, lowering the percentage of fat increases the percentage of carbohydrates. In reality, as long as the diet achieves the target number of calories, many different dietary approaches are effective (Raynor & Champagne, 2016).

Evidence of low to moderate quality from a meta-analysis of randomized controlled trials showed that both low-carbohydrate and low-fat diets are associated with an estimated 8-kg weight loss at 6-month follow-up compared to no diet (Johnston et al., 2014). At 12-month follow-up, approximately 1 to 2 kg of this loss was regained. Small statistical differences existed among several of the diets, but it was likely unimportant in people who want to lose weight. These results support the idea that most low-calorie diets lead to clinically important weight loss *if the diet is followed* (Johnston et al., 2014). The "best" diet is the one the patient will adhere to. Table 15.2 summaries the 15 evidence-based diets associated with weight loss *if* a reduction in calorie intake is achieved (Jensen et al., 2014). A comparison of various weight loss plans and sample menus appears in Table 15.3.

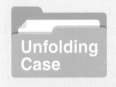

Recall Emma. In an effort to lose weight, she has been weighing and measuring her food and tracking her total daily intake, which averages between 900 to 1100 cal/day. Her food records show she eats grains and protein foods but no vegetables, fruits, or dairy. What would you tell Emma about appropriate calories and weight loss diets? What would you tell her about healthy eating?

Low-Fat Approach

The low-fat diet craze began during the 1990s with the hope it would ensure weight loss and improve cardiometabolic risk factors such as serum cholesterol and triglycerides. Because fat has more than twice the calories as an equivalent amount of protein or carbohydrate, in theory lowering fat intake lowers total calorie intake. The percentage of calories from fat in a diet classified as low fat may be ≤20% to <30% of total calories. The Ornish diet, at ≤20% of calories from fat, is a low-fat diet approach.

Table 15.2	Evidence-Based Dietary Approaches Associated with Weight Loss if Low-Calorie Intake Is Achieved
Dietary Approach	**Description***
Diet from the European Association for the Study of Diabetes Guidelines	Food group approach without formal prescribed calorie restriction
Higher protein diet	Prescribed calorie restriction of 25% protein, 30% fat, and 45% carbohydrate
Higher protein Zone-type diet	Five meals a day, each composed of 30% protein, 30% fat, and 40% carbohydrate without prescribed calorie restriction
Lacto-ovo vegetarian-style diet	Prescribed calorie restriction
Low-calorie diet	Prescribed calorie restriction
Low-carbohydrate diet	Initial carbohydrate intake of <20 g/day without prescribed calorie restriction
Low-fat vegan-style	10%–25% of calories from fat without prescribed calorie restriction
Low-fat diet	20% of calories from fat without prescribed calorie restriction
Low–glycemic load diet	With or without prescribed calorie restriction
Lower-fat, high-dairy diet	≤30% fat, four servings of dairy per day, with or without increased fiber and/or low-glycemic index foods with prescribed calorie restriction
Macronutrient-targeted diets	Prescribed calorie restriction with 15%–25% protein, 20%–40% fat, and 35%, 45%, 55%, or 65% carbohydrates
Mediterranean-style diet	Prescribed calorie restriction
Moderate-protein diet	12% protein, 30% fat, 58% carbohydrates without prescribed calorie restriction
High–glycemic load or low–glycemic load meals	Prescribed calorie restriction
The American Heart Association-style Step 1 diet	Prescribed calorie restriction of 1500–1800 cal/day with <30% fat, <10% saturated fat

*In diets without a prescribed calorie restriction, calorie deficits result from restricting or eliminating specific foods or food groups.

Source: Jensen, M., Ryan, D., Apovian, C., Ard, J., Comuzzie, A. G., Donato, K. A., . . . Yanovski, S. Z. (2014). 2013 AHA/ACC/TOS guideline for the management of overweight and obesity in adults. A report of the American College of Cardiology/American Heart Association Task Force on Practice Guidelines and the Obesity Society. *Circulation, 129,* S102–S138.

Although the amount of weight loss has not been shown to be greater with low fat (<30% total calories) versus a higher fat intake (>40% total calories), the cardiometabolic outcomes are different: With moderate weight loss, low-fat diets produce a greater decrease in LDL cholesterol but are not as effective at lowering serum triglycerides or raising high-density lipoprotein (HDL) cholesterol (Jensen et al., 2014). Because of this, a low-fat diet approach may not be best suited to people with metabolic syndrome or diabetes.

Low-Carbohydrate Approach

Low-carbohydrate diets have become a popular weight loss strategy in recent years. A low-carbohydrate diet is commonly defined as being limited to no more than 20 g of carbohydrate per day without a restriction on the total calorie intake. This level of carbohydrate intake results in ketone formation, which helps dampen hunger. Carbohydrate content is liberalized to 50 g/day after desired weight is achieved. An example of a low-carbohydrate diet is the Atkins Diet.

As stated earlier, over 12 months or longer, the amount of weight loss from a low-carbohydrate diet is not different than that achieved by a calorie-restricted, low-fat diet (Jensen et al., 2014). However, not all researchers agree. A study by Bazzano et al. (2014) found that at 12 months follow-up, participants on the low-carbohydrate diet had greater decreases in weight and fat mass. In addition, the low-carbohydrate diet resulted in a greater decrease in triglyceride levels and a greater increase in HDL level than those on the low-fat diet.

High-Protein Approach

High-protein diets provide 25% to 30% of calories from protein without defined proportions of carbohydrate and fat. For weight loss, high-protein diets must also restrict calories. Weight loss

Table 15.3   A Comparison of Weight Loss Diet Plans and Sample Menus

	Low Fat (20% of total calories)	Balanced (Moderate Fat/ Moderate Protein)	Low Carbohydrate (20 g/day)
Approximate composition of sample plans and menus			
Total calories	1490	1490	1481
Carbohydrate	45%	50%	5%
Protein	35%	20%	30%
Fat	20%	30%	65%
Intake patterns			
Total servings from each group per day			
Grains	4	7	0
Nonstarchy vegetables	5	2	1
Fruits	3	3	1
Milk or yogurt	3 fat-free	2 fat-free	0
Protein foods	12 oz lean protein	5 oz lean protein	16 oz medium fat protein
Fats	2	5	5
Sample menu			
Breakfast	½ cup orange juice ¾ cup scrambled egg beaters 1 slice whole wheat toast 1 tsp butter	½ cup orange juice 1 oz shredded wheat 2 slices whole wheat toast 1 cup skim milk 2 tsp butter	½ cup orange juice 4 scrambled eggs cooked in 2 tsp butter 1 oz pork sausage
Snack	⅔ cup plain yogurt with ¾ cup blueberries		
Lunch	Salad greens topped with 2 cups (total) of raw vegetables (carrots, cucumber, onions, mushrooms, tomatoes, and peppers) 4 oz grilled chicken breast Fat-free dressing 5 whole wheat baked crackers 1 ¼ cup diced watermelon 1 cup fat-free milk	2 slices whole wheat bread 2 oz deli turkey 1 tsp mayonnaise 1 cup salad made with greens, carrots, onions, and mushrooms 1 tbsp Italian dressing	6 oz grilled hamburger (without bun) topped with lettuce, ketchup, and mustard
Snack		1 small apple	20 peanuts (counts as 2 fats)
Dinner	5 oz baked haddock ½ cup steamed broccoli ½ cup baked sweet potato 1 tbsp light lower fat margarine spread ½ cup fat-free, sugar-free pudding	3 oz baked haddock ⅓ cup brown rice ½ cup steamed broccoli 1 tsp butter 1 ¼ cup strawberries	5 oz fried haddock ½ cup steamed broccoli 1 tsp butter
Snack	3 cups no-fat-added popcorn	1 oz whole wheat crackers	

resulting from high-protein diets (25% of calories) is the same as that from a typical protein diet (15% of calories) when the diets provide the same number of total calories (Jensen et al., 2014). High-protein weight loss diets do not result in better cardiometabolic outcomes than normal protein weight loss diets.

Dietary Pattern Approach

Pattern-based approaches, such as the Mediterranean diet, Dietary Approaches to Stop Hypertension (DASH) diet, and vegan diet, generally lower calorie intake and result in at least a 3% decrease in body weight (Jensen et al., 2014). With these approaches, calorie intake is either reduced because a restricted calorie level is specified (e.g., a 1500-calorie Mediterranean or 1800-calorie DASH diet) or because specific foods and/or food groups are eliminated or restricted (e.g., vegan diet).

Dietary pattern approaches emphasize the overall diet by providing guidance on the types of food to consume rather than prescribing specific levels of macronutrients or calories. This approach may not produce greater weight loss than other approaches but tends to result in improved overall diet quality due to the emphasis on foods that are commonly underconsumed, such as fruits and vegetables.

Meal Replacement Approach

Consuming liquid meal replacements or prepackaged foods is one approach that may promote more weight loss than standard low-calorie diets and behavior counseling (Rock et al., 2016). Prepacked foods overcome several barriers to dietary adherence, including portion control, convenience, and reduced decision making. Commercial diet programs, such as Jenny Craig and Nutrisystem, feature one to two meals per day of vitamin- and mineral-fortified, low-calorie "meals," which may be in the form of a shake, frozen entrée, or meal bar.

In overweight and obese women, the use of liquid and bar meal replacements is associated with greater weight loss at up to 6 months compared to a balanced low-calorie diet of conventional food (Jensen et al., 2014). Rock et al. (2016) found that incorporating portion-controlled prepackaged entrees in the context of intensive behavioral weight loss counseling promotes greater weight and fat loss than a standard self-selected diet with comparable meal satisfaction. Long-term studies are needed to determine how meal replacements impact weight loss maintenance.

Very-Low-Calorie Diet

Very-low-calorie diets (VLCDs) provide less than 800 cal/day, usually in the form of a liquid shake that is enriched with high biologic value protein and 100% of the Daily Value for micronutrients. Initial weight loss is quick and substantial, but VLCDs are associated with gallstones and sudden death and greater weight regain compared with weight loss achieved through a more moderate calorie restriction (Hemmingsson et al., 2012). A meta-analysis of randomized controlled trials shows anti-obesity drugs and meal replacements are the most effective strategies for maintaining weight loss maintenance after a VLCD (Johansson, Neovius, & Hemmingsson, 2014).

VLCDs should be used only in limited circumstances in a medical care setting with the provision of medical supervision and high-intensity lifestyle intervention (Jensen et al., 2014). VLCDs are often used prior to bariatric surgery to reduce overall surgical risk in people with severe obesity (Faria, Faria, de Almeida Cardeal, & Ito, 2015). They have also been shown to be safe, well tolerated, and effective in reducing preoperative weight and operative time when used 2 weeks prior to elective laparoscopic cholecystectomy in obese patients (Burnand, Lahiri, Burr, Jansen van Rensburg, & Lewis, 2016).

Eating Strategies

As previously stated, any number of dietary approaches will result in weight loss as long as a calorie deficit is achieved. Eating strategies frequently used to implement dietary approaches are featured in the following sections.

Portion Control

The increasing size of portions observed in the United States over the last few decades is one factor that promotes higher calorie intake and likely contributes to the increase in obesity prevalence over this time period (Piernas & Popkin, 2011). Evidence from randomized controlled trials supports portion control as a weight loss approach (Raynor & Champagne, 2016). Providing clients with common household equivalents to estimate portion sizes is a useful tool. Proportioned 100-calorie packages and smaller dinner plates, serving utensils, and glassware may also help "right size" portions.

Eliminating Sugar-Sweetened Beverages

It has been proposed that "small changes" in intake that result in a daily decrease in calorie intake by 100 to 200 calories may be a useful strategy for promoting weight management (Hills, Byrne, Lindstrom, & Hill, 2013). If reducing or eliminating sugar-sweetened beverage (SSB) intake does not result in a compensatory increase in calories from other sources, this approach should promote weight loss. A randomized controlled trial found that replacing SSB with water or artificially sweetened beverages leads to a 2% to 2.5% weight loss over a 6-month period (Tate et al., 2012).

Eating Frequency

A common belief is that regular, frequent meals and snacks may help control hunger and thereby promote weight management. The few randomized controlled trials that have examined the impact of eating frequency on weight loss have not found that high eating frequency leads to greater weight loss (Kulovitz et al., 2014).

Breakfast

Another commonly held belief is that eating breakfast helps achieve and maintain healthy weight. Observational evidence suggests an association between breakfast and body weight and weight loss, but evidence to support this idea is lacking (Dhurandhar et al., 2014). Only three randomized controlled trials, all of short duration, examined the impact of eating breakfast on weight loss, and none found that breakfast promotes greater weight loss (Raynor & Champagne, 2016).

Physical Activity

It is clear that reducing calorie intake is more likely to result in clinically significant weight loss compared to increasing physical activity (Swift, Johannsen, Lavie, Earnest, & Church, 2014). However, the combination of a lower calorie diet with increasing physical activity produces greater weight loss over 12 months than interventions based on diet or physical activity alone (Johns, Hartmann-Boyce, Jebb, & Aveyard, 2014). Increasing activity during weight loss helps preserve or increase lean body mass, which favorably impacts metabolic rate. Other benefits of high levels of physical activity and cardiorespiratory fitness are lowered risks of cardiovascular disease, type 2 diabetes, and all-cause mortality (Swift et al., 2013). High cardiovascular fitness level is associated with greater survival in all BMI categories (McAuley, Kokkinos, Oliveira, Emerson, & Myers, 2010).

Research has consistently demonstrated that a high level of physical activity is crucial for maintaining weight loss (Donnelly et al., 2009). High calorie expenditure allows a higher calorie intake to be consumed while still achieving calorie balance.

Regardless of weight loss goals, increasing physical activity should be an integral part of any obesity treatment plan. Current physical activity guidelines recommend the following (Donnelly et al., 2009):

- Approximately 30 minutes of moderate to vigorous physical activity (MVPA) 5 to 7 days per week to prevent weight gain
- 150 to 420 minutes/week of MVPA for weight loss
- 200 to 400 minutes/week of MVPA to maintain weight loss

Moderate-intensity aerobic activity (e.g., walking, cycling, swimming) is most commonly recommended for weight loss and maintenance. Clients with severe obesity may struggle to achieve levels of aerobic exercise that are sufficient to reap health benefits (Blackburn, Wollner, & Heymsfield, 2010). A better option may be progressive strength training, a safe and effective form of exercise that improves insulin sensitivity and increases muscle strength.

Promoting Exercise Adherence

Unlike dietary adherence, exercise adherence seems to improve with less structure, possibly by eliminating the barriers of lack of time or financial expense. Strategies that may promote exercise adherence include encouraging clients to

- Exercise at home rather than at on-site or supervised exercise sessions.
- Exercise in multiple short bouts (10 minutes each) instead of one long session.
- Adopt a more active lifestyle, such as taking the stairs instead of the elevator or pacing while on the phone instead of sitting down.

Behavior Change

Behavior change theories and models provide an evidence-based approach for changing eating and exercise behaviors for obesity treatment (Raynor & Champagne, 2016). Behavior change focuses on changing eating and exercise behaviors thought to contribute to obesity and closely monitoring those behaviors. Key behavior change strategies for weight loss and maintenance are described in Box 15.2. Behavior change ideas are outlined in Box 15.3.

BOX 15.2   Key Behavior Change Strategies

- *Self-monitoring* involves keeping a detailed record of the time, amount, description, preparation, and calorie content of all foods and beverages consumed. Recording additional information, such as the client's emotional state, intensity of hunger, and activities at the time of eating, may help identify "problem" behaviors. The primary purpose of using food records is to increase awareness of how often and under what circumstances the client engages in behaviors that support or sabotage weight loss efforts. The act of recording food eaten causes people to alter their intake. Self-monitoring of activity establishes a record of the type and amount (in minutes) of daily programmed activity. Lifestyle activity can be monitored with the use of a fitness tracker. Self-monitoring is often considered one of the most essential components of behavior change.
- *Goal setting* may involve specific goals, such as minutes of physical activity per day or grams of carbohydrate per day or involve specific eating behaviors in need of improvement, such as putting utensils down between mouthfuls or eating only in one place. Goals should be realistic, specific, and measurable so that success can be achieved, thereby engendering a sense of accomplishment and bolstering motivation. Instead of a goal to "eat better," a goal may be to "eat oatmeal and fruit for breakfast 5 days per week."
- *Stimulus control* involves restructuring the environment to avoid or change cues that trigger undesirable behaviors (e.g., keeping "problem" foods out of sight or out of the house) or instituting new cues to elicit positive behaviors (e.g., putting walking shoes by the front door as a reminder to go walking).
- *Problem solving* involves identifying eating problems or high-risk situations, planning alternative behaviors, implementing the alternative behaviors, and evaluating the plan to determine whether or not it reduces problem eating behaviors.
- *Cognitive restructuring* involves reducing negative self-talk, increasing positive self-talk, setting reasonable goals, and changing inaccurate beliefs.
- *Relapse prevention* focuses on teaching clients how to prevent lapses from becoming relapses.

Comprehensive Lifestyle Programs

Overweight and obese adults who want to lose weight should be advised to participate in a comprehensive lifestyle program provided by a skilled professional team for ≥6 months; such programs help participants adhere to a lower calorie diet and increase physical activity through the use of behavioral strategies (Jensen et al., 2014). Longer duration programs (>1 year) result in greater weight loss and are more effective in preventing weight regain (Millen, Wolongevicz, Nonas, & Lichtenstein, 2014). Electronically delivered weight loss programs may result in smaller weight loss than in-person interventions (Raynor & Champagne, 2016). Commercial weight loss diets that include comprehensive lifestyle intervention, such as Weight Watchers, can be used provided there is peer-reviewed published evidence of their safety and efficacy (Raynor & Champagne, 2016).

Weight Maintenance After Loss

Although losing weight may be difficult, keeping it off is even harder. The majority of obese and overweight patients have been shown to regain about one-third of the weight lost with treatment within 1 year and return to their original weight in 3 to 5 years after conclusion of the weight loss program (Castelnuovo et al., 2011). It is recommended that overweight and obese people who have lost weight participate in a long-term (≥1 year) weight loss maintenance program (Jensen et al., 2014).

Calorie expenditure is lower after weight loss because a lighter/smaller body requires fewer calories than a heavier/larger body when performing the same activity. Metabolic changes that occur during weight loss may also contribute to the risk of regain. Evidence shows that weight loss causes an adaptive thermogenesis which is a lowering of calorie expenditure beyond what can be predicted by changes in body weight and composition (Camps, Verhoef, & Westerterp, 2013). This metabolic adaptation is a survival mechanism to conserve energy during periods of famine. After weight loss, adaptive thermogenesis may be responsible for a decrease in calorie expenditure of 20 to 200 cal/day—meaning someone who has lost significant weight may burn up to 200 fewer calories per day compared to someone of the same weight who has not experienced weight

BOX 15.3 Behavior Change Ideas

Think Thin

- Make a list of reasons why you want to lose weight.
- Set long-term goals; avoid crash dieting based on getting into a particular dress or weighing a certain weight for an upcoming event or occasion.
- Give yourself a nonfood reward (e.g., new clothes, a night of entertainment) for losing weight.
- Enlist the support of family and friends.
- Learn to distinguish hunger from cravings.

Plan Ahead

- Keep food only in the kitchen, not scattered around the house.
- Stay out of the kitchen except when preparing meals and cleaning up.
- Avoid tasting food while cooking; don't take extra portions to get rid of a food.
- Place the low-calorie foods in the front of the refrigerator; keep the high-calorie foods hidden.
- Remove temptation to better resist it: "Out of sight, out of mind."
- Plan meals, snacks, and grocery shopping to help eliminate hasty decisions and impulses that may sabotage dieting.

Eat Wisely

- Wait 10 minutes before eating when you feel the urge; hunger pangs may go away if you delay eating.
- Never skip meals.
- Eat before you're starving and stop when satisfied, not stuffed.
- Eat only in one designated place and devote all your attention to eating. Activities such as reading and watching television can be so distracting that you may not even realize you ate.
- Serve food directly from the stove to the plate instead of family style, which can lead to large portions and second helpings.

- Eat the low-calorie foods first.
- Drink water with meals.
- Use a small plate to give the appearance of eating a full plate of food.
- Chew food thoroughly and eat slowly.
- Put utensils down between mouthfuls.
- Leave some food on your plate to help you feel in control of food rather than feeling that food controls you.
- Eat before attending a social function that features food; while there, select low-calorie foods to nibble on.
- Eat satisfying foods and do not restrict particular foods.

Shop Smart

- Never shop while hungry.
- Shop only from a list; resist impulse buying.
- Buy food only in the quantity you need.
- Don't buy foods you find tempting.
- Stock on fruits and vegetables for low-calorie snacking.

Change Your Lifestyle

- Keep busy with hobbies or projects that are incompatible with eating to take your mind off eating.
- Brush your teeth immediately after eating.
- Trim recipes of extra fat and sugar.
- Keep food and activity records.
- Keep hunger records.
- Give yourself permission to enjoy an occasional planned indulgence and do so without guilt; don't let disappointment lure you into a real eating binge.
- Exercise.
- Get more sleep if fatigue triggers eating.
- Weigh yourself regularly.

---

loss. Camps et al. (2013) found that people with a larger weight loss show a greater decrease in resting metabolic rate and that adaptive thermogenesis may persist for up to 44 weeks after weight loss. Adaptive thermogenesis was no longer observed when weight was regained to preloss or higher weight. The disproportionate decrease in calorie expenditure after weight loss could be one of the factors contributing to the high rate of regain (Camps et al., 2013).

Similarly, a study by Rosenbaum, Hirsch, Gallagher, and Leibe (2008) found that total calorie expenditure, especially calorie expenditure at low levels of physical activity, is lower after weight loss than is predicted by actual changes in body weight and composition and persists well beyond the period of weight loss. This lower calorie expenditure at low levels of physical activity supports findings that show people who are able to successfully maintain weight loss over prolonged periods of time engage in high levels of physical activity (Wing & Hill, 2001).

In fact, high levels of physical activity are characteristic of people enrolled in the National Weight Control Registry (NWCR), which was founded in 1994 to identify and investigate behavioral and psychological characteristics of people who are successful in maintaining significant weight loss (NWCR, 2016). Registered enrollees must be at least 18 years old and have maintained at least a 30-pound weight loss for 1 year or longer. The NWCR is currently tracking more than 10,000 people in the registry; the average participant has lost an average of 66 pounds and kept it off for 5½ years. Participants are surveyed annually to examine the behavioral and psychological characteristics of weight maintainers and to identify the strategies they use to maintain their weight loss. Most enrollees exercise approximately 1 hour/day. Other characteristics of successful weight maintainers appear in Box 15.4.

BOX 15.4   Successful Weight Maintenance

Participants in the National Weight Control Registry (NWCR) employ a variety of strategies to successfully maintain weight loss.

- Most maintain a low-calorie, low-fat diet and report high levels of physical activity.
- 78% eat breakfast every day.
- 90% exercise, on average, approximately 1 hour per day. Walking is the exercise of choice for most people.
- 75% weigh themselves at least once a week.
- 62% watch fewer than 10 hours of TV a week.

Source: National Weight Control Registry facts. (2016). Available at http://nwcr.ws/Research/default.htm. Accessed on 6/3/16.

Better long-term weight maintenance is associated with larger initial weight loss and longer duration of maintenance (Thomas, Bond, Phelan, Hill, & Wing, 2014). Weight regain is most likely to occur in people who ease up on physical activity, increase their fat intake, use less dietary restraint, and weigh themselves less often. Long-term weight loss maintenance is possible but requires sustained behavior change (Thomas et al., 2014).

Medications

In conjunction with comprehensive lifestyle intervention, medications may be considered for adults with a BMI ≥30 or in adults with a BMI ≥27 with comorbid conditions such as hypertension, type 2 diabetes, or dyslipidemia. There are five U.S. Food and Drug Administration (FDA)-approved long-term drugs for the treatment of obesity (Table 15.4), three of which were approved before 2014.

- Orlistat reduces the absorption of dietary fat; side effects are due to fat in the stool. Because the malabsorption of fat impairs the absorption of fat-soluble vitamins, a vitamin supplement should be taken separately from administration of the medication and ideally with some fat. A low-calorie diet containing 30% of calories from fat should be consumed. Over-the-counter Alli is a lower dose of the prescription version of orlistat.
- Lorcaserin works by enhancing the feeling of satiety, although some patients report a decrease in appetite or decrease in cravings (Kahan & Brown, 2016). It is generally very well tolerated. Patients who respond to the medication do so relatively quickly; therefore, if a patient fails to lose 5% of their weight after 12 weeks, lorcaserin is generally discontinued because it is unlikely that continued treatment would be successful (Smith et al., 2014).
- Phentermine/topiramate together produces impressive weight loss at quite low doses (Kahan & Brown, 2016). If it fails to produce a 3% weight loss after 12 weeks on the recommended dose, the FDA recommends it be discontinued or increased to the highest dose for another 12 weeks. If weight loss is not 5%, the drug should be gradually discontinued (FDA, 2015).

A systematic and clinical review of the three medications listed earlier found (Yanovski & Yanovski, 2014)

- When combined with lifestyle treatment, obesity medications produce greater weight loss and an increased likelihood of achieving clinically meaningful 1 year weight loss compared to placebo.
- The proportion of patients who lost ≥5% of weight ranged from 37% to 47% for lorcaserin, 35% to 73% for orlistat, and 67% to 70% for top-dose phentermine/topiramate ER.
- All three medications improve cardiometabolic risk factors more than placebo, but none have been shown to lower cardiovascular morbidity or mortality.

Table 15.4 | **U.S. Food and Drug Administration-Approved Drugs for Long-Term Obesity Treatments**

Generic Name/Trade Name	Year Approved	Drug Type	Administration	Common Side Effects
Orlistat/Xenical	1999	Pancreatic lipase inhibitor	Oral; with food	Gastrointestinal issues (cramping, diarrhea, oily spotting, fecal incontinence), rare cases of severe liver injury reported
Lorcaserin/Belviq	2012	Serotonin receptor agonist	Oral	Headache, hypoglycemia, dizziness, fatigue, nausea, dry mouth, cough, and constipation
Phentermine-topiramate/ Qsymia	2012	Phentermine is an appetite suppressant; topiramate is an antiepileptic.	Oral	Paraesthesia, dizziness, altered taste sensation, insomnia, constipation, dry mouth
Liraglutide 3.0 mg/Saxenda	2014	Glucagon-like 1 receptor agonist	Injectable	Nausea, hypoglycemia, diarrhea, constipation, vomiting, headache
Naltrexone-bupropion ER/ Contrave	2014	Naltrexone is an opioid receptor blocker; bupropion is a dopamine and norepinephrine reuptake inhibitor.	Oral; with food	Nausea, constipation, headache, vomiting, dizziness, insomnia, dry mouth, diarrhea

Source: U.S. Food and Drug Administration. (2015). *Medications target long-term weight control.* Available at http://www.fda.gov/forconsumers/consumerupdates /ucm312380.htm. Accessed 6/2/16 and Kahan, S., & Brown, N. (2016). Pharmacotherapy options for obesity. *Weight Management Matters, 14*(3), 1, 7–13.

The following obesity medications were approved in 2014; studies on the long-term effectiveness are not yet available.

- Liraglutide was initially approved in 2010 for diabetes treatment and, after study, approved in 2014 for obesity treatment (Kahan & Brown, 2016). It is believed to promote weight loss by impairing appetite and increasing satiety. Liraglutide is injected subcutaneously into the abdomen, arm, or thigh. Response to treatment should be evaluated 12 weeks after the target dose is attained; failure to achieve at least a 4% weight loss warrants discontinuing the medication. During drug testing, liraglutide was found to cause thyroid tumors in rats and mice, some of which were cancers. It is not known if it will cause thyroid tumors in people (www.saxenda.com).
- Naltrexone-bupropion SR combination leads to an impressive and synergistic weight loss (Kahan & Brown, 2016). Subjectively, patients report decreased appetite and fewer cravings. Target dose is typically achieved 16 weeks from initiation. After 12 weeks on the target dose, the medication should be stopped if weight loss is <5%.

Evidence is generally lacking on the usefulness of dietary supplements in promoting weight loss (Box 15.5).

Bariatric Surgery

Bariatric surgery is the most effective way to achieve significant and lasting weight loss and can lead to amelioration or resolution of most obesity-related comorbidities (Buchwald et al., 2004; Hutter et al., 2011). It is an option for obese patients at high medical risk and for patients who, despite comprehensive lifestyle treatment, are unable to lose weight or maintain weight loss that improves health. The criteria for bariatric surgery used by Medicare and most private insurers are outlined in Box 15.6. Weight loss surgeries are considered both bariatric and metabolic surgeries because in addition to leading to significant weight loss, they treat type 2 diabetes as well as lower cardiometabolic risk factors (Mechanick et al., 2013).

Surgical procedures for obesity work by restricting the stomach's capacity or combining a reduced stomach capacity with gastric manipulation. The most common types of bariatric surgery procedures are laparoscopic adjustable gastric banding (LAGB), Roux-en-Y gastric bypass (RYGB), and sleeve gastrectomy (SG). The biliopancreatic diversion with duodenal switch (BPD-DS) is not popular in the United States; it involves both restriction and malabsorption

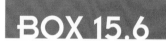

BOX 15.5   Selected Weight Loss Supplements

Acai: no definitive evidence that it promotes weight loss; little information regarding its safety when consumed in supplement form.

Ephedra (ma huang): shown to promote a modest but significant increase in weight loss when used for 6 months or less; long-term efficacy untested. Associated with serious adverse events, such as seizures, stroke, and death. Sale banned in the United States since 2004.

Bitter orange: claims state bitter orange is a substitute for ephedra. Evidence is insufficient to support its use for any health purpose. Safety concerns have been raised.

Caffeine: may aid weight loss to small extent or help lower weight gain. Tolerance develops and may lower effectiveness over time. Can cause nausea, vomiting, tachycardia, and seizures at high doses.

Calcium: probably not effective in promoting weight loss or limiting gain, whether from food sources of supplements. Excess calcium alters mineral balance; calcium supplements may increase the risk of kidney stones.

Chromium picolinate: little evidence that it increases lean body mass or decreases body fat; may cause watery stools, headache, weakness, nausea, vomiting, constipation, and hives at high doses.

Coleus forskohlii: no evidence of benefit on weight or appetite; no long-term safety trials in humans.

Conjugated linoleic acid: may help promote a very small weight loss and body fat; appears to be fairly safe.

Chitosan: little evidence of benefit; there are no long-term safety trials in humans.

Glucomannan: little to no effect on weight loss; appears to be safe.

Guar gum: no evidence of effectiveness; safe when consumed with adequate fluid.

Green tea extract: not enough reliable data to assess its effect on weight loss. A few, small studies suggest that regular consumption of green tea/extract may promote weight control. Moderate amounts are safe for most adults.

Hoodia: no reliable evidence supports its use for any health condition. Safety has not been studied.

L-Carnitine: studies are limited and do no support its use for weight loss.

Yohimbe: not effective in promoting weight loss; can cause severe side effects including heart failure and death.

Yohimbine: insufficient evidence on efficacy and safety to support its use in weight loss.

Sources: National Institutes of Health, National Center for Complementary and Integrative Health. (2015). *Weight control and complementary and integrative approaches: What the science says*. Available at https://nccih.nih.gov/health /providers/digest/weightloss-science#acai. Accessed on 6/6/16 and National Institutes of Health, Office of Dietary Supplements. (2016). *Dietary supplements for weight loss. Fact sheet for consumers*. Available at https://ods.od.nih.gov /pdf/factsheets/WeightLoss-Consumer.pdf. Accessed on 6/6/16.

BOX 15.6   Criteria for Determining Appropriateness of Bariatric Surgery

Inclusion Criteria

- BMI ≥40 or BMI ≥35 with comorbidities
- Failure to lose weight by nonsurgical means
- Absence of contraindications
- Well-informed, compliant, motivated patient

Exclusion Criteria

- Endocrine or other disorder that, when treated, will resolve obesity
- Current drug or alcohol abuse
- Uncontrolled, severe psychiatric illness
- Pregnancy

Source: Weight Management Dietetic Practice Group, Cummings, S., & Isom, K. (Eds.). (2015). *Academy of Nutrition and Dietetics Pocket Guide to Bariatric Surgery* (2nd ed.). Chicago, IL: Academy of Nutrition and Dietetics.

BOX 15.7 Recommended Supplements for Bariatric Patients

Patients with Laparoscopic Adjustable Gastric Banding

- One multivitamin and mineral supplement
- 1200–1500 mg calcium
- At least 3000 IU vitamin D

Patients with Roux-en-Y Gastric Bypass and Laparoscopic Sleeve Gastrectomy

- Two adult multivitamin and mineral supplements
- 1200–1500 mg calcium
- At least 3000 IU of vitamin D
- Vitamin B_{12} in the form of sublingual, subcutaneous, or intramuscular preparations if absorption of oral Vitamin B_{12} is inadequate
- Total iron, through multivitamin and mineral supplements and additional supplements, should be 45–60 mg.

Source: Mechanick, J., Youdin, D., Jones, D., Garvey, W., Hurley, D. L., Molly McMahon, M., . . . Brethauer, S. (2013). Clinical practice guidelines for the perioperative nutritional, metabolic, and nonsurgical support of the bariatric surgery patient—2013 update: Cosponsored by American Association of Clinical Endocrinologists, the Obesity Society, and American Society for Metabolic & Bariatric Surgery. *Surgery for Obesity and Related Diseases, 9,* 159–191.

and has higher nutritional risks. All procedures are performed laparoscopically, if possible. At this time, there is insufficient evidence to generalize which procedure is "best" for the severely obese population. The choice of procedure depends on individual goals, risk profile, patient preference, and local expertise (Mechanick et al., 2013).

Vitamin and micronutrients deficiencies are one of the disadvantages of bariatric surgery; they are most likely to develop after the first year of surgery. Recommended minimal daily nutritional supplementation, in chewable form, is outlined in Box 15.7. Patients take vitamin and mineral supplements for the rest of their lives.

Laparoscopic Adjustable Gastric Banding

LAGB works purely by restricting the capacity of the stomach. An inflatable band encircles the uppermost stomach to create a 15- to 30-mL capacity gastric pouch with a limited outlet between the pouch and the main section of the stomach (Fig. 15.4). The outlet diameter can be adjusted

Figure 15.4 ▶

Adjustable gastric banding.

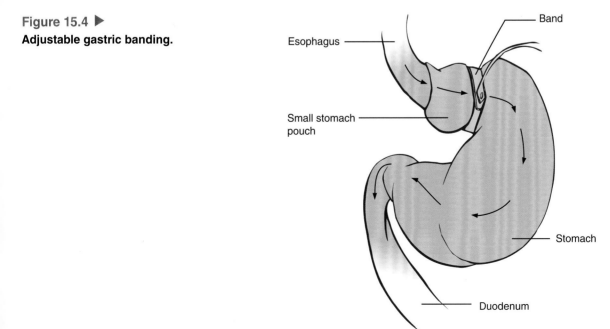

by inflating or deflating a small bladder inside the "belt" through a small subcutaneous reservoir. The size of the outlet can be repeatedly changed as needed. Clients must understand the importance of eating small meals, eating slowly, chewing food thoroughly, and progressing the diet gradually from liquids, to pureed foods, to soft foods.

LAGB is less invasive than RYGB, but its results are less reliable and less effective. Ten-year follow-up of LAGB shows a maximum weight loss of approximately 20% at 1 to 2 years, with 15% weight loss at 10 years (Sjöström et al., 2007). The popularity of LAGB has decreased in the United States, primarily due to inferior weight loss, complex follow-up, a lower remission rate of diabetes, and a high rate of reoperation due to complications (Raynor and Champagne, 2016). Common micronutrient deficiencies after LAGB include calcium, iron, thiamin, and vitamin D.

Roux-en-Y Gastric Bypass

> **Dumping Syndrome**
> symptoms (e.g., nausea, abdominal cramping, diarrhea, hypoglycemia) that occur from rapid emptying of an osmotic load from the stomach into the small intestine.

RYGB has long been considered the gold standard procedure for obesity (Raynor & Champagne, 2016). The GI tract is permanently altered as a small pouch is created at the top of the stomach and the jejunum is attached via a small hole in the pouch. Food bypasses most of the stomach, the entire duodenum, and a small portion of the proximal jejunum (Fig. 15.5). Removal of the pyloric sphincter increases the risk of **dumping syndrome**.

Typical weight loss is 35% at 1 to 2 years and 30% at 10 years (Sjöström, et al, 2007). Part of the effectiveness of RYGB is attributed to its impact on gut hormones that induce satiety, inhibit food intake, increase insulin sensitivity, and slow gastric emptying (Weight Management Dietetic Practice Group, Cummings, & Isom, 2015). In the 1990s, RYGB in morbidly obese clients was found to improve type 2 diabetes within days of the procedure, suggesting that improved insulin sensitivity occurred independently of weight loss (Pories et al., 1995).

Mortality rate, rate of complications, and rate of severe metabolic abnormalities is highest in RYGB of all three surgeries (Raynor & Champagne, 2016). The most common micronutrient deficiencies after RYGB include calcium, iron, folate, vitamin B_{12}, thiamin, and vitamin D (Weight Management Dietetic Practice Group et al., 2015).

Sleeve Gastrectomy

SG removes approximately 80% of the stomach longitudinally, resulting in a small pouch resembling a sleeve (hence the name) or long thin banana (Fig. 15.6). The pyloric sphincter and

Figure 15.5 ▶
Roux-en-Y gastric bypass.

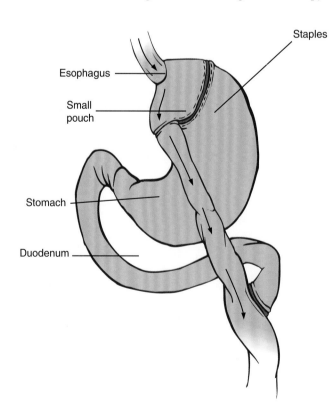

Figure 15.6 ▶
Sleeve gastrectomy.

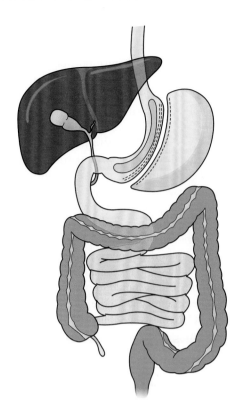

intestines remain intact so the food pathway is not altered. As in RYGB, removal of most of the stomach results in increases in gut hormone levels that induce satiety, inhibit food intake, increase insulin sensitivity, and slow gastric emptying (Weight Management Dietetic Practice Group et al., 2015). SG is gaining in popularity because it produces similar weight loss and remission of type 2 diabetes patients as RYGB (5 years of follow-up are now available) but at lower cost, lower morality, lower rates of complications, and fewer metabolic complications (Raynor & Champagne, 2016). Common micronutrient deficiencies after SG include calcium, iron, vitamin B_{12}, thiamin, and vitamin D (Weight Management Dietetic Practice Group et al., 2015).

Nutrition Therapy for Bariatric Surgery

Bariatric surgery is not a magical cure for weight loss but rather an adjunct to comprehensive lifestyle treatment, namely, diet, physical activity, and behavior change. Bariatric surgery requires dramatic and dynamic changes in intake. Nutrition therapy is important presurgically, postsurgically, and long term for weight management and overall health.

Presurgical Phase

Surgeons and insurance companies commonly require clients lose 5% to 10% of excess body weight prior to surgery for the purpose of improving surgical outcomes (Weight Management Dietetic Practice Group et al., 2015). Patients may be given a choice between a VLCD of protein shakes and a standard diet using ordinary foods. Schouten, van der Kaaden, van't Hof, and Feskens (2015) found that although protein shakes produce comparable preoperative weight loss, patient compliance, tolerance, and acceptance were all significantly better when a standard diet was used.

Preoperative nutrition counseling addresses presurgical weight loss and behavior change. Nutrition goals may be to decrease or eliminate fast food, eliminate SSBs, decrease processed foods, and drink 48 to 64 oz of noncarbonated, no-calorie fluids throughout the day. Behavior goals may be to eat a structured eating pattern, practice mindful eating, and self-monitor eating and physical activity (Weight Management Dietetic Practice Group et al., 2015). Patients are screened for problematic eating behaviors that are barriers to postsurgical success, such as binge eating, emotional eating, and boredom eating (Tempest, 2012).

Preoperative counseling also gives patients a realistic expectation of the postoperative phase, dispelling any notions that the surgery guarantees success. Topics to address include the need to drastically reduce portion sizes, the unpredictability of food intolerances, and the necessity of regular physical activity (Tempest, 2012). Patients should be given educational materials on hydration, texture progression, vitamin supplements, protein supplements, meal planning, mindful eating, and portion control for use after hospital discharge.

Initial Postsurgical Phase: The First 3 Months After Surgery

Nutrition care after bariatric surgery has two distinct phases: the early postoperative phase that occurs through the first 3 months and the remaining 3 months to 1 year after surgery (Weight Management Dietetic Practice Group et al., 2015). Although there is no evidence to support a specific protocol of postsurgical diet stages, sample diet advancement through the first 3 postoperative months is outlined in Box 15.8. Although nutrition complications can occur any time after bariatric surgery, they are most likely in the initial 3 months (Table 15.5).

The diet progresses from clear and full liquids to a soft/pureed diet in stage 3 (Box 15.9). Patients are advised to take small bites and thoroughly chew foods until they are the consistency of applesauce. The patient should stop eating when he or she feels full. Fluids can be consumed right up to mealtime because they leave the stomach quickly, and there is no evidence to support the notion that fluids before meals speed gastric emptying, increase the risk of dumping syndrome, or cause satiety before eating (Weight Management Dietetic Practice Group et al., 2015). However, fluids should not be consumed with meals or for at least 30 minutes after meals to decrease the risk of dumping syndrome.

Table 15.5   Potential Nutrition Complications After Bariatric Surgery

Complication	Possible Causes	Possible Interventions
Dehydration	Inadequate intake Excessive losses through vomiting or severe diarrhea	Intravenous hydration Encourage fluid intake even when patients deny thirst Antiemetics
Diarrhea	Lactose intolerance Drinking fluids with meals Infection Dumping syndrome Intake of sugar alcohols (LAGB, RYGB, and SG do not cause diarrhea)	Vary with cause If lactose intolerant, use full liquids composed of whey protein isolates, soy-based protein, or other lactose-free, protein-containing liquids
Dumping syndrome	Rapid emptying of hyperosmolar load (high-sugar and high-carbohydrate foods) into the jejunum	Avoid hypertonic foods and fluids such as juice, soda, frosting, concentrated sweets, foods with added sugars. Limit foods that provide ≥25 g total sugar per serving. Avoid added sugars such as white and brown sugar, honey, high-fructose corn syrup. Avoid liquids with meals.
Protein malnutrition (uncommon in bariatric surgery)	Poor oral intake Prolonged vomiting or diarrhea	Exact protein requirements after bariatric surgery are unknown. Suggested goals may be 60–80 g protein per day or 1–1.5 g protein per kilogram ideal body weight/d.
Constipation	Use of narcotics Inadequate fluid intake Low fiber intake Calcium or iron supplementation	Assess fluid and fiber intake for adequacy. Reduce iron dosage to the lowest possible dose. Stool softener or laxative may be needed.
Eating issues Food intolerances Regurgitation without nausea or true vomiting Food gets "stuck"	Altered taste Eat or drink too much or too rapidly Failure to chew food thoroughly Inadequate chewing Improperly moistened food	Avoid foods not tolerated. Remind patient to eat and drink mindfully and slowly. Avoid problem foods until tolerance improves.

Source: Weight Management Dietetic Practice Group, Cummings, S., & Isom, K. (Eds.). (2015). *Academy of Nutrition and Dietetics Pocket Guide to Bariatric Surgery* (2nd ed.). Chicago, IL; American Academy of Nutrition and Dietetics.

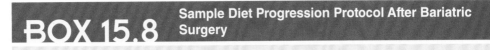

BOX 15.8 Sample Diet Progression Protocol After Bariatric Surgery

Stage 1: Initiated within 24 hours after surgery

- Clear liquid diet consisting of liquids that have no carbonation, sugar, caffeine, or alcohol.
- Liquids should be sipped throughout the day; straws should not be used initially.

Stage 2: Begins POD 2 to 3 and lasts until approximately POD 14; includes clear liquids for hydration and full liquids for nutrition

- Fluid goals should be met with 50% full liquids and 50% clear liquids. Women should consume at least 48 oz fluid per day; men should consume at least 60 oz. Fluid should be sipped throughout the day to improve tolerance.
- Clear liquids continue as identified above. Solid clear liquids, such as sugar-free ice pops and gelatin, may be better tolerated in patients with nausea. Salty liquids, such as broth or bouillon, are encouraged in patients having problems staying hydrated.
- Full liquids should provide <25 g sugar per serving, such as low-fat or fat-free milk, whey, whey isolate, or soy protein powder (limit protein powders to 25 to 30 g protein per serving); light yogurt, plain yogurt, Greek yogurt, sugar-free pudding made with fat-free or low-fat milk.
- Added sugars are avoided because they can lead to dumping syndrome.
- Liquid or chewable vitamin supplementation begins.

Stage 3: Soft/pureed food diet

- Begins on POD 14 and lasts approximately 3 weeks
- Increase clear liquids and replace full liquids with soft, moist protein sources (diced, ground, or pureed) as tolerated. Fat-free gray or light mayonnaise may be used to moisten ground meats, moist fish, or poultry; other protein sources include eggs, fat-free or low-fat cottage cheese, cooked beans.
- Full liquids containing protein may be used as meal replacements.
- Slow mindful eating is vital.
- Stop eating when satisfied.
- Eat three meals a day or five small meals a day.
- Fluids should not be consumed with meals or within 30 minutes after eating.
- Protein should be eaten first at every meal/snack.
- Avoidance of high-fat and high-sugar foods continues.
- Around 3½ to 4 weeks postop, soft fruits and well-cooked vegetables are added as tolerated.
- Protein should continue to be eaten first at every meal/snack.
- Advance texture of fruit and vegetables as tolerated.
- Around 5 weeks postop, some patients may tolerate salad.
- Patients must view the diet as a prescription to meet nutrient needs while healing and losing weight.
- 2 to 3 oz protein sources three to five times a day with fruit and or vegetables
- Grains are avoided until patient comfortably consumes adequate daily protein and fruits and vegetables.
- Whole grains are introduced as patient weight stabilizes and hunger increases if protein, fruit, and vegetable intake is adequate.
- Hydration remains important.

Stage 4: Regular solid food diet

- Amount of food consumed will vary meal to meal and day to day.
- Intake should be guided by hunger and satiety cues; mindful eating is encouraged.
- Calorie allowance is based on patient's weight, age, and activity.
- Whole grains and starchy vegetables are added slowly.
- Stringy vegetables, fruits with skins or membranes, dry or fibrous meat, untoasted breads, pasta, and rice may need to be avoided because they may cause obstruction or may not be tolerated.

POD, postoperative day.
Source: Weight Management Dietetic Practice Group, Cummings, S., & Isom, K. (Eds.). (2015). *Academy of Nutrition and Dietetics Pocket Guide to Bariatric Surgery* (2nd ed.). Chicago, IL; American Academy of Nutrition and Dietetics.

BOX 15.9   Sample Menu for Soft/Pureed Diet*

After Gastric Bypass Surgery

Before breakfast	¼ cup sugar-free instant breakfast made with fat-free milk
	¼ cup sugar-free gelatin
Breakfast	Plain Greek yogurt
30 minutes later until lunch	16 oz fluid sipped, such as 1 cup sugar-free decaffeinated tea and 1 cup fat-free milk
Lunch	Tuna salad made with nonfat mayonnaise
30 minutes later until dinner	16 oz of fluid sipped, such as 1 cup liquid protein supplement, 4 oz low sodium tomato juice, and 4 oz sugar-free popsicle
Dinner	3 tbsp nonfat cottage cheese
30 minutes later until bedtime	8 to 16 oz fluid sipped, such as 1 cup skim milk and 1 cup high-protein cream of chicken soup

*All beverages should be sipped slowly at a rate of 2 oz every 15 minutes.

Patients are encouraged to eat three scheduled meals a day and not "graze." Protein is needed after surgery to minimize the loss of lean body mass, but guidelines for protein intake have not been defined. Many programs encourage 1.0 to 1.5 g protein/kg/day. Added sugars are eliminated to reduce the risk of dumping syndrome after RYGB and because they are a source of empty calories.

Later Postsurgical Phase: 3 Months to 1 Year After Surgery

Around 3 months after surgery, patients are ready to follow a lifelong healthy eating pattern to promote weight maintenance. Eating nutrient-dense foods helps patients distinguish between physical and emotional hunger. Three meals with one to two snacks daily comprise the structured pattern. Food portions and speed of eating are monitored to promote weight loss and maintenance (Weight Management Dietetic Practice Group et al., 2015). Fluid goals should continue to be met with low-calorie or noncalorie, noncarbonated, caffeine-free beverages. Fluids are avoided with meals and for at least 30 minutes afterward. Alcohol should be avoided.

Success of Bariatric Surgery

Patients experience periods of weight loss and weight plateaus after bariatric surgery. Typically, patients who have had RYGB and SG reach maximum weight loss 12 to 18 months after surgery. For most patients, weight stabilizes within 18 months after surgery. Factors that influence the

BOX 15.10   Calculating Excess Body Weight (EBW) and Percentage of Excess Body Weight (%EBW)

Excess body weight = current weight − weight corresponding to BMI of 25

Example: A 5 ft 5 in tall patient weighs 234 pounds

As listed in Table 7.5, weight corresponding to a BMI of 25 for a 5 ft 5 in tall person is 150 pounds.

234 pounds − 150 pounds = 84 pounds excess weight

% Excess body weight loss = (current excess weight / initial excess weight) × 100

Example: Patient listed above now weighs 190 pounds after losing 44 pounds following surgery.

Determine current excess weight: 190 pounds current weight − 150 pounds = 40 pounds excess body weight

(40 pounds current excess weight / 84 pounds previous excess weight) × 100 = 47.6% excess body weight loss

BOX 15.11	**Factors that May Contribute to Weight Regain After Bariatric Surgery**

Physiologic

Levels of gut hormones that cause anorexia are initially elevated after surgery but fall to normal levels over time.

Ghrelin increases, which promotes appetite

Stoma or pouch dilation

Behavioral

Resumption of presurgery eating habits, such as emotional eating, food cravings, and the intake of calorie-dense foods

"Grazing" instead of regular scheduled meals can contribute to excess calorie intake

Soft foods provide short-term but not long-term satiety and may lead to overeating

Improved tolerance to a greater variety of foods

Eating too quickly

Ignoring satiety signals

Exercise noncompliance

Alcohol intake or abuse

Poor self-monitoring or education

Source: Page, M. (2016). The Instinct Diet: An alternative approach to post-operative weight regain. *Weight Management Matters, 14*(3), 2–4.

amount of weight lost after bariatric surgery include the type of surgery, the length of time since the surgery, and adherence to dietary and behavioral recommendations. A study by Moizé et al. (2013) found that the only significant independent variables affecting the percentage of excess weight loss over time are total daily calorie intake, baseline weight, and time.

Although there is no agreed on definition of success after bariatric surgery, patient progress can be assessed by percentage of extra weight lost (%EWL) (Box 15.10), total weight loss (e.g., losing 20%–30% of initial weight), or BMI (e.g., achieving a BMI of <35) (Scinta, 2012). Some studies consider <50% EWL or <20% total weight loss to be inadequate (Sjöström et al., 2007). Weight regain after bariatric surgery is complex and multifactorial (Box 15.11).

Nutrition for Weight Maintenance

For successful weight maintenance, lifelong periodic medical nutrition therapy visits are recommended to reinforce healthy eating and behaviors (Weight Management Dietetic Practice Group et al., 2015). Weight maintenance requires that patients eat mindfully with attention to hunger and satiety cues. Factors associated with successful weight maintenance after bariatric surgery include compliance to nutrition recommendations, realistic expectations, regular moderate aerobic physical activity, tracking food intake, monitoring weight, adequate sleep, meal planning, limiting fluids with and immediately after meals, and periodic assessment to identify and treat eating or other psychiatric disorders. Studies show participation in postoperative behavioral support groups is valuable for enhancing weight loss (Nijamkin et al., 2012).

An example of a post-bariatric weight loss program designed to help patients continue to lose weight and develop positive habits is a modified version of the "iDiet" (Instinct Diet). The 12-week-long program, based on social cognitive theory and cognitive behavioral theory, has shown impressive results for both weight loss and reduction of cravings for high-calorie food during weight loss (Page, 2016). The program incorporates a structured diet with group support and web-based tools. The original iDiet is high-fiber, moderate-protein, high volume of nutrient-dense foods to promote satiety and encourages fluid with food, especially high-fiber cereals to promote satiety (Page, 2016). Compared to the original iDiet, the iDiet for bariatric patients (Box 15.12)

- Provides lower amounts of high-fiber foods
- Recommends protein foods be eaten first at every meal and snack
- Recommends fluids not be consumed with meals or up to 30 minutes after eating
- Is adjusted downward in calories if the patient is intolerant to the high volume of nutrient dense food. Available calorie levels are 1000, 1200, 1500, 1800, and 2000.

BOX 15.12   Sample Meal Plans—Standard iDiet and Bariatric Diet Modifications

Meal	Standard iDiet Meal Plan	Bariatric Meal Plan
		Be sure to have a calorie-free drink between meals/snacks. Try to eat your protein FIRST (marked in bold).
Breakfast	1–½ slices iDiet legal toast (50 calories/slice) + 1 egg fried/boiled/poached + 1 tsp butter + 1 cup fresh fruit	**1 egg fried/boiled/poached** + 1–½ slices iDiet legal toast (50 calories/slice) with 1 tsp butter + ½ cup fresh fruit
Snack	½ cup 0% plain Greek yogurt + 1/4 cup high-fiber cereal and 1/4 cup fresh fruit	**½ cup 0% plain Greek yogurt** + ¼ cup high-fiber cereal and ¼ cup fresh fruit
Lunch	Soup and sandwich: 1 cup broth vegetable soup + 1 ham **sandwich made with 2 slices iDiet bread (50 cal per slice)**, 2 thin slices ham, 1 slice fat free cheese, 1 tsp low-calorie mayo, mustard, lettuce, tomato, onion, hot peppers	Salad plate: **⅓ cup legumes + 2 slices (2 oz) turkey breast or 1 egg + 1 tsp bacon bits or sunflower seeds** + 2–3 cups salad greens and nonstarchy veggies + 1½ tbsp low-calorie dressing + 1 sugar-free gelatin dessert
Snack	½ cup high-fiber cereal + ¼ cup milk + ¼ cup berries	**Small protein shake** (≤100 calories, ≥10 g protein) Example: EAS AdvantEdge, Designer Whey, Unjury
Dinner	2½ oz (raw weight) fiber gourmet pasta (cooked), ½ cup tomato sauce (65 calories), 2 tbsp grated parmesan cheese, and 2 cups green salad with 2 tsp low-calorie dressing	**2–3 oz plain grilled fish or shellfish** with 2 tbsp low-calorie sauce + 1½ cups cooked green or red vegetables, 1 sliced tomato with drizzle of olive oil and vinegar or 1 tsp of low-cal dressing
Dessert	Chocolate-tipped strawberries	Yogurt parfait: **½ cup 0% plain Greek yogurt** with ¼ cup high fiber cereal + ¼ cup fresh fruit.*
Total	**Calories: 1196** **Protein: 50 g** **Fiber: 67 g**	**Calories: 1080** **Protein: 80 g** **Fiber: 45 g**

*High protein dessert!
Source: Page, M. (2016). The Instinct Diet: An alternative approach to post-operative weight regain. *Weight Management Matters, 14*(3), 2–4.

NURSING PROCESS   Obesity

Rosa is 37 years old, 5 ft 4 in tall, and the mother of two children. Before her first child was born 10 years ago, her normal weight was 140 pounds. She gained 35 pounds during pregnancy and didn't regain her normal weight before her second pregnancy a year later. She is now at her heaviest weight of 180 pounds. She complains of fatigue and thinks her weight contributes to her asthma. She admits to "out of control eating" and has tried several diets but has been unable to take weight off and keep it off. Her doctor told her she has prehypertension and encouraged her to lose weight to lower both her blood pressure and serum glucose levels. The fear of needing medication for hypertension or diabetes has motivated her to lose weight.

Assessment

Medical–Psychosocial Data	• Medical history and comorbidities such as hypertension, dyslipidemia, cardiovascular disease, diabetes, sleep apnea, osteoarthritis, and esophageal reflux • Medications that may promote weight gain or interfere with weight loss, such as insulin and other antidiabetes agents, steroid hormones, psychotropic drugs, mood stabilizers, antidepressants, and antiepileptic drugs • Motivation to lose weight including previous history of successful and unsuccessful attempts to lose weight, social support, and perceived barriers to success
Anthropometric Assessment	• Height, current weight, BMI • Weight history; heaviest adult weight, usual body weight • Waist circumference

NURSING PROCESS

Obesity

Biochemical and Physical Assessment
- Lab values related to comorbidities, such as total cholesterol, LDL cholesterol, HDL cholesterol, triglycerides, glucose, hemoglobin A1c
- Triiodothyronine (T_3) and thyroxine (T_4) for thyroid function
- Blood pressure

Dietary Assessment
- How many daily meals and snacks do you usually eat?
- What is a typical day's intake?
- How do you think your usual intake needs to change to be healthier or to help you lose weight?
- How often do you eat breakfast?
- How many servings of fruits and vegetables do you eat daily?
- How much sweetened soda do you drink daily?
- Do you watch your fat intake? If so, what do you do to limit fat?
- Do you watch your carbohydrate intake? If so, what do you do to limit carbohydrates?
- How many meals per week do you eat out?
- In regard to diet, what is your "weakness"?
- Do you know if you eat for reasons other than hunger, for example, when you are bored, sad, lonely, or anxious?
- Do you take vitamins, minerals, or supplements to help with weight loss? If so, what?
- What is your goal weight?
- How much moderate-intensity exercise do you do on a daily basis? How active is your lifestyle? How easy would it be for you to become more active?
- How much alcohol do you consume?
- Do you have any cultural, religious, or ethnic food preferences?
- Do you have any food allergies or intolerances?

Diagnosis

Possible Nursing Diagnosis Obesity related to excess calorie intake as evidence by a BMI of 31

Planning

Client Outcomes

The client will
- Gradually increase physical activity to a total of 60 minutes of moderate-intensity activity on most days of the week
- Explain the relationship between calorie intake, physical activity, and weight control
- Consume a nutritionally adequate, hypocaloric diet consisting of healthy carbohydrates, healthy fats, and lean protein
- Eat at least three meals per day
- Practice behavior change to modify undesirable eating habits
- Lose 1 to 2 pounds/week on average until 10% of initial weight is lost
- Improve health status as evidenced by a decrease in total cholesterol, LDL cholesterol, and glucose; an increase in HDL cholesterol; and improved blood pressure, as appropriate

Nursing Interventions

Nutrition Therapy
- Decrease calorie intake to 1200 a day in three meals.
- Provide a 1200-calorie eating plan that specifies portion sizes and number of servings from each food group recommended for each meal.
  The daily plan will include
  4 grains, preferably all of them whole grains
  1½ cups of vegetables
  1 cup of fruit
  3 oz of protein foods
  2 cups of fat-free milk
  4 tsp of oil
- Encourage ample fluid intake, preferably water and other noncalorie drinks, to promote excretion of metabolic wastes.

| NURSING PROCESS | Obesity |

Client Teaching

Instruct the client on

The interrelationship between a hypocaloric diet, increased physical activity, and behavior change in managing weight

The eating plan essentials, including
- The emphasis on high-satiety foods, such as whole grains, fruit and vegetables, low fat or non-fat dairy, and lean protein
- Tips for eating out (see Chapter 10), food preparation techniques, and the basics of food purchasing and label reading

Behavioral matters, including
- Eating only in one place while sitting down
- Putting utensils down between mouthfuls
- Monitoring hunger on a scale of 1 to 10 with 1 corresponding to "famished" and 10 corresponding to "stuffed." Encourage clients to eat when the hunger scale is at about 3 and to stop when satisfied (not full) at about 6 or 7.
- Weighing oneself at least once a week
- Periodically keeping a record of food intake and activity
- "Planning" splurges instead of eating on impulse. Planned splurges involve making a conscious decision to eat something, enjoying every mouthful of the food, and then moving on from the experience without feelings of guilt or failure.

Changing eating attitudes by
- Replacing negative self-talk with positive talk
- Replacing the attitude of "always being on a diet" with an acceptance of eating healthier and less as a way of life
- Consulting a physician or dietitian if questions concerning the eating plan or weight loss arise

Evaluation

Evaluate and Monitor
- Monitor weight.
- Evaluate food and activity records to assess adherence; suggest changes in the meal plan as needed.
- Provide periodic feedback and reinforcement.
- Monitor biochemical data for improvements attributable to weight loss.

EATING DISORDERS: ANOREXIA NERVOSA, BULIMIA NERVOSA, BINGE-EATING DISORDER, AND EATING DISORDERS NOT OTHERWISE SPECIFIED

Body Dysmorphic Disorder
excessive preoccupation with a real or imagined defect in physical appearance.

Anorexia Nervosa (AN)
a condition of self-imposed fasting or severe self-imposed dieting.

Bulimia Nervosa (BN)
an eating disorder characterized by recurrent episodes of bingeing and purging.

Eating disorders are clinically defined as psychological disorders. They are characterized by severe disturbances in eating behaviors, which can have a profound effect on health and/or psychosocial functioning. Other characteristics include obsessive ideation about body size and weight and **body dysmorphic disorder** or distorted body image. Table 15.6 compares **anorexia nervosa (AN)** and **bulimia nervosa (BN)**. Binge-eating disorder (BED) is the other eating disorders defined in the newest edition of the *Diagnostic and Statistical Manual of Mental Disorders* (*DSM-5*) (American Psychiatric Association, 2013).

Eating disorders result from complex interaction of genetic, biologic, behavioral, psychological, and social factors; however, the etiology of eating disorders in not known. Studies indicate that genetic heritability may account for 50% to 80% of the risk of developing an eating disorder (Bulik et al., 2006) and contributes to the neurobiological factors underlying eating disorders (Kaye, Fudge, & Paulus, 2009).

Table 15.6 A Comparison of Anorexia Nervosa and Bulimia Nervosa

	Anorexia Nervosa	Bulimia Nervosa
Major characteristics	Compulsive pursuit of thinness Intense fear of gaining weight or becoming fat Self-worth based on size and shape	Binge eating accompanied by a lack of sense of control Self-worth based on size and shape
Onset and population	Usually develops during adolescence or young adulthood; 90%–95% are female	Usually develops during adolescence or young adulthood; is more likely to occur in men than anorexia
Typical eating and exercise behaviors	Semi-starvation with compulsive exercise; onset of disorder is usually preceded by dieting behavior	Gorging (e.g., 1200–11,500 calories in a short amount of time) followed by purging, such as self-induced vomiting, excessive exercise, abuse of laxatives, emetics, diuretics, or fasting; "dieting" is a way of life but bingeing may occur several times per day and may be planned
Weight	Significantly low body weight compared to what is minimally expected for age, gender, developmental trajectory, and physical health	Fluctuations are normal; weight may be normal or slightly above normal.
Emotional symptoms	Vicarious enjoyment of food; denial of the condition can be extreme; body image disturbance; pronounced emotional changes; low self-esteem	Displays mood swings; full recognition of the behavior as abnormal; ongoing feelings of isolation, self-deprecating thoughts, depression, and low self-esteem
Physical symptoms	Lanugo hair on the face and trunk; brittle listless hair; dry skin, brittle nails, intolerance of cold	May appear normal Swollen salivary glands in cheeks Sores, scars, or calluses on knuckles or hands
Cardiovascular effects	Bradycardia, hypotension, orthostatic hypotension	Arrhythmias; palpitations; weakness
GI effects	Delayed gastric emptying, decreased motility, severe constipation	Bloating, constipation, flatulence; gastric dilation with rupture is a risk
Endocrine/metabolic imbalances	Cold sensitivity; fatigue; hypercholesterolemia, hypoglycemia; amenorrhea or menstrual irregularities	Menstrual irregularities, dehydration, and electrolyte imbalances may occur secondary to vomiting and laxative abuse; rebound fluid retention with edema
Musculoskeletal	Osteopenia, osteoporosis, muscle wasting and weakness	Dental erosion; muscular weakness
Growth status	Arrested growth and maturation	Usually not affected
Nutrient deficiencies	Protein–calorie malnutrition; various micronutrient deficiencies	Varies

Source: Eating disorders. (2016). Available at www.nutritioncaremanual.org. Accessed on 5/29/16 and Laureate Eating Disorders Program. (n.d.). Available at www.eatingdisorders.laureate.com. Accessed on 5/29/16.

Risk factors that precede the diagnosis of an eating disorder include dieting, early childhood eating and GI problems, increased concern about weight and size, negative self-evaluation, sexual abuse, and other traumas (Ozier & Henry, 2011). Major stressors, such as the onset of puberty, parents' divorce, death of a family member, and ridicule of being or becoming fat may be precipitating factors. Athletes (e.g., dancers, gymnasts) may develop eating disorders to improve their performance. People with eating disorders often have coexisting mood, anxiety, impulse control, or substance use disorders (Hudson, Hiripi, Pope, & Kessler, 2007). Each person's recovery process is unique; therefore, treatment plans are highly individualized.

A multidisciplinary approach that includes nutrition counseling, behavior change, psychotherapy, family counseling, and group therapy is most effective. Antidepressant drugs effectively reduce the frequency of problematic eating behaviors but do not eliminate them. Most eating disorders are treated on an outpatient basis; however, life-threatening consequences of malnutrition in severe cases of AN may necessitate inpatient treatment (Rocks, Pelly, & Wilkinson, 2014). Treatment can be complex and protracted.

Figure 15.7 ▶

A woman suffering from anorexia sees herself as overweight.

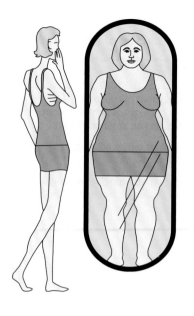

Anorexia Nervosa

AN is characterized by a significantly lower than expected body weight, intense fear of becoming overweight or persistent behavior that interferes with weight gain, and a distorted body image (Fig. 15.7) (American Psychiatric Association, 2013). Feeding issues include self-imposed starvation, avoidance of social eating, disassociation from internal hunger cues, and food rituals that delay or extend a meal, such as repeated cutting or reheating of food. Denial of the condition can be extreme.

There is no proven treatment for AN and the rates of relapse and chronicity are high (Kaye, Wierenga, Bailer, Simmons, & Bischoff-Grethe, 2013). Although "full" and "partial" recovery are not clearly defined, it is estimated that 50% of people diagnosed with AN have a full recovery with treatment, 30% achieve partial recovery, and 20% have lifelong problems and maintain dieting and food fears (Academy of Nutrition and Dietetics, 2016). The overall mortality rate is reported to range from 5% to 20% (Academy of Nutrition and Dietetics, 2016).

Nutrition Therapy for Anorexia Nervosa

Symptoms of starvation are treated before any psychological treatment can be successful. Restoring weight through gradual increases in calorie intake is one of the priorities in the initial stages of inpatient care and is a vital step in overall recovery (Cockfield & Philpot, 2009). In some patients, a more realistic initial goal may be to simply halt weight loss.

Refeeding Syndrome
a potentially life-threatening condition characterized by severe shifts in fluid and electrolytes, especially phosphorus, from the extracellular to intracellular fluid when refeeding begins in a person who is severely malnourished and depleted in total body phosphorus. Thiamin deficiency may also occur secondary to increased metabolism of carbohydrates.

Consistent evidence-based recommendations for how to achieve weight restoration in people with AN are lacking (Rocks et al., 2014). Most nutrition prescriptions start with 1200 to 1400 cal/day and gradually increase in 100- to 200-calorie increments with a goal weight gain of 1 to 2 pounds/week (Academy of Nutrition and Dietetics, 2016). Young patients may be given an initial intake of 800 to 1000 cal/day (Ebeling et al., 2003). A lower-than-needed calorie intake as treatment begins is intended to reduce the risk **refeeding syndrome**, even though it is a rare complication. Patients who weigh <70% of expected body weight are at greatest risk, particularly during the first week of treatment (Golden & Meyer, 2004).

An opposing viewpoint is to begin weight restoration treatment with a diet providing 2000 cal/day while closely monitoring vital signs, so that recovery is not delayed (Kohn, Madden, & Clarke, 2011). Although both approaches lead to weight gain during hospitalization, it is not possible to draw conclusions as to the most safe and preferential calorie prescription or method of nutrient delivery (Rocks et al., 2014).

Strategies to promote compliance and feelings of trust include involving the client in formulating individualized goals and meal plans; offering rewards linked to the quantity of calories

> ## BOX 15.13 — Nutrition Strategies for Anorexia Nervosa
>
> - Eat a meal or snack every 3 to 4 hours even if not hungry during initial phase of treatment. Eat sources of protein, fat, and complex carbohydrates, preferably whole grains, at every meal and snack.
> - Eat attractive meals based on individual food preferences. Foods that are nutritionally dense help to minimize the volume of food needed. Finger foods served cold or at room temperature help to minimize satiety sensations.
> - Never force the client to eat and minimize the emphasis on food. Initially, clients may respond to nutrition therapy better if they are allowed to exclude high-risk binge foods from their diet. However, the binge foods should be reintroduced later so that the "feared food" (trigger food) idea is not promoted.
> - Gradually increase portion sizes.
> - Gradually increase variety of foods consumed. Introduce feared or forbidden foods gradually based on individual progress.
> - Because gastrointestinal intolerance may exist, limit gassy foods in the early stages of treatment, such as cruciferous vegetables (broccoli, cauliflower, cabbage), dried peas and beans, dried prunes and raisins, carbonated beverages, garlic, onions, melon, and products containing sorbitol. It may also be prudent to limit fatty and fried foods.
> - A multivitamin and mineral supplement may be prescribed until intake is adequate.
> - Use a hunger scale to identify internal cues for hunger, satiety, and fullness (see Box 15.1).
>
> **Source:** Academy of Nutrition and Dietetics. (2016). *Nutrition care manual. Anorexia nervosa meal planning tips.* Available at https://www.nutritioncaremanual.org/client_ed.cfm?ncm_client_ed_id=64. Accessed on 6/7/16.

Calorie Density
the amount of calories in a given weight of food.

consumed, not to weight gain; and having the client record food intake and exercise activity. A study by Schebendach et al. (2008) showed that among clients who achieved restoration of weight through treatment for AN, those who consumed diets low in **calorie density** and limited in variety had increased risk of relapse. Box 15.13 lists nutrition strategies for AN.

Bulimia Nervosa

BN is characterized by binge-eating episodes followed by purging to prevent weight gain. Binge and purge episodes occur at least once a week for 3 months but may occur several times a day. An episode of binge eating is characterized by eating a large amount of food within any 2-hour period that is accompanied by a feeling of lack of control over eating. Binge foods tend to be soft, easy to swallow, easy to regurgitate, and composed of high-fat or high-sugar foods that the client normally restricts from the diet. Binges lead to guilt and self-disgust. Purging is accomplished by self-induced vomiting; laxative, diuretic, or diet pill abuse; or excessive exercise. Unlike AN, people who have BN usually recognize that their eating behaviors are abnormal.

Nutrition Therapy for Bulimia Nervosa

People with BN associate body shape and weight with self-worth. They tend to have fewer serious medical complications than do people with AN because their undernutrition is less severe. Treatment approaches are similar for BN and AN, except the goal is weight maintenance, not weight restoration. Treatment may include cognitive behavioral therapy and medication, such as antidepressants or mood stabilizers. Nutritional counseling focuses on identifying and correcting food misinformation and fears and includes discussing normal weight fluctuations, planning meals, establishing a normal pattern of eating, and identifying the dangers of dieting. People with bulimia must understand that gorging is only one aspect of a complex pattern of altered behavior; in fact, excessive dietary restriction is a major contributor to the disorder. Although most clients with BN want to lose weight, dieting and recovery from an eating disorder are incompatible. Normalization of eating behaviors is a primary goal. Nutrition strategies for BN are listed in Box 15.14.

BOX 15.14   Nutrition Strategies for Bulimia Nervosa

- Preplan all meals and snacks.
- To increase awareness of eating and satiety, eat while seated at the table, avoid finger foods, and the meal duration should be of appropriate length.
- Avoid dieting and skipping meals.
- Eat balanced meals at regular intervals.
- A high-protein and/or high-fiber snack slightly before the times of the day when the binge is most likely to occur may help promote satiety and keep blood glucose levels within normal range.
- Eat protein, fat, and high-fiber foods for satiety and bulk.
- Consume adequate fluid, preferably water.
- Gradually introduce forbidden binge foods. This is a key step in changing the all-or-none behavior of bingeing and purging.
- Consume foods in appropriate portion sizes. Choosing proportioned foods may be helpful.
- A daily multivitamin may be appropriate if intake or variety is low.
- When relapse occurs, the structured meal plan should be resumed immediately.
- Engage in 30 minutes of physical activity per day. Exercise may help reduce bulimia.

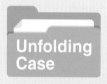

Unfolding Case

Recall Emma. She admits that she has seen a counselor for an eating disorder and that she binges and purges when she's "bad." She recognizes that bingeing and purging are not normal behaviors and admits to feeling out of control when a binge begins. Her restrictive dieting practices always proceed her periods of bingeing. She purges with vomiting and laxatives, which caused her to be hospitalized for hypokalemia. Is counting calories a good strategy for Emma? What strategies would you recommend to help Emma normalize her eating behaviors?

Binge-Eating Disorder

BED was included as its own category of eating disorder in the *DSM-5*. Previously, it was not recognized as a separate disorder and was diagnosable only under the catch-all category of eating disorder not otherwise specified. BED is defined as "recurring episodes of eating significantly more food in a short period of time than most people would eat under similar circumstances, with episodes marked by feelings of lack of control" (American Psychiatric Association, 2013). By definition, binge eating occurs, on average, at least once a week over 3 months. People with BED eat even when they are not hungry; eat until uncomfortably full; may eat too fast or binge eat alone to hide the behavior; and feel guilty, embarrassed, or disgusted after overeating. Unlike BN, people with BED do not purge.

BED differs from common overeating in that it is more severe, is associated with more subjective distress regarding the eating behavior, and is accompanied with physical and psychological problems. People with BED may be of normal weight, but most are obese (Westerberg & Waitz, 2013). BED is associated with a history of dieting and with other psychological issues, such as depression. Risk factors include childhood obesity, parental obesity, high degree of body dissatisfaction, poor self-esteem, and impaired social functioning (Academy of Nutrition and Dietetics, 2016).

Psychotherapy, particularly cognitive behavior therapy, and medication are the main treatment modalities for BED (Westerberg & Waitz, 2013). The focus of nutrition therapy is to normalize eating behaviors with emphasis on recognizing internal hunger and satiety cues (Box 15.15). Reducing binge eating may be followed by participation in a weight control program.

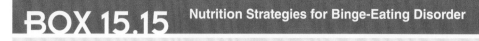

BOX 15.15   Nutrition Strategies for Binge-Eating Disorder

- Use a hunger rating scale to identify hunger, satiety, and fullness. For instance, on a scale of 1 to 10, 1 represents "starving," 10 represents "stuffed," and satiety may be 6 or 7. A workable range may be to eat at a 3 or 4 and stop at 6 or 7.
- Eat slowly, allowing 20 to 30 minutes for each meal to allow the brain to signal that the body has eaten enough.
- Make eating its own activity; avoid TV and other electronics, reading, cooking, and driving while eating.
- Eat seated and avoid eating alone.
- Enjoy the food.
- Know that you can have more when hunger returns.
- Do not label any foods "forbidden."

Source: Academy of Nutrition and Dietetics. (n.d.). *Nutrition care manual. Binge eating disorder meal planning tips.* Available at https://www.nutritioncaremanual.org/client_ed.cfm?ncm_client_ed_id=63. Accessed on 6/7/16.

Eating Disorders Not Otherwise Specified

The prevalence of eating disorders not otherwise specified (EDNOS) is unknown because there is no simple definition of EDNOS. This group represents subacute cases of AN or BN, such as people of normal weight who purge without bingeing.

How Do You Respond?

If 1200 calories can promote a 1- to 2-pound loss per week, will a more drastic calorie reduction speed the weight loss process?

People often think that the greater the calorie deficit, the quicker the weight loss. In reality, cutting calories too much may result in higher proportions of lean tissue loss. This leads to a lowering of basal energy expenditure and reduced exercise tolerance, making weight loss and maintenance more difficult (Blackburn et al., 2010).

REVIEW CASE STUDY

"I hate being fat."

Client history: CC is a 43-year-old mother of three who has experienced gradual weight gain after the birth of each of her children. She is 5 ft 7 in tall, weighs 189 pounds, works full-time, and does not engage in regular exercise. She is considered prediabetic and has prehypertension and appears eager to make lifestyle changes to improve her health and be a better nutritional role model for her children. She has successfully lost weight in the past through Weight Watchers but eventually got bored and regained all of the weight she lost. She wants to try a low-carbohydrate diet because she heard it is the best and easiest way to lose weight. Her usual intake is as follows: no breakfast, snacks at a vending machine twice a day, fast food for lunch, and dinner with the family. Her dinner usually consists of about 6 oz of meat, potatoes, some- times a vegetable, bread with butter, and dessert. CC admits to a weakness for "sweets."

- What is CC's weight status based on her BMI?
- What additional information about her eating behaviors would be helpful?
- What would you tell her about the "best and easiest" way to lose weight?
- What foods does she eat that provide carbohydrates? Compared to the low-carbohydrate eating plan outlined in Table 15.3, what food groups would she need to increase? Decrease?
- What other lifestyle changes would you recommend for her?
- Create a nursing care plan complete with nursing diagnosis, client goal, interventions, and monitoring recommendations.

STUDY QUESTIONS

1 The client asks if it is okay for her to follow a low-carbohydrate, Atkins-type diet in the short term to get her started on her weight loss efforts. Which of the following would be the nurse's best response?
   a. "No, low-carbohydrate diets are not healthy and would only sabotage your weight loss efforts."
   b. "An Atkins-type diet can help you lose weight as can many other types of diets. The important factor that determines whether you lose weight is the number of calories you eat, not the proportion of carbohydrates, protein, and fat you eat."
   c. "A low-carbohydrate diet is better than any other type of diet and is a good choice for you to use."
   d. "A low-fat diet is easier. Try that instead."

2 A major reason why it becomes increasing difficult to keep losing weight on a weight loss diet is that
   a. The loss of fat tissue lowers metabolic rate.
   b. A lighter body expends fewer calories than a heavier body when doing activity.
   c. Fluid retention becomes an issue over time.
   d. A decrease in food intake means that fewer calories are used to metabolize food.

3 The client asks if meal replacements, such as Jenny Craig products, are a good idea to help with weight loss. Which of the following would be the nurse's best response?
   a. "They are a great way to control portions and can help you adhere to your diet when used as suggested."
   b. "They are gimmicks that fail to teach you how to control your own intake. They are not recommended."
   c. "Most people gain weight while using them. You should stay away from them."
   d. "They are not nutritionally balanced so you actually have to overeat in order to meet your nutritional requirements if you use them."

4 Which of the following strategies promotes adherence to exercise? Select all that apply.
   a. Promote structure by encouraging the client to exercise at on-site or supervised exercise sessions.
   b. Encourage the client to exercise in multiple short bouts (10 minutes each), instead of one long session.
   c. Encourage a more active lifestyle, such as parking far away from the door when going to the mall or work.
   d. Encourage the client to exercise at home.

5 Which of the following calorie level ranges is considered appropriate for weight loss diets for most women?
   a. 1800 to 2000 cal/day
   b. 1200 to 1500 cal/day
   c. 1000 to 1200 cal/day
   d. 800 to 1000 cal/day

6 Which of the following increases the risk of dumping syndrome after bariatric surgery?
   a. Consuming high-sugar foods or fluids with meals
   b. Not chewing food thoroughly
   c. Inadequate protein intake
   d. Eating too frequently

7 When instituting nutrition therapy for a client diagnosed with BN, the priority is to
   a. Teach the client about nutrient and calorie requirements.
   b. Halt weight loss.
   c. Normalize eating behaviors.
   d. Provide sufficient calories for weight gain.

8 When instituting nutrition therapy for a client diagnosed with AN, the priority is to
   a. Teach the client about nutrient and calorie requirements.
   b. Halt or restore weight lost.
   c. Normalize eating behaviors.
   d. Halt purging behaviors.

KEY CONCEPTS

- Approximately 36% of American adults are obese. The prevalence of obesity has increased in both genders, in all age groups, and among all races and ethnicities.
- Obesity is a chronic disease of multifactorial origin. It is likely that an obesogenic environment, behavior, and genetics are involved in its development.
- Obesity is resistant to treatment when success is measured by achieving healthy BMI alone. Rather than concentrating solely on weight loss to measure success, other health benefits, such as lowered blood pressure and lowered serum glucose levels, should also be considered.
- A modest weight loss of 5% to 10% of initial body weight usually effectively lowers health risks. For some people, a reasonable goal may be to halt weight gain, not to lose weight.
- A hypocaloric intake, increased physical activity, and behavior therapy are the cornerstones to weight loss therapy. Medication and surgery are additional options for some people.
- In theory, a calorie deficit of 500 to 1000 cal/day results in a loss of 1 to 2 pounds/week. In practice, biologic adaptations occur, making it increasingly difficult to continue losing weight without a further reduction in calories.
- Generally, weight loss diets range from 1200 to 1500 cal/day for most women and 1500 to 1800 cal/day for men.
- A number of evidence-based diets perform equally well in promoting short- and long-term weight loss in adults as long as calorie intake is low enough to cause weight loss. What matters is the relationship between calorie intake and calorie output, not the source of calories consumed.

- Because portion sizes have grown over the last few decades, people's perception of what a normal portion size is may be distorted. Estimating portion sizes using common household items may help people "right size." Other recommendations include using a smaller dinner plate, smaller utensils, and prepackaged 100-calorie products.
- Meal replacements eliminate choices in what to eat and how much to eat and have been shown to effectively promote weight loss and weight maintenance after loss.
- Behavior therapy promotes lifelong changes in eating and activity habits. It is a process that involves identifying behaviors that need improvement, setting specific behavioral goals, modifying "problem" behaviors, and reinforcing the positive changes.
- An increase in activity helps to burn calories and has a favorable impact on body composition and weight distribution. Even without weight loss, exercise lowers blood pressure and improves glucose tolerance and blood lipid levels.
- To achieve weight loss, 150 to 420 minutes/week of MVPA may be needed. Even greater amounts of activity may be necessary to maintain weight after weight loss.
- People who are severely obese may not be able to achieve the recommended intensity and duration of aerobic benefits to reap weight loss benefits. Progressive strength training may be a better option for physical activity for this population.
- Clients may be more likely to adhere to a physical activity program if they are encouraged to participate in physical activity at home and in short bouts, if that is preferred. Moving more throughout the day by reducing sedentary activities is also recommended.
- Weight maintenance after loss may be more difficult to achieve than weight loss itself. Common characteristics of people who are able to maintain long-term weight loss include consuming a low-calorie diet, eating consistently from day to day, eating breakfast, becoming very physically active, weighing themselves frequently, watching TV for a limited period of time, and not letting a small weight gain become a big weight gain.

- Medication is adjunctive therapy in the treatment of obesity. Drugs are not effective in all people, and they are only effective for as long as they are used.
- Surgery to promote weight loss therapy involves limiting the capacity of the stomach. Gastric bypass also circumvents a portion of the small intestine to cause malabsorption of calories. Both types effectively promote weight loss but are tools, not magic strategies.
- Bariatric surgeries require lifelong changes in eating behaviors to ensure continued success. The postsurgical diet progresses from clear liquids to pureed food to a soft diet. Fluid is avoided with meals and for at least 30 minutes afterward because fluid drinking with meals may contribute to dumping syndrome. Sugars are avoided to decrease the risk of dumping syndrome. Nutritional deficiencies are a lifelong risk, requiring preventive supplementation.
- AN, BN, and BED are characterized by abnormal eating behaviors and are usually preceded by dieting or restrictive eating. Although their cause is unknown, they are considered to be multifactorial in origin.
- AN is a condition of severe self-imposed starvation, often accompanied by a frantic pursuit of exercise. Although they appear to be severely underweight, anorexics have a distorted self-perception of weight and see themselves as overweight. They may have numerous physical and mental symptoms. Anorexia can be fatal.
- Bulimia, which occurs more frequently than anorexia, is characterized by binge eating (consuming large amounts of food in a short period) and purging (e.g., self-induced vomiting, laxative abuse). Foods consumed tend to be soft and easily regurgitated. People with bulimia usually appear to be of normal or slightly above normal weight, and they experience less severe physical symptoms than anorexic individuals do. Bulimia is rarely fatal.
- BED is similar to bulimia except that it is not accompanied by purging behaviors. A nondieting approach may be used to help normalize eating behaviors.
- Eating disorders are best treated by a team approach that includes nutritional intervention and counseling to restore normal eating behaviors and adequate nutritional status.

Check Your Knowledge Answer Key

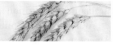

1 **FALSE** Comprehensive lifestyle treatment is the foundation of any treatment for obesity, even when other therapies are used, such as medication and bariatric surgery.
2 **FALSE** People who need to lose weight but are not ready to make lifestyle changes to achieve weight loss should be advised to employ strategies to avoid weight gain. Medications are used only in conjunction with comprehensive lifestyle treatment, not in place of it.
3 **TRUE** Metabolic changes that occur with weight loss, such as adaptive thermogenesis, make it more difficult to maintain weight loss, especially in the short term.

4 **TRUE** People who successfully lose weight are advised to participate in a long-term comprehensive weight loss maintenance program to improve their chances of maintaining their new lower weight.
5 **FALSE** An initial weight loss of as little as 3% to 5% of body weight results in improvements in risk factors for cardiovascular disease.
6 **TRUE** Reducing calories is more effective at promoting weight loss than is increasing physical activity. Ideally, both approaches combined with behavior change are employed to manage weight.

7 **TRUE** Micronutrient deficiencies are common after bariatric surgery. Patients are advised to take specific supplements for the rest of their lives.

8 **FALSE** A general calorie target for weight loss for men is 1500 to 1800 cal/day. For women, the recommended target is 1200 to 1500 cal/day.

9 **FALSE** Neither cutting carbohydrates nor cutting fat grams ensures weight loss unless total calories are reduced. There is no magic combination of nutrients that causes weight loss independent of reducing calories.

10 **TRUE** People affected by bulimia tend to have fewer medical complications than those affected by anorexia because the undernutrition is less severe.

Student Resources on thePoint®
For additional learning materials, activate the code in the front of this book at
http://thePoint.lww.com/activate

Websites

For reliable information on weight, dieting, physical fitness, and obesity

Obesity Society at www.obesity.org

Calorie Control Council at www.caloriecontrol.org

Division of Nutrition, Physical Activity, and Obesity, National Center for Chronic Disease Prevention and Health Promotion at www.cdc.gov/nccdphp/dnpa

National Heart, Lung, and Blood Institute Obesity Education Initiative at www.nhlbi.nih.gov/about/oei/index.htm

Shape Up America! at www.shapeup.org

Weight-Control Information Network at http://www.niddk.nih.gov/health-information/health-communication-programs/win/Pages/default.aspx

For free intake/diet analysis

FitDay at www.fitday.com

FoodCount at www.foodcount.com (offers both free and fee-based subscriptions)

SuperTracker at www.supertracker.usda.gov

For eating disorders

Anorexia Nervosa & Related Eating Disorders (ANRED) at www.anred.com

National Eating Disorders Association at www.nationaleatingdisorders.org

Overeaters Anonymous, Inc. at www.oa.org

The Renfrew Center at www.renfrew.org

References

Academy of Nutrition and Dietetics. (2016). *Nutrition care manual.* Available at www.nutritioncaremanual.org. Accessed 6/3/16.

American Psychiatric Association. (2013). *Diagnostic and Statistical Manual of Mental Disorders* (5th ed.). Arlington, VA: American Psychiatric Association.

Bazzano, L., Hu, T., Reynolds, K., Yao, L., Bunol, C., Liu, Y., . . . He, J. (2014). Effects of low-carbohydrate and low-fat diets. A randomized trial. *Annals of Internal Medicine, 161,* 309–318.

Blackburn, G., Wollner, S., & Heymsfield, S. (2010). Lifestyle interventions for the treatment of class III obesity: A primary target for nutrition medicine in the obesity epidemic. *The American Journal of Clinical Nutrition, 91*(Suppl.), 289S–292S.

Briggs, D., Lockie, S., Wu, Q., Lemus, M. B., Stark, R., & Andrews, Z. B. (2013). Calorie restricted weight loss reverses high-fat diet-induced ghrelin resistance, which contributes to rebound weight gain in a ghrelin-dependent manner. *Endocrinology, 154,* 709–717.

Buchwald, H., Avidor, Y., Braunwald, E., Jensen, M. D., Pories, W., Fahrbach, K., & Schoelles, K. (2004). Bariatric surgery: A systematic review and meta-analysis. *JAMA, 292,* 1724–1737.

Bulik, C., Sullivan, P., Tozzi, F., Furberg, H., Lichtenstein, P., & Pedersen, N. L. (2006). Prevalence, heritability, and prospective risk factors for anorexia nervosa. *Archives of General Psychiatry, 63,* 305–321.

Burnand, K., Lahiri, R., Burr, N., Jansen van Rensburg, L., & Lewis, M. P. (2016). A randomised, single blinded trial, assessing the effect of a two week preoperative very low calorie diet on laparoscopic cholecystectomy in obese patients. *HPB (Oxford), 18,* 456–461.

Camps, S., Verhoef, S., & Westerterp, K. (2013). Weight loss, weight maintenance, and adaptive thermogenesis. *The American Journal of Clinical Nutrition, 97,* 990–994.

Castelnuovo, G., Manzoni, G., Villa, V., Cesa, G., Pietrabissa, G., & Molinari, E. (2011). The STRATOB study: Design of a randomized controlled clinical trial of Cognitive Behavior Therapy and Brief Strategic Therapy with telecare in patients with obesity and binge-eating disorder referred to residential nutritional rehabilitation. *Trials, 12,* 114. doi:10.1186/1745-6215-12-114

Chaput, J., Klingenberg, L., Astrup, A., & Sjodin, M. (2011). Modern sedentary activities promote overconsumption of food in our current obesogenic environment. *Obesity Reviews, 12,* e12–e20.

Cockfield, A., & Philpot, U. (2009). Feeding size 0: The challenges of anorexia nervosa. Managing anorexia from a dietitian's perspective. *The Proceedings of the Nutrition Society, 68,* 281–288.

Corsica, J., & Hood, M. (2011). Eating disorders in an obesogenic environment. *Journal of the American Dietetic Association, 111,* 996–1000.

Demaria, A. (2013). The multiple challenges of obesity. *Journal of the American College of Cardiology, 61,* 784–786.

Dhurandhar, E., Dawson, J., Alcorn, A., Larsen, L., Thomas, E. A., Cardel, M., . . . Allison, D. B. (2014). The effectiveness of breakfast recommendations on weight loss: A randomized controlled trial. *The American Journal of Clinical Nutrition, 100,* 507–513.

Donnelly, J., Blair, S., Jakicic, J., Manore, M. M., Rankin, J. W., & Smith, B. K. (2009). American College of Sports Medicine position stand: Appropriate physical activity intervention strategies for weight loss and prevention of weight regain for adults. *Medicine and Science in Sports and Exercise, 41,* 459–471.

Ebeling, H., Tapanainen, P., Joutsenoja, A., Koskinen, M., Morin-Papunen, L., Järvi, L., . . . Wahlbeck, K. (2003). A practice guideline for treatment of eating disorders in children and adolescents. *Annals of Medicine, 35,* 488–501.

Faria, S., Faria, O., de Almeida Cardeal, M., & Ito, M. K. (2015). Effects of a very low calorie diet in the preoperative stage of bariatric surgery: A randomized trial. *Surgery for Obesity and Related Diseases, 11,* 230–237.

Farias, M., Cuevas, A., & Rodriguez, F. (2011). Set-point theory and obesity. *Metabolic Syndrome and Related Disorders, 9,* 85–89.

Farooqi, I., & O'Rahilly, S. (2009). Leptin: A pivotal regulator of human energy homeostasis. *The American Journal of Clinical Nutrition, 89,* 980S–984S.

Finkler, E., Heymsfield, S., & St-Onge, M. (2012). Rate of weight loss can be predicted by patient characteristics and intervention strategies. *Journal of the Academy of Nutrition and Dietetics, 112,* 75–80.

Fock, K., & Khoo, J. (2013). Diet and exercise in management of obesity and overweight. *Journal of Gastroenterology and Hepatology, 28*(Suppl. 4), 59–63.

Fryar, C., Carroll, M., & Ogden, C. (2014). Prevalence of overweight, obesity, and extreme obesity among adults: United States, 1960–1962 through 2011–2012. Available at http://www.cdc.gov/nchs/data /hestat/obesity_adult_11_12/obesity_adult_11_12.htm. Accessed on 5/19/16.

Golden, N., & Meyer, W. (2004). Nutritional rehabilitation of anorexia nervosa. Goals and dangers. *International Journal of Adolescent Medicine and Health, 16,* 131–144.

Hemmingsson, E., Johansson, K., Eriksson, J., Sundström, J., Neovius, M., & Marcus, C. (2012). Weight loss and dropout during a commercial weight-loss program including a very-low-calorie diet, a low-calorie diet, or restricted normal food: Observational cohort study. *The American Journal of Clinical Nutrition, 96,* 953–961.

Herrera, B., & Lindgren, C. (2010). The genetics of obesity. *Current Diabetes Reports, 10,* 498–505.

Hills, A., Byrne, N., Lindstrom, R., & Hill, J. (2013). 'Small changes' to diet and physical activity behaviors for weight management. *Obesity Facts, 6,* 228–238.

Hooper, L., Abdelhamid, A., Moore, H., Douthwaite, W., Skeaff, C. M., & Summerbell, C. D. (2012). Effect of reducing total fat intake on body weight: Systematic review and meta-analysis of randomised controlled trials and cohort studies. *BMJ, 345,* e7666.

Hudson, J., Hiripi, E., Pope, H., Jr., & Kessler, R. (2007). The prevalence and correlates of eating disorders in the National Comorbidity Survey Replication. *Biological Psychiatry, 61,* 348–358.

Hutter, M., Schirmer, B., Jones, D., Ko, C. Y., Cohen, M. E., Merkow, R. P., . . . Nguyen, N. T. (2011). First report from the American College of Surgeons—Bariatric Surgery Center Network: Laparoscopic sleeve gastrectomy has morbidity and effectiveness position between the band and the bypass. *Annals of Surgery, 254,* 410–422.

Iepsen, E., Lundgren, J, Holst, J., Madsbad, S., & Torekov, S. S. (2016). Successful weight loss maintenance includes long-term increased meal responses of GLP-1 and PYY 3-36. *European Journal of Endocrinology, 174,* 775–784.

Jensen, M., Ryan, D., Apovian, C., Ard, J. D., Comuzzie, A. G., Donato, K. A., . . . Yanovski, S. Z. (2014). 2013 AHA/ACC/TOS guideline for the management of overweight and obesity in adults. A report of the American College of Cardiology/American Heart Association Task Force on Practice Guidelines and the Obesity Society. *Circulation, 129,* S102–S138.

Johansson, K., Neovius, M., & Hemmingsson, E. (2014). Effects of anti-obesity drugs, diet, and exercise on weight-loss maintenance after a very-low-calorie diet or low-calorie diet: A systematic review and meta-analysis of randomized controlled trials. *The American Journal of Clinical Nutrition, 99,* 14–23.

Johns, D., Hartmann-Boyce, J., Jebb, S., & Aveyard, P. (2014). Diet or exercise interventions vs combined behavioral weight management programs: A systematic review and meta-analysis of direct comparisons. *Journal of the Academy of Nutrition and Dietetics, 114,* 1557–1568.

Johnston, B., Kanters, S., Bandayrel, K., Wu, P., Naji, F., Siemieniuk, R. A., . . . Mills, E. J. (2014). Comparison of weight loss among named diet programs in overweight and obese adults: A meta-analysis. *JAMA, 312,* 923–933.

Kahan, S., & Brown, N. (2016). Pharmacotherapy options for obesity. *Weight Management Matters, 14*(3), 1, 7–13.

Kaye, W., Fudge, J., & Paulus, M. (2009). New insights into symptoms and neurocircuit function of anorexia nervosa. *Nature Reviews. Neuroscience, 19,* 573–584.

Kaye, W., Wierenga, C., Bailer, U., Simmons, A. N., & Bischoff-Grethe, A. (2013). Nothing tastes as good as skinny feels: The neurobiology of anorexia nervosa. *Trends in Neuroscience, 36*(2), doi:10.1016 /j.tins.2013.01.003

Kohn, M., Madden, S., & Clarke, S. (2011). Refeeding in anorexia nervosa: Increased safety and efficiency through understanding the pathophysiology of protein calorie malnutrition. *Current Opinion in Pediatrics, 23,* 390–394.

Kulovitz, M., Ktavitz, L., Mermier, C., Gibson, A. L., Conn, C. A., Kolkmeyer, D., & Kerksick, C. M. (2014). Potential of meal frequency as a strategy for weight loss and health in overweight or obese adults. *Nutrition, 30,* 386–392.

Loos, R., & Rankinen, T. (2005). Gene-diet interactions on body weight changes. *Journal of the American Dietetic Association, 105*(Suppl. 1), S29–S34.

Masters, R., Reither, E., Powers, D., Yang, Y., Burger, A. E., & Link, B. G. (2013). The impact of obesity on US mortality levels: The importance of age and cohort factors in population estimates. *American Journal of Public Health, 103,* 1895–1901.

McAuley, P., Kokkinos, P., Oliveira, R., Emerson, B. T., & Myers, J. N. (2010). Obesity paradox and cardiorespiratory fitness in 12,417 male veterans aged 40 to 70 years. *Mayo Clinic Proceedings, 85,* 115–121.

Mechanick, J., Youdin, D., Jones, D., Garvey, W., Hurley, D. L., Molly McMahon, M., . . . Brethauer, S. (2013). Clinical practice guidelines for the perioperative nutritional, metabolic, and nonsurgical support of the bariatric surgery patient—2013 Update: Cosponsored by American Association of Clinical Endocrinologists, the Obesity Society, and American Society for Metabolic & Bariatric Surgery. *Surgery for Obesity and Related Diseases, 9,* 159–191.

Millen, B., Wolongevicz, D., Nonas, C., & Lichtenstein, A. (2014). 2013 American Heart Association/American College of Cardiology/The Obesity Society Guideline for the management of overweight and obesity in adults: Implications and new opportunities for registered dietitian nutritionists. *Journal of the Academy of Nutrition and Dietetics, 114,* 1730–1735.

Moizé, V., Andreu, A., Flores, L., Torres, F., Ibarzabal, A., Delgado, S., . . . Vidal, J. (2013). Long-term dietary intake and nutritional deficiencies following sleeve gastrectomy or Roux-En-Y gastric bypass in a Mediterranean population. *Journal of the Academy of Nutrition and Dietetics, 113,* 400–410.

Nabi, T., Rafiq, N., & Qayoom, O. (2016). Leptin dysfunction: A cause for obesity. *International Journal of Health Sciences and Research, 6*(1), 498–505.

National Weight Control Registry. (2016). *The National Weight Control Registry.* Available at http://www.nwcr.ws/. Accessed on 6/3/16.

Nijamkin, M., Campa, A., Sosa, J., Baum, M., Himburg, S., & Johnson, P. (2012). Comprehensive nutrition and lifestyle education improves weight loss and physical activity in Hispanic Americans following gastric bypass surgery: A randomized controlled trial. *Journal of the Academy of Nutrition and Dietetics, 112,* 382–390.

Ogden, C., Carroll, M., Fryar, C., & Fiegal, K. (2015). *Prevalence of obesity among adults and youth: United States, 2011–2014* (NCHS Data Brief No. 219). Available at http://www.cdc.gov/nchs/data /databriefs/db219.pdf. Accessed on 6/8/16.

Ozier, A., & Henry, B. (2011). Position of the American Dietetic Association: Nutrition intervention in the treatment of eating disorders. *Journal of the American Dietetic Association, 1111,* 1236–1241.

Page, M. (2016). The Instinct Diet: An alternative approach to postoperative weight regain. *Weight Management Matters, 14*(3), 2–4.

Piernas, C., & Popkin, B. (2011). Increased portion sizes from energy-dense foods affect total energy intake at eating occasions in the US children and adolescents: Patterns and trends by age group and sociodemographic characteristics, 1977-2006. *The American Journal of Clinical Nutrition, 94,* 1324–1332.

Pories, W. J., Swanson, M. S., MacDonald, K. G., Long, S. B., Morris, P. G., Brown, B. M., . . . Dolezal, J. M. (1995). Who would have thought it? An operation proves to be the most effective therapy for adult-onset diabetes mellitus. *Annals of Surgery, 222,* 339–352.

Prospective Studies Collaboration. (2009). Body-mass index and cause-specific mortality in 900,000 adults: Collaborative analyses of 57 prospective studies. *The Lancet, 373,* 1083–1096.

Raynor, H., & Champagne, C. (2016). Position of the Academy of Nutrition and Dietetics: Interventions for the treatment of overweight and obesity in adults. *Journal of the Academy of Nutrition and Dietetics, 116,* 129–147.

Rhee, K., McEachern, R., & Jelalian, E. (2014). Parent readiness to change differs for overweight child dietary and physical activity behaviors. *Journal of the Academy of Nutrition and Dietetics, 114,* 1601–1610.

Rock, C., Flatt, S., Pakiz, B., Barkai, H. S., Heath, D. D., & Krumhar, K. C. (2016). Randomized clinical trial of portion-controlled prepackaged foods to promote weight loss. *Obesity, 24,* 1230–1237.

Rocks, T., Pelly, F., & Wilkinson, P. (2014). Nutrition therapy during initiation of refeeding in underweight children and adolescent inpatients with anorexia nervosa: A systematic review of the evidence. *Journal of the Academy of Nutrition and Dietetics, 114,* 897–907.

Rosenbaum, M., Hirsch, J., Gallagher, D., & Leibel, R. (2008). Long-term persistence of adaptive thermogenesis in subjects who have maintained a reduced body weight. *The American Journal of Clinical Nutrition, 88,* 906–912.

Ross, S., Flynn, J., & Pate, R. (2015). What is really causing the obesity epidemic? A review of reviews in children and adults. *Journal of Sports Sciences, 32*(12), 1148–1153. doi:10.1080/02640414.2015.1093650.

Schebendach, J., Mayer, L., Devlin, M., Attia, E., Contento, I. R., Wolf, R. L., & Walsh, B. T. (2008). Dietary energy density and diet variety as predictors of outcome in anorexia nervosa. *The American Journal of Clinical Nutrition, 87,* 810–816.

Schouten, R., van der Kaaden, I, van't Hof, G., & Feskens, P. (2016). Comparison of preoperative diets before bariatric surgery: A randomized, single-blinded, non-inferiority trial. *Obesity Surgery, 26*(8), 1743–1749. doi:10.1007/s11695-015-1989-8

Scinta, W. (2012). Measuring success: A comparison of weight loss calculations. *Bariatric Times, 9*(7), 18–20.

Silventoinen, K., Rokholm, B., Kaprio, J., & Sorensen, T. (2010). The genetic and environmental influences on childhood obesity: A systematic review of twin and adoption studies. *International Journal of Obesity, 34,* 29–40.

Sjöström, L., Narbo, K., Sjöström, D., Karason, K., Larsson, B., Wedel, H., . . . Carlsson, L. M. (2007). Effects of bariatric surgery on mortality in Swedish obese subjects. *The New England Journal of Medicine, 357,* 741–752.

Smith, S., O'Neil, P., Astrup, A., Finer, N., Sanchez-Kam, M., Fraher, K., . . . Shanahan, W. R. (2014). Early weight loss while on lorcaserin, diet and exercise as a predictor of week 52 weight-loss outcomes. *Obesity, 22,* 2137–2146.

Swift, D., Johannsen, N., Lavie, C., Earnest, C. P., & Church, T. S. (2014). The role of exercise and physical activity in weight loss and maintenance. *Progress in Cardiovascular Diseases, 56,* 441–447.

Swift, D., Lavie, C., Johannsen, N., Arena, R., Earnest, C. P., O'Keefe, J. H., . . . Church, T. S. (2013). Physical activity, cardiorespiratory fitness, and exercise training in primary and secondary coronary prevention. *Circulation Journal, 77,* 281–292.

Tate, D., Turner-McGrievy, G., Lyons, E., Stevens, J., Erickson, K., Polzien, K., . . . Popkin, B. (2012). Replacing caloric beverages with water or diet beverages for weight loss in adults: Main results of the Choose Healthy Options Consciously Everyday (CHOICE) randomized clinical trial. *The American Journal of Clinical Nutrition, 95,* 555–563.

Tchernof, A., & Després, J. P. (2013). Pathophysiology of human visceral obesity: An update. *Physiological Reviews, 93,* 359–404.

Tempest, M. (2012). Counseling the outpatient bariatric client. *Today's Dietitian, 14,* 38–41.

Thomas, J., Bond, D., Phelan, S., Hill, J. O., & Wing, R. R. (2014). Weight-loss maintenance for 10 years in the National Weight Control Registry. *American Journal of Preventive Medicine, 46,* 17–23.

U.S. Food and Drug Administration. (2015). *Medications target long-term weight control.* Available at http://www.fda.gov/forconsumers/consumerupdates/ucm312380.htm. Accessed 6/2/16.

Wardle, J., Carnell, S., Haworth, C., & Plomin, R. (2008). Evidence for a strong genetic influence on childhood adiposity despite the force of the obesogenic environment. *The American Journal of Clinical Nutrition, 87,* 398–404.

Wee, C., Davis, R., & Phillips, R. (2005). Stage of readiness to control weight and adopt weight control behaviors in primary care. *Journal of General Internal Medicine, 20,* 410–415.

Weight Management Dietetic Practice Group, Cummings, S., & Isom, K. (Eds.). (2015). *Academy of Nutrition and Dietetics Pocket Guide to Bariatric Surgery* (2nd ed.). Chicago, IL; American Academy of Nutrition and Dietetics.

Westerberg, D., & Waitz, M. (2013). Binge-eating disorder. *Osteopathic Family Physician, 5,* 230–233.

Wing, R., & Hill, J. (2001). Successful weight loss maintenance. *Annual Review of Nutrition, 21,* 323–341.

Yanovski, S., & Yanovski, J. (2014). Long-term treatment for obesity: A systematic and clinical review. *JAMA, 311,* 74–86.

Chapter 16

Nutrition for Patients with Metabolic or Respiratory Stress

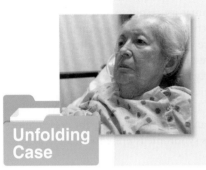

Unfolding Case

Franny Werts

Franny is a 70-year-old female recently admitted to the hospital after sustaining five thoracic spine compression fractures from falling backward down the stairs. She is confused and a neurologic consult is ordered. Shortly after admission, she developed a fever and tachycardia. Pneumonia was suspected, and she was diagnosed with sepsis and transferred to the intensive care unit (ICU). She is 5 ft tall and weighs 112 pounds with a body mass index (BMI) of 22.

Check Your Knowledge

True	False		
☐	☐	**1**	Enteral nutrition (EN) is the preferred method of nutrition support in critically ill patients if the gastrointestinal (GI) tract is functional.
☐	☐	**2**	Stress hormones promote the breakdown of stored nutrients and lean body mass.
☐	☐	**3**	Underfeeding may be adequate to maintain gut integrity in critically ill patients who are at low to moderate nutrition risk.
☐	☐	**4**	Serum levels of the proteins albumin and prealbumin are used to identify malnutrition in critically ill patients.
☐	☐	**5**	In critically ill patients, bowel sounds must be present before EN support can begin.
☐	☐	**6**	Predictive formulas are just as accurate as indirect calorimetry in determining a patient's calorie requirements.
☐	☐	**7**	In previously well-nourished patients, it is better to overfeed than underfeed when initiating feedings during critical illness.
☐	☐	**8**	For most critically ill patients, protein requirements are proportionately higher than calorie requirements.
☐	☐	**9**	Patients with burns covering 10% of total body surface area have calorie and protein requirements that are too high to be met with an oral intake alone.
☐	☐	**10**	High-fat, low-carbohydrate EN formulas are recommended for patients with acute respiratory failure because they yield less carbon dioxide (CO_2) when metabolized than standard formulas.

Learning Objectives

Upon completion of this chapter, you will be able to

1 Explain how the hormonal response to severe acute stress affects metabolism.
2 Explain why enteral nutrition, when feasible, is a superior to parenteral nutrition in patients who are critically ill.

3 Calculate a patient's calorie and protein requirements.
4 Discuss the cause and signs of refeeding syndrome.
5 Teach a client how to increase protein and calorie intake.
6 Devise a high-calorie, high-protein menu with small frequent meals.

Critical illness generally refers to any acute, life-threatening illness or injury, such as trauma (e.g., gunshot wounds, motor vehicle accidents, severe burns), certain diseases (e.g., pancreatitis, acute renal failure), extensive surgery, or infection. It is typically associated with a state of catabolic stress characterized by a systemic inflammatory response and carries the risk of increased infectious morbidity, multiple-organ dysfunction, prolonged hospitalization, and disproportionate mortality (McClave et al., 2016). Once considered adjunct therapy, nutrition support is now thought to help mitigate the metabolic response to stress, prevent oxidative cellular injury, and favorably dampen immune responses. Early enteral nutrition (EN), appropriate macro- and micronutrient delivery, and tight glycemic control may reduce the severity of the illness, reduce complications, decrease length of stay in the ICU, and improve outcomes (McClave et al., 2016).

This chapter discusses the stress response and nutrition therapy for critical illness. Nutrition therapy for burns and acute respiratory distress syndrome is presented.

STRESS RESPONSE

Disruptions to homeostasis elicit a body-wide stress response characterized by physical and hormonal changes to promote healing and resolve inflammation. The intensity of the stress response depends to some extent on the cause and/or severity of the initial injury; for instance, the larger the body surface area burned, the greater is the intensity of the stress response that follows. Hormonal and inflammatory responses account for the changes in metabolic rate, heart rate, blood pressure, and nutrient metabolism that characterize metabolic stress.

Hormonal Response to Stress

Stress Response
a complex series of hormonal and metabolic changes that occur to enable the body to adapt to stressors.

Hypercatabolism
higher than normal breakdown of large molecules into smaller ones, such as muscle protein into amino acids.

Hypermetabolism
higher than normal metabolism.

The **stress response** has three phases: the ebb phase, the flow phase, and the recovery or resolution phase. The ebb phase typically lasts for 12 to 24 hours postinjury. It is characterized by shock with hypovolemia and diminished tissue oxygenation. Cardiac output, oxygen consumption, urinary output, and body temperature fall, and glucagon and catecholamine levels rise. Treatment goals are to restore blood flow to organs, maintain adequate oxygenation to all tissues, and stop bleeding. This initial phase ends when the patient is hemodynamically stable.

The flow phase follows and is marked by metabolic abnormalities. A spike in circulating levels of hormones that direct the "fight or flight response" (e.g., glucagon, catecholamines, cortisol) promotes the breakdown of stored nutrients (e.g., glucose from glycogen, amino acids from skeletal muscle tissue, fatty acids from adipose) to meet immediate energy needs. As stored nutrients and tissues are catabolized, energy expenditure and metabolic rate increase. **Hypercatabolism** and **hypermetabolism** cause oxygen consumption, cardiac output, carbon dioxide (CO_2) production, and body temperature to increase. The length of this phase depends on the severity of injury or infection and the development of complications.

Resolution of the stress leads to the recovery phase, which is marked by anabolism and a return to normal metabolic rate.

Inflammatory Response to Stress

Acute-Phase Response
trauma- or inflammation-induced release of inflammatory mediators that cause changes in the levels of plasma proteins and clinical symptoms of inflammation.

C-reactive Protein
an acute-phase protein that is produced by the liver and released into circulation during acute inflammation.

Cytokines
a group name for more than 100 different proteins involved in immune responses. Prolonged production of proinflammatory cytokines promotes hypercatabolism.

In reaction to infection or tissue injury, the immune system mounts a quick, **acute-phase response** to destroy infections agents, prevent further tissue damage, and promote healing. Inflammation causes positive acute-phase proteins, such as **C-reactive protein**, to increase in concentration. Negative acute-phase proteins, such as albumin, prealbumin, and transferrin, decrease in response to inflammation. **Cytokines** and

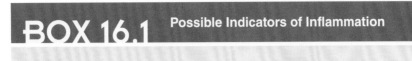

BOX 16.1   Possible Indicators of Inflammation

Laboratory

- Decreased serum albumin
- Decreased serum transferrin
- Decreased serum prealbumin
- Increased C-reactive protein
- Increased blood glucose
- Increased or decreased WBC count
- Increased percentage of neutrophils in the cell differential
- Decreased platelet count
- Negative nitrogen balance

Clinical

- Fever
- Hypothermia
- Presence of infection
- Urinary tract infection
- Pneumonia
- Blood stream infection
- Wound or incision infection
- Abscess

Source: White, J., Guenter, P., Jensen, G., Malone, A., & Schofield, M. (2012). Consensus statement: Academy of Nutrition and Dietetics and the American Society for Parenteral and Enteral Nutrition: Characteristics recommended for the identification and documentation of adult malnutrition (undernutrition). *Journal of Parenteral and Enteral Nutrition, 36,* 275–283.

other immune system molecules are responsible for regulating acute-phase proteins; they also produce changes in other cells that cause systemic symptoms of inflammation, such as anorexia, fever, lethargy, and weight loss. Clinical and laboratory findings used to identify the presence of inflammation are listed in Box 16.1.

The inflammatory response is a desired reaction and is generally self-limiting. However, when the response is exaggerated and prolonged the beneficial response becomes damaging. **Sepsis** is a life-threatening syndrome where an abnormal systemic response to infection causes organ dysfunction (Singer et al., 2016). Sepsis is the primary cause of death from infection (Singer et al., 2016). Septic shock differs from sepsis in the severity of complications and the heightened risk of death.

Sepsis
an abnormal systemic host response to infection that causes life-threatening organ dysfunction.

It is now well understood that inflammation related to critical illness is a potent contributor to malnutrition (Malone & Hamilton, 2013). Malnutrition is associated with impaired immune function, weakened respiratory muscles, prolonged ventilator dependence, and increased infectious complications in critically ill patients (Charles et al., 2014). However, it is difficult to actually define malnutrition in critically ill people. For instance, albumin and prealbumin have been used as diagnostic markers of malnutrition, but these negative acute phase proteins decrease in response to inflammation and physiologic stress and do not accurately reflect nutrition status in the ICU setting (Davis, Sowa, Keim, Kinnare, & Peterson, 2012). Proposed guideline for diagnosing moderate malnutrition in acutely ill or injured patients is the presence of two or more of the following characteristics (Malone & Hamilton, 2013):

- Weight loss, such as 1% to 2% of usual body weight in 1 week
- Calorie intake of <75% for >7 days
- Mild depletion of body fat
- Mild depletion of muscle mass
- Mild fluid accumulation

The same characteristics are used to identify severe malnutrition, but the thresholds are more severe, such as calorie intake of ≤50% for ≥5 days and moderate to severe fluid accumulation.

NUTRITION THERAPY

Nutrition therapy in critical illness largely means **nutrition support**. Oral intake is established as soon as possible, but anorexia is common and may preclude oral intake for days to months (Casaer & Van den Berghe, 2014). Nutrition support is used until the patient is able to orally consume 66% to 75% of estimated needs (Brantley & Mills, 2012). The goal of nutrition support is to improve outcomes, namely, infectious morbidity, ventilator-dependent days, and length of stay in ICU (McClave et al., 2016).

Nutrition Support
the provision of nutrition via enteral feeding tubes or parenteral catheters.

BOX 16.2	Summary of Nutrition Support Guidelines in Critical Illness

Method of Feeding

- EN is strongly recommended over PN when appropriate.
- EN should start within 24 to 48 hours following admission.
- Either gastric or small bowel feedings are appropriate; consider small bowel feedings if patient is at high risk for aspiration or has intolerance to gastric feedings.

Calories

- Calorie needs can be determined by indirect calorimetry, predictive equations, or by a simple weight-based formula:
  - 25 to 30 cal/kg/day of *admission weight* for patients with BMI <30
  - 11 to 14 cal/kg of *actual body weight* per day for patients with BMI in the range of 30–50
  - 22 to 25 cal/kg of *ideal body weight* per day for patients with BMI >50

Protein

- Positive outcomes in critical illness may be more dependent on adequate protein than adequate total calorie intake.
- Protein recommendations are
  - 1.2 to 2.0 g/kg/actual weight for adults with BMI <30; higher amounts may be necessary for certain illnesses, such as burns
  - ≥2.0 g/kg ideal body weight per day for patients with BMI of 30 to 40
  - Up to 2.5 g/kg ideal body weight per day for patients with BMI ≥40

Other

- Supplemental glutamine added to an EN formula not already containing glutamine is not recommended.
- Antioxidant micronutrients, such as vitamins E and C, selenium, zinc, and copper, may improve outcomes for patients with burns, trauma, and those requiring mechanical ventilation.
- Fluid requirements are highly individualized according to losses that occur through exudates, hemorrhage, emesis, diuresis, diarrhea, and fever.
- Patients with persistent diarrhea may benefit from the use of the fiber-containing formula, a semi-elemental formula in place of a polymeric formula, or a soluble fiber supplement.

Source: McClave, S., Taylor, B., Martindale, R., Warren, M. M., Johnson, D. R., Braunschweig, C., . . . Compher, C. (2016). Guidelines for the provision and assessment of nutrition support therapy in the adult critically ill patient: Society of Critical Care Medicine (SCCM) and American Society for Parenteral and Enteral Nutrition (A.S.P.E.N.). *Journal of Parenteral and Enteral Nutrition, 40*, 159–211.

Minimizing body protein catabolism is a secondary goal. Box 16.2 summarizes current guidelines for nutrition support in critically ill patients.

Nutrition Support

For most critically ill patients, EN is a safe and more practical feeding route than PN. EN is preferred because it helps maintain gut integrity, modulates stress and the systemic immune response, and lessens disease severity (McClave et al., 2016). It is recommended that EN be initiated as soon as fluid resuscitation is complete and the patient is hemodynamically stable, preferably within the first 24 to 48 hours (McClave et al., 2016). However, not all studies agree that early nutrition support through PN is more harmful than through EN (Harvey et al., 2014). Guidelines for when to use PN are outlined in Box 16.3.

Studies support the idea that bowel sounds and passing flatus or stool are not required before EN can begin in critically ill patients based on the rationale that bowel sounds are only indicative of contractility and do not necessarily relate to mucosal integrity, barrier function, or absorptive capacity (McClave et al., 2016). In most critically ill patients, delivery into the stomach is acceptable; however, lower gastrointestinal (GI) feedings are recommended for patients

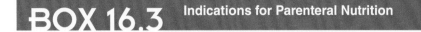

BOX 16.3 Indications for Parenteral Nutrition

- Initiate PN after 7 days of hospitalization when EN is not feasible in patients at low nutrition risk.
- Initiate PN as soon as possible after admission to the ICU when EN is not feasible in patients at high nutrition risk or those who are malnourished.
- Consider supplemental PN after 7 to 10 days in patients who are unable to meet >60% of their calorie and protein requirements via EN regardless of the patients' level of nutrition risk.
- Initiate EN as soon as possible in patients on PN. PN is discontinued when EN provides >60% of the patient's estimated calorie requirements.

Source: McClave, S., Taylor, B., Martindale, R., Warren, M. M., Johnson, D. R., Braunschweig, C., . . . Compher, C. (2016). Guidelines for the provision and assessment of nutrition support therapy in the adult critically ill patient: Society of Critical Care Medicine (SCCM) and American Society for Parenteral and Enteral Nutrition (A.S.P.E.N.). *Journal of Parenteral and Enteral Nutrition, 40,* 159–211.

at high risk for aspiration or those who are intolerant to gastric feedings. Volume-based feeding protocols that specify total amount per 24 hours provide more nutrition than hourly rates (McClave et al., 2016).

Regarding enteral formula selection,

- For most patients, a standard polymeric (intact macronutrients) formula may be used to initiate nutrition support in the ICU.
- For obese patients, a low-caloric density formula with a reduced nonprotein calorie-to-nitrogen ratio (NPC:N) is suggested (proportionately lower in calories from carbohydrates and fats than in protein content).
- For patients in the surgical ICU or with severe trauma, an immune-modulating formula that provides arginine, fish oils, and/or glutamine may be considered.
- No benefit has been shown for routine use of other specialty formulas and disease-specific formulas in the ICU, such as pulmonary formulas for acute respiratory failure and hepatic formulas for critically ill patients with acute or chronic liver disease.

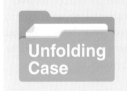

Unfolding Case

Recall Franny. She was given intravenous (IV) fluids and is hemodynamically stable. A nasoduodenal feeding tube is inserted for EN to begin immediately. Is this the best feeding method and route for Franny?

Calories

Indirect Calorimetry (IC)
an indirect estimate of resting energy expenditure that measures the ratio of CO_2 expired to the amount of oxygen inspired and uses those values in a mathematical equation.

Indirect calorimetry (IC) is considered the gold standard for determining calorie requirements, but it is not routinely performed because it is difficult and impractical (Peake et al., 2014). IC is not widely available and cannot be performed on all patients, such as on patients with a chest tube, those using supplemental oxygen, or patients who are uncooperative.

When IC is not an option, calorie needs can be estimated by either a predictive equation or a simple weight-based equation (see Box 16.2). Although there are more than 200 predictive equations, their accuracy rates range from 40% to 75% when compared to IC and none stand out as being the most accurate for ICU patients (McClave et al., 2016). Regardless of the method used to estimate calorie requirements, calorie expenditure should be reevaluated more than once a week so that intake can be optimized (McClave et al., 2016).

EN during critical illness has consistently been shown to provide substantially less than the full-recommended calorie requirement, mostly because of GI dysmotility, especially delayed gastric emptying (Peake et al., 2014). Frequent interruption of EN delivery for procedures or surgery contributes to the typical provision of approximately 60% of estimated calorie needs. A study by Peake et al. (2014) found that substituting routine formula that provides 1.0 cal/mL with a 1.5-cal/mL formula resulted in 46% greater delivery of calories without adverse effects when administered at the same rate. Studies are needed to determine if increasing the delivery of calories affects patient outcomes.

Calorie Targets

Traditionally, it has been recommended that patients receive 80% of calorie and protein goals in the first week of ICU to optimize outcomes (Heyland, Cahill, & Day, 2011). However, randomized controlled trials have not unequivocally proven that early aggressive nutrition support actually prevents or lessens muscle catabolism or speeds recovery in immobilized critically ill patients with systemic inflammation (Schetz, Casaer, & Van den Berghe, 2013).

Trophic Enteral Feeding
usually defined as 10 to 20 mL/hour or 10 to 20 cal/hour or up to 500 cal/day.

Some available evidence shows that in patients without severe prior malnutrition, **trophic enteral feeding**, or permissive underfeeding, in the first ICU week is at least as good as full EN and that early addition of PN to inadequate EN does not provide any benefit and increases morbidity (Schetz et al., 2013). A recent systematic review and meta-analysis found no difference in the risk of acquired infections, hospital mortality, ICU length of stay, or ventilator-free days between patients receiving an intentionally hypocaloric intake compared to a full calorie target (Marik & Hooper, 2016). Potential mechanisms by which underfeeding benefits patients include less hyperglycemia, lower production of proinflammatory cytokines, less nutrient oxidation, and less hypermetabolism leading to less CO_2 production (Zaloga, 2012). A study by Charles et al. (2014) found no difference in infection rates between critically ill study participants in surgical ICU who received 25 to 30 cal/kg/day and those who received 50% of that amount. Researchers speculate that optimizing nutrition support is more about how much protein is provided than the amount of calories consumed. Recommendations are as follows (McClave et al., 2016):

- Low-risk patients who have normal baseline nutrition status and low disease severity that cannot maintain volitional intake do not require EN over the first week of hospitalization. In this population, aggressive EN may provide little, if any, benefit during this time. Daily monitoring is necessary to detect deterioration in patient status.
- Either trophic or full nutrition EN is appropriate for patients with acute respiratory distress syndrome/acute lung injury and those expected to need mechanical ventilation ≥72 hours because these two strategies yield similar outcomes over the first week of hospitalization.
- Patients who are severely malnourished or at high nutrition risk should be advanced toward goal as quickly as tolerated over 24 to 48 hours and should be monitored for refeeding syndrome. EN should provide more than 80% of estimated or calculated calorie and protein goals within 48 to 72 hours.

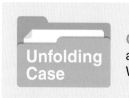

Unfolding Case   **Consider Franny.** Calculate her estimated calorie needs. What is an appropriate calorie target for her as the tube feeding begins? What is an appropriate protein intake for her?

Refeeding Syndrome

Refeeding syndrome is an ill-defined disorder that generally occurs when carbohydrate is reintroduced into the diet of severely malnourished patients (Box 16.4). It may also develop in critically ill patients who receive aggressive nutrition repletion, either via PN, EN, or an oral diet (Academy of Nutrition and Dietetics [AND], 2012). The sudden availability of carbohydrate stimulates insulin secretion and increases the need for thiamin and minerals involved in carbohydrate metabolism. Hypophosphatemia, hypokalemia, and hypomagnesemia can occur as cells rapidly remove these minerals from the bloodstream. Edema and heart failure can result from sodium and fluid retention. Thiamin deficiency can cause acidosis, hyperventilation, and neurologic impairments.

Refeeding Syndrome
a potentially fatal complication that occurs from an abrupt change from a catabolic state to an anabolic state and increase in insulin caused by a dramatic increase in carbohydrate intake.

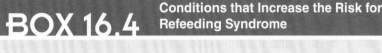

BOX 16.4 Conditions that Increase the Risk for Refeeding Syndrome

Chronic alcoholism
Chronic undernutrition or malnutrition of calories and/or protein
Morbid obesity with recent massive weight loss
Prolonged fasting
Long-term use of simple IV hydration
Cardiac and cancer cachexia

Refeeding syndrome symptoms range from a mild decrease in serum electrolytes that respond quickly to repletion to life-threatening changes in metabolic and organ systems (AND, 2012). For mild refeeding syndrome, initiation of EN is not affected as long as electrolyte abnormalities are corrected. In severe refeeding syndrome, thiamin supplementation, ongoing electrolyte replacement, and slower advancement of EN may be needed.

Protein

Protein is the most important macronutrient for wound healing, supporting immune function, and maintaining lean body mass (McClave et al., 2016). For most critically ill patients, the increased need for protein is proportionately higher than the increased need for calories. Yet, as with calories, the recommendations for protein are not universally agreed upon, and there may be more uncertainty over protein requirements than calorie needs. Protein recommendations vary according to the patient's BMI and severity of critical illness (see Box 16.2). Supplemental protein in the form of protein modules may be considered for patients who are unable to meet their needs due to frequent interruptions in EN support. Glutamine is a nonessential amino acid but is considered a conditionally essential amino acid, particularly during catabolic and stress states (Wischmeyer, Dhaliwal, McCall, Ziegler, & Heyland, 2014). Studies suggest that after illness and injury, glutamine helps modulate the inflammatory response and helps prevent organ injury (Wischmeyer, 2008). Glutamine added to PN has been associated with a decrease in hospital mortality and length of hospital stay (Wischmeyer et al., 2014). However, data from five randomized controlled trials showed no significant benefit on mortality, infections, or hospital length of stay when glutamine is added to an EN regimen (McClave et al., 2016).

Micronutrients

Micronutrients, namely, trace elements, vitamins, and electrolytes, are administered to critically ill patients to prevent deficiencies and associated complications (Casaer & Van den Berghe, 2014). Routine IV administration of micronutrients during the acute phase of critical illness may help prevent refeeding syndrome where deficiencies of thiamine, potassium, and phosphate can cause potentially fatal complications. The use of pharmacologic doses of trace elements (selenium, copper, manganese, zinc, and iron) and antioxidant vitamins (E, C, and beta-carotene) has been proposed as a means to reduce organ failure in critical illness, but a high-quality randomized controlled trial showed no benefit (Heyland et al., 2013). The usefulness of nutrient supplementation may depend on the type of critical illness and whether or not a deficiency was present before the onset of critical illness (Alhazzani et al., 2013). Antioxidant vitamins and trace minerals may improve patient outcomes, especially in burns, trauma, and critical illness requiring mechanical ventilation (McClave et al., 2016).

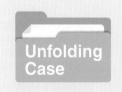

Think of Franny. As her signs and symptoms of inflammation and infection begin to resolve, her appetite improves but only for tea and toast. She wants the feeding tube removed but isn't hungry enough to eat a whole tray of food. What steps will you take to help maximize Franny's oral intake? How many calories should she be consistently consuming before the feeding tube can be removed?

Unfolding Case

Recovery

Patients are typically transitioned to an oral diet as soon as possible, usually following extubation. The goal of nutrition therapy is to maximize intake to preserve lean body mass. However, a study on the adequacy of oral intake in the 7 days following extubation revealed that the mean calorie and protein intake for the entire study group never exceeded 55% of daily requirements (Peterson et al., 2010). A number of contributing factors are likely, including residual pain after endotracheal tube removal, delays in ordering a diet, restrictive diets, patient fatigue, anorexia, GI upset, and nothing by mouth (NPO) orders for tests or procedures.

Monitoring oral intake and individualizing nutrition therapy are vital to optimize recovery. A high-calorie, high-protein diet with small frequent meals may help maximize intake (Box 16.5). A nutrient-dense diet provides nutrients important for wound healing and recovery (Table 16.1). Oral nutrition supplements can provide significant protein, calories, and nutrients. Supplemental EN may be necessary.

Table 16.1   Nutrients Important for Wound Healing and Recovery

Nutrient	Rationale for Increased Need	Possible Deficiency Outcome
Protein	To replace lean body mass lost during the catabolic phase after stress To restore blood volume and plasma proteins lost during exudates, bleeding from the wound, and possible hemorrhage To replace losses resulting from immobility (increased excretion) To meet increased needs for tissue repair and resistance to infection	Significant weight loss Impaired/delayed wound healing Shock related to decreased blood volume Edema related to decreased serum albumin Diarrhea related to decreased albumin Anemia Increased risk of infection related to decreased antibodies, impaired tissue integrity Increased mortality
Calories	To replace losses related to lack of oral intake and hypermetabolism during catabolic phase after stress To spare protein To restore normal weight	Signs and symptoms of protein deficiency due to use of protein to meet energy requirements Extensive weight loss
Water	To replace fluid lost through vomiting, hemorrhage, exudates, fever, drainage, diuresis To maintain homeostasis	Signs, symptoms, and complications of dehydration such as poor skin turgor, dry mucous membranes, oliguria, anuria, weight loss, increased pulse rate, decreased central venous pressure
Vitamin C	Important for capillary formation, tissue synthesis, and wound healing through collagen formation Needed for antibody formation	Impaired/delayed wound healing related to impaired collagen formation and increased capillary fragility and permeability Increased risk of infection related to decreased antibodies
Thiamin, niacin, riboflavin	Requirements increase with increased metabolic rate	Decreased enzymes available for energy metabolism
Folic acid, vitamin B_{12}	Needed for cell proliferation and, therefore, tissue synthesis Important for maturation of red blood cells Impaired folic acid synthesis related to some antibiotics; impaired vitamin B_{12} absorption related to some antibiotics	Decreased or arrested cell division Megaloblastic anemia
Vitamin A	Important for immune function	Decreased immune function and increased risk of infectious morbidity and mortality
Vitamin K	Important for normal blood clotting Impaired intestinal synthesis related to antibiotics	Prolonged prothrombin time
Iron	To replace iron lost through blood loss	Signs, symptoms, and complications of iron deficiency anemia such as fatigue, weakness, pallor, anorexia, dizziness, headaches, stomatitis, glossitis, cardiovascular and respiratory changes, possible cardiac failure
Zinc	Needed for protein synthesis and wound healing Needed for normal lymphocyte and phagocyte response	Impaired/delayed wound healing Impaired immune response

BOX 16.5   A Sample High-Calorie, High-Protein Menu

Breakfast

Orange juice
Cheese and mushroom omelet
Wheat toast with butter and jelly
Milk
Coffee with whipped cream added

Snack

Smoothie made with Greek yogurt, instant breakfast mix, whole milk, and strawberries

Lunch

New England clam chowder
Chicken salad sandwich on a croissant
Milk
Ice cream with chocolate sauce and whipped cream

Snack

Greek yogurt

Dinner

Meat loaf with gravy
Baked potato with sour cream
Broccoli with cheese sauce
Spinach salad with hard-cooked eggs, onions, walnuts, and vinaigrette dressing
Milk
Carrot cake with cream cheese frosting

Snack

Melon topped with fruited Greek yogurt

BURNS

Extensive burns are a severe form of metabolic stress. Loss of lean body mass can be significant. The extensive inflammatory response causes rapid fluid shifts and large losses of fluid, electrolytes, protein, and other nutrients from the wound. Fluid and electrolyte replacement to maintain adequate blood volume and blood pressure is the priority of the initial postburn period. Paralytic ileus, anorexia, pain, infection or other complications, emotional trauma, and medical–surgical procedures may complicate nutrition support.

Nutrition Therapy for Burn Patients

Patients with more than 20% total body surface area (TBSA) or inhalation injuries that require ventilator support should receive EN if the GI tract is functional (AND, 2012). If possible, EN is initiated within 4 to 6 hours of injury; early initiation is associated with improved structure and function of the GI tract and fewer episodes of infection and may also blunt the hypermetabolic response to burns. Early initiation may be facilitated by placing a nasoenteric tube into the small bowel. PN is used only when EN is not feasible or tolerated (McClave et al., 2016).

Historically, calorie requirements for burns have been estimated at >5000 per day (Gottschlich & Irenton-Jones, 2001). However, changes in burn care, such as excision of nonviable tissue and grafting, have lowered hypermetabolic calorie expenditure (McClave et al., 2016). Estimates of calorie needs have also decreased in response to the dangers associated with overfeeding (AND, 2012). IC is recommended as the most accurate method to assess calorie requirements in burn patients. No predictive equations have found to be precise in estimating calorie needs of patients with >20% TBSA burns. If IC is not available or feasible, calorie needs may be estimated by the weight-based formula of 25 to 30 cal/kg (AND, 2012). A weight loss goal may be to prevent >10% loss of admission weight.

Recommended protein intake is 1.5 to 2.0 g/kg/day (McClave et al., 2016). Adequacy of protein intake is evaluated by wound healing and adherence of skin grafts.

Calorie and protein needs increase if complications develop or if there were preexisting conditions and lessen as wound healing progresses. However, wound closure does not result in an immediate decrease in calorie needs, and elevated requirements may persist for many months after a burn.

For burns covering less than 20% of TBSA, an oral high-protein, high-calorie diet can adequately meet protein and calorie requirements of most patients. Small frequent meals of calorie- and protein-dense foods (Box 16.6) and oral nutrition supplements help maximize intake. Daily calorie counts may be used to monitor intake. When calorie and protein intake is less than

---

BOX 16.6   Ways to Increase Protein and Calorie Density of Foods

Ways to Increase Protein Density

- Add skim milk powder to milk.
- Substitute milk for water in recipes.
- Melt cheese on sandwiches, casseroles, hot vegetables, or potatoes.
- Spread peanut butter on apples or crackers or mix into hot cereals.
- Sprinkle nuts on cereals, desserts, or salads; mix into casseroles or stir-fry.
- Coat breaded meats with eggs first; add chopped hard-cooked eggs to casseroles.
- Top fruit with yogurt or Greek yogurt.
- Use plain yogurt or plain Greek yogurt in place of sour cream.
- Add commercially available whey protein powder to water, milk, shakes, or smoothies.

Ways to Increase Calorie Density

- Spread cream cheese on hot bread.
- Add butter or margarine to hot foods: potatoes, vegetables, cooked cereal, rice, pasta, pancakes, and soups.
- Use gravy over potatoes, meat, or vegetables.
- Use mayonnaise in place of salad dressing.
- Use whipped cream on desserts and in coffee and tea.
- Add honey to cooked cereals, fruit, coffee, or tea.
- Add marshmallows to hot chocolate.

75% of estimated need for more than 3 days, EN should be used for supplemental or total nutrition (AND, 2012). Supplemental EN given during the night is useful when nutritional needs are not met through food alone. If oral intake is negligible, EN can provide 100% of need.

Although it is generally agreed that vitamin needs increase in burn patients because of losses from wounds, the need for healing, and changes in metabolism, the exact requirements are not known (AND, 2012). Supplements may be most important for patients consuming an oral diet because EN and PN formulas generally provide more than the Dietary Reference Intakes for vitamins and minerals in the volume necessary to meet the high calorie requirement (AND, 2012). Supplements of vitamin C, vitamin A, and zinc plus a multivitamin are recommended by the Shriners Burn Hospital for patients with burns on more than 20% of TBSA (AND, 2012).

ACUTE RESPIRATORY DISTRESS SYNDROME

Acute respiratory distress syndrome (ARDS) is a severe lung disease; acute lung injury (ALI) is a less severe form of lung disease. Both diseases are characterized by inflammation of the lung parenchyma and increased pulmonary capillary permeability leading to impaired gas exchange. Pulmonary edema interferes with ventilation and damages the alveoli. Oxygen levels fall in the blood and tissues, leading to impaired cellular function and possibly cell death. Hypercapnia can cause acidosis. Breathing is labored and heart rate increases. Cyanosis, confusion, and drowsiness may develop. Heart arrhythmias and coma may result.

Nutrition Therapy for Acute Respiratory Distress Syndrome Patients

ARDS and ALI are most often observed as part of systemic inflammatory processes, such as sepsis, pneumonia, trauma, burn, aspiration, and pancreatitis (AND, 2012). The underlying inflammatory condition increases calorie and protein requirements and the risk for malnutrition. Average duration of mechanical ventilation in patients with ARDS or ALI is 10 to 14 days, making nutrition support necessary. EN is used if the GI tract is functional; intestinal feedings may be preferred because they lower the risk of aspiration.

Overfeeding is avoided because it increases CO_2 production and may complicate respiratory function and ventilator weaning. However, weight loss should be prevented even in overweight patients (AND, 2012). Calorie requirements may be estimated by IC or predictive equations, or by the weight-based formula of 25 to 35 cal/kg. Either trophic or full nutrition is appropriate because these two strategies yield similar outcomes over the first week of hospitalization in patients with ARDS (McClave et al., 2016). Protein requirements generally range from 1.5 to 2.0 g/kg/day. Generally, standard formulas are recommended. Of note,

- EN products specially formulated for patients with respiratory disease are high in fat and low in carbohydrate based on the assumption that lesser amounts of carbohydrate yield less CO_2. However, it is recommended these formulas not be used in ICU patients with acute respiratory failure based on the results of uncontrolled studies that show that increasing the ratio of fat to carbohydrate only lowers CO_2 production in the ICU patient who is overfed (Radrizzani & Iapichino, 1998). When the appropriate amount of calories is provided, the macronutrient composition of the formula is much less likely to affect CO_2 production.
- Acute respiratory failure patients who require fluid restriction may benefit from a calorie-dense EN formulas (e.g., those providing 1.5–2.0 cal/mL) that provide more nutrition in less volume than standard formulas (McClave et al., 2016).
- Due to conflicting data, McClave et al. (2016) did not make a recommendation regarding the use of EN formulas with anti-inflammatory lipid profiles (such as those containing omega-3 fish oils and borage oil) and antioxidants for patients with ARDS.

NURSING PROCESS

Metabolic Stress

Yin is a frail, 74-year-old man admitted to the hospital with multiple serious but non–life-threatening injuries resulting from a car accident. He weighs 122 pounds and is 5 ft 6 in tall.

Assessment

Medical–Psychosocial History	• Current diagnoses and medications • Medical history, including hyperlipidemia, hypertension, cardiovascular disease, renal impairments, diabetes, GI complaints • Medications that affect nutrition, such as lipid-lowering medications, cardiac drugs, antihypertensives • Extent of injuries; significance of GI trauma, if appropriate • Hemodynamic status; signs and symptoms of hemorrhaging • Neurologic status (e.g., confusion, disorientation); ability to eat, ability to self-feed • GI functions such as hypoactive bowel sounds, distention, complaints of nausea, anorexia • Psychosocial and economic issues prior to injury, such as whether finances, loneliness, or isolation impaired his food intake; determine who does food shopping and preparation and whether the client is a candidate for the Meals on Wheels program.
Anthropometric Assessment	• Height, current weight • Recent weight history; usual weight • BMI
Biochemical and Physical Assessment	• Complete blood count • Blood chemistry, including major electrolytes • Serum glucose • Input and output • Clinical symptoms of malnutrition such as wasted appearance

NURSING PROCESS | Metabolic Stress

Dietary Assessment

- Do you have any difficulty chewing or swallowing?
- Do you have nausea or any other symptoms that interfere with your ability to eat?
- Are you able to feed yourself?
- Do you follow a special diet at home?
- Do you have enough food to eat at home?
- Do you have any food intolerances or allergies?
- Do you have any cultural, religious, or ethnic food preferences?
- Do you take vitamins, minerals, or supplements? If so, what?
- How much alcohol do you consume?

Diagnosis

Possible Nursing Diagnoses

Imbalanced nutrition: eating less than the body requires related to anorexia and increased requirements related to injuries

Planning

Client Outcomes

The client will
- Maintain normal fluid and electrolyte balance
- Meet 75% of his goal calories and protein via oral diet with supplements
- Describe the principles and rationale of a high-calorie, high-protein diet
- Avoid complications of undernutrition, such as weight loss, poor wound healing, infections

Nursing Interventions

Nutrition Therapy

- Initially, give IV fluid and electrolytes as ordered.
- When oral intake begins, encourage the intake of calorie- and protein-dense foods first; encourage intake of between-meal supplements.

Client Teaching

Instruct the client on
- The importance of protein and calories in promoting wound healing and recovery and overall health
- The eating plan essentials, including
  - How to increase calories and protein in the diet (Box 16.6)
  - To eat small frequent meals to maximize intake

Evaluation

Evaluate and Monitor

- Monitor fluid and electrolyte balance and other biochemical values.
- Monitor percentage of food consumed.
- Monitor weight.
- Monitor for complications, such as delayed wound healing or infection.
- Observe for tolerance to oral diet.
- Suggest changes in the meal plan as needed.
- Provide periodic feedback and reinforcement.

How Do You Respond?

Do flavored waters marketed to improve immune function really work? There are several flavored waters available on grocery store shelves that feature descriptive terms such as "defend," "protect," or "immunity" on the label. All of these products contain added vitamins and/or minerals, such as vitamins A, C, D, or E; B vitamins; or zinc. Some provide calories from sweeteners; others are calorie-free. Although certain vitamins and minerals *are* important for normal immune system functioning, it is a huge leap to conclude that any of these products provide health benefits beyond those obtained from a normal mixed diet. Consuming more than required of any nutrients necessary for immune system functioning does not boost immune function—unless the immune system was impaired because of a nutrient deficiency. Manufacturers are free to put in whatever nutrients they desire in whatever amounts they choose; scientific evidence of benefit or need is not required to make a function claim.

REVIEW CASE STUDY

Samuel was recently discharged after being hospitalized for burns he suffered in an industrial accident that covered 18% TBSA. He is 38 years old, 5 ft 9 in tall, and currently weighs 134 pounds. His pre-burn weight was 150 to 155 pounds. He received 3 meals a day plus three high-protein shakes while in the hospital. He is motivated to regain weight, but he refuses to drink any more of the shakes—they are too sweet and taste artificial. The dietitian told him he should be eating at least 2000 calories and include protein-dense foods at each meal and snack, but he lives alone and doesn't have the appetite for that amount of food.

His usual pre-burn intake appears in the box on the right.

- Evaluate Samuel's current BMI and normal adult weight. Calculate his weight loss percentage over the past month. Is it significant? What would be an appropriate goal weight?

- What specific strategies would you recommend he implement to improve his overall intake?
- Is 2000 calories an appropriate amount of daily calories for him? What sources of protein did he usually consume?
- Devise a sample menu for him that takes into account the calories and protein he needs, living arrangements, and lack of appetite.

Breakfast: Coffee with creamer; 2 doughnuts
Lunch: 2 hot dogs on buns, French fries; Diet soft drink
Dinner: Frozen pizza; Ice cream; Beer

STUDY QUESTIONS

1 When should nutrition support be initiated in a critically ill patient who is at high nutrition risk upon admission to the ICU?
   a. Within 24 hours
   b. Within 24 to 48 hours
   c. Within 3 days
   d. Within the first week

2 Which of the following strategies will increase protein density?
   a. Using whipped cream in place of milk in coffee
   b. Spreading cream cheese on hot bread
   c. Using plain yogurt in place of sour cream
   d. Using mayonnaise in place of salad dressing

3 In a burned patient with a functional GI tract, why is EN preferred over PN?
   a. Because EN can provide higher amounts of calories and protein
   b. Because EN is less likely to interfere with oral intake
   c. Because EN is less expensive
   d. Because EN has a lower risk of infectious complications

4 Why may underfeeding critically ill patients be beneficial?
   a. Because it provides less work for the GI tract to do
   b. Because all methods of measuring a person's energy expenditure overestimate their needs so a lower calorie load is a prudent approach
   c. Because it provides fewer substrates for the body to make proinflammatory molecules and has a positive effect on hyperglycemia
   d. Because it causes stress hormone levels to drop

5 What is the primary intervention in the initial postburn period?
   a. PN
   b. Supplements of trace elements
   c. Fluid and electrolytes
   d. A low-carbohydrate diet to decrease CO_2 production

6 What does a spike in C-reactive protein indicate in people with acute metabolic stress?
   a. Protein needs are not being met.
   b. Protein intake is adequate.
   c. An inflammatory response is occurring.
   d. The inflammatory response has ended.

7 What causes refeeding syndrome in patients who are fed after being in a catabolic state?
   a. A dramatic increase in fluid intake
   b. A dramatic increase protein intake
   c. A dramatic increase in fat intake
   d. A dramatic increase in carbohydrate intake

8 Which of the following metabolic abnormalities are associated with refeeding syndrome?
   a. Hyperphosphatemia
   b. Thiamin deficiency
   c. Hypocalcemia
   d. Hyponatremia

KEY CONCEPTS

- Once considered adjunct therapy, nutrition support is now thought to help mitigate the metabolic response to stress, prevent oxidative cellular injury, and favorably dampen immune responses.
- The ebb phase following acute illness or injury lasts approximately 24 hours and is resolved when the patient is hemodynamically stable.
- The metabolic response to acute stress is characterized by hormonal and inflammatory responses that change the body's chemistry. The duration of this phase varies with the severity of the stress and whether complications develop.
- Stress hormones increase blood glucose levels, metabolism, and body protein catabolism.
- The inflammatory response is mediated by immune system components that alter the concentration of certain plasma proteins that were historically used to assess for malnutrition, namely, albumin, prealbumin, and transferrin.
- Early EN, appropriate macro- and micronutrient delivery, and tight glycemic control may reduce the severity of the illness, reduce complications, decrease length of stay in the ICU, and improve outcomes. EN is preferred if the GI tract is functional.
- PN is used when the GI tract is not functional, when there is intolerance to EN, and to supplement EN when EN is unable to fully meet the patient's needs. PN is discontinued when 60% of calorie needs are met with EN.
- Calorie needs can be determined by IC, predictive equations, or weight-based formulas. The validity of predictive equations varies.
- During the first week of hospitalization, permissive underfeeding, called tropic feeds, in low to moderate risk critically ill patients may be preferred over full nutrition. Tropic feeds may help reduce hyperglycemia, lower the production of proinflammatory cytokines, and produce less CO_2.
- Refeeding syndrome may develop when carbohydrates are reintroduced into the diet of people who have adapted to starvation by burning fat. Hypophosphatemia, hypokalemia, hypomagnesemia, and thiamin deficiency can occur. Symptoms range from mild to life-threatening.
- For most critically ill patients, protein requirements are proportionately higher than calorie requirements. For nonobese patients, protein recommendation is 1.2 to 2.0 cal/kg of actual weight, although patients with burns may require even higher amounts of protein.
- Routine IV administration of micronutrients during the acute phase may help reduce the risk of refeeding syndrome. The usefulness of micronutrient supplements depends on the type of critical illness and the patient's nutritional status prior to critical illness.
- Oral intake is resumed when possible. Small, frequent meals help achieve a high-calorie, high-protein intake. Initially, supplemental nocturnal EN may be necessary to meet calorie and protein requirements.
- Extensive burns are a severe form of stress. Nutritional support may be complicated by stress ulcers, anorexia, pain, and the consequences of medical–surgical treatments.
- An oral high-calorie, high-protein diet with various vitamin and mineral supplements may be adequate for burns covering less than 20% of TBSA. For more extensive burns, EN support is necessary, and early feedings are recommended. PN support may be needed due to high nutritional needs or EN intolerance.
- Overfeeding is avoided in patients with ARDS. Calorie needs may be estimated by using the weight-based formula of 25 to 35 cal/kg; full or trophic feedings yield the same result over the first week of hospitalization. Standard intact formulas are recommended, although a calorie-dense formula that provides 1.5 to 2.0 cal/mL may be used for patients who require a fluid restriction. High-fat, low-carbohydrate formulas are not recommended in the ICU; avoiding overfeeding is more effective at lowering CO_2 production than is lowering carbohydrate intake.

Check Your Knowledge Answer Key

1 **TRUE** EN is the preferred route of nutrition support in critically ill patients if the GI tract is functional because it is more practical, less invasive, and helps support gut integrity.

2 **TRUE** Stress hormones have catabolic actions in the body; that is, they stimulate the breakdown of glycogen, adipose tissue, and lean body mass. They function opposite to insulin, which lowers blood glucose levels.

3 **TRUE** Underfeeding may be adequate to maintain gut integrity in critically ill patients who are at low to moderate nutrition risk.

4 **FALSE** Serum levels of the proteins albumin and prealbumin change in response to inflammation and so are not used to diagnose malnutrition.

5 **FALSE** Feeding into the GI tract is safe even before bowel sounds or passing of flatus/stool is observed. It is considered safe and appropriate to feed patients with mild to moderate ileus as long as they remain hemodynamically stable.

6 **FALSE** IC is the gold standard for determining calorie requirements; however, it is not routinely performed. Predictive formulas are not as accurate as IC. A simple weight-based formula, such as 25 to 30 cal/kg is often used.

7 **FALSE** Overfeeding is avoided in all critically ill patients. In patients who were previously well nourished and at low nutrition risk and disease severity, providing full nutrition may offer no benefits to permissive underfeeding.

8 **TRUE** For most critically ill patients, protein requirements are proportionately higher than calorie requirements.

9 **FALSE** Patients with burns at 10% of TBSA should be able to consume enough protein and calories orally. When TBSA of burns exceeds 20%, EN is needed.

10 **FALSE** High-fat, low-carbohydrate formulas are not recommended for critically ill ICU patients with acute respiratory failure even though they are intended to yield less CO_2 than standard formulas. Avoiding excess calories, not manipulating the proportion of macronutrients, is the most important element for controlling CO_2 production.

Student Resources on thePoint®
For additional learning materials, activate the code in the front of this book at
http://thePoint.lww.com/activate

Websites

American Association of Critical-Care Nurses at www.aacn.org

American Burn Association at www.ameriburn.org

American Society for Parenteral and Enteral Nutrition at https://www.nutritioncare.org/

Society of Critical Care Medicine at www.sccm.org

Surviving Sepsis Campaign at www.survivingsepsis.org

References

Academy of Nutrition and Dietetics. (2012). *Nutrition care manual.* Available at http://www.nutritioncaremanual.org/. Accessed on 6/15/16.

Alhazzani, W., Jacobi, J., Sindi, A., Hartog, C., Reinhart, K., Kokkoris, S., . . . Jaeschke, R. Z. (2013). The effect of selenium therapy on mortality in patients with sepsis syndrome: A systematic review and meta-analysis of randomized controlled trials. *Critical Care Medicine, 41,* 1555–1564.

Brantley, S., & Mills, M. (2012). Overview of enteral nutrition. In C. M. Mueller (Ed.), *The A.S.P.E.N. adult nutrition support core curriculum* (2nd ed., pp. 170–184). Silver Spring, MD: American Society for Parenteral and Enteral Nutrition.

Casaer, M., & Van den Berghe, G. (2014). Nutrition in the acute phase of critical illness. *The New England Journal of Medicine, 370,* 1227–1236.

Charles, E., Petroze, R., Metzger, R., Hranjec, T., Rosenberger, L. H., Riccio, L. M., . . . Sawyer, R. G. (2014). Hypocaloric compared with eucaloric nutritional support and its effect on infection rates in a surgical intensive care unit: A randomized controlled trial. *The American Journal of Clinical Nutrition, 100,* 1337–1343.

Davis, C., Sowa, D., Keim, K., Kinnare, K., & Peterson, S. (2012). The use of prealbumin and C-reactive protein for monitoring nutrition support in adult patients receiving enteral nutrition in an urban medical center. *Journal of Parenteral Enteral Nutrition, 36,* 197–204.

Gottschlich, M., & Irenton-Jones, C. (2001). The Curreri formula: A landmark process for estimating the caloric needs of burn patients. *Nutrition in Clinical Practice, 16,* 172–173.

Harvey, S., Parrott, F., Harrison, D., Bear, D., Segaran, E., Beale, R., . . . Rowan, K. M. (2014). Trial of the route of early nutritional support in critically ill adults. *The New England Journal of Medicine, 371,* 1673–1684.

Heyland, D., Cahill, N., & Day, A. (2011). Optimal amount of calories for critically ill patients: Depends on how you slice the cake? *Critical Care Medicine, 39,* 2619–2626.

Heyland, D., Muscedere, J., Wischmeyer, P., Cook, D., Jones, G., Albert, M., . . . Day, A. G. (2013). A randomized trial of glutamine and antioxidants in critically ill patients. *The New England Journal of Medicine, 368,* 1489–1497.

Malone, A., & Hamilton, C. (2013). The Academy of Nutrition and Dietetics/The American Society for Parenteral and Enteral Nutrition consensus malnutrition characteristics: Application in practice. *Nutrition in Clinical Practice, 28,* 639–650.

Marik, P., & Hooper, M. (2016). Normocaloric versus hypocaloric feeding on the outcomes of ICU patients: A systematic review and meta-analysis. *Intensive Care Medicine, 42,* 316–323.

McClave, S., Taylor, B., Martindale, R., Warren, M. M., Johnson, D. R., Braunschweig, C., . . . Compher, C. (2016). Guidelines for the provision and assessment of nutrition support therapy in the adult critically ill patient: Society of Critical Care Medicine (SCCM) and American Society for Parenteral and Enteral Nutrition (A.S.P.E.N.). *Journal of Parenteral Enteral Nutrition, 40,* 159–211.

Peake, S., Davies, A., Deane, A., Lange, K., Moran, J. L., O'Connor, S. N., . . . Chapman, M. J. (2014). Use of a concentrated enteral nutrition solution to increase calorie delivery to critically ill patients: A randomized, double-blind, clinical trial. *The American Journal of Clinical Nutrition, 100,* 616–625.

Peterson, S., Tsai, A., Scala, C., Sowa, D. C., Sheean, P. M., & Braunschweig, C. L. (2010). Adequacy of oral intake in critically ill patients 1 week after extubation. *Journal of the American Dietetic Association, 11,* 427–433.

Radrizzani, D., & Iapichino, G. (1998). Nutrition and lung function in the critically ill patients. *Clinical Nutrition, 17,* 7–10.

Schetz, M., Casaer, P., & Van den Berghe, G. (2013). Does artificial nutrition improve outcome of critical illness? *Critical Care, 17,* 302.

Singer, M., Deutschman, C. S., Seymour, C. W., Shankar-Hari, M., Annane, D., Bauer, M., . . . Angus, D. C. (2016). The third international consensus definitions for sepsis and septic shock (Sepsis-3). *JAMA, 315,* 801–810.

Wischmeyer, P. (2008). Glutamine: Role in critical illness and ongoing clinical trials. *Current Opinion in Gastroenterology, 24,* 190–197.

Wischmeyer, P., Dhaliwal, R., McCall, M., Ziegler, T. R., & Heyland, D. K. (2014). Parenteral glutamine supplementation in critical illness: A systematic review. *Critical Care, 18,* R76.

Zaloga, P. (2012). *Permissive underfeeding of critically ill patients. Nestle nutrition.* Available at http://www.nestle-nutrition.com/topics. Accessed on 5/22/12.

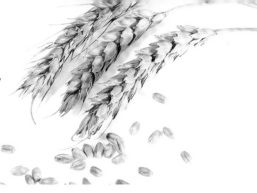

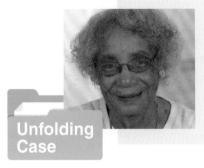

Bertha Parker

Bertha is an 84-year-old female who was diagnosed with type 2 diabetes 30 years ago. She has multiple chronic health problems including mild to moderate dementia and gastroparesis. During a recent hospitalization for uncontrolled diabetes, she was given a swallowing evaluation after nurses observed hoarseness and coughing during and after swallowing.

Check Your Knowledge

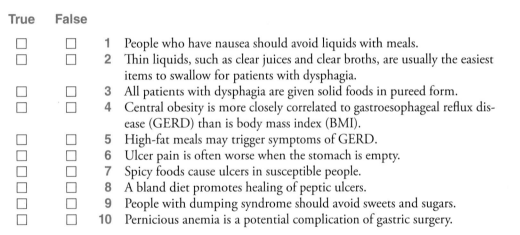

True	False		
☐	☐	1	People who have nausea should avoid liquids with meals.
☐	☐	2	Thin liquids, such as clear juices and clear broths, are usually the easiest items to swallow for patients with dysphagia.
☐	☐	3	All patients with dysphagia are given solid foods in pureed form.
☐	☐	4	Central obesity is more closely correlated to gastroesophageal reflux disease (GERD) than is body mass index (BMI).
☐	☐	5	High-fat meals may trigger symptoms of GERD.
☐	☐	6	Ulcer pain is often worse when the stomach is empty.
☐	☐	7	Spicy foods cause ulcers in susceptible people.
☐	☐	8	A bland diet promotes healing of peptic ulcers.
☐	☐	9	People with dumping syndrome should avoid sweets and sugars.
☐	☐	10	Pernicious anemia is a potential complication of gastric surgery.

Learning Objectives

Upon completion of this chapter, you will be able to

1 Give examples of ways to promote eating in people with anorexia.
2 Describe nutrition interventions that may help maximize intake in people who have nausea.
3 Compare the three levels of solid food textures included in the National Dysphagia Diet.
4 Compare the four liquid consistencies included in the National Dysphagia Diet.
5 Describe nutrition therapy recommendations for someone with gastroesophageal reflux disease (GERD).
6 Teach a patient about the role of nutrition therapy in the treatment of peptic ulcer disease.
7 List possible nutrition strategies for patients with gastroparesis.
8 Give examples of nutrition therapy recommendations for people experiencing dumping syndrome.

Table 17.1	The Role of the Upper Gastrointestinal Tract in the Mechanical and Chemical Digestion of Food

Site	Mechanical Digestion	Chemical Digestion
Mouth	Chewing breaks down food into smaller particles. Food mixes with saliva for ease in swallowing.	Saliva contains lingual lipase, which has a limited role in the digestion of fat, and salivary amylase, which begins the process of starch digestion. Food is not held in the mouth long enough for significant digestion to occur there.
Esophagus	Propels food downward into the stomach Lower esophageal sphincter relaxes to move food into stomach.	None
Stomach	Churns and mixes food with digestive enzymes to reduce it to a thin liquid called chyme Forward and backward mixing motion at the pyloric sphincter pushes small amounts of chyme into the duodenum.	Secretes pepsin, which begins to break down protein into polypeptides Secretes gastric lipase, which has a limited role in fat digestion Secretes intrinsic factor, necessary for the absorption of vitamin B_{12} Absorbs some water, electrolytes, certain drugs, and alcohol

Nutrition therapy is used in treating many digestive system disorders. For many disorders, diet merely plays a supportive role in alleviating symptoms rather than altering the course of the disease. For other gastrointestinal (GI) disorders, nutrition therapy is the cornerstone of treatment. Frequently, nutrition therapy is needed to restore nutritional status that has been compromised by dysfunction or disease.

This chapter begins with disorders that affect eating and covers disorders of the upper GI tract (mouth, esophagus, and stomach) that have nutritional implications. Table 17.1 outlines the roles these sites play in the mechanical and chemical digestion of food. Problems with the upper GI tract affect nutrition mostly by affecting food intake and tolerance to particular foods or textures. Nutrition-focused assessment criteria for upper GI tract disorders are listed in Box 17.1.

BOX 17.1	Nutrition-Focused Assessment for Upper Gastrointestinal Disorders

- GI symptoms that interfere with intake such as anorexia, early satiety, difficulty chewing and swallowing, nausea and vomiting, heartburn
- Changes in eating made in response to symptoms
- Complications that affect nutritional status, such as weight loss, aspiration pneumonia, diarrhea
- Usual pattern of eating and frequency of meals and snacks
- Adequacy of intake according to MyPlate recommendations, including fluid intake
- Use of tobacco, over-the-counter drugs for GI symptoms, and alcohol
- Food allergies or intolerances, such as high-fat foods, citrus fruits, spicy food
- Use of nutritional supplements including vitamins, minerals, fiber, and herbs
- Client's willingness to change his or her eating habits

DISORDERS THAT AFFECT EATING

Anorexia

Anorexia
lack of appetite; it differs from anorexia nervosa, a psychological condition characterized by denial of appetite.

Anorexia is a common symptom of many physical conditions and a side effect of certain drugs. Emotional issues, such as fear, anxiety, and depression, frequently cause anorexia. The aim of nutrition therapy is to stimulate the appetite to maintain adequate nutritional intake. The following interventions may help:

- Serve food attractively and season according to individual taste. If decreased ability to taste is contributing to anorexia, enhance food flavors with tart seasonings (e.g., orange juice, lemonade, vinegar, lemon juice) or strong seasonings (e.g., basil, oregano, rosemary, tarragon, mint).
- Schedule procedures and medications when they are least likely to interfere with meals, if possible.
- Control pain, nausea, or depression with medications as ordered.
  - Provide small, frequent meals.
  - Withhold beverages for 30 minutes before and after meals to avoid displacing the intake of more nutrient-dense foods.
  - Offer liquid supplements between meals for additional calories and protein if meal consumption is low.
  - Limit fat intake if fat is contributing to early satiety.

Quick Bite High-fat foods

- "Fats"—nuts, nut butters, oils, margarine, butter, salad dressings, creams (liquid, sour, whipped)
- Fatty meats, including many processed meats (bologna, pastrami, hard salami), bacon, sausage
- Milk and milk products containing whole or 2% milk
- Rich desserts, such as cakes, pies, cookies, pastries
- Many savory snacks, such as potato chips, cheese puffs, tortilla chips

Nausea and Vomiting

Nausea and vomiting may be related to a decrease in gastric acid secretion, a decrease in digestive enzyme activity, a decrease in GI motility, gastric irritation, or acidosis. Other causes include bacterial and viral infection; increased intracranial pressure; equilibrium imbalance; liver, pancreatic, and gallbladder disorders; and pyloric or intestinal obstruction. Drugs and certain medical treatments may also contribute to nausea.

Intractable Vomiting
vomiting that is difficult to manage or cure.

The short-term concern of nausea and vomiting is fluid and electrolyte balance, which can be maintained by intravenous (IV) administration until an oral intake resumes. With prolonged or **intractable vomiting**, dehydration and weight loss are concerns.

Nutrition intervention for nausea is a commonsense approach. Food is withheld until nausea subsides. When the patient is ready to eat, clear liquids are offered and progressed to a regular diet as tolerated. Small, frequent meals of low-fat, readily digested carbohydrates are usually best tolerated. Other strategies that may help are to

Quick Bite Readily digested low-fat carbohydrates

Dry toast
Saltine crackers
Plain rolls
Pretzels
Angel food cake
Oatmeal
Canned peaches and canned pears
Banana

- Encourage the patient to eat slowly and not to eat if he or she feels nauseated
- Promote good oral hygiene with mouthwash and ice chips
- Limit liquids with meals because they can cause a full, bloated feeling
- Encourage a liberal fluid intake between meals with whatever liquids the patient can tolerate, such as clear soup, juice, gelatin, ginger ale, and popsicles
- Serve foods at room temperature or chilled; hot foods may contribute to nausea
- Avoid high-fat and spicy foods if they contribute to nausea

DISORDERS OF THE ESOPHAGUS

Dysphagia
impaired ability to swallow.

Symptoms of esophageal disorders range from difficulty swallowing and the sensation that something is stuck in the throat to heartburn and reflux. **Dysphagia** and gastroesophageal reflux disease are discussed next.

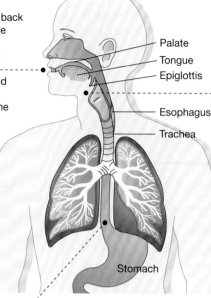

Figure 17.1 ▶

Swallowing phases and symptoms of impairments.

Oral Phase
    solid food is chewed and mixed with saliva to form bolus
    the tongue propels liquids and food to the back of the mouth to start the swallowing process
    possible symptoms of impairments:
• difficulty chewing solid food
• "pocketing" food in the cheek
• loss of food from the lips
• delayed swallowing

Palate
Tongue
Epiglottis

Esophagus

Trachea

Pharyngeal Phase
    food and liquid bolus passes through the pharynx into the esophagus
    possible symptoms of impairments:
• food sticking in the throat; choking sensation
• drooling
• coughing before, during, or after swallowing
• aspiration; repeated pneumonia
• hoarseness after swallowing
• weight loss

Stomach

Esophageal Phase
    bolus passes through esophagus into the stomach via peristaltic movements
    possible symptoms of impairments:
• difficulty with solid food (can handle pureed food)
• heartburn
• vomiting
• burping

Dysphagia

Swallowing is a complex series of events characterized by three basic phases (Fig. 17.1). Dysphagia is an impairment in the swallowing process. It can have a profound impact on intake, hydration status, and nutritional status and greatly increases the risk of aspiration and its complications of bacterial pneumonia and bronchial obstruction.

Although aging causes natural changes in the ability to swallow, dysphagia is often related to neurologic impairments, such as cerebral vascular accident, dementia, amyotrophic lateral sclerosis (ALS), myasthenia gravis, brain tumor, traumatic brain injury, cerebral palsy, Parkinson disease, and multiple sclerosis. Mechanical causes include obstruction, inflammation, edema, and surgery of the throat. Refer patients with actual or potential swallowing impairments to the speech pathology department for a swallowing evaluation.

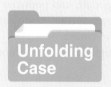

Unfolding Case

Consider Bertha. Based on her symptoms, which phase of swallowing is impaired? What may be the cause of Bertha's impairment? What other symptoms may she display?

Viscosity
the condition of being resistant to flow; having a heavy, gluey quality.

Nutrition Therapy for Dysphagia

The goal of nutrition therapy for dysphagia is to modify the texture of foods and/or **viscosity** of liquids to enable the patient to achieve adequate nutrition and hydration while decreasing the risk of aspiration. Solid foods may be minced, mashed, ground, or pureed, and thin liquids may be thickened to facilitate swallowing, but these measures often dilute the nutritional value of the diet and make food and beverages less appealing. Emotionally, dysphagia can affect quality of life; patients with dysphagia may feel panic at mealtime, avoid eating with others, and stop eating even when they still feel hungry. Meeting nutritional needs is a challenge, and in some instances, enteral nutrition may be necessary.

The National Dysphagia Diet, developed through consensus by a group of dietitians, speech-language pathologists (SLP), and researchers, standardized nutrition therapy for dysphagia on a national level (National Dysphagia Diet Task Force, 2002). The National Dysphagia Diet is composed of three levels of solid textures and four liquid consistencies (Table 17.2).

The levels of solid food and liquids are ordered separately to allow maximum flexibility and safety in meeting the patient's needs. The patient may start at any of the levels. The solid food consistencies include pureed, mechanically altered, and a more advanced consistency of mixed

Table 17.2 National Dysphagia Diet

Level of Diet	Description	Foods Allowed
Three levels of solid textures		
Level 1: Pureed	Foods are totally pureed to a smooth, homogenous, and cohesive consistency. Eliminates sticky foods, such as peanut butter, and coarse-textured foods, such as nuts and raw fruits and vegetables	Smooth cooked cereals; slurried or pureed bread products; milk; smooth desserts such as yogurt, pudding, custard, and applesauce; pureed fruits, vegetables, meats, scrambled eggs, and soups
Level 2: Mechanically altered	Soft-textured, moist foods that are easily formed into a bolus. Eliminates coarse textures, nuts, and raw fruits and vegetables (except bananas)	Cooked cereals may have a little texture; some well-moistened, ready-to-eat cereals; well-moistened pancakes with syrup; slurried bread; moist well-cooked potatoes, noodles, and dumplings; soft poached or scrambled eggs; soft canned or cooked fruit; soft, well-cooked vegetables with ½ pieces (except no corn, peas, and other fibrous vegetables). Moist ground or minced tender meat in pieces no larger than ¼ in, soft casseroles, cottage cheese, tofu; moist cobblers and moist soft cookies; soups with easy-to-chew meat or vegetables
Level 3: Advanced	Near-normal textured foods; excludes crunchy, sticky, or very hard foods. Food is bite-sized and moist.	All breads are allowed except for those that are crusty; moist cereals; most desserts except those with nuts, seeds, coconut, pineapple, or dried fruit; soft, peeled fruit without seeds; moist tender meats or casseroles with small pieces of meat; moist potatoes, rice, and stuffing; all soups except those with chewy meats or vegetables; most cooked, tender vegetables, except corn; shredded lettuce. No nuts, seeds, coconut, and chewy candy.
Four standard liquid consistencies		
Thin	All regular unthickened beverages and supplements	Clear juices, frozen yogurt, ice cream, milk, water, coffee, tea, soda, broth, plain gelatin, liquidy fruits such as watermelon
Nectar-like	Liquids thicker than water but thin enough to sip through a straw	Nectars, vegetable juices, chocolate milk, buttermilk, thin milkshakes, cream soups, other properly thickened beverages
Honey-like	Liquids that are too thick to sip through a straw; can be eaten with a spoon but do not hold their shape	Honey, tomato sauce, yogurt
Spoon-thick	Liquids thickened to pudding consistency that need to be eaten with a spoon	Pudding, custard, hot cereal

Source: National Dysphagia Diet Task Force. (2002). *The national dysphagia diet: Standardization for optimal care.* Chicago, IL: American Dietetic Association.

textures. The liquids are described as "thin," "nectar-like," "honey-like," or "spoon-thick," which means they are thick enough to require the use of a spoon.

Generally, a SLP performs a swallowing evaluation on the patient to determine the appropriate consistency of food and liquids and recommends feeding techniques based on the patient's individual status. Changes to the diet prescription are made as the patient's ability to swallow improves or deteriorates.

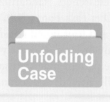
Unfolding Case

Recall Bertha. The SLP has recommended Bertha be placed on a pureed diet with honey-like thickened liquids. She refuses to eat "baby" food. What foods are the appropriate texture in their normal state? Can Bertha meet her nutrient requirements without consuming foods in pureed form?

Solid Textures

Generally, moist, semisolid foods are easiest to swallow, such as pudding, custards, scrambled eggs, and yogurt, because they form a cohesive bolus that is more easily controlled. Dry, crumbly, and sticky foods are avoided. Some foods, such as bread, are **slurried** to create a texture easily swallowed while retaining the appearance of "regular" bread.

Pureed food is often described as having poor sensory appeal with items indistinguishable from one another (Keller & Duizer, 2014). Commercial thickeners added to pureed foods can allow pureed foods to be molded into the appearance of "normal" food (Fig. 17.2). However, a study comparing the acceptability of molded pureed meats and vegetables to the same items but in scooped form found the scooped pureed food was more acceptable and identifiable (Lepore, Sims, Gal, & Dahl, 2014). Although no one chooses to eat a pureed diet, many patients are grateful they can consume food orally.

Liquid Consistencies

Thickened liquids are more cohesive than thin liquids and are easier to control. Commercial thickening agents provide instructions on how to mix the product with liquids to achieve the desired consistency, yet wide variations in consistency occur depending on the beverage type,

Slurried
a slurry is a thickener dissolved in liquid that is added to dry or pureed foods to produce a texture that is soft and cohesive.

Figure 17.2 ▶

Examples of pureed and molded foods.

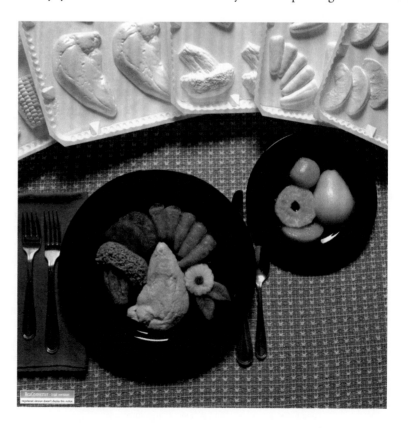

type of thickener (e.g., starch based or gum based), temperature of the liquid, and time between thickened fluid preparation and service to the patient (Adeleye & Rachal, 2007). Commercially prepared thickened beverages eliminate issues related to quality control.

Thickened beverages are often poorly accepted, making it difficult to maintain an adequate fluid intake. Potential complications include dehydration, decreased compliance with swallowing guidelines, increased risk of aspiration pneumonia due to aspiration of thickened liquids, and decreased quality of life (Panther, 2005). Although thickened liquids may reduce the risk of aspiration in some patients, research suggests that drinking plain water alone is less likely to cause problems if it is aspirated than if it is consumed with food or other liquids. Consequently, free water protocols (FWP), such as the Frazier Free Water Protocol, are being used to permit patients with documented aspiration to drink plain water between meals (Garcia & Chambers, 2010). A randomized controlled trial of an FWP showed no adverse events from using the FWP and identified increased fluid intake and reported high quality of life outcomes among the FWP participants (Carlaw et al., 2011).

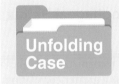

Unfolding Case

Think of Bertha. She is refusing thickened liquids. She desperately wants a cup of black tea. How would you respond to her request for tea?

Feeding Techniques

In addition to modifying the texture of solids and liquids, various feeding techniques may be used to facilitate safe swallowing:

- Serve small, frequent meals to help maximize intake.
- Encourage patients with dysphagia to rest before mealtime. Postpone meals if the patient is fatigued.
- Give mouth care immediately before meals to enhance the sense of taste.
- Instruct the patient to think of a specific food to stimulate salivation. A lemon slice, lemon hard candy, or dill pickles may also help to trigger salivation, as may moderately flavored foods.
- Reduce or eliminate distractions at mealtime so that the patient can focus his or her attention on swallowing. Limit disruptions, if possible, and do not rush the patient; allow at least 30 minutes for eating.
- Place the patient in an upright or high Fowler's position. If the patient has one-sided facial weakness, place the food on the other side of the mouth. Tilt the head forward to facilitate swallowing.
- Use adaptive eating devices, such as built-up utensils and mugs with spouts, if indicated. Syringes should never be used to force liquids into the patient's mouth because this can trigger choking or aspiration. Unless otherwise directed, do not allow the patient to use a straw.
- Encourage small bites and thorough chewing.
- Discourage the patient from consuming alcohol because it reduces cough and gag reflexes.

Gastroesophageal Reflux Disease

Gastroesophageal Reflux Disease (GERD)
gastroesophageal reflux is the backflow of gastric acid into the esophagus; GERD occurs when symptoms of reflux happen two or more times a week.

Gastroesophageal reflux disease (GERD) occurs when gastric contents back up into the esophagus producing the common symptoms of indigestion, "heartburn," and regurgitation. GERD is a chronic relapsing disease of unknown etiology. Up to 20% of the adult population in Western countries experiences reflux symptoms on a weekly basis (Dent, El-Serag, Wallander, & Johansson, 2005), and at least 50% of people remain on continuous drug therapy (Caselli et al., 2014). Proton pump inhibitors (PPIs) are not always completely effective in managing GERD symptoms.

Chronic untreated GERD may cause reflux esophagitis, esophageal ulcers with bleeding, esophageal stricture, dysphagia, pulmonary disease, Barrett esophagus, and esophageal cancer. The amount of acid refluxed, the severity of heartburn, and the damage to the esophagus do not always

Concept Mastery Alert

The patient with GERD should not lie down for at least 3 hours after eating. Instead, the patient should be encouraged to eat small meals as a way to help control his or her GERD symptoms.

BOX 17.2 — Lifestyle and Nutrition Therapy Modifications for Gastroesophageal Reflux Disease

Weight loss is strongly recommended for patients with BMI >25 or patients with recent weight gain.
Avoid meals within 3 hours of lying down.
Avoid high-fat meals.
Eliminate foods that the individual correlates with GERD symptoms.
Elevate the head of the bed during sleep.

Source: Katz, P., Gerson, L., & Vela, M. (2013). Guidelines for the diagnosis and management of gastroesophageal reflux disease. *The American Journal of Gastroenterology, 108,* 308–328.

correlate: Severe pain can occur in the absence of esophageal damage and severe damage may occur with minimal heartburn (Stenson, 2006). Lifestyle and nutrition therapy are considered important adjunct therapies in the treatment of GERD (Box 17.2).

Nutrition Therapy for Gastroesophageal Reflux Disease

Patients with GERD are often advised to

- *Lose weight if overweight.* GERD is recognized as an obesity-related comorbidity (Prachand & Alverdy, 2010); however, there is a greater correlation between GERD and central obesity than between GERD and body mass index (BMI) (Corley, Kubo, & Zhao, 2007). All types of bariatric surgeries have been shown to improve GERD (Pallati et al., 2014). Interestingly, new onset GERD is associated with weight gain even in people with a normal BMI (Jacobson, Somers, Fuchs, Kelly, & Camargo, 2006).
- *Eliminate coffee, caffeine, chocolate, spicy foods, citrus, carbonated beverages, fatty foods, and mint.* Citrus and tomato-based products may also aggravate symptoms. However, there have been no studies conducted to date that have shown clinical improvement in GERD symptoms or complications with eliminating any of these foods (Katz, Gerson, & Vela, 2013). Because individual tolerance varies, patients should always be advised to avoid foods that provoke symptoms. Keeping a 3-day food diary may help identify problematic foods.

Caselli et al. (2014) conducted a randomized controlled pilot trial to investigate whether an elimination diet could improve GERD symptoms in patients who do not respond at all or completely to PPIs. Based on moderate to severe reactions identified by leukocytotoxic testing, researchers observed significant improvement in GERD symptoms in PPI non- or partial responders compared with controls after 1 month of an exclusion diet. In descending order, the top food offenders were milk, lettuce, Brewer's yeast, pork, coffee, rice, sole, asparagus, and tuna. Interestingly, with the exception of coffee, none of these foods are those that patients are most often advised to avoid. The results of this trial suggest a possible role of food intolerance in the cause of GERD symptoms and point to a possible use of an exclusion diet when PPIs are not effective.

Quick Bite Obsolete approaches for GERD and peptic ulcer disease

Bland diet
Increased milk intake

DISORDERS OF THE STOMACH

Peptic ulcer disease (PUD), gastroparesis, and gastrectomy are disorders of the stomach that use nutrition therapy to help control symptoms.

Peptic Ulcer Disease

Peptic Ulcer
erosion of the GI mucosal layer caused by an excess secretion of, or decreased mucosal resistance to, hydrochloric acid and pepsin.

The majority of **peptic ulcers** occur in the duodenum; other sites include the lower end of the esophagus, the stomach, and jejunum. *Helicobacter pylori* infection is a major cause of ulcers, yet most people infected with *H. pylori* do not develop the disease. *H. pylori* appears to secrete an enzyme that depletes gastric mucus, making the mucosal layer more susceptible to erosion. For these patients, eradicating the bacteria—typically with a combination of antibiotics and acid-suppressing drugs—generally cures the ulcer. Some studies suggest that using probiotics along with eradication therapy may increase the rate of eradication and lower the incidence of side effects (Zhen-Hua, Gao, & Fang, 2013). The second leading cause of peptic ulcers is the use of non-steroidal anti-inflammatory drugs (NSAIDs) and/or aspirin. Eating spicy food does not cause ulcers.

The most common symptom of peptic ulcers is epigastric pain, which is described as gnawing or burning that is usually worse at night or when the stomach is empty. However, not all people with peptic ulcers experience epigastric pain. Less frequent symptoms include bloating, early satiety, and nausea. The most common and severe complication of PUD is GI bleeding, which can be life-threatening. From a nutritional standpoint, pain or early satiety may impair intake and lead to weight loss. Blood loss can lead to iron deficiency. Long-term use of medications to decrease gastric acid production may impair the absorption of calcium, iron, and vitamin B_{12}.

Nutrition Therapy for Peptic Ulcer Disease

Quick Bite Foods high in soluble fiber

Dried peas and beans
Lentils
Oats
Certain fruits and vegetables, such as oranges, potatoes, carrots, apples

Nutrition therapy may play a supportive role in treatment by helping to minimize symptoms of PUD. Eating strategies that may be helpful include eating smaller, more frequent meals and not eating for at least 2 hours before bedtime. Although patients may be told to avoid pepper, caffeine, tea, coffee, and chocolate, there is no evidence that diet causes or prevents PUD or speeds ulcer healing. For instance, Shimamoto et al. (2013) found no association between coffee consumption and gastric or duodenal ulcers. As with GERD, patients should be advised to avoid any foods not individually tolerated.

Gastroparesis

Gastroparesis, or delayed gastric emptying, is a chronic motility disorder of the stomach that can cause nausea, vomiting, bloating, early satiety, and abdominal pain (Parrish & McCray, 2011). Symptoms vary greatly among individuals and can come and go over time. Potentially life-threatening complications include electrolyte imbalances, dehydration, malnutrition, and poor glycemic control. Quality of life can be greatly affected. Although gastroparesis is most commonly associated with diabetes, it may also occur secondary to gastric bypass surgery, Parkinson disease, multiple sclerosis, scleroderma, and post–viral syndrome or may be idiopathic.

Nutrition Therapy for Gastroparesis

There are no clinical or randomized prospective trials available to provide data to establish evidence-based practice guidelines (Parrish & McCray, 2011). Based on limited data available and experience, Parrish and McCray (2011) recommend that patients

- Consume smaller, more frequent meals. Six to 8 meals/day may be necessary to achieve an adequate intake.
- Consume more liquids. Some patients do not experience impairments in liquid emptying, only solids. Solids may be best tolerated in the morning, with tolerance decreasing as the day progresses. Liquid calorie intake should increase as tolerance to solids decreases.
- Decrease fiber intake, such as legumes, whole grain cereals, nuts, seeds, dried fruit, and skins and seeds of fruits and vegetables because certain types of fiber slow gastric emptying.
- Consume fat in liquids if fat in solids is not tolerated. As an important source of calories, fat should not be restricted unless not tolerated in any form.
- Chew foods thoroughly.
- Sit upright for 1 to 2 hours after eating.
- Control blood glucose levels if patient has diabetes.

Unfolding Case

Consider Bertha. She has had gastroparesis on and off for years. Nausea, vomiting, and pain are her most common symptoms. She continues to have symptoms of gastroparesis while on a pureed diet with honey-like liquids. What other nutrition therapy interventions may help reduce Bertha's symptoms? What are nutritional concerns with prolonged vomiting related to gastroparesis?

Gastrectomy

Gastrectomy is the surgical removal of part or all the stomach which may be done to treat malignancy, refractory PUD, or GI bleeding. Similar components of gastrectomy surgeries are used in bariatric surgeries, which are surgeries to treat obesity (see Chapter 15). Partial gastrectomies leave a portion of the stomach that is then surgically connected to the duodenum or jejunum. Total gastrectomies remove all of the stomach so that the lower esophagus connects directly to the small intestine. With either type of gastrectomy, a smaller or absent stomach increases the risk of maldigestion and malabsorption due to rapid gastric emptying and shortened transit time.

A common complication after gastric surgery is dumping syndrome. Rapid emptying of stomach contents into the intestine causes fluid from the plasma and extracellular fluid to shift into the intestines to dilute the hyperosmolar bolus. The large volume of hypertonic fluid in the jejunum and an increase in peristalsis leads to cramping, diarrhea, and abdominal pain. Weakness, dizziness, and tachycardia occur as the volume of circulating blood decreases. These symptoms occur within 10 to 20 minutes after eating and characterize the early dumping syndrome.

An intermediate dumping reaction occurs 20 to 30 minutes after eating as undigested food is fermented in the colon, producing gas, abdominal pain, cramping, and diarrhea (Academy of Nutrition and Dietetics, 2016). Malabsorption of calories and nutrients produces weight loss and increases the risk of malnutrition. Other potential nutritional complications are outlined in Table 17.3.

Late dumping syndrome occurs 1 to 3 hours after eating and is especially common after consuming simple sugars (Academy of Nutrition and Dietetics, 2016). The rapid absorption of carbohydrate causes a quick spike in blood glucose levels; the body compensates by oversecreting insulin. Blood glucose levels drop rapidly, and symptoms of hypoglycemia develop, such as shakiness, sweating, confusion, and weakness.

Nutrition Therapy for Patients with Dumping Syndrome

Nutrition intervention can control or prevent symptoms of dumping syndrome. Unlike most initial postoperative feedings, clear liquid diets are not used because sugars contribute to the concentration of particles entering the intestine. Patients begin oral feedings with sips of water and broth. After tolerance is established,

- Patients are started on small, frequent meals consisting of only one or two foods per meal or snack, one of which is a protein.

Table 17.3   Potential Nutritional Complications of Dumping Syndrome

Potential Complication	Possible Contributing Factors	Possible Treatment
Iron deficiency anemia	Decreased food intake A decrease in hydrochloric acid secretion impairs the conversion of iron to its absorbable form. If the duodenum is bypassed or food moves through it too quickly, iron absorption cannot occur (the duodenum is the site of iron absorption).	Iron supplementation is necessary.
Steatorrhea (excess fat in the stools)	Rapid intestinal time does not allow enough time for fat to be exposed to digestive enzymes. If the duodenum is bypassed, less pancreatic lipase is available to digest fat. Bacterial overgrowth (excessive growth of intestinal bacteria) can develop from low gastric acidity or altered motility; it interferes with the action of bile, which is important for the emulsification of fat.	Supplemental pancreatic enzymes may be necessary. Medium-chain triglycerides may be used for additional calories (but lack the essential fatty acids). Supplements of fat-soluble vitamins may be prescribed; their absorption is dependent on the absorption of fat.
Pernicious anemia	Intrinsic factor, necessary for the absorption of vitamin B_{12} from the intestine, is produced by the stomach. It may be absent after gastric surgery. It may take years for a deficiency to develop.	Injections of vitamin B_{12} may be necessary.
Bone disease (osteomalacia and osteoporosis)	Calcium is normally absorbed in the duodenum; if it is bypassed or the transit time is too rapid, calcium malabsorption can occur. Fat malabsorption causes calcium and vitamin D to be malabsorbed. Lower calcium intake related to lactose intolerance	Supplements of calcium and vitamin D may be necessary.

Quick Bite Sources of sugar alcohols

Dietetic candy
Sugarless gum, cough drops, and mints
Certain fruits: apples, pears, peaches, prunes

Functional Fiber
fiber that has been isolated from food that
has beneficial physiologic effects.

- Food must be thoroughly chewed.
- Liquids are provided 30 minutes to 1 hour after consuming solids, not with meals, because they promote quick movement through the GI tract.
- Simple sugars and sugar alcohols are avoided to limit the hypertonicity of the mass as it reaches the jejunum.
- Lactose may be restricted because lactose intolerance is common.
- Patients are advised to lie down after eating.
- **Functional fibers**, such as pectin and guar gum, may be used to delay gastric emptying and treat diarrhea (Academy of Nutrition and Dietetics, 2016).
- Liquid multivitamin and mineral supplements are recommended, and vitamin B_{12} injections may be necessary depending on the extent of surgery.
  - Over time, the diet is liberalized as the remaining portion of the stomach or duodenum hypertrophies to hold more food and allow for more normal digestion. Box 17.3 features antidumping syndrome diet guidelines.
  - Patients who are unable to tolerate the normal diet progression may require nutrition support.

BOX 17.3   Antidumping Syndrome Diet Guidelines

Eating Strategies

- Eat small, frequent meals.
- Consume beverages 30 minutes or later after a meal, not with meals.
- Avoid sugar, honey, syrup, sorbitol, and xylitol and all food and beverages that have any of those listed as one of the first three ingredients on the label.
- Eat a source of protein at each meal because it helps slow gastric emptying.
- Choose low-fiber grains; mostly canned, not fresh fruit; non-gassy, well-cooked vegetables without seeds or skins.
- Adding soluble fibers like pectin or guar gum to meals may slow gastric emptying and reduce the risk of diarrhea.
- Avoid carbonated beverages if they cause bloating.

Recommended Foods

- Breads and cereals: refined plain breads, crackers, rolls, unsweetened cereal, rice, and pasta that provide less than 2 g fiber per serving
- Vegetables: well-cooked or raw vegetables without seeds or skins, strained vegetable juice, lettuce; avoid "gassy" vegetables such as broccoli, cauliflower, cabbage, and corn.
- Fruits: banana, soft melons, unsweetened canned fruit
- Milk and milk products: 1% or fat-free milk (if not lactose intolerant); choose yogurt, soy milk, and ice cream without sugar added.
- Meat and meat alternatives: tender, well-cooked meat, fish, poultry, egg, and soy without added fat; smooth nut butters. Avoid all of the following: fried meats, fish, and poultry; high-fat luncheon meats, sausage, hot dogs, and bacon; tough or chewy meats; dried peas and beans; nuts.
- Fats: oils, butter, margarine, cream cheese, mayonnaise
- Beverages: decaffeinated coffee and tea; sugar-free soft drinks; avoid caffeinated beverages, alcohol.
- Other: allowed foods made with artificial sweeteners such as NutraSweet, sucralose, acesulfame potassium

Sample Menu (When Recovered Enough to Eat Six Times a Day)

Breakfast

1 poached egg
1 slice white toast with butter
1 hour later: 1 cup decaffeinated coffee with half and half

Midmorning Snack

1 cup yogurt without added sugar
1 hour later: 1 cup plain unsweetened soy milk

Lunch

½ cup cottage cheese with two unsweetened, canned peach halves
Dinner roll with butter
1 hour later: 8 oz sugar-free ginger ale

Midafternoon Snack

2 oz cheddar cheese
4 saltine crackers

Dinner

3 oz baked chicken
½ cup white rice with butter
½ cup cooked carrots with butter
1 hour later: caffeine-free tea

Bedtime Snack

1 cup yogurt without added sugar

NURSING PROCESS

Gastroesophageal Reflux Disease

Jason is 28 years old and complains of frequent painful heartburn. He takes antacids on a daily basis and has lost 14 pounds over the last few months. His strategy to avoid pain is to avoid eating. He is 5 ft 8 in tall, currently weighs 170 pounds, and has an appointment to see his doctor. In the meantime, he has come to you, the corporate nurse on staff where he works, to see what he can do to help control his heartburn.

Assessment

Medical–Psychosocial History

- Medical history that would contribute to GERD, such as hiatal hernia
- Symptoms that may affect nutrition, such as difficulty swallowing or nausea and vomiting
- Use of medications that may decrease lower esophageal sphincter (LES) pressure, such as anticholinergic agents, diazepam, or theophylline
- Use of medications that may damage the mucosa, such as NSAIDs or aspirin
- History of smoking
- Level of activity

Anthropometric Assessment

BMI, weight loss percentage

Biochemical and Physical Assessment

Abnormal lab values, if available, especially hemoglobin and hematocrit because low values may indicate bleeding

Dietary Assessment

- How many meals do you eat daily?
- Would you say your meals are small, medium, or large in size?
- Are there any particular foods that cause heartburn, especially alcohol, coffee, tea, caffeine, pepper, mint, chocolate, or fatty foods?
- What foods do you avoid?
- Can you correlate your symptoms to
  - Lying down after eating?
  - Wearing tight clothes?
  - Eating right before bed?
- Do you take vitamins, minerals, herbs, or other supplements?
- Do you have ethnic, religious, or cultural food preferences?

Diagnosis

Possible Nursing Diagnoses

Imbalanced nutrition: eating less than the body requires as evidenced by weight loss related to inadequate intake secondary to heartburn

Planning

Client Outcomes

The client will
- Report relief from symptoms
- Consume adequate calories and nutrients
- Use less medication to control symptoms
- Explain nutrition and lifestyle modifications for controlling GERD symptoms
- Exhibit normal laboratory values

Nursing Interventions

Nutrition Therapy

- Lose weight to achieve BMI <25.
- Avoid high fat meals.
- Eliminate any foods not tolerated.
- Eat small frequent meals to avoid increasing intra-abdominal pressure.
- Avoid eating within 3 hours of bedtime.

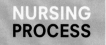

NURSING PROCESS
Gastroesophageal Reflux Disease

Client Teaching

Instruct the client
- That nutrition interventions may help control symptoms but do not treat the underlying problem
- To avoid high-fat meals, large meals, and any foods not tolerated
- To lose weight gradually to achieve a healthy weight of <25 BMI
- On lifestyle modifications that may help improve symptoms, such as elevating the head of the bed and not eating within 3 hours of bedtime

Evaluation

Evaluate and Monitor
- Monitor for improvement in symptoms.
- Monitor weight.
- Monitor for medication usage.

How Do You Respond?

Are there any foods that can treat heartburn? The chronic nature of heartburn, the high prevalence of PPI use in the United States, and recent reports about the risks of long-term use of PPIs (Wilhelm, Riater, & Kale-Pradhan, 2013) fuel the interest in natural heartburn remedies. Evidence linking the use of specific foods with relief of heartburn is largely anecdotal, but as long as the use of natural remedies does not preclude necessary medical treatment, there is little risk in trying unproven food remedies. Such unproven remedies include consuming probiotics, vinegar, coconut water, almonds, and teas such as ginger and persimmon. Patients who are on long-term PPI therapy should not suddenly discontinue drug treatment; gradual tapering and doctor supervision are advised.

REVIEW CASE STUDY

Barbara is a 72-year-old woman with a "Type A" personality who was diagnosed with a peptic ulcer more than 40 years ago. At that time, her doctor told her to follow a bland diet and eat three meals per day with three snacks per day of whole milk to "quiet" her stomach. She meticulously complied with the diet to the point of becoming obsessive about eating anything that may not be "allowed." She lost 15 pounds by following the bland diet because her intake was so restricted. She recently began experiencing ulcer symptoms and has put herself back on the bland diet, convinced it is necessary in order to recover from her ulcer.

Yesterday, she ate the following as shown on the right:

- Barbara's 1600-calorie MyPlate plan calls for 1.5 cups of fruit, 2 cups of vegetables, 5 grains, 5 oz of meat/beans, 3 cups of milk, and 5 teaspoons of oils. How does her intake compare? What food groups is she undereating? Overeating? What are the potential nutritional consequences of her current diet?

- What other information would be helpful for you to know in dealing with Barbara?
- Barbara clearly wants to be on a bland diet; what would you tell her about diet recommendations for PUD? What recommendations would you make to improve her symptoms and meet her nutritional requirements while respecting her need to follow a "diet"?

Breakfast: 1 poached egg; 2 slices dry white toast; 1 cup whole milk
Morning Snack: 1 cup whole milk
Lunch: ¾ cup cottage cheese with ½ cup canned peaches
Afternoon snack: 1 cup whole milk
Dinner: 3 oz boiled chicken; ½ cup boiled plain potatoes; ½ cup boiled green beans; ½ cup gelatin
Evening snack: 1 cup whole milk

STUDY QUESTIONS

1   The patient asks if coffee is bad for his peptic ulcer. Which of the following would be the nurse's best response?
a. "Coffee does not cause ulcers, and drinking it probably does not interfere with ulcer healing. You may try eliminating it from your diet to see what impact it has on your symptoms and then decide whether or not to avoid it."
b. "Both caffeinated and decaffeinated coffee can cause ulcers and interfere with ulcer healing. You should eliminate both from your diet."
c. "You need to eliminate caffeinated coffee from your diet, but it is safe to drink decaffeinated coffee."
d. "You can drink all the coffee you want; it does not affect ulcers."

2   Which statement indicates the patient needs further instruction about GERD?
a. "I know a bland diet will help prevent the heartburn I get after eating."
b. "Lying down after eating can make GERD symptoms worse."
c. "High-fat meals can make GERD symptoms worse."
d. "Losing excess weight can help prevent symptoms of GERD."

3   Which of the following snacks would be best for a patient who wants to eat who has nausea?
a. Cheese
b. Peanuts
c. Banana
d. A milkshake

4   The nurse knows her instructions have been effective when the patient with dumping syndrome verbalizes she should
a. Avoid lying down after eating.
b. Drink liquids between, not with, meals.
c. Eat simple sugars in place of starches.
d. Avoid protein.

5   A patient with dumping syndrome asks why it is so important to avoid sugars and sweets. Which of the following is the nurse's best response?
a. "Sugars and sweets provide empty calories, so they should be limited in everyone's diet."
b. "Sugars draw water into the intestines and cause cramping and diarrhea."
c. "Sugar makes blood glucose levels increase; hyperglycemia is a complication of dumping syndrome."
d. "Avoiding sugars and sweets helps ensure that they will not displace the intake of protein, which you need for healing."

6   Which of the following is an appropriate breakfast for a patient on a level 1 dysphagia diet?
a. Poached egg
b. Cream of wheat
c. Granola with milk
d. Toast cut into small pieces

7   A patient who develops pernicious anemia after gastric surgery needs supplemental
a. Protein
b. Iron
c. Folic acid
d. Vitamin B_{12}

8   The best dessert for a patient with GERD is
a. Chocolate cake
b. Peppermint ice cream
c. Cheesecake
d. Applesauce

KEY CONCEPTS

- Nutrition therapy for GI disorders may help minimize or prevent symptoms. For some GI disorders, nutrition therapy is the cornerstone of treatment.
- Small, frequent meals may help to maximize intake in patients who have anorexia. Avoiding high-fat foods may lessen the feeling of fullness.
- After nausea and vomiting subside, low-fat, easily digested carbohydrate foods, such as crackers, toast, oatmeal, and bland fruit, usually are well tolerated. Patients should avoid liquids with meals because liquids can promote the feeling of fullness.
- The National Dysphagia Diet has three different solid food textures and four different liquid consistencies. A SLP recommends the appropriate level for solids and liquids based on a swallowing evaluation.
- Pureed foods are less calorically dense than normal textured foods. They are also less visually appealing. Patients with dysphagia are monitored for poor intakes and weight loss.

- People with GERD should lose weight if overweight, avoid large meals and bedtime snacks, eliminate individual intolerances, and avoid fatty foods.
- There is no evidence that diet causes ulcers or promotes their healing. Patients are commonly advised to avoid any foods not tolerated.
- Patients with gastroparesis may benefit from consuming small, frequent meals; using more liquid calories to compensate for the decreased tolerance to solids; chewing foods thoroughly; sitting up for 1 to 2 hours after eating; reducing fiber intake; and consuming fat calories mostly in liquid form if solid fats are not tolerated.
- Nutrition therapy for dumping syndrome consists of eating small, frequent meals; eating protein at each meal; avoiding concentrated sugars and sugar alcohols; and adding pectin or guar gum to meals to slow gastric emptying. Liquids should be consumed 30 minutes to 1 hour or longer after eating instead of with meals.

Check Your Knowledge Answer Key

1 **TRUE** Drinking liquids with meals may promote a bloated feeling and contribute to nausea. Encourage patients to drink fluids between meals, especially clear liquids such as water, clear juices, gelatin, ginger ale, and popsicles.

2 **FALSE** Thin liquids are the most difficult consistency to control for people who have swallowing difficulties. Thickened liquids have a more cohesive consistency that is easier to manage.

3 **FALSE** The degree of texture modification for dysphagia is determined by the individual's ability to chew and swallow. There are three levels of solid textures: pureed, mechanically altered, and an advanced consistency of mixed textures.

4 **TRUE** GERD is a comorbidity of obesity, but central obesity is more closely correlated to GERD than is BMI.

5 **TRUE** Fat lowers LES pressure, so high-fat meals may cause symptoms of GERD.

6 **TRUE** Ulcer pain is often worse when the stomach is empty.

7 **FALSE** There is no evidence that any particular foods cause ulcers.

8 **FALSE** A bland diet is considered obsolete. It does not promote ulcer healing, and eating moderate amounts of nonbland foods has not been shown to irritate peptic ulcers.

9 **TRUE** People with dumping syndrome should avoid sugars and sweets because they contribute to a high osmolar load when the gastric contents enter the intestine. Over time, the diet is liberalized to allow sugars and sweets as the remaining stomach and intestine accommodate to the change in the stomach's holding capacity.

10 **TRUE** Because intrinsic factor is produced in the stomach and is necessary for the intestinal absorption of vitamin B_{12}, people who have had a gastrectomy are at risk of developing pernicious anemia. The symptoms may take years to develop because the body stores vitamin B_{12}.

Student Resources on thePoint®

For additional learning materials, activate the code in the front of this book at
http://thePoint.lww.com/activate

Websites

American College of Gastroenterology at www.acg.gi.org

American Gastroenterological Association at www.gastro.org

National Digestive Diseases Information Clearinghouse (NDDIC), a service of the National Institute of Diabetes and Digestive and Kidney Diseases (NIDDK), National Institutes of Health at http://digestive.niddk.nih.gov

The Helicobacter Foundation at www.helico.com

References

Academy of Nutrition and Dietetics. (2016). *Nutrition care manual.* Available at http://www.nutritioncaremanual.org. Accessed on 7/12/16.

Adeleye, B., & Rachal, C. (2007). Comparison of the rheological properties of ready-to-serve and powdered instant food-thickened beverages at different temperatures for dysphagic patients. *Journal of the American Dietetic Association, 107,* 1176–1182.

Carlaw, C., Finlayson, H., Beggs, K., Visser, T., Marcoux, C., Coney, D., & Steele, C. M. (2011). Outcomes of a pilot water protocol project in a rehabilitation setting. *Dysphagia, 27,* 297–306.

Caselli, M., Zuliani, G., Cassol, F., Fusetti, N., Zeni, E., Lo Cascio, N., . . . Gullini, S. (2014). Test-based exclusion diets in pastor-esophageal reflux disease patients: A randomized controlled pilot trial. *World Journal of Gastroenterology, 20,* 17190–17195.

Corley, D., Kubo, A., & Zhao, W. (2007). Abdominal obesity, ethnicity and gastro-oesophageal reflux symptoms. *Gut, 56,* 756–762.

Dent, J., El-Serag, H., Wallander, M., & Johansson, S. (2005). Epidemiology of gastro-oesophageal reflux disease: A systematic review. *Gut, 54,* 710–717.

Garcia, J., & Chambers, E. (2010). Managing dysphagia through diet modifications. *The American Journal of Nursing, 110,* 26–33.

Jacobson, B., Somers, S., Fuchs, C., Kelly, C. P., & Camargo, C. A., Jr. (2006). Body-mass index and symptoms of gastroesophageal reflux in women. *The New England Journal of Medicine, 354,* 2340–2348.

Katz, P., Gerson, L., & Vela, M. (2013). Guidelines for the diagnosis and management of gastroesophageal reflux disease. *The American Journal of Gastroenterology, 108,* 308–328.

Keller, H., & Duizer, L. (2014). What do consumers think of pureed food? Making the most of the indistinguishable food. *Journal of Nutrition in Gerontology and Geriatrics, 33,* 139–159.

Lepore, J., Sims, C., Gal, N., & Dahl, W. (2014). Acceptability and identification of scooped versus molded pureed foods. *Canadian Journal Dietetic Practice and Research, 75,* 145–147.

National Dysphagia Diet Task Force. (2002). *The national dysphagia diet: Standardization for optimal care.* Chicago, IL: American Dietetic Association.

Pallati, P., Shaligram, A., Shostrom, V., Oleynikov, D., McBride, C. L., & Goede, M. R. (2014). Improvement in gastroesophageal reflux disease symptoms after various bariatric procedures: Review of the bariatric outcomes longitudinal database. *Surgery for Obesity and Related Diseases, 19*, 502–507.

Panther, K. (2005). The Frazier Free Water Protocol. *Perspectives, Dysphagia, 14*, 4–9.

Parrish, C., & McCray, S. (2011). Gastroparesis and nutrition: The art. *Practical Gastroenterology, 9*, 26–41.

Prachand, V., & Alverdy, J. (2010). Gastroesophageal reflux disease and severe obesity: Fundoplication or bariatric surgery? *World Journal of Gastroenterology, 16*, 3757–3761.

Shimamoto, T., Yamamichi, N., Kodashima, S., Takahashi Y., Fujishiro, M., Oka, M., . . . Koike, K. (2013). No association of coffee consumption with gastric ulcer, duodenal ulcer, reflux esophagitis, and non-erosive reflux disease: A cross-sectional study of 8,013 healthy subjects in Japan. *PLoS One, 8*(6), e65996. doi:10.1371/journal.pone.0065996

Stenson, W. (2006). The esophagus and the stomach. In M. E. Shils, M. Shike, A. C. Ross, B. Caballero, & R. J. Cousins (Eds.), *Modern nutrition in health and disease* (10th ed., pp. 1179–1188). Philadelphia, PA: Lippincott Williams & Wilkins.

Wilhelm, S., Riater, R., & Kale-Pradhan, P. (2013). Perils and pitfalls of long-term effects of proton pump inhibitors. *Expert review of Clinical Pharmacology, 6*, 443–451.

Zhen-Hua, W., Gao, Q. Y., & Fang, J. Y. (2013). Meta-analysis of the efficacy and safety of *Lactobacillus*-containing and *Bifidobacterium*-containing probiotic compound preparation in Helicobacter pylori eradication therapy. *Journal of Clinical Gastroenterology, 47*, 25–32.

Chapter 18

Nutrition for Patients with Disorders of the Lower GI Tract and Accessory Organs

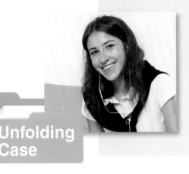

Unfolding Case

Stephanie Schlau

Stephanie is an 18-year-old college freshman who was diagnosed with type 1 diabetes 12 years ago. She has an insulin pump, is of healthy weight, and has no other significant medical history. She went to the student health center on campus with complaints of fatigue, abdominal cramping, and diarrhea.

Check Your Knowledge

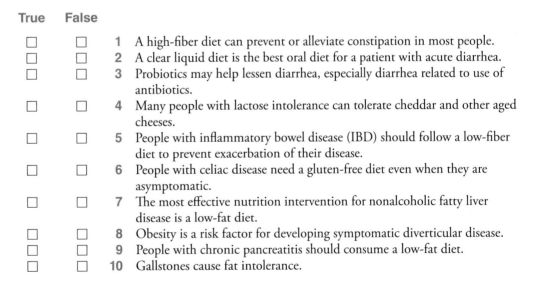

True	False		
☐	☐	**1**	A high-fiber diet can prevent or alleviate constipation in most people.
☐	☐	**2**	A clear liquid diet is the best oral diet for a patient with acute diarrhea.
☐	☐	**3**	Probiotics may help lessen diarrhea, especially diarrhea related to use of antibiotics.
☐	☐	**4**	Many people with lactose intolerance can tolerate cheddar and other aged cheeses.
☐	☐	**5**	People with inflammatory bowel disease (IBD) should follow a low-fiber diet to prevent exacerbation of their disease.
☐	☐	**6**	People with celiac disease need a gluten-free diet even when they are asymptomatic.
☐	☐	**7**	The most effective nutrition intervention for nonalcoholic fatty liver disease is a low-fat diet.
☐	☐	**8**	Obesity is a risk factor for developing symptomatic diverticular disease.
☐	☐	**9**	People with chronic pancreatitis should consume a low-fat diet.
☐	☐	**10**	Gallstones cause fat intolerance.

Learning Objectives

Upon completion of this chapter, you will be able to

1. Modify a regular diet to be high in fiber.
2. Instruct a patient on the nutrition therapy recommendations for diarrhea.
3. Give examples of appropriate nutrition interventions for various symptoms and complications of malabsorption syndrome.
4. Modify a regular diet to be low in lactose.
5. Identify sources of gluten.
6. Instruct a patient with an ileostomy on appropriate diet modifications.
7. Describe nutrition interventions for a nonalcoholic liver disease.
8. Compare a low-fat diet to a regular diet.

Figure 18.1 ▶

The sites of nutrient absorption.

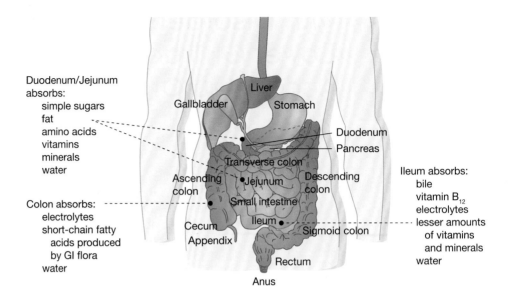

The lower gastrointestinal (GI) tract consists of the small and large intestines, rectum, and anus. Ninety to 95% of nutrient absorption occurs in the first half of the small intestine (Fig. 18.1). The large intestine absorbs water and electrolytes and promotes the elimination of solid wastes. The accessory organs—liver, gallbladder, and pancreas—play vital roles in nutrient digestion. With many disorders of the lower GI tract and accessory organs, nutrition therapy is used to improve or control symptoms; replenish losses; and promote healing, if applicable. For one GI disorder, celiac disease, nutrition therapy is the sole mode of treatment.

This chapter presents nutrition therapy for altered bowel elimination, malabsorption syndromes, disorders of the large intestine, and disorders of the accessory organs. Box 18.1 lists nutrition-focused assessment criteria for lower GI disorders.

ALTERED BOWEL ELIMINATION

Constipation

Criteria for diagnosing constipation include having fewer than three bowel movements per week, passing stools that are hard, and excessive straining during defecation. Inadequate fiber intake, physical inactivity, and low food intake increase the risk of constipation. Constipation can occur secondary to irregular bowel habits, psychogenic factors, chronic laxative use, metabolic and endocrine disorders, and bowel abnormalities (e.g., tumors, hernias, strictures). Certain medications, such as analgesics that contain opiates, antidepressants, diuretics, aluminum hydroxide, and iron and calcium supplements cause constipation. Contrary to popular belief, daily bowel movements are not necessary provided the stools are not hard and dry.

BOX 18.1	**Nutrition-Focused Assessment for Lower Gastrointestinal (GI) Disorders**

- GI symptoms that interfere with intake, such as anorexia, early satiety, pain, abdominal distention
- Changes in eating made in response to symptoms
- Complications that affect nutritional status, such as weight loss, diarrhea, blood loss
- Usual pattern of eating and frequency of meals and snacks
- Adequacy of intake according to MyPlate recommendations, including fluid intake
- Use of tobacco, over-the-counter drugs for GI symptoms, alcohol, and caffeine
- Food allergies or intolerances, such as high-fat foods, milk, high-fiber foods
- Use of nutritional supplements including vitamins, minerals, fiber, and herbs
- Client's willingness to change his or her eating habits

Nutrition Therapy for Constipation

To treat constipation, it is standard practice to recommend that fiber intake be increased. Although a goal of 25 to 38 g/day, which is the Adequate Intake for fiber, may be recommended, those levels are based on the amount of fiber needed to protect against coronary heart disease not for optimal bowel function. The amount of fiber needed to alleviate constipation varies among individuals and is usually determined by trial and error.

Fiber increases stool weight, bulk, and fecal water content and stimulates peristalsis to promote a more rapid transit time. Insoluble fiber is more effective at treating constipation than soluble fiber. Foods with the highest proportion of insoluble fiber are whole grains, wheat bran, and the skins and seeds of fruit and vegetables. Fiber intake is increased by adding fiber-rich foods (e.g., vegetables) and replacing low-fiber foods with higher fiber versions (e.g., replacing white pasta with whole wheat pasta) (Box 18.2). However, most fruits, vegetables, and whole wheat breads provide only 1 to 3 g of fiber per serving. Foods with the highest amount of fiber per serving are high fiber cereals and legumes, which may provide 10 g/serving or up to 8 g/serving, respectively. Fiber supplements may be necessary if adequate fiber cannot be consumed through food.

A gradual increase in fiber is recommended to avoid symptoms of intolerance such as gas, cramping, and diarrhea. If these side effects do occur, they are usually temporary and subside within several days. To achieve maximum benefit, fiber intake should be spread throughout the day.

Other interventions to promote bowel regularity include

- Ensuring an adequate fluid intake of at least 64 oz/day; without enough water, a high-fiber diet can worsen constipation, abdominal pain, bloating, and gas (Academy of Nutrition and Dietetics [AND], 2016).
- Increasing aerobic exercise
- Consuming **probiotics** or **prebiotics** daily, such as yogurt containing live bacterial cultures, acidophilus milk, and kefir

Quick Bite **Fiber supplements**

Promoted for regularity
Metamucil
Fiberall
Fiber-Lax
Ready Fiber
Citrucel

Probiotics
live microorganisms found in food that, when consumed in adequate amounts, are beneficial to health.

Prebiotics
nondigestible food components that stimulate the growth of probiotic bacteria within the large intestine.

Diarrhea

Diarrhea is a common symptom of many GI disorders and infectious diseases and is a frequent side effect of chemotherapy and radiation. It is characterized by an increase in the frequency of bowel movements and/or water content of stools, which alters either the consistency or volume of fecal output. A rapid transit time decreases the time available for water, sodium, and potassium to be absorbed through the colon; the result is more water and electrolytes in the stools and the potential for dehydration, hyponatremia, hypokalemia, acid–base imbalance, and metabolic acidosis. Chronic diarrhea can lead to malnutrition related to impaired digestion, absorption, and intake.

Osmotic diarrhea occurs when there is an increase in particles in the intestine, which draws water in to dilute the high concentration. The causes of osmotic diarrhea include maldigestion of nutrients (e.g., lactose intolerance), excessive intake of sorbitol or fructose, dumping syndrome, tube feedings, and some laxatives. It is cured by treating the underlying cause.

Secretory diarrhea is related to an excessive secretion of fluid and electrolytes into the intestines. Bacterial, viral, protozoan, and other infections cause secretory diarrhea, as do some medications and some GI disorders, such as Crohn disease and celiac disease. An excessive amount of bile acids or unabsorbed fatty acids in the colon can also cause secretory diarrhea. If the cause is infection, antibiotics are the primary component of treatment. Symptoms may be treated with medications that decrease GI motility or thicken the consistency of stools, such as the soluble fiber psyllium (Metamucil).

Antibiotic-acquired diarrhea is caused by the disruption in GI microbiota as a side effect of antibiotic therapy. Symptoms range from mild and self-limiting to severe, particularly in *Clostridium difficile* infections (Hempel et al., 2012).

BOX 18.2 High-Fiber Diet

- A high-fiber diet is a regular diet that substitutes whole grains for refined grains and is high in other fiber-rich foods—namely, fresh fruits, vegetables, and dried peas and beans.
- Unprocessed bran may be added as tolerated.
- At least eight 8-oz glasses of fluid are recommended daily.
- A high-fiber diet is used for constipation and diverticulosis. It may also promote weight loss and helps lower serum cholesterol levels and improve glucose tolerance in diabetes. All healthy Americans are urged to increase their intake of fiber.
- The diet should not be used in cases of intestinal inflammation or stenosis, postgastrectomy, or pseudo-obstruction.

Guidelines to Achieve a High-Fiber Diet

- Substitute whole grains for refined grains.

Use	In place of
Whole wheat bread	White bread
Brown rice	White rice
Whole wheat pasta	White pasta
Bran or whole grain cereal	Refined cereals
Whole wheat flour	White flour

- Eat more dried peas or beans.
- Eat more fresh fruit; leave the skin on whenever possible. Apples, blackberries, blueberries, figs, dates, kiwifruit, mango, oranges, pears, prunes, strawberries, and raspberries are high in fiber.
- Eat more vegetables. Cooked asparagus, green beans, broccoli, Brussels sprouts, cabbage, carrots, celery, corn, eggplant, parsnips, peas, snow peas, Swiss chard, and turnips are good choices.
- Other foods with fiber include popcorn, nuts, sunflower seeds, and sesame seeds.

Sample Menu

Breakfast	Lunch	Dinner	Snacks
Prune juice	Split pea soup	Roast chicken	Low-fat popcorn
Bran flakes with milk	Ham sandwich on	Brown rice	Dried fruit and nuts
Whole wheat toast with jelly	whole wheat bread with lettuce and	Tossed salad with fresh vegetables	Raw carrots and celery with dip
Fresh orange sections	tomato	Steamed broccoli	
	Fresh strawberries	Whole wheat roll	
	Date cookie	with butter	
	Milk	Milk	
		Blueberries over ice cream	

Potential Problems

Flatus, distention, cramping, and osmotic diarrhea related to increasing fiber content of the diet too much or too quickly

Recommended Interventions

Initiate a high-fiber diet gradually to develop the patient's tolerance. If symptoms of intolerance persist, reduce fiber content to maximum amount tolerated by the patient.

Patient Teaching

Instruct the patient that

- A high-fiber diet increases stool bulk and speeds passage of food through intestines.
- Increasing fiber intake gradually may be better tolerated than increasing fiber intake quickly.
- Fiber intake may be increased by making subtle changes in eating and cooking habits such as eating more fresh fruits and vegetables, especially with the skin on.
- Switching to high-fiber breads and cereals can significantly increase fiber intake; the first ingredient on the label should be "whole wheat" or "100% whole wheat," not just "wheat."

BOX 18.2 High-Fiber Diet (continued)

- A variety of foods high in fiber should be eaten; numerous forms of fiber exist, and each performs a different action in the body (see Chapter 2).
- A meatless main dish made with dried peas and beans is a high-fiber alternative to traditional entrées.
- Fresh or dried fruit, nuts, and seeds make high-fiber snacks.
- Coarse, unprocessed wheat bran is most effective as a laxative; it can be incorporated into the diet by mixing it with juice or milk; by adding it to muffins, quick breads, casseroles, and meat loaves before baking; or by sprinkling it over cereal, applesauce, eggs, or other foods.
- Bran should be added to the diet slowly (up to 3 tbsp/day) to decrease the likelihood of developing flatus and distention.
- Certain foods (in addition to being high in fiber) have laxative effects: prunes and prune juice, figs, and dates.
- At least eight 8-oz glasses of fluid should be consumed daily.

Quick Bite High-potassium foods include

Apricot nectar	Orange juice
Avocado	Papaya
Banana	Potatoes
Canned apricots and peaches	Tomato juice
Cantaloupe	Yogurt

Quick Bite Items that stimulate GI motility

Diarrhea may improve by avoiding foods that stimulate GI motility, such as the following:

- Alcohol
- Caffeine
- Items high in simple sugars, such as milk (lactose), fruit (fructose), and carbonated beverages (sucrose)
- High-fiber and gas-producing foods, such as nuts, beans, corn, broccoli, and cabbage
- Sugar alcohols (e.g., sorbitol in "dietetic" products)

Lactose
the disaccharide (double sugar) in milk composed of glucoses and galactose.

Nutrition Therapy for Diarrhea

Nutrition therapy for diarrhea is largely supportive and depends on the severity of diarrhea and the underlying cause. Maintaining or restoring fluid and electrolyte balance is the primary focus. Mild diarrhea lasting 24 to 48 hours usually requires no nutrition intervention other than encouraging a liberal fluid intake to replace losses. Oral rehydration solutions, such as Pedialyte and Rehydralyte, may be used. Clear liquids are avoided because they have high osmolality related to their high sugar content, which may promote osmotic diarrhea. For more serious cases, intravenous (IV) therapy is used to replace fluid and electrolytes.

On a short-term basis, a low-fiber diet (Box 18.3) that is also low in fat and **lactose** may help decrease bowel stimulation. Food and beverages that stimulate GI motility are avoided. High-potassium foods are encouraged. Banana flakes, apple powder, or other sources of pectin may be added to foods to help thicken the consistency of stools (AND, 2016).

Probiotics may help lessen diarrhea, especially diarrhea related to use of antibiotics. A systematic review and meta-analysis found moderate quality evidence that suggests probiotics are safe and effective for preventing *C. difficile*–associated diarrhea (Goldenberg et al., 2013). Because it is not known which strains or doses of probiotics may be most beneficial, it may be prudent to obtain probiotics from food sources, such as yogurt, kefir, and acidophilus milk, instead of supplements. Patients with intractable diarrhea may need complete bowel rest (i.e., total parenteral nutrition or TPN).

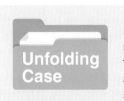

Unfolding Case

Recall Stephanie. Her vital signs and temperature are within normal limits. The physician assistant diagnoses viral gastritis and advises her to eat a bland diet until her symptoms abate. Is a bland diet the best option for Stephanie? What specific foods would you recommend she consume? What foods should she avoid?

BOX 18.3   Low-Fiber Diet

- This diet restricts fiber to decrease the volume and frequency of stools.
- This diet is a short-term diet to be used when the bowel is inflamed, such as in the acute stages of diverticulitis, ulcerative colitis, and Crohn disease. It may also be used for esophageal and intestinal stenosis, in preparation for or after bowel surgery, or for new colostomy or ileostomy.

General Guidelines to Achieve a Low-Fiber Diet

- Use refined white flour products, such as white bread and rolls, white pasta, white rice, refined, low-fiber cereals.
- Eat only vegetables that are canned, do not have skins or seeds, and are well cooked.
- Choose canned, soft, or cooked fruit and fruit juices without pulp (except prune juice); ripe bananas, citrus sections without membranes.
- Eat plain desserts made without nuts or coconut, such as plain cakes, puddings (rice, bread, plain), cookies, and ice cream.
- Avoid foods high in fiber.
  - Whole grain breads and cereals
  - Most raw vegetables, vegetables with seeds, gassy vegetables, cooked greens or spinach
  - Fresh fruit with skins or seeds, dried fruits, prune juice
  - Dried peas and beans
  - Anything containing nuts, seeds, or coconut; popcorn

Additional Recommendations

- Avoid milk and milk products that contain lactose if lactose intolerance is suspected. Low-lactose and lactose-free alternatives include acidophilus milk, yogurt, soy milk, and almond milk.
- Avoid high-fat protein foods (sausage, bacon, many cold cuts).
- Avoid items that stimulate GI motility: alcohol, caffeine, sorbitol, and xylitol.
- Probiotic foods may help, such as yogurt with live bacterial cultures, acidophilus milk, and kefir.

Sample Menu

Breakfast	**Lunch**	**Dinner**	**Snacks**
Pulp-free orange juice	Tomato juice	Roast chicken	Saltine crackers
Poached egg	Turkey sandwich on	White rice	Rice cakes
White toast with jelly	white bread with	Cooked carrots	Tomato juice
	salad dressing	Italian bread with olive	Fresh banana
	Canned peach halves	oil	Milk
		Gelatin made with ripe	
		bananas	
		Soy milk	

Potential Problems

Constipation related to low fiber content of diet; insufficient fiber intake causes decrease in stool bulk and slowing of intestinal transit time.

Persistent diarrhea related to poor tolerance of even small amounts of fiber contained in a low-fiber diet; tolerance of fiber varies among patients and conditions.

Recommended Interventions

Liberalize diet to allow more fiber; this diet is intended to be short-term.

Further reduce fiber content by eliminating all fruits and vegetables except strained fruit juice.

Patient Teaching

Instruct the patient that

- Reducing fiber slows passage of food through the bowel.
- Fiber is a component of plants and, therefore, is found in fruits, vegetables, whole grains, dried peas and beans, and nuts.
- Diet is intended to be short-term.
- Food preparation techniques to reduce fiber include removing skins, seeds, and membranes of fruits and vegetables that are high in fiber and cooking allowed vegetables until they are very tender.

MALABSORPTION DISORDERS

Malabsorption
a broad term that describes altered or inadequate nutrient absorption from the GI tract.

Malabsorption occurs secondary to nutrient maldigestion or from alterations to the absorptive surface of the intestinal mucosa. Generally, malabsorption related to maldigestion involves one or few nutrients, whereas malabsorption that stems from an altered mucosa is more generalized, resulting in multiple nutrient deficiencies and weight loss.

Symptoms of malabsorption vary with the underlying disorder, ranging from minimal to widespread and serious. Malabsorption may be suspected in patients who have weight loss, growth failure, postprandial abdominal pain, bloating, and flatulence. Watery diarrhea and distention are symptoms of malabsorption from carbohydrate maldigestion (e.g., lactose intolerance), whereas the passage of less frequent stools that are oily, bulky, and foul-smelling is a symptom of malabsorption related to fat maldigestion (e.g., pancreatitis). The excretion of fat in the stools means that essential fatty acids, fat-soluble vitamins, calcium, and magnesium are also lost through the stools. Nutrient deficiencies can cause metabolic complications, such as osteomalacia and bone pain related to the deficiencies of calcium, vitamin D, and magnesium. Appetite may be poor and nutrient needs may be elevated for healing. The risk for malnutrition can be high.

Steatorrhea
excess fat in the stools that are loose, foamy, and foul-smelling.

The goal of nutrition therapy for malabsorption syndromes is to control **steatorrhea**, promote normal bowel elimination, restore optimal nutritional status, and promote healing, when applicable. Nutrition therapy is individualized according to symptoms and complications; possible diet modifications appear in Table 18.1. Specific malabsorption syndromes are discussed in the following sections—namely, lactose intolerance, inflammatory bowel disease (IBD), celiac disease, and short bowel syndrome.

Lactose Malabsorption

Lactose Malabsorption
incomplete digestion of lactose.

Lactase Nonpersistence
reduced activity of lactase at the jejunal brush border, which is common in the majority of human adults. Low lactase activity may cause symptoms after lactose is consumed.

Lactose Intolerance
GI symptoms of lactose malabsorption that occur after a blinded, placebo-controlled lactose challenge.

Lactase Persistence
persistence of a high level of lactase into adulthood which enables adequate digestion of larger amounts of lactose.

Lactose malabsorption refers to impaired lactose digestion related to reduced activity of lactase, the enzyme that splits lactose into its component simple sugars glucose and galactose. Without adequate lactase, lactose reaches the large intestine where microbiota ferment the sugar, which may produce bloating, cramping, flatulence, and diarrhea. Particles of undigested lactose increase the osmolality of intestinal contents, increasing the likelihood of osmotic diarrhea. Symptoms range from mild to severe, depending on the amount of lactase actually produced and the amount of lactose consumed.

Lactose malabsorption caused by a complete lack of lactase—congenital lactase deficiency—is rare. The most frequent cause of lactose malabsorption is **lactase nonpersistence**, a common condition in which lactase activity is low in most of the world's adults, particularly in adults of Asian, Native American, and African descent (Heaney, 2013). Lactase nonpersistence is not synonymous with **lactose intolerance**, which by definition requires evidence of lactose malabsorption and the development of symptoms, which is not currently done in practice (Misselwitz et al., 2013).

In comparison to lactase nonpersistence, Caucasians from Northern Europe or Northern European descent retain high lactase levels during adulthood, which is termed **lactase persistence**. Both lactase persistence and nonpersistence are normal human conditions (Misselwitz et al., 2013).

Lactose malabsorption may also occur secondary to GI disorders that alter the integrity and function of intestinal villi cells, where lactase is secreted. For instance, people with IBD lose lactase activity when the disease is active and sometimes for a prolonged period afterward. The loss of lactase may also develop secondary to malnutrition because the rapidly growing intestinal cells that produce lactase are reduced in number and function. Symptoms tend to be more severe and occur more quickly after eating lactose than when lactose malabsorption is caused by lactase nonpersistence.

Nutrition Therapy for Lactose Malabsorption

Nutrition therapy for lactose malabsorption is to reduce lactose to the maximum amount tolerated by the individual, which is dose-related (Box 18.4). People with lactose nonpersistence may be asymptomatic when they consume doses less than 4 to 12 g of lactose (e.g., 1/3 to 1 cup of milk) or when lactose is consumed as part of a meal. Chocolate milk may be better tolerated than plain milk, although the reason is unclear (Heaney, 2013). A proven way to improve lactose tolerance is to gradually increase milk intake: Add a half-glass of milk to 1 meal on the first day, a half-glass to each of 2 meals on the second day, and continue the gradual daily increase

Table 18.1   Nutrition Therapy for Malabsorption Symptoms

Symptoms	Dietary Interventions	Rationale
Anorexia	Small, frequent meals	To maximize intake
	Oral nutrition supplements	Liquid supplements are easy to consume, are nutritionally dense, and leave the stomach quickly.
	Enteral nutrition if anorexia is severe and/or prolonged	To meet calorie and nutrient needs until the patient is able to consume an adequate oral intake
Diarrhea	Low-fiber diet	To minimize stimulation to the bowel
	Ensure adequate fluid and electrolytes.	Increased losses of fluid and electrolytes in the stool
	Avoid lactose.	Lactase activity may be lost during acute episodes of malabsorption due to altered integrity and function of intestinal villi cells; lactase deficiency may persist into remission.
Nutrient deficiencies	Nutrient-dense diet	To replenish losses, facilitate healing, and meet increased needs related to the metabolism of a high-calorie, high-protein diet.
	Vitamin supplements; may need water-soluble forms of the fat-soluble vitamins	Dietary sources may not be adequate to meet need. Water-soluble forms do not require normal fat absorption to be absorbed, as do fat-soluble vitamins in their natural form.
	Oral or parenteral vitamin B_{12}	Bacterial overgrowth, pancreatic insufficiency, and ileal disease or resection impair vitamin B_{12} absorption.
	Calcium supplements	Serum calcium may be low related to low serum albumin or calcium malabsorption related to poor vitamin D absorption or the binding of calcium with unabsorbed fats to form unabsorbable soaps.
	Other mineral supplements	Magnesium levels are often low in some malabsorption syndromes; losses of zinc are high in patients with fistulas.
Steatorrhea	Limit fat.	To avoid aggravating fat malabsorption
	MCT oil may be used for calories.	MCT oil is absorbed without undergoing digestion.
Tissue damage (e.g., resulting from inflammation or surgery) and/or weight loss	Increase calories (2000–3500 cal/day). Increase protein (1.0–1.5 g/kg/day).	Calories and protein are needed to facilitate healing and restore weight.
Formation of calcium oxalate kidney stones related to binding of calcium to fat instead of oxalate, leaving increased amount of oxalate available for absorption into the blood	Increase fluids.	To dilute the urine

TFN, medium chain triglycerides.

(Hertzler & Savaiano, 1996). This strategy promotes the development of intestinal microbiota that contains its own lactase, thereby building tolerance over time. Another strategy that may improve tolerance is to use probiotics that favor colonization with lactase-containing organisms (Heaney, 2013). For people who want to consume milk or lactose-containing foods beyond their limit, lactose-reduced milk and lactase enzyme tablets or liquid may be used.

For patients with GI disorders, a lactose-restricted diet is indicated at least until the disorder is resolved and sometimes for a prolonged period thereafter. Because lactose is used as an ingredient in many foods and drugs, a lactose-free diet is not realistic.

Unfolding Case

Recall Stephanie. Her symptoms resolved when she limited her intake to chicken broth, Gatorade, and tomato juice, but when she resumed her normal eating pattern, her symptoms returned. She has unintentionally lost a few pounds. She decided to keep a food diary to see if her symptoms correlated to food. She concluded that milk is a problem and has eliminated all milk and dairy products from her eating pattern. What nutrients may she be lacking in by eliminating all dairy? Is it appropriate for her to eliminate all dairy? Does eliminating dairy effectively eliminate all sources of lactose?

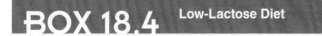

BOX 18.4 Low-Lactose Diet

- Lactose is the sugar in milk; limit or avoid milk and foods made with milk.
- Individual tolerance varies; eat dairy foods as tolerance allows.
- Lactose tolerance may improve by introducing a small serving of a lactose-containing food and increasing the amount consumed daily.
- Lactose is better tolerated with meals, not alone. Chocolate milk may be better tolerated than plain milk.
- These ingredients are derived from milk but are lactose-free: casein, lactate, lactalbumin, lactic acid.
- Avoid products whose ingredient list contains butter, cream, milk, milk solids, or whey.
- Choose nondairy sources of calcium to ensure an adequate intake, such as canned salmon with bones, calcium-fortified tofu, orange juice, and soy milk; shellfish; "greens" such as turnip, collard, and kale; dried peas and beans; broccoli; and almonds.

Lactose-Free Milk and Nondairy Foods	Low-Lactose Dairy Foods	Possible Hidden Sources of Lactose
Lactose-free milk	Aged cheese, such as cheddar, Swiss, and parmesan	Bread
Almond, rice, or soy milk	Cream cheese	Baked goods
Soy yogurt, soy cheese	Ricotta cheese	Breakfast cereals
Soy sour cream	Cottage cheese	Instant potatoes and soups
	Yogurt	Margarine
		Lunch meats
		Salad dressings
		Mixes for pancakes, biscuits and cookies
		Powdered meal replacement supplements

Inflammatory Bowel Disease

IBD, including Crohn disease (CD) and ulcerative colitis (UC), is a group of chronic immune disorders of unclear etiology, although a combination of genetic and environmental factors may be involved (Massironi et al., 2013). CD and UC are characterized by cycles that alternate between active and quiescent states; they share common symptoms and treatments (Table 18.2). Very limited data suggest diet plays a role in the onset and course of IBD; however, the association has not been clearly demonstrated (T. Yamamoto, 2013).

Malnutrition occurs in both CD and UC patients, during active or quiescent states (Alastair, Emma, & Emma, 2011). Malnutrition may be caused by poor intake, poor digestion, increased requirements related to systemic inflammation, malabsorption due to chronic inflammation, drug–nutrient interactions, and, in patients with CD, previous surgical resection of the bowel (Massironi et al., 2013). Evidence-based diet recommendations do not exist for patients with IBD, other than to follow a healthy and varied diet (Massironi et al., 2013).

Nutrition Therapy for Crohn Disease

Because CD primarily affects the small bowel, it is more likely than UC to cause nutritional complications, such as protein-calorie malnutrition and micronutrient deficiencies. Nutrition plays a pivotal role in treatment, even though there is a lack of solid evidence to formulate strong dietary recommendations (A. Cohen et al., 2013). Nutrition interventions are based on the presence and severity of symptoms, the presence of complications, and the nutritional status of the patient (see Table 18.1). Restrictions are kept to a minimum to encourage an adequate intake. Nutrition therapy varies over the course of the disease.

When CD is active, patients may benefit from

- A low-fiber diet to minimize bowel stimulation (see Box 18.3)
- Limiting fat if steatorrhea is present
- Increasing protein and calories to facilitate healing
- Restricting the intake of lactose, fructose, and sorbitol if diarrhea is present
- Consuming small, frequent meals to help maximize intake

Table 18.2	Comparison Between Crohn Disease and Ulcerative Colitis	
	Crohn Disease	**Ulcerative Colitis**
Area affected	Can occur anywhere along the GI tract but most commonly occurs in the ileum and colon	Confined to the rectum and colon
Disease pattern	Inflammation is discontinuous, with normal tissue between patches of inflamed tissue. All layers of the bowel are affected.	Inflammation is continuous, beginning at rectum and usually extending into the colon. Affects only the mucosal layer
Main symptoms	Diarrhea, abdominal pain, weight loss	Diarrhea, abdominal pain, rectal bleeding Weight loss, fever, and weakness are common when most of the colon is involved.
Complications	Fistulas, abscesses Stricture of the ileum Bowel perforation Bowel obstructions may occur from scar tissue formation. Toxic megacolon Increased risk of intestinal cancer	Tissue erosion and ulceration Toxic megacolon Greatly increased risk of cancer
Nutritional complications	Impaired bile acid reabsorption may cause malabsorption of fat, fat-soluble vitamins, calcium, magnesium, and zinc. Malnutrition may occur from nutrient malabsorption, decreased intake, or intestinal resections. Anemia related to blood loss or malabsorption Vitamin B_{12} deficiency related to B_{12} malabsorption from the ileum due to inflammation	Anemia related to blood loss Dehydration and electrolyte imbalances related to diarrhea Protein depletion from losses through inflamed tissue
Medical treatment	Antidiarrheals, immunosuppressants, immunomodulators, biologic therapies, and anti-inflammatory agents	Antidiarrheals, immunosuppressants, and anti-inflammatory agents
Surgical intervention	Most common procedure is ileostomy; disease often recurs in the remaining intestine.	Most common procedure is total colectomy; surgery prevents recurrence.

Patients are often reluctant to eat because they associate eating with pain and diarrhea. Enteral nutrition (EN) may be used for supplemental or complete nutrition. Because EN is at least as effective as parenteral nutrition (PN) but with lower costs and fewer side effects, the use of PN is limited to a small group of IBD patients for whom EN has failed or is contraindicated (Massironi et al., 2013).

Nutrition Therapy for Ulcerative Colitis

Dietary modifications for UC are based on symptoms and complications. When the disease is active, symptoms of bleeding and diarrhea are treated with an increased intake of fluid, electrolytes, protein, and calories. A low-fiber diet minimizes stimulation to the bowel. Other diet modifications that may be appropriate depending on symptoms and complications are outlined in Table 18.1.

Nutrition Therapy During Inflammatory Bowel Disease Remission

For both CD and UC, dietary restrictions are liberalized during periods of remission. Patients tend to have strong beliefs about the role of diet in the cause of IBD and in improving or worsening their symptoms (Hou, Lee, & Lewis, 2014). Box 18.5 lists food items that patients commonly believe worsen or improve their IBD (A. Cohen et al., 2013). Unfortunately, items from each of the food groups have been noted to worsen symptoms and so the list does not provide generalizable information to benefit others (Hou et al., 2014). Keeping a food diary to monitor tolerance and identify specific triggers may help manage symptoms.

A number of defined dietary regimens are promoted in lay literature as being beneficial in managing IBD based on theories of how food interacts with the body (Hou et al., 2014). The Specific Carbohydrate Diet (SCD), the Fermentable Oligo-, Di-, and Monosaccharides (FODMAP) diet, and the Paleolithic (Paleo) diet are among the regiments advocated for IBD.

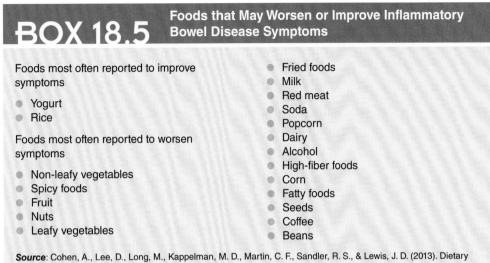

BOX 18.5 Foods that May Worsen or Improve Inflammatory Bowel Disease Symptoms

Foods most often reported to improve symptoms

- Yogurt
- Rice

Foods most often reported to worsen symptoms

- Non-leafy vegetables
- Spicy foods
- Fruit
- Nuts
- Leafy vegetables

- Fried foods
- Milk
- Red meat
- Soda
- Popcorn
- Dairy
- Alcohol
- High-fiber foods
- Corn
- Fatty foods
- Seeds
- Coffee
- Beans

Source: Cohen, A., Lee, D., Long, M., Kappelman, M. D., Martin, C. F., Sandler, R. S., & Lewis, J. D. (2013). Dietary patterns and self-reported associations of diet with symptoms of inflammatory bowel disease. *Digestive Diseases and Science, 5–8*, 1322–1328.

Little evidence exists for the efficacy of these diets. Prospective randomized controlled trials are needed to clarify the role of diet in IBD.

Celiac Disease

Celiac disease is a genetic autoimmune disorder characterized by chronic inflammation of the proximal small intestine mucosa related to a permanent intolerance to certain gluten-forming proteins found in wheat, barley, and rye. When ingested, these proteins trigger an immune response that damages the villi that line the mucosa of the small intestine. Loss of absorptive surface area and a decrease in digestive enzymes lead to malabsorption of macro- and micro-nutrients, resulting in diarrhea, flatulence, weight loss, vitamin and mineral deficiencies, iron deficiency anemia, and loss of bone. People at risk of celiac disease are those who have an autoimmune disease (e.g., type 1 diabetes), Down syndrome, or a first-degree relative with celiac disease.

Dermatitis Herpetiformis
a chronic inflammatory skin disease characterized by groups of red, raised blisters that itch and burn.

Symptoms and their severity vary widely among individuals, depending on the patient's age and the duration and extent of the disease. Children typically exhibit GI symptoms such as chronic diarrhea, steatorrhea, flatulence, abdominal pain, bloating, weight loss, irritability, and failure to thrive. Adults may also present with GI symptoms and with non-GI symptoms such as abnormal liver function tests, unexplained iron deficiency anemia, bone disease, **dermatitis herpetiformis**, and peripheral neuropathy.

GI symptoms alone cannot accurately differentiate celiac disease from other common GI disorders (Rubio-Tapia, Hill, Kelly, Calderwood, & Murray, 2013). A positive celiac disease-specific serology in patients with villous atrophy identified by small intestine biopsy is needed to confirm the diagnosis (Leffler & Schuppan, 2010). Ideally, testing for celiac disease occurs before a gluten-free diet is implemented. However, because of media attention on gluten-free diets, people often adopt the diet without an objective celiac disease diagnosis (Oxentenko & Murray, 2015).

Nonceliac gluten sensitivity (NCGS) is a condition in which people do not have the diagnostic features of celiac disease but develop celiac-like symptoms in response to eating gluten. Symptoms alone cannot reliably differentiate celiac disease from NCGS because symptoms overlap between the two conditions (Lundin & Aladini, 2012). Although knowledge about NCGS is still growing, it appears that it does not have a strong genetic basis, is not associated with malabsorption or nutritional deficiencies, and is not associated with an increased risk for autoimmune disorders or intestinal malignancy (Rubio-Tapia et al., 2013). Treatment is a gluten-free diet, although it is not known if long-term strict avoidance of all gluten is necessary because NCGS may be transient (Fasano, Sapone, Zevallos, & Schuppan, 2015).

Nutrition Therapy for Celiac Disease

The only effective treatment for celiac disease is a life-long gluten-free diet (Box 18.6). "Gluten-free" actually means gluten intake so low it does not cause harm because complete elimination is not possible due to contamination of foods with small amounts of gluten. Although the exact daily amount of gluten that poses no harm is not known, less than 10 mg/day is probably unlikely to cause damage in most patients (Oxentenko & Murray, 2015). The U.S. Food and Drug Administration (FDA) requires that foods labeled as "gluten-free" contain less than 20 ppm of gluten (FDA, 2013).

Over time, a gluten-free diet leads to repair of intestinal damage and resolution of symptoms and increases in body weight and bone mineralization. Failure to adhere to the diet increases the risk for malignancies such as small bowel adenocarcinoma, cancer of the esophagus, and B-cell and T-cell non-Hodgkin lymphomas, especially T-cell lymphomas (Ludvigsson, 2012). Biopsies are the only way to confirm healing of the intestine. In a U.S. study, the median time from beginning the gluten-free diet to achieving mucosal healing was 3 years (Rubio-Tapia et al., 2013). In some patients, intestinal healing does not occur despite the absence of symptoms and normal serology (Rubio-Tapia et al., 2013).

Some people have nonresponsive celiac disease, defined as having persistent symptoms, signs, or laboratory abnormalities typical of celiac disease despite adhering to a gluten-free diet for 6 to 12 months (Rubio-Tapia et al., 2013). The most common cause is inadvertent gluten intake. Other potential causes include other food intolerances, bacterial overgrowth, microscopic colitis, and pancreatic insufficiency.

Gluten
a general name for the storage proteins gliadin (in wheat), secalin (in rye), and hordein (in barley).

Gluten is found in wheat, rye, and barley—grains that form the foundation of a healthy diet in many cultures. Pure or specially produced oats containing ≤20 ppm gluten can be safely consumed by most people with celiac disease, and there is no evidence that daily intake should be limited to a specific amount (La Vieille, Pulido, Abbott, Koerner, & Godefroy, 2016). In contrast, there is a high likelihood that commercial oats may be contaminated with gluten from other grains (Koerner et al., 2011) and that a small number of people with celiac disease seem to be clinically intolerant to pure oats (La Vieille et al., 2016). Therefore, even if confirmed to be pure, people with celiac disease who introduce oats in their diets should be monitored clinically and via serological testing to determine safety (Rubio-Tapia et al., 2013).

A gluten-free diet requires a major lifestyle change, so compliance is a challenge. Gluten-free products (e.g., breads, pastry) made with rice, corn, or potato flour have different textures and tastes than "normal" products and may not be well accepted. They may also be expensive. Even patients who are willing to comply have difficulty following the diet because of the pervasiveness of gluten in processed foods and medications and confusion over identifying sources of gluten on food labels. The diet is very restrictive, requires conscientious label reading, and is difficult to adhere to while eating out.

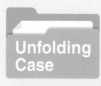

Think of Stephanie. Despite conscientiously following a low-lactose eating pattern, her symptoms persisted, and her weight loss continued. She is eventually seen by a gastroenterologist who diagnoses celiac disease and iron deficiency anemia. Is there a connection between type 1 diabetes and celiac disease? Should she continue to restrict lactose from her eating pattern? How will nutrition counseling for a college student who lives in a dorm differ from counseling for an adult living in her own home? Stephanie knows she should eat fiber to help regulate her blood glucose levels; what sources of fiber would be appropriate on a gluten-free diet?

BOX 18.6 Gluten-Free Diet

- Gluten, a protein fraction found in wheat, rye, and barley, is eliminated. Oats are at high risk of gluten contamination, so only oats labeled gluten-free are suitable. All products made from these grains or their flours are eliminated.
- Many foods are naturally gluten free: milk, butter, cheese; fresh, frozen, and canned fruits and vegetables; fresh meat, fish, poultry, eggs; dried peas and beans; nuts; corn; and rice.

Allowed Grains and Related Foods	Grains to Eliminate	Questionable Foods (may contain wheat, barley, or rye)
Amaranth	Wheat–all forms including	Bouillon cubes
Arrowroot	• Wheat flours, such as	Brown rice syrup
Buckwheat	bromated flour, durum flour,	Chips/potato chips
Cassava	enriched flour, graham	Candy
Corn, cornstarch	flour, phosphated flour,	Cold cuts, hot dogs, salami,
Flax	plain flour, self-rising flour,	sausage
Gums	semolina, white flour	Communion wafer
Acacia (gum Arabic)	• Wheat starch, wheat bran,	Flavored or herbal coffee
Carob bean gum	wheat germ, cracked	Flavored or herbal tea
Carrageenan	wheat, hydrolyzed wheat	French fries
Cellulose	protein, farina	Gravy
Guar	• Einkorn, emmer, spelt,	Imitation fish
Locust bean	kamut	Meat substitutes
Xanthan	Barley	Matzo
Indian rice grass	Rye	Rice and corn cereals (may contain barley malt)
Job's tears	Malt	
Legumes, legume	Triticale (a cross between	Rice mixes
flours	wheat and rye)	Sauces
Millet		Seasoned or dry roasted nuts
Nut flours		Seasoned tortilla chips
Oats (uncontaminated)		Self-basting turkey
Potatoes, potato flour		Soups
Quinoa		Soy sauce
Rice, all plain; rice flour		Vegetables in sauce
Sago		
Seeds		
Soy		
Sorghum		
Tapioca		
Teff		
Wild rice		
Yucca		

Sample Menu

Breakfast	Lunch	Dinner	Snacks
Orange juice	Cuban black beans with brown rice	Tomato juice	Plain nuts
Gluten-free cornflakes	Pure corn tortilla	Roast chicken	Rice cake
Milk	Milk	Quinoa pilaf	Banana
Coffee	Plain yogurt topped with chopped almonds	Steamed broccoli	Apple slices with peanut butter
	Coffee/tea	Corn bread made without wheat flour	
		Blueberries over ice cream made without gluten stabilizers	

Additional Considerations

- Patients may be discouraged and overwhelmed when faced with a lifelong restricted diet. Provide support, encouragement, and thorough diet instructions.
- The patient may have temporary lactose malabsorption and may require a lactose-restricted diet.

(continued)

BOX 18.6   Gluten-Free Diet (continued)

Potential Problems

Increased expense related to buying special gluten-free foods

Inadequate intake of several nutrients (B vitamins, calcium, zinc, and iron) related to the lower content of these nutrients in gluten-free products compared to the enriched and fortified grains and cereals they replace

Inadequate intake of fiber related to the absence of whole wheat products

Recommended Interventions

Encourage the patient to use as many "normal" items as possible such as grits, rice, and rice cereals; they are easy to obtain and less expensive than special products.

Encourage a varied diet of allowed foods and enriched gluten-free products over non-enriched; recommend a gluten-free, age-appropriate multivitamin and mineral supplement.

Encourage fiber from legumes, nuts, fruit, vegetables, and gluten-free whole grains such as flax seed, millet, uncontaminated oats, quinoa, brown rice, and amaranth.

Patient Teaching

Instruct the patient on the importance of adhering to the diet even when no symptoms are present. "Cheating" on the diet can damage intestinal villi even if no symptoms develop. To permanently eliminate all flours and products containing wheat, rye, barley, triticale, and malt, the patient should

- Read labels. As per the Food Allergen Labeling and Consumer Protection Act of 2004, all food products must be clearly labeled to indicate the presence of wheat. This Act simplifies label reading to identify wheat gluten, but less obvious sources of gluten from barley (e.g., malt flavorings and extracts) require more careful reading. Patients should check with the manufacturer *before* using products of questionable composition.
- Use corn, potato, rice, arrowroot, and soybean flours and their products.
- Use the following as thickening agents: arrowroot starch, cornstarch, tapioca starch, rice starch, and sweet rice flour.
- Eat an otherwise normal, well-balanced diet adequate in nutrients and calories. Lactose is restricted only if not tolerated. Weight gain may be slowly achieved.

  Provide the patient with the following aids:

- A detailed list of foods allowed and not allowed
- Information regarding support groups; see "Websites" section at the end of this chapter
- Gluten-free recipes

Short Bowel Syndrome

Short Bowel Syndrome (SBS)
a complex condition resulting from extensive surgical resection of the intestinal tract resulting in an inadequate absorptive surface that may lead to maldigestion and malabsorption.

Intestinal Failure
the inability to maintain protein-calorie, fluid, electrolyte, or micronutrient balance when on a conventional diet.

Short bowel syndrome (SBS) is one of the most common forms of **intestinal failure**. It occurs when the small bowel is surgically shortened to the extent that the remaining bowel is unable to absorb adequate levels of nutrients to meet the individual's needs. The severity of SBS depends on the length, anatomy, and health of the remaining bowel (Matarese, 2013). Symptoms include diarrhea, steatorrhea, electrolyte imbalances, weight loss, dehydration, and malnutrition related to maldigestion and malabsorption. The most common causes of SBS in adults are small bowel resections from strangulated bowel, CD, ischemia, malignancy, trauma, or malabsorptive bariatric surgery (Wall, 2013).

Nutrition Therapy for Short Bowel Syndrome

Nutrition therapy varies with the length, location, and health of the remaining bowel and over time. Adaptation, a process that increases the absorptive capacity of the remaining small bowel, begins shortly after intestinal resection and may continue for 2 years or longer (Matarese, 2013). In the early months after bowel surgery, PN is the major source of nutrition and hydration until the remaining bowel adapts.

- Patients with an ileocecal valve and colon, even with as little as 50 cm of small bowel, are often able to survive without artificial nutrition support because they are able to adequately absorb fluid and electrolytes and utilize calories from short-chain fatty acids generated by colonic fermentation of unabsorbable carbohydrates. The amount of calories absorbed is proportional to the length of the remaining colon and may increase with adaptation.
- Patients with a small bowel <100 cm that ends in a jejunostomy or ileostomy may need permanent PN and hydration to survive. Loss of the ileum, especially the terminal ileum, is more detrimental than loss of jejunum because it is the only site for absorption of intrinsic factor–bound vitamin B_{12} and bile salts. Disruption of enterohepatic circulation of bile salts leads to severe fat malabsorption and steatorrhea. Rapid gastric emptying and rapid small bowel transit time also occur (Wall, 2013). Patients without a colon are at greater risk of dehydration.

As appropriate, patients should consume a whole-food diet or an intact EN formula as soon as possible for maximum bowel stimulation and adaptation (Matarese, 2013). Continuously infused EN increases macronutrient absorption more than oral feeding alone. When the patient can consume oral nutrition without excessive stool or ostomy output and can maintain or gain weight, the amount of PN is gradually decreased.

In general, calorie needs increase by at least 50% over normal (Matarese, 2013). Table 18.3 outlines medical nutrition therapy for SBS based on the amount of bowel remaining. Other diet modifications are made according to the patient's symptoms/complications (see Table 18.1). Food should be chewed thoroughly, and patients should eat slowly. Fluids should be limited to ½ cup with meals; fluid should be consumed throughout the day but not within an hour before or after eating. A sample menu appears in Box 18.7. Patients are able to return to a 3-meal-per-day eating pattern after adaption occurs.

Table 18.3 Medical Nutrition Therapy for Short Bowel Syndrome

Nutrient	Small Bowel Ostomy	Colonic Continuity
Carbohydrates	50% of total energy; complex carbohydrates including soluble fiber, limit simple sugars	50%–60% of total energy; complex carbohydrates, including soluble fiber
Proteins	20%–30% of total energy	20%–30% of total energy
Fats	≤40% of total energy	20%–30% of total energy
Fluids	ORS important; minimize fluids with meals, sipping of fluids between meals	Minimize fluids with meals, sipping of fluids between meals
Vitamins	Daily multiple vitamin with minerals; monthly vitamin B_{12}; possibly vitamins A, D,* and E supplements	Daily multiple vitamin with minerals; possibly vitamin B_{12}; possibly vitamins A, D, and E supplements
Minerals	Generous use of sodium chloride on food; calcium 1000–1500 mg daily; possibly iron, magnesium, and zinc supplements	400–600 mg calcium with meals; possibly iron, magnesium, and zinc supplements; reduced oxalate
Meals	4–6 small meals	3 small meals plus 2–3 snacks

ORS, oral rehydration solution.
*25-hydroxy vitamin D.
Source: Wall, E. A. (2013). An overview of short bowel syndrome management: Adherence, adaptation, and practical recommendations. *Journal of the Academy of Nutrition and Dietetics, 113*(9), 1200–1208.

BOX 18.7   Sample Menu for Patient with Short Bowel Syndrome

Breakfast

1 slice of white toast with 1 tsp butter and sugar-free jelly
Poached egg
¼ cup orange juice diluted with ¼ cup water

Midmorning Snack

8 oz plain or artificially sweetened Greek yogurt
At least 1 hour later
8 oz Promote (low-fat, lactose-free, high-protein oral formula)

Lunch

2 oz deli turkey with mayonnaise on a ½ white hamburger roll
½ cup canned peaches
½ cup water

Midafternoon Snack

6 saltine crackers
1 oz cheese
At least 1 hour later
8 oz Promote

Dinner

2 oz lean roast beef
½ cup mashed potatoes
½ cup cooked carrots
2 tsp butter
½ cup water
After dinner snack
Rice cake with 1 tbsp creamy peanut butter

Note: Throughout the day, at least 1 hour after eating, an additional 1.5 L fluid or more as needed.

CONDITIONS OF THE LARGE INTESTINE

Irritable Bowel Syndrome

Irritable bowel syndrome (IBS), one of the most frequently diagnosed GI conditions, is a symptom-based disorder defined by the presence of abdominal pain with diarrhea, constipation, or both in the absence of any other disease that may cause these symptoms (Chey, Kurlander, & Eswaran, 2015). Bloating and distention are other common complaints. In the United States, symptoms are 1.5 to 2 times more prevalent in women than in men, with women more commonly reporting abdominal pain and men more commonly reporting diarrhea (Lovell & Ford, 2012). In the United States, there is even distribution in the prevalence of IBS with constipation, IBS with diarrhea, and IBS with a mixed bowel pattern (Guilera, Balboa, & Mearin, 2005). IBS can greatly impair quality of life and work productivity.

IBS may be treated with a variety of therapies, including nutrition therapy. Traditional nutrition therapy strategies have been less than ideal. Anecdotal strategies have been to avoid large meals, alter fiber intake, eat less fat, avoid caffeine and gas-producing foods, and follow an elimination diet to identify potential food intolerances or allergies. Of late, lifestyle and nutrition therapy have become increasingly important treatment options (Chey et al., 2015). For instance, exercise has been shown to improve overall IBS symptoms more than usual treatment (Johannesson, Simrén, Strid, Bajor, & Sadik, 2011). Patients should be encouraged to increase their level of physical activity as tolerated.

Nutrition Therapy for Irritable Bowel Syndrome

As many as 90% of patients with IBS restrict their intake to prevent or improve symptoms (Hayes, Fraher, & Quigley, 2014). True food allergies contribute to only a small number of IBS cases; however, food intolerances are common (Chey et al., 2015). Emerging evidence suggests an **elimination diet** low in fermentable oligosaccharides, disaccharides, monosaccharides, and polyols (FODMAP) (Box 18.8) and a gluten-free diet may be beneficial.

Incomplete digestion of fructose and other short-chain carbohydrates distends the bowel via osmotic effects and rapid fermentation and leads to the production of short-chain fatty acids and gas. In some people with IBS, FODMAPs may result in IBS symptoms (Staudacher, Whelan, Irving, & Lomer, 2011). Tolerance to FODMAPs is dose related; small amounts of FODMAPs may be tolerated, whereas eating beyond a person's threshold causes symptoms to develop. After a period of 6 to 8 weeks, patients

Elimination Diet
a diet that eliminates foods suspected of producing symptoms of intolerance or allergies; suspected foods are added back to the diet individually to identify offending foods.

BOX 18.8 Low-FODMAP Diet

- A low-FODMAP diet limits fruits and fruit juices with high levels of fructose. Fruits and juices that have more glucose and less fructose may be tolerated in measured amounts.
- Because high-fructose corn syrup (HFCS) is half glucose and half fructose, it may be tolerated by some people when consumed in limited amounts.
- Sugar alcohols (polyols) are sorbitol, mannitol, xylitol, and maltitol. Sorbitol is found naturally in certain fruits and fruit juices; this and other sugar alcohols are used as artificial sweeteners in sugar-free gums, mints, and other "diet" foods.

Guidelines to Achieve a Low-FODMAP Diet

- Avoid products that list fructose, crystalline fructose (not HFCS), honey, and sorbitol on the label.
- Avoid sugar alcohols found in "diet" or "dietetic" foods.
- Limit beverages with HFCS to 12 oz or less per day. Consume with food for improved tolerance.
- Fresh or frozen fruit may be better tolerated than canned fruit.
- Cooked vegetables may be better tolerated than raw.
- Fructose and sorbitol may be ingredients in medications. Check with the pharmacist.
- Tolerance is affected by the dose eaten at any one time.
- Avoid lactose if lactose intolerant.

	Foods Low in FODMAP	High-FODMAP Foods to Avoid	Questionable Foods/Foods to Limit
Fruit	Bananas, blackberries, blueberry, grapefruit, honeydew, kiwifruit, lemons, limes, mandarin orange, melons (except watermelon), oranges, passion fruit, pineapple, raspberries, rhubarb, strawberries, tangelos	Fruit: apples, pear, guava, honeydew melon, mango, Asian pear, papaya, quince, star fruit, watermelon Stone fruit: apricots, peaches, cherries, plums, nectarines Fruits high in sugar: grapes, persimmon, lychee Dried fruit Fruit juice Dried fruit bars Fruit pastes and sauces: tomato paste, chutney, plum sauce, sweet and sour sauce, barbecue sauce Fruit juice concentrate	Fruit canned in heavy syrup, other fruits
Vegetables	Bamboo shoots, bok choy, carrots, cauliflower*, celery, cucumber*, eggplant*, green beans*, green peppers*, leafy greens, parsnip, pumpkin, spinach, sweet potatoes, white potatoes, other root vegetables	Onion, leek, garlic, shallots, asparagus, artichokes, cabbage, Brussels sprouts, cauliflower, mushrooms, sugar snap peas, snow peas Legumes and lentils	Avocado, corn, mushrooms, tomatoes, other beans

(continued)

BOX 18.8   Low-FODMAP Diet (continued)

	Foods Low in FODMAP	High-FODMAP Foods to Avoid	Questionable Foods/Foods to Limit
Other	All meats All fats Oats Rice Yogurt and hard cheeses Eggs Aspartame (Equal, NutraSweet) Saccharin (Sweet'N Low) Sugar Glucose Maple syrup	Wheat and wheat products Rye and rye products Pasta made from wheat Cereal made from wheat Cakes, cookies, crackers made from wheat Fortified wines: sherry, port, etc. Chicory-based coffee substitute Honey Certain additives identified on food labels, such as inulin (often labeled as chicory root extract), fructo-oligosaccharides, sorbitol, mannitol, xylitol, maltitol, isomalt Desserts sweetened with fructose or sorbitol (e.g., ice cream, cookies, popsicles)	Items containing HFCS if not tolerated Milk and other sources of lactose if not tolerated

*Possible gas-forming foods that may need to be avoided.

who are able to control their symptoms with complete exclusion of FODMAPs are encouraged to gradually reintroduce eliminated foods so keep restrictions to a minimum.

FODMAPs are found in

- Honey and certain fruits that are high in free fructose. Although eating free fructose causes symptoms, consuming fructose with a near equal concentration of glucose is likely to be well tolerated because glucose promotes the absorption of fructose. That is why fructose from white sugar (composed of equal parts of glucose and fructose) is generally completely absorbed, but fructose from a pear, which contains approximately 4 times more fructose than glucose, is poorly absorbed.
- Wheat, onions, garlic, and inulin (fructans)
- Milk, yogurt, and ice cream (lactose)
- Legumes (galacto-oligosaccharides)
- Certain fruits and sugarless gums, mints, and dietetic foods containing sugar alcohols such as sorbitol, mannitol, or xylitol

Through a randomized clinical trial, Halmos, Power, Shepherd, Gibson, and Muir (2014) found 70% of IBS patients experienced symptom improvement while following a low-FODMAP diet compared to a typical Australian diet regardless of the IBS subtype. Not all FODMAP-containing foods worsen IBS symptoms in all patients, and because there are no defined cutoff values for high- and low-FODMAP foods, there are discrepancies in identifying foods to avoid. Although data are promising, more evidence is needed before a strong recommendation can be made in support of the FODMAP diet (Moayyedi et al., 2015).

A randomized, double-blind, placebo-controlled rechallenge trial of IBS patients with a history of gluten sensitivity found that a gluten-free diet improved symptoms in 40% of patients (Biesiekierski et al., 2011). However, gluten-free means wheat-free, and wheat contains fructans (a FODMAP), which may have been the source of the intolerance. In an Australian study of IBS patients with wheat sensitivity, FODMAPs were more closely associated with symptoms than was gluten (Biesiekierski et al., 2013).

Other nutrition therapy interventions are often used for IBS with varying effectiveness. Soluble fiber (psyllium), but not insoluble fiber (wheat bran), has been associated with improved IBS symptoms, especially in patients with IBS-constipation (Moayyedi et al., 2014). Wheat bran contains FODMAPs, which may aggravate symptoms. Probiotics may be effective in improving overall IBS symptoms and quality of life, but more studies are needed to determine what type, strain, dose, and treatment duration are optimal (Zhang et al., 2016). Peppermint oil improves cramping but may cause GERD or constipation (Chey et al., 2015).

Diverticular Disease

Diverticular disease is a spectrum of conditions in which there are complications from diverticula, such as hemorrhage, inflammation, abscesses, strictures, and fistulas. The most common manifestation of diverticular disease is acute uncomplicated diverticulitis, characterized by inflammation of one or more colonic diverticula without abscess of perforation (Peery, 2016). Even after inflammation from acute diverticulitis is resolved, many patients report that symptoms persist for months to years. Chronic abdominal pain and altered bowel habits occurring after resolution of acute diverticulitis have been termed postdiverticulitis IBS (E. Cohen et al., 2013).

Diverticula
pouches that protrude outward from the muscular wall of the intestine usually in the sigmoid colon.

Diverticulosis
an asymptomatic condition characterized by diverticula.

Diverticulitis
inflammation and infection that occurs when fecal matter gets trapped in the diverticula.

It was a long-standing belief that low-fiber diets caused diverticular disease by increasing pressure within the intestinal lumen leading to mucosal herniation and the formation of **diverticula**. Newer cross-sectional studies suggest low fiber intakes are not associated with an increased risk of **diverticulosis** (Peery et al., 2013). A high intake of red meat has been implicated in the development of symptomatic diverticular disease, possibly by way of altering gut microbiota (De Filippo et al., 2010). Obesity has been shown to increase the risk of **diverticulitis** by 80% (Strate et al., 2009).

Nutrition Therapy for Diverticular Disease

Despite the lack of solid evidence on the role of fiber in its etiology, a high-fiber diet (see Box 18.2) is recommended to prevent diverticular disease based on the theory that soft, bulky stools that are easily passed decrease pressure within the colon. Crowe et al. (2014) observed that a higher intake of fiber is associated with a lower risk of diverticular disease and that cereal and fruit fiber had a stronger effect on reducing risk than did fiber from vegetables or potatoes. Once the diverticula develop, a high-fiber diet cannot make them disappear. A high fiber intake may reduce the risk of hospital admission for diverticular disease (Crowe et al., 2014).

Guidelines for preventing recurrent diverticulitis are extrapolated from what is known about first occurrence risk and incudes the recommendation to consume a high-fiber diet (Stollman, Smalley, & Hirano, 2015). It is common practice for patients to be told to avoid nuts, seeds, and popcorn based on the theory that these can become trapped in diverticula and cause inflammation; yet there is no scientific evidence to support this practice (Strate, Liu, Syngal, Aldoori, & Giovannucci, 2008).

During an acute phase of diverticulitis, patients are given nothing by mouth (NPO) until bleeding and diarrhea subside. Oral intake resumes with clear liquids and progresses to a low-fiber diet until inflammation and bleeding are no longer a risk (AND, 2016). A high-fiber diet is recommended unless symptoms of diverticulitis recur. A daily intake of probiotic and prebiotic foods, such as yogurt, miso, or kefir, may be helpful. Patients who are treated with a low-fiber diet in the hospital may be reluctant to switch to a high-fiber diet on discharge. Diet compliance depends on the patient's understanding of the rationale and benefits of a high-fiber diet for long-term treatment of diverticulosis and prevention of diverticulitis.

Ileostomies and Colostomies

Ileostomy
a surgically created opening (stoma) on the surface of the abdomen from the ileum.

Colostomy
a surgically created opening on the surface of the abdomen from the colon.

An **ileostomy** and a **colostomy** are performed after part or all of the colon, anus, and rectum are removed, usually for treatment of severe IBD, intestinal lesions, obstructions, or colon cancer.

Potential nutritional problems arise because large amounts of fluid, sodium, and potassium are normally absorbed in the colon. The smaller the length of remaining

Effluent
flowing discharge.

colon, the greater is the potential for nutritional problems. For that reason, ileostomies create more problems than colostomies, in which some of the colon is retained.

Effluent from an ileostomy is liquidy; fluid and electrolyte losses are considerable, and the absorption of fat, fat-soluble vitamins, bile acid, and vitamin B_{12} is decreased. Effluent through a colostomy varies from liquid to formed stools, depending on the length of colon that remains. Over time, adaptation occurs.

Nutrition Therapy for Ileostomies and Colostomies

The goals of nutrition therapy for ileostomies and colostomies are to promote healing postoperatively; minimize symptoms; and prevent nutrient deficiencies, dehydration, and electrolyte imbalances. Initially, only clear liquids that are low in simple sugars (e.g., diluted fruit juice, broth, tea) are given to reduce the risk of osmotic diarrhea. The diet is advanced to a low-fiber diet (see Box 18.3) to reduce stool output. Patients need extra protein and calories to promote healing and may have experienced weight loss prior to surgery related to diarrhea or the underlying disease. Fear of eating is common. Within 6 weeks after surgery, the patient should be consuming a near-regular diet. Nutrition therapy guidelines focus on minimizing symptoms (Box 18.9.) Foods not tolerated initially can be reintroduced in a few months.

BOX 18.9 Nutrition Therapy Guidelines for Colostomies and Ileostomies

Colostomies

- Begin with a clear liquid diet; progress to a low-fiber diet. A near-normal diet is generally achieved within 6 weeks.
- Avoid any food not tolerated; reintroduce item after a couple of weeks, 1 at a time.
- Consume adequate fluid: 8–10 cups/day or more.
- Chew food thoroughly because improperly chewed food can cause a stomal blockage.
- Eat meals on a schedule to help promote a regular bowel pattern. Eating the largest meal in the middle of the day and a small evening meal helps to reduce nighttime stool output.
- Avoid practices that may contribute to swallowed air and gas formation.
  - Chewing gum, using a straw, carbonated beverages, smoking, chewing tobacco, eating quickly
- Avoid foods that can cause diarrhea.
  - Foods that are acidic, spicy, fried, greasy, or high in sugar
- Avoid odor and/or gas-causing foods.
  - Alcohol, apples, asparagus, bananas, dried peas and beans, broccoli, Brussels sprouts, cabbage, cauliflower, eggs, fish, dairy products, fatty foods, melons
- Avoid foods that may cause blockage.
  - Bean sprouts, cabbage, celery, coconut, corn, cucumber, dried fruit, grapes, nuts, peas, popcorn, salad greens, seeds, vegetable and fruit skins, whole grains, pineapple
- Add foods that may thicken stool.
  - Applesauce, bananas, banana flakes, cheese, pasta, pectin, potatoes, rice, saltines, tapioca, yogurt, white bread
- Add foods that may decrease odor.
  - Buttermilk, parsley, yogurt, kefir, cranberry juice

Ileostomies: All of the Above Plus

- Initially eat small, frequent meals.
- Avoid beverages with meals if experiencing high output; consume before or after eating.
- Encourage higher salt intake to replenish losses.
- Use oral rehydration beverages to help maintain fluid and electrolyte balance.
- Limit fat if the patient has steatorrhea or diarrhea from a significant ileal resection. MCT oil may be used for calories because it is absorbed without the aid of bile salts.
- Provide supplemental nutrients as needed. Because vitamin B_{12} is normally absorbed in the distal ileum, anemia related to vitamin B_{12} malabsorption can occur in patients with ileostomies, necessitating lifelong parenteral injections or nasal sprays of vitamin B_{12}.

Obtaining adequate fluid and electrolytes is a major concern. A high fluid intake (8–10 cups daily) is needed to replenish losses. A high fluid intake is especially important for ileostomy patients to maintain a normal urine output and minimize the risk of renal calculi. Many patients inaccurately assume that a high fluid intake contributes to diarrhea. Reassure the patient that excess fluid is excreted through the kidneys, not the stoma.

DISORDERS OF THE ACCESSORY GASTROINTESTINAL ORGANS

The liver, pancreas, and gallbladder are known as accessory organs of the GI tract. Although food does not come in direct contact with these organs, they play vital roles in the digestion of macronutrients. Liver disease, pancreatitis, and gallbladder disease are discussed next.

Liver Disease

The liver is a highly active organ involved in the metabolism of almost all nutrients. After absorption, almost all nutrients are transported to the liver, where they are "processed" before being distributed to other tissues. The liver synthesizes plasma proteins, blood clotting factors, and nonessential amino acids and forms urea from the nitrogenous wastes of protein. Triglycerides, phospholipids, and cholesterol are synthesized in the liver, as is bile, an important factor in the digestion of fat. Glucose is synthesized, and glycogen is formed, stored, and broken down as needed. Vitamins and minerals are metabolized, and many are stored in the liver. Finally, the liver is vital for detoxifying drugs, alcohol, ammonia, and other poisonous substances.

Liver damage can have profound and devastating effects on the metabolism of almost all nutrients. It can range from mild and reversible (e.g., fatty liver) to severe and terminal (e.g., hepatic coma). Liver failure can occur from chronic liver disease or secondary to critical illnesses.

The objectives of nutrition therapy for liver disease are to avoid or minimize permanent liver damage, restore optimal nutritional status, alleviate symptoms, and avoid complications. Adequate protein and calories are needed to promote liver cell regeneration. However, regeneration may not be possible if liver damage is extensive.

Fatty Liver Disease

Steatohepatitis
fat accumulation in the liver with inflammation.

Cirrhosis
liver disease that occurs when damaged liver cells are replaced by functionless scar tissue, seriously impairing liver function and disrupting normal blood circulation through the liver.

Fatty liver disease is characterized by abnormal fat deposition in the liver. Fatty liver occurs in the majority of patients with alcoholic liver disease. Nonalcoholic fatty liver disease (NAFLD) is a spectrum of diseases ranging in severity from simple steatosis, which is often asymptomatic and benign, to nonalcoholic **steatohepatitis** (NASH), its progressive subtype. First described in 1980, it is now the leading cause of liver disease in developed nations, affecting an estimated 30% of the adult U.S. population (Rinella, 2015). An estimated 20% of the patients with NAFLD have NASH, which can progress to **cirrhosis** necessitating liver transplantation (McCarthy & Rinella, 2012).

NAFLD is strongly associated with obesity and metabolic syndrome—a cluster of symptoms that include central obesity, insulin resistance, type 2 diabetes, hypertension, and abnormal blood lipid levels. Other causes include exposure to drugs and toxic metals, long-term PN, and GI bypass surgery.

Sustained weight loss is the most effective treatment for NAFLD and should serve as the cornerstone of treatment. Studies show that even a modest weight loss of 5% to 10% of body weight can be enough to improve NAFLD and metabolic syndrome (Naniwadekar, 2010). Modest weight loss of less than 2 pounds per week is associated with a decrease in metabolic syndrome and improvement in the histologic features of NASH in >80% of cases (Kim & Younossi, 2008). A decrease of as little as ~200 cal/day has been shown to improve liver enzymes, fasting glucose, body mass index (BMI), and the degree of hepatic steatosis (M. Yamamoto et al., 2007). The long-term goals are to achieve and maintain healthy body weight.

Although weight loss is the primary goal of nutrition therapy for NAFLD, rapid weight loss (>2.5 pounds per week) should be avoided: Rapid breakdown of adipose tissue can deliver an excessive load of fatty acids to the liver which may worsen liver damage and clinical symptoms (Kargulewicz, Stankowiak-Kulpa, & Grzymishawski, 2014).

Bariatric surgery is considered for patients who are unable to lose weight. Studies show that bariatric surgery can improve or reverse NAFLD, NASH, and fibrosis (Taitano et al., 2015).

Studies indicate the proportion of macronutrients consumed is important. Animal data and observational studies suggest that a high-carbohydrate diet worsens liver injury from NAFLD (McCarthy & Rinella, 2012). A Mediterranean diet, which is recommended for patients with metabolic syndrome, is prudent for patients with NAFLD. A summary of proposed lifestyle guidelines for NAFLD/NASH appears in Table 18.4.

Hepatitis

Hepatitis
inflammation of the liver that may be caused by viral infections, alcohol abuse, and hepatotoxic chemicals such as chloroform and carbon tetrachloride.

Although fatty liver can cause **hepatitis**, the most frequent causes are infection from hepatitis viruses A, B, and C. Early symptoms of hepatitis include anorexia, nausea and vomiting, fever, fatigue, headache, and weight loss. Later, symptoms such as dark-colored urine, jaundice, liver tenderness, and, possibly, liver enlargement may develop. In many cases, particularly those caused by hepatitis A, liver cell damage that occurs from acute hepatitis is reversible with proper rest and adequate nutrition.

Patients with acute hepatitis may have difficulty consuming an adequate intake because of anorexia, early satiety, and fatigue. Generally, patients need 30 to 35 cal/kg of body weight and 1.0 to 1.2 g protein/kg body weight (AND, 2016). A balanced pattern with between-meal feedings of oral nutrition supplements may help ensure an adequate intake. Sodium is restricted for patients with ascites, and fat is limited to <30% of total calories if steatorrhea is present.

Sometimes, acute hepatitis advances to chronic hepatitis, especially when hepatitis is caused by hepatitis C. For people with chronic hepatitis, dietary restrictions are usually not necessary unless symptoms interfere with nutrient intake or utilization.

Table 18.4   Proposed Lifestyle Guidelines for Patients with Nonalcoholic Fatty Liver Disease/Nonalcoholic Steatohepatitis

Guidelines	Rationale
Limit calories to 1200–1500 cal/day.	Promotes gradual weight loss which lowers liver enzymes and improves metabolic syndrome risks and the degree of hepatic steatosis
Lower total carbohydrate intake to 40%–50% of total calories.	Improves levels of circulating insulin, fasting triglycerides, and hepatic fat
Avoid high-fructose corn syrup.	HFCS, primarily from soft drinks, is associated with complications of metabolic syndrome and an increase in liver enzymes
Consider a Mediterranean-style eating pattern rich in monounsaturated fat.	May reduce the risks of metabolic syndrome and NAFLD
Increase omega-3 fatty acid intake through food and/or supplements.	May improve dyslipidemia
Consider vitamin E supplement of 800 IU/day.	Shown to improve liver histology; however, some studies show increased all-cause mortality from ≥400 IU vitamin E per day. Caution is advised.
Increase moderate-vigorous physical activity to at least 150 minute/week; aerobic exercise 5 times per week, resistance training ≥2 times per week.	Improves liver enzymes independent of weight loss; should be part of any healthy lifestyle

HFCS, high-fructose corn syrup; NAFLD, nonalcoholic fatty liver disease.
Source: McCarthy, E., & Rinella, M. (2012). The role of diet and nutrient composition in nonalcoholic fatty liver disease. *Journal of the Academy of Nutrition and Dietetics, 112,* 401–409.

Cirrhosis

Scarring from chronic hepatitis can lead to cirrhosis. Liver damage progresses slowly, and some patients are asymptomatic. Early nonspecific symptoms include fever, anorexia, weight loss, and fatigue. Glucose intolerance is common. Later, portal hypertension, dyspepsia, diarrhea or constipation, jaundice, esophageal varices, hemorrhoids, ascites, edema, bleeding tendencies, anemia, hepatomegaly, and splenomegaly may develop. Malnutrition is common and a major risk factor for mortality (Bajaj, 2010). It may be related to impaired intake, impaired absorption, altered metabolism, or iatrogenic causes.

Nutrition therapy recommendations are to

- Increase calories
- Provide 0.8 to 1.2 g protein/kg/day
- Limit fat to <30% of total calories if the patient has steatorrhea
- Control carbohydrates if the patient is glucose intolerant
- Small frequent meals may help maximize intake. Oral nutrition supplements may improve overall intake.
- Provide a soft, low fiber, or liquid texture if the patient has esophageal varices
- Limit sodium to <2000 mg/day if the patient has ascites or edema
- A fluid restriction may be necessary based on serum sodium level
- Vitamin and mineral supplements may be needed
- EN support may be necessary

The liver "fails" when liver cell loss is extensive. Ominous changes in mental function, such as impaired memory and concentration, slow response time, drowsiness, irritability, flapping tremor, and fecal odor of the breath, signal **hepatic encephalopathy**, which may progress to **hepatic coma**. Although the exact cause of these central nervous system (CNS) changes is unknown, a high serum ammonia level plays a major role because it affects cerebral edema and neurotransmitter function (Caruana & Shah, 2011).

Hepatic Encephalopathy
the CNS manifestations of advanced liver disease characterized by irritability, short-term memory loss, and impaired ability to concentrate.

Hepatic Coma
unconsciousness caused by severe liver disease.

Historically, protein restriction was used to reduce the risk from hepatic encephalopathy; however, restricting protein may worsen nutrition status, decrease lean muscle mass, and lead to less ammonia removal (McClave et al., 2016). Therefore, protein recommendations are the same as for other critically ill patients: 1.2 to 2.0 g/kg actual body weight per day. There is no evidence that using a hepatic enteral formula enriched with branch chain amino acids improves mental status in patients with hepatic encephalopathy who are already receiving antibiotics and lactulose.

Liver Transplantation

Nutrition Therapy for Liver Transplantation

Liver transplantation is a treatment option for patients with severe and irreversible liver disease. Many patients awaiting a transplant are malnourished. Moderate to severe malnutrition increases the risk of complications and death after transplantation. Whenever possible, nutrient deficiencies and imbalances are corrected before the transplantation to promote a positive outcome.

There is not one specific posttransplant diet. Nutrient recommendations vary with the posttransplant stage and are individualized according to the patient's nutritional status, weight, tolerance, and laboratory values. Eating resumes as soon as possible after surgery. Calorie and protein needs are increased from the stress of surgery. Small, frequent meals and commercial supplements may help maximize intake. Vitamin and mineral supplements are ordered. Although oral nutrition is the preferred route, EN support is used if the patient is unable to consume adequate nutrition for 5 to 7 days.

After the initial hypermetabolic period, the patient's calorie and protein needs return toward normal. Long-term complications associated with immunosuppressive therapy, such as excessive weight gain, hypertension, hyperlipidemia, osteopenic bone disease, and diabetes, may require nutrition therapy. The use of immunosuppressant drugs elevates the importance of safe food handling practices to avoid foodborne illness.

Pancreatitis

The pancreas is responsible for secreting enzymes needed to digest dietary carbohydrates, protein, and fat. Until they are needed, these enzymes are held in the pancreas in their inactive form. Inflammation of the pancreas causes digestive enzymes to be retained in the pancreas and converted to their active form, so they literally begin to digest the pancreas. Because the pancreas also produces insulin, people with **pancreatitis** may also develop hyperglycemia related to insufficient insulin secretion.

Pancreatitis
inflammation of the pancreas.

Acute Pancreatitis

Acute pancreatitis, a potentially life-threatening disease, is a leading cause of hospitalization worldwide (Zhao et al., 2015). Alcohol abuse and gallstones account for more than 70% of cases of acute pancreatitis (Owyang, 2008). Other causes include hypertriglyceridemia ($\geq$1000 mg/dL), cystic fibrosis, renal failure, and the use of certain medications. Many cases are iatrogenic. Patients present with acute abdominal pain in the upper quadrant, nausea, and vomiting. Levels of serum **amylase** and **lipase** are elevated. Mild acute pancreatitis usually resolves in a few days without permanent damage. Severe acute pancreatitis occurs in 15% to 20% of acute pancreatitis cases and carries a high mortality rate (Tenner, Baillie, DeWitt, & Vege, 2013)

Amylase
a class of enzymes that split starch molecules.

Lipase
an enzyme that splits fat molecules.

Nutrition Therapy for Acute Pancreatitis

Traditionally, initial treatment of mild acute pancreatitis included fasting for the first few days with IV fluids followed by a clear liquid diet after abdominal pain resolved and serum levels of pancreatic enzymes normalized. Clear liquids were then gradually advanced to a soft or solid low-fat diet over 3 to 7 days to avoid pain and relapse. The patient's tolerance to solid food was the basis for hospital discharge. However, there is little evidence to support this feeding strategy.

Emerging data suggest that it is not necessary to delay feedings until pancreatic enzyme levels normalize and abdominal pain is resolved. A randomized controlled trial by Li et al. (2013) found that early oral refeeding based on hunger in patients with mild acute pancreatitis was safe and reduced the length of hospital stay. It is recommended oral feedings begin when pain is decreasing and inflammatory markers are improving (Working Group International Association of Pancreatology [IAP]/American Pancreatic Association [APA], 2013). EN is considered when an oral diet is not instituted within 7 days (McClave et al., 2016).

Likewise, the necessity of initiating feedings with a clear liquid diet has also been challenged: Studies show that in patients with mild acute pancreatitis, a soft diet as the initial meal is well tolerated and leads to a shorter total length of hospitalization without an increase in adverse effects (Rajkumar, Karthikeyan, Ali, Sistla, & Kate, 2013). Moraes et al. (2010) found that an initial feeding of a full solid diet is safe and reduces length of hospitalization when compared to a clear liquid or soft diet.

For patients with severe acute pancreatitis, recommendations are to (McClave et al., 2016)

- Initiate EN at a trophic rate and advance to goal as fluid volume resuscitation is completed, within 24 to 48 hours. Delaying initiating of EN beyond the first 72 to 96 hours increases the risk of rapid deterioration in nutritional status and its complications. Compared to PN, EN has a better risk/benefit ratio, including lower infectious morbidity, length of hospital stay, and mortality.
- Use either the gastric or jejunal route for feeding. Tolerance and clinical outcomes do not vary between these two routes.
- Select a standard polymeric formula. Studies are needed to determine whether an immune-modulating formula would be beneficial.
- Consider PN after 1 week when EN is contraindicated or not feasible.

The optimal criteria for initiating oral feedings in patients with severe acute pancreatitis are not known. As with mild acute pancreatitis, studies in patients with severe acute pancreatitis have demonstrated that initiating feeding based on the patient's hunger, not the resolution of abdominal pain or normalization of pancreatic enzyme levels, decreased the duration of fasting and the length of hospitalization (Zhao et al., 2015). In addition, there was no difference in

BOX 18.11 Low-Fat Diet (continued)

Food preparation techniques to reduce fat content

- Trim fat from meat and remove skin from chicken before cooking.
- Place meats to be baked or roasted on a rack to allow the fat to drain.
- Bake, broil, steam, or sauté foods in a vegetable cooking spray or allowed fats.
- Cook with bouillon, lemon, vinegar, wine, herbs, and spices instead of adding fat.
- Make fat-free soup stock by preparing the stock a day ahead and refrigerating it overnight. The fat will harden and can easily be removed from the surface. Make fat-free gravies also by this method.
- Purchase "select" grade meats because they are lower in fat than "choice" and "prime" grades.

Cholecystitis
inflammation of the gallbladder.

symptoms; for others, symptoms develop during sleep. Gallstones that obstruct the cystic duct can lead to **cholecystitis**, causing abdominal pain, nausea and vomiting, jaundice, fever, fat intolerance, and flatulence. Surgical removal of the gallbladder may be used to treat symptomatic gallstones. After the gallbladder is removed, the common bile duct collects and holds bile until mealtime when it is released into the duodenum.

No diet modifications are necessary for healthy people with asymptomatic gallstones. Patients with symptomatic gallstones may be advised to consume a low-fat diet (<30% total calories from fat) based on the rationale that limiting fat intake reduces stimulation to the gallbladder and minimizes pain. Although some patients' symptoms are aggravated by consuming fat, it is not known if patients with gallstones are any more intolerant of fat than the general population. Patients are encouraged to avoid individual food intolerances.

There is not a standard guideline for nutrition therapy after a cholecystectomy (Marcason, 2014). Total fat intake and the amount of fat at each meal should be limited for several months to allow the body time to adapt to the gallbladder's absence (Box 18.11). Fat intake is gradually increased as tolerated. Increasing fiber may help normalize bowel function in patients with diarrhea that may occur from the laxative effect of nonconcentrated bile continuously draining into the intestines. Increasing soluble fiber intake may help prevent gastritis related to the presence of bile in the stomach. Sources of soluble fiber include canned fruit; fresh fruit without skins, peels, membranes, and/or seeds; oatmeal; and barley. Small meals are recommended if reflux is a problem.

NURSING PROCESS

Crohn Disease

Andrew is a 20-year-old man who is admitted to the hospital for suspected CD. His chief complaints are crampy abdominal pain, diarrhea, weight loss, fatigue, and anorexia. He has lost 15 pounds since his symptoms began 2 weeks ago. He is prescribed IV fluids, sulfasalazine, prednisone, an antidiarrheal medication, and a diet as tolerated.

Assessment

Medical–Psychosocial History
- Medical and surgical history
- Use of prescribed and over-the-counter medications
- Support system

Anthropometric Assessment
- Height, current weight, usual weight; percentage weight loss; body mass index (BMI)

NURSING PROCESS   Crohn Disease

Biochemical and Physical Assessment	• Hemoglobin (Hgb), hematocrit (Hct) • Serum electrolyte levels • Blood pressure • Signs of dehydration (poor skin turgor, dry mucous membranes, etc.)
Dietary Assessment	• How has your intake changed since you began experiencing symptoms? • Do you know if any particular foods cause problems? Did you have any food intolerances or allergies before your symptoms began? • How many meals per day are you eating? • How much fluid are you drinking in a day? • Have you ever followed any kind of diet before? • Do you take vitamins, minerals, or other supplements? • Do you use alcohol? • Who prepares your meals?

Diagnosis

Possible Nursing Diagnoses	Imbalanced nutrition: eating less than the body needs related to diarrhea and altered ability to digest and absorb nutrients.

Planning

Client Outcomes	The client will • Consume adequate calories and protein to restore normal weight • Experience improvement in symptoms (diarrhea, abdominal pain, fatigue, anorexia) • Restore normal fluid balance • Describe the principles and rationale of nutrition therapy for CD and implement the appropriate interventions

Nursing Interventions

Nutrition Therapy	• Provide a low-fat, low-fiber, high-protein, lactose-restricted diet as tolerated. • Provide lactose-free commercial supplements between meals to enhance protein and calorie intake. • Encourage high fluid intake, especially of fluids high in potassium such as tomato juice, apricot nectar, and orange juice. • Promote gradual return to normal diet as tolerated.
Client Teaching	Instruct the client • On the purpose and rationale of a low-fat, low-fiber, lactose-restricted diet; advise the patient that he may be able to tolerate fiber and milk after the disease goes into remission • On the importance of consuming adequate protein, calories, and fluid to promote healing and recovery • To maximize intake by eating small, frequent meals • To avoid colas and other sources of caffeine because they stimulate peristalsis • To eliminate individual intolerances • To chew food thoroughly and avoid swallowing air • On the importance of consuming adequate fluid while taking sulfasalazine • That prednisone should improve his appetite but may cause fluid retention and gastrointestinal upset • To communicate any side effects he experiences from the medications

Evaluation

Evaluate and Monitor	• Intake and output; fluid and electrolyte status • Percentage of food consumed • Tolerance to fat (may need to reduce fat level) • Diarrhea (if patient does not tolerate an oral diet, determine whether a defined formula EN feeding is appropriate) and other symptoms • Weight changes and BMI

How Do You Respond?

Is it a good idea to detox or cleanse the gut? Not only is it unnecessary to detox or cleanse the gut, it is also potentially harmful based on the regimen used, such as consuming only juices or water for several days, fasting, taking specific supplements, irrigating the colon, or using enemas or laxatives. The body eliminates toxins through the lungs, kidneys, colon, lymph system, and the liver. There is no convincing evidence that detox or cleansing actually removes toxins from the body or improves health.

Are "live active cultures" the same thing as probiotics? Live active cultures are microorganisms associated with foods that are often used to ferment food. For instance, live active cultures in yogurt refer to the mixture of bacterial species, such as *Lactobacillus acidophilus*, *Lactobacillus bulgaricus*, and *Lactobacillus casei*, that ferment milk into yogurt. Some live active cultures do not survive the fermentation process. By definition, probiotics are live microorganisms that have been shown to benefit health when consumed in adequate amounts. Some yogurts contain therapeutic doses of probiotics to provide a health benefit, such as to prevent or treat acute diarrhea.

REVIEW CASE STUDY

Brittany is a 33-year-old woman who was recently diagnosed with IBS. She alternates between episodes of diarrhea and constipation and complains of distention and abdominal pain. Her doctor suggested she eat more fiber and take Metamucil. She dislikes whole wheat bread. She is reluctant to take a fiber supplement; she knows fiber helps people with constipation, and because she also has diarrhea, she believes it will only make her problem worse. She is thinking about adding yogurt to her usual diet to see if that helps. She drinks an "irritable bowel syndrome–friendly tea" that is supposed to help, but she hasn't noticed any improvement.

Her usual intake is as follows:

Breakfast: Orange juice; white toast with peanut butter; coffee
Snacks: Small bag of chips from the vending machine
Lunch: Fast-food hamburger on a bun; small French fries; diet coke
Snacks: Cheese and crackers; glass of wine
Dinner: Beef or chicken; mashed potatoes; broccoli; tossed salad with Italian dressing; ice cream; coffee
Snacks: Milk and cookies, apples

- What does Brittany need to know about fiber and bowel function? What would you say to her about eating more fiber? About taking a fiber supplement? About yogurt? And about "irritable bowel syndrome–friendly tea"?
- What else do you need to know about Brittany to help relieve her symptoms?
- What other diet interventions could she implement to try to improve her symptoms?
- What foods does Brittany consume that are high in FODMAPs?

STUDY QUESTIONS

1 When developing a teaching plan for a patient who has chronic diarrhea, which of the following foods would the nurse suggest as an appropriate source of potassium?
   a. Tomato juice
   b. Pinto beans
   c. Milk
   d. Broccoli

2 Which statement indicates the patient with an ileostomy needs further instruction about what to eat?
   a. "Drinking lots of water increases the output from my ileostomy."
   b. "It is best to eat a small evening meal."
   c. "Oatmeal and bananas may help control diarrhea."
   d. "A regular eating schedule will help regulate my bowel pattern."

3 The client asks if yogurt with probiotics will relieve her symptoms of irritable bowel syndrome. Which of the following would be the nurse's best response?
   a. "Unfortunately, there isn't anything that will help relieve irritable bowel syndrome."
   b. "Although it is not guaranteed to help, probiotics may help and do not pose a health risk in healthy people."
   c. "Because little is known about the effects of probiotics on health, you should avoid consuming them."
   d. "Probiotics are the only dietary intervention known to help irritable bowel syndrome."

4 The nurse knows his or her instructions have been effective when the client with celiac disease verbalizes that an appropriate breakfast is
   a. Eggs and toast
   b. Grits with berries
   c. Bran flakes cereal with milk
   d. Buttermilk pancakes with syrup

5 Which of the following would be most appropriate in modifying a regular diet to a high-fiber diet?
   a. Ice cream in place of gelatin
   b. Apple in place of apple juice
   c. Rice in place of mashed potatoes
   d. Cream of wheat in place of cream of rice

6 Which of the following may be an appropriate source of calcium for a client who is lactose intolerant?
   a. Aged cheddar cheese
   b. Pudding
   c. Lean meats
   d. Refined breads and cereals

7 A client with fat malabsorption is at risk for which of the following?
   a. Calcium oxalate kidney stones
   b. Constipation
   c. Deficiencies of essential amino acids
   d. Type 2 diabetes

8 Which of the following strategies would help a client achieve a low-fat diet?
   a. Substitute margarine for butter.
   b. Limit portion sizes of meat.
   c. Substitute whole wheat bread for white bread.
   d. Eat more fruit in place of vegetables.

KEY CONCEPTS

- The first half of the small intestine is the site where most nutrients are absorbed. Conditions that affect the small intestine can impair the absorption of one or many nutrients.
- The large intestine absorbs water and electrolytes. Disorders of the colon can cause major problems with fluid and electrolyte balance.
- Most cases of constipation can be alleviated or prevented by increasing fiber and fluid intake. The amount of fiber needed to promote bowel regularity varies among people.
- To achieve a high-fiber diet, high-fiber foods are eaten in place of those low in fiber, such as whole wheat bread for white bread, high-fiber cereal for refined cereal, and whole fruits for fruit juices. Other sources of fiber include dried peas and beans, vegetables, nuts, and seeds.

- Other than encouraging fluids and foods high in potassium, nutrition therapy usually is not necessary for acute diarrhea of short-term duration. Because many clear liquids are hyperosmolar and may contribute to osmotic diarrhea, they should be avoided until diarrhea subsides. Foods that help thicken stools, such as bananas and oatmeal, are encouraged. Patients should avoid items that stimulate peristalsis, such as caffeine; alcohol; and high-fiber, gassy foods.
- A low-fiber diet is appropriate only for short-term use. Its effect is to decrease stimulation to the bowel and slow intestinal transit time.
- Lactase nonpersistence is common in much of the world's adult population; tolerance varies considerably among individuals. Some people tolerate milk with food, whereas

others tolerate only lactose-reduced milk. Lactose malabsorption that occurs secondary to intestinal disorders is usually more symptomatic than lactase nonpersistence and requires a more restrictive intake.

- During exacerbation of IBDs, patients need increased amounts of calories and protein and may not tolerate fiber and lactose. Patients are often reluctant to eat, fearing that food will cause pain and diarrhea. Some patients with CD require EN or PN for bowel rest. During remission, the diet is liberalized as tolerated.
- A gluten-free diet prevents intestinal villi changes, steatorrhea, and other symptoms in patients with celiac disease. All forms and sources of wheat, rye, and barley must be permanently eliminated from the diet, even in patients who are asymptomatic. Pure oats may or may not be tolerated. A gluten-free diet requires major lifestyle changes and is difficult to follow. Some patients do not respond to a gluten-free diet, but that may be because they have not closely adhered to the diet.
- People with NCGS develop celiac-like symptoms in response to eating gluten even though they do not have the diagnostic features of celiac disease. It is not known how long or how strictly they should adhere to a gluten-free diet.
- SBS occurs in patients who have a significant portion of the small intestine removed. Maldigestion and associated diarrhea causes an excessive loss of nutrients and fluid and may lead to malnutrition and chronic dehydration. PN is usually used until adaptation begins, although some patients need PN permanently. Patients need to eat as soon as possible to stimulate the bowel and promote adaptation. Tolerance to fat, lactose, and sugar is impaired.
- IBS is a common but not serious disorder. Soluble fiber and/or low-lactose diet may help relieve symptoms in some people. Research on the benefits of probiotics and prebiotics is encouraging but not conclusive. A low-FODMAP diet may offer the most significant and sustained improvement in IBS symptoms but more research is needed.

- Obesity and a high intake of red meat are implicated in the development of symptomatic diverticular disease. During acute diverticulitis, patients may be given a low-fiber diet to reduce bowel stimulation. A high-fiber diet may be recommended to prevent diverticular disease.
- Fluid and electrolytes are of primary concern for patients with ileostomies and colostomies. Low-fiber foods may help to reduce stoma discharge and irritation. Additional calories and protein are needed to promote healing.
- Gradual and sustained weight loss is the most effective treatment of NAFLD. A Mediterranean diet can improve abnormalities of the metabolic syndrome and reduce hepatic steatosis.
- Adequate calories and protein promote liver cell regeneration in patients with hepatitis and cirrhosis. Sodium and fluid may be restricted if ascites develop. A liquid or soft diet is recommended if regular textured foods irritate esophageal varices.
- People who have undergone liver transplantation have high protein and calorie needs. Glucose intolerance may occur, and sodium intake may be restricted depending on the individual's profile. Immunosuppressant drugs may interfere with intake and appetite.
- It is safe and beneficial for patients with mild acute pancreatitis to consume an oral intake when pain begins to subside and enzyme levels begin to normalize. A soft or even regular diet is preferred over a clear liquid diet.
- Patients with severe acute pancreatitis should receive EN as soon as possible to avoid rapid deterioration in their nutritional status.
- People with CP should consume a normal fat intake, which is an important source of calories. PERT taken with meals and snacks allows for a normal fat intake. Patients who develop glucose intolerance may benefit from a carbohydrate-controlled diet.
- A common practice is to recommend a low-fat diet for patients with symptomatic gallstones and for people who have had a cholecystectomy.

Check Your Knowledge Answer Key

1 **TRUE** For most people, consuming more fiber and fluid prevents or alleviates constipation.

2 **FALSE** A clear liquid diet contains items that are hyperosmolar, such as sweetened carbonated beverages, fruit juice, and flavored ices; consuming them may contribute to osmotic diarrhea.

3 **TRUE** Probiotics may help lessen diarrhea, especially diarrhea related to use of antibiotics.

4 **TRUE** Because most of the lactose in cheddar and other natural, aged cheeses has been converted to lactic acid or removed in the cheese-making process, most people who are lactose intolerant can tolerate cheddar and other aged cheeses.

5 **FALSE** Eating a low-fiber diet is not necessary for people with IBD except during acute exacerbation or if there are strictures.

6 **TRUE** For a patient with celiac disease, the long-term effects of eating even small amounts of gluten are harmful, even when patients are asymptomatic.

7 **FALSE** The most beneficial nutrition intervention for NAFLD is to promote gradual, sustained weight loss, which improves fasting glucose, BMI, and the degree of hepatic steatosis.

8 **TRUE** Obesity is an important risk factor for developing symptomatic diverticular disease.

9 **FALSE** A normal fat intake of 30% to 40% of total calories is usually well tolerated and is important for total calorie intake. PERT enables patients with CP to tolerate fat.

10 **FALSE** Gallstones may be asymptomatic. It is not certain that people with symptomatic gallstones are more intolerant of fat than the general population.

Websites

Celiac Disease Foundation at www.celiac.org

Celiac Sprue Association/USA at http://csaceliacs.org

Crohn's and Colitis Foundation of America at www.ccfa.org

Gluten Intolerance Group at www.gluten.net

Information on prebiotics and probiotics is available at www.usprobiotics .org, a nonprofit research and educational website made possible by the California Dairy Research Foundation and Dairy & Food Culture Technologies.

National Digestive Diseases Information Clearinghouse at http:// digestive.niddk.nih.gov

United Ostomy Associations of America, Inc. at www.uoa.org

References

Academy of Nutrition and Dietetics. (2016). *Nutrition care manual.* Available at https://www.nutritioncaremanual.org/. Accessed on 6/25/16.

Alastair, F., Emma, G., & Emma, P. (2011). Nutrition in inflammatory bowel disease. *Journal of Parenteral and Enteral Nutrition, 35,* 571–580. doi:10.1177/0148607111413599

Bajaj, J. (2010). Review article: The modern management of hepatic encephalopathy. *Alimentary Pharmacology & Therapeutics, 31,* 537–547.

Biesiekierski, J., Newnham, E., Irving, P., Barrett, J. S., Haines, M., Doecke, J. D., . . . Gibson, P. R. (2011). Gluten causes gastrointestinal symptoms in subjects without celiac disease: A double-blind randomized placebo-controlled trial. *The American Journal of Gastroenterology, 106,* 508–514.

Biesiekierski, J., Peters, S., Newnham, E., Rosella, O., Muir, J. G., & Gibson, P. R. (2013). No effects of gluten in patients with self-reported non-celiac gluten sensitivity after dietary reduction of fermentable, poorly absorbed, short-chain carbohydrates. *Gastroenterology, 145,* 320.e1–e3–328.e1–e3

Caruana, P., & Shah, N. (2011). Hepatic encephalopathy: Are NH_4 levels and protein restriction obsolete? *Practical Gastroenterology, 95,* 6–18.

Chey, W., Kurlander, J., & Eswaran, S. (2015). Irritable bowel syndrome: A clinical review. *JAMA, 313,* 949–958.

Cohen, A., Lee, D., Long, M., Kappelman, M. D., Martin, C. F., Sandler, R. S., & Lewis, J. D. (2013). Dietary patterns and self-reported associations of diet with symptoms of inflammatory bowel disease. *Digestive Diseases and Sciences, 58,* 1322–1328.

Cohen, E., Fuller, G., Bolus, R., Modi, R., Vu, M., Shahedi, K., . . . Spiegel, B. (2013). Increased risk for irritable bowel syndrome after acute diverticulitis. *Clinical Gastroenterology and Hepatology, 11,* 1614–1619.

Crowe, F., Balkwill, A., Cairns, B., Appleby, P. N., Green, J., Reeves, G. K., . . . Beral, V. (2014). Source of dietary fibre and diverticular disease incidence: A prospective study of UK women. *Gut, 63,* 1450–1456.

De Filippo, C., Cavalieri, D., Di Paola, M., Ramazzotti, M., Poullet J. B., Massart, S., . . . Lionetti, P. (2010). Impact of diet in shaping gut microbiota revealed by a comparative study in children from Europe and rural Africa. *Proceedings of the National Academy of Sciences of the United States of America, 107,* 14691–14696.

Fasano, A., Sapone, A., Zevallos, V., & Schuppan, D. (2015). Nonceliac gluten sensitivity. *Gastroenterology, 148,* 1195–1204.

Gheorghe, C., Seicean, A., Saftoiu, A., Tantau, M., Dumitru, E., Jinga, M., . . . Diculescu, M. (2015). Romanian guidelines on the diagnosis and treatment of exocrine pancreatic insufficiency. *Journal of Gastrointestinal and Liver Diseases, 24,* 117–123.

Goldenberg, J., Ma, S. S. Y., Saxton, J., Martzen, M. R., Vandvik, P. O., Thorlund, K., . . . Johnston, B. C. (2013). Probiotics for the prevention of *Clostridium difficile*-associated diarrhea in adults and children. *Cochrane Database of Systematic Reviews,* (5), CD006095.

Guilera, M., Balboa, A., & Mearin, F. (2005). Bowel habit subtypes and temporal patterns in irritable bowel syndrome: Systematic review. *The American Journal of Gastroenterology, 100,* 1174–1184.

Halmos, E., Power, V., Shepherd, S., Gibson, P. R., & Muir, J. G. (2014). A diet low in FODMAPs reduces symptoms of irritable bowel syndrome. *Gastroenterology, 146,* 67.e5–75.e5.

Hayes, P., Fraher, M., & Quigley, E. (2014). Irritable bowel syndromes: The role of food in pathogenesis and management. *Gastroenterology & Hepatology, 10,* 164–174.

Heaney, R. (2013). Dairy intake, dietary adequacy, and lactose intolerance. *Advances in Nutrition, 4,* 151–156.

Hempel, S., Newberry, S., Maher, A., Wang, Z., Miles, J. N., Shanman, R., . . . Shekelle, P. G. (2012). Probiotics for the prevention and treatment of antibiotic-associated diarrhea: A systematic review and meta-analysis. *JAMA, 307,* 1959–1969.

Hertzler, S., & Savaiano, D. (1996). Colonic adaptation to daily lactose feeding in lactose maldigesters reduces lactose intolerance. *The American Journal of Clinical Nutrition, 64,* 232–236.

Hou, J., Lee, D., & Lewis, J. (2014). Diet and inflammatory bowel disease: Review of patient-targeted recommendations. *Clinical Gastroenterology and Hepatology, 12,* 1592–1600.

Johannesson, E., Simrén, M., Strid, H., Bajor, A., & Sadik, R. (2011). Physical activity improves symptoms in irritable bowel syndrome: A randomized controlled trial. *The American Journal of Gastroenterology, 106,* 915–922.

Kargulewicz, A., Stankowiak-Kulpa, H., & Grzymishawski, M. (2014). Dietary recommendations for patients with nonalcoholic fatty liver disease. *Przegląd Gastroenterologiczny, 9,* 18–23.

Kim, C., & Younossi, Z. (2008). Nonalcoholic fatty liver disease: A manifestation of the metabolic syndrome. *Cleveland Clinic Journal of Medicine, 75,* 721–728.

Koerner, T., Cléroux, C., Poirier, C., Cantin, I., Alimkulov, A., & Elamparo, H. (2011). Gluten contamination in the Canadian commercial oat supply. *Food Additives & Contaminants. Part A, Chemistry, Analysis, Control, Exposure & Risk Assessment, 28,* 705–710.

La Vieille, S., Pulido, O., Abbott, M., Koerner T. B., & Godefroy, S. (2016). Celiac disease and gluten-free oats: A Canadian position based on a literature review. *Canadian Journal of Gastroenterology & Hepatology, 2016,* 1870305. doi:10.1155/2016/1870305

Leffler, D., & Schuppan, D. (2010). Update on serologic testing in celiac disease. *The American Journal of Gastroenterology, 105,* 2520–2524.

Li, J., Xue, G., Liu, Y., Javed, M. A., Zhao, X. L., Wan, M. H., . . . Tang, W. F. (2013). Early oral refeeding wisdom in patients with mild acute pancreatitis. *Pancreas, 42*, 88–91.

Lovell, R., & Ford, A. (2012). Effect of gender on prevalence of irritable bowel syndrome in the community: Systematic review and meta-analysis. *The American Journal of Gastroenterology, 107*, 991–1000.

Ludvigsson, J. (2012). Mortality and malignancy in celiac disease. *Gastrointestinal Endoscopy Clinics of North America, 22*, 705–722.

Lundin, K., & Alaedini, A. (2012). Non-celiac gluten sensitivity. *Gastrointestinal Endoscopy Clinics of North America, 22*, 723–734.

Marcason, W. (2014). What medical nutrition therapy guideline is recommended post-cholecystectomy? *Journal of the Academy of Nutrition and Dietetics, 114*, 1136.

Massironi, S., Rossi, R., Cavalcoli, F., Della Valle, S., Fraquelli, M., & Conte, D. (2013). Nutritional deficiencies in inflammatory bowel disease: Therapeutic approaches. *Clinical Nutrition, 32*, 904–910.

Matarese, L. (2013). Nutrition and fluid optimization for patients with short bowel syndrome. *Journal of Parenteral and Enteral Nutrition, 37*, 161–170.

McCarthy, E., & Rinella, M. (2012). The role of diet and nutrient composition in nonalcoholic fatty liver disease. *Journal of the Academy of Nutrition and Dietetics, 112*, 401–409.

McClave, S., Taylor, B., Martindale, R., Warren, M. M., Johnson, D. R., Braunschweig, C., . . . Compher, C. (2016). Guidelines for the provision and assessment of nutrition support therapy in the adult critically ill patient: Society of Critical Care Medicine (SCCM) and American Society for Parenteral and Enteral Nutrition (A.S.P.E.N.). *Journal of Parenteral and Enteral Nutrition, 40*, 159–211.

Misselwitz, B., Pohl, D., Frühauf, H., Fried, M., Vavricka, S. R., & Fox, M. (2013). Lactose malabsorption and intolerance: Pathogenesis, diagnosis and treatment. *United European Gastroenterology Journal, 1*(3), 151–159.

Moayyedi, P., Quigley, E., Lacy, B., Lembo, A. J., Saito, Y. A., Schiller, L. R., . . . Ford, A. C. (2014). The effect of fiber supplementation on irritable bowel syndrome: A systematic review and meta-analysis. *The American Journal of Gastroenterology, 109*, 1367–1374.

Moayyedi, P., Quigley, E., Lacy, B., Lembo, A. J., Saito, Y. A., Schiller, L. R., . . . Ford, A. C. (2015). The effect of dietary intervention on irritable bowel syndrome: A systematic review. *Clinical and Translational Gastroenterology, 6*, e107. doi:10.1038/ctg.2015.21

Moraes, J., Felga, G., Chebli, L., Franco, M. B., Gomes, C. A., Gaburri, P. D., . . . Chebli. (2010). A full solid diet as the initial meal in mild acute pancreatitis is safe and result in a shorter length of hospitalization: Results from a prospective, randomized, controlled, double-bind clinical trial. *Journal of Clinical Gastroenterology, 44*, 517–522.

Naniwadekar, A. (2010). Nutritional recommendations for patients with non-alcoholic fatty liver disease: An evidence-based review. *Practical Gastroenterology, 34*, 8–16.

Owyang, C. (2008). Pancreatitis. In L. Goldman & D. Ausiello (Eds.), *Cecil medicine* (23rd ed., pp. 1070–1078). Philadelphia, PA: Saunders.

Oxentenko, A., & Murray, J. (2015). Celiac disease: Ten things that every gastroenterologist should know. *Clinical Gastroenterology and Hepatology, 13*, 1396–1404.

Peery, A. (2016). Colonic diverticula and diverticular disease: 10 Facts clinicians should know. *North Carolina Medical Journal, 77*, 220–222.

Peery, A., Sandler, R., Ahnen, D., Galanko, J. A., Holm, A. N., Shaukat, A., . . . Baron, J. A. (2013). Constipation and a low-fiber diet are not associated with diverticulosis. *Clinical Gastroenterology and Hepatology, 11*, 1622–1627.

Rajkumar, N., Karthikeyan, V., Ali, S., Sistla, S. C., & Kate, V. (2013). Clear liquid diet vs soft diet as the initial meal in patients with mild acute pancreatitis: A randomized interventional trial. *Nutrition in Clinical Practice, 28*, 365–370.

Rasmussen, H., Irtun, O., Olesen, S., Drewes, A. M., & Holst, M. (2013). Nutrition in chronic pancreatitis. *World Journal of Gastroenterology, 19*, 7267–7275.

Rinella, M. (2015). Nonalcoholic fatty liver disease: A systematic review. *JAMA, 313*, 2263–2273.

Rubio-Tapia, A., Hill, I., Kelly, C., Calderwood, A. H., & Murray J. A. (2013). ACG clinical guidelines: Diagnosis and management of celiac disease. *The American Journal of Gastroenterology, 108*, 656–676.

Sikkens, E., Cahen, D., van Eijck, C., Kuipers E. J., & Bruno, M. J. (2012). Patients with exocrine insufficiency due to chronic pancreatitis are undertreated: A Dutch national survey. *Pancreatology, 12*, 71–73.

Staudacher, H., Whelan, K., Irving, P., & Lomer, M. (2011). Comparison of symptom response following advice for a diet low in fermentable carbohydrates (FODMAPs) versus standard dietary advice in patients with irritable bowel syndrome. *Journal of Human Nutrition and Dietetics, 24*, 487–495.

Stollman, N., Smalley, W., & Hirano, I. (2015). American Gastroenterological Association Institute guideline on the management of acute diverticulitis. *Gastroenterology, 149*, 1944–1949.

Strate, L., Liu, Y., Aldoori, W., Aldoori, W. H., Syngal, S., & Giovannucci, E. L. (2009). Obesity increases the risks of diverticulitis and diverticular bleeding. *Gastroenterology, 136*, 115–122.

Strate, L., Liu, Y., Syngal, S., Aldoori, W. H., & Giovannucci, E. L. (2008). Nut, corn, and popcorn consumption and the incidence of diverticular disease. *JAMA, 300*, 907–914.

Taitano, A., Markow, M., Finan, J., Wheeler, D. E., Gonzalvo, J. P., & Murr, M. M. (2015). Bariatric surgery improves histological features of nonalcoholic fatty liver disease and liver fibrosis. *Journal of Gastrointestinal Surgery, 19*, 429–436.

Tenner, S., Baillie, J., DeWitt, J., & Vege, S. S. (2013). American College of Gastroenterology guideline: Management of acute pancreatitis. *American Journal of Gastroenterology, 108*, 1400–1415.

U.S. Food and Drug Administration. (2013). Food labeling: Gluten-free labeling of foods. Final rule. *Federal Register, 78*(15), 47154–47179.

Wall, E. (2013). An overview of short bowel syndrome management: Adherence, adaptation, and practical recommendations. *Journal of the Academy of Nutrition and Dietetics, 113*, 1200–1208.

Working Group International Association of Pancreatology/American Pancreatic Association. (2013). IAP/APA evidence-based guidelines for the management of acute pancreatitis. *Pancreatology, 13*(4 Suppl. 2), e1–e15.

Yamamoto, M., Iwasa, M., Iwata, K., Kaito, M., Sugimoto, R., Urawa, N., . . . Adachi, Y. (2007). Restriction of dietary calories, fat and iron improves non-alcoholic fatty liver disease. *Journal of Gastroenterology and Hepatology, 22*, 1563–1568.

Yamamoto, T. (2013). Nutrition and diet in inflammatory bowel disease. *Current opinion in Gastroenterology, 29*, 216–221.

Zhang, Y., Li, L., Guo, C., Mu, D., Feng, B., Zuo, X., & Li, Y. (2016). Effects of probiotic type, dose and treatment duration on irritable bowel syndrome diagnosed by Rome III criteria: A meta-analysis. *BMC Gastroenterology, 16*, 62. doi:10.1186/s12876-016-0470-z

Zhao, X., Zhu, S., Xue, G., Li, J., Liu, Y. L., Wan, M. H., . . . Tang, W. F. (2015). Early oral refeeding based on hunger in moderate and severe acute pancreatitis: A prospective controlled, randomized clinical trial. *Nutrition, 31*, 171–175.

Zhou, D., Wang, W., Cheng, X., Wei, J., & Zheng, S. (2015). Antioxidant therapy for patients with chronic pancreatitis: A systematic review and meta-analysis. *Clinical Nutrition, 34*, 627–634.

Chapter 19

Nutrition for Patients with Diabetes Mellitus

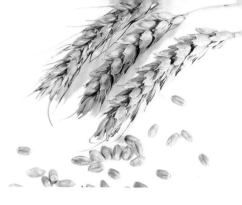

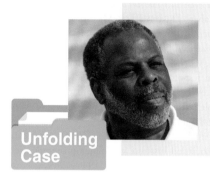

Unfolding Case

Darius Jackson

Darius is the first male in his family to reach the age of 60 years without having a stroke or myocardial infarction. He has had hypertension for decades and was recently diagnosed with type 2 diabetes with a hemoglobin A1c of 9.2%. He was immediately prescribed metformin and a basal insulin regimen of 10 units/day and told to lose weight.

Check Your Knowledge

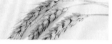

True	False		
☐	☐	1	The progression of prediabetes to diabetes is inevitable.
☐	☐	2	The cornerstone of nutrition therapy for diabetes is to eat a low-carbohydrate diet.
☐	☐	3	Weight loss lowers the risk of type 2 diabetes only when it achieves a weight within an individual's healthy body mass index (BMI) range.
☐	☐	4	Alcohol is more likely to cause hypoglycemia when consumed without food rather than with food.
☐	☐	5	People with diabetes should avoid fruit because fructose produces a higher postprandial rise in glucose than sucrose.
☐	☐	6	People with diabetes are not allowed to eat sweetened foods because sugar raises blood glucose levels faster than other types of carbohydrates.
☐	☐	7	All people with diabetes should consume a bedtime snack to avoid hypoglycemia.
☐	☐	8	People who practice carbohydrate counting do not have to pay attention to protein or fat intake.
☐	☐	9	A chocolate candy bar is a good choice for treating mild hypoglycemia.
☐	☐	10	People with diabetes should limit their intake of saturated fat and trans fat.

Learning Objectives

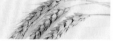

Upon completion of this chapter, you will be able to

1 Discuss strategies recommended to prevent diabetes.
2 Describe the nutrition recommendations for managing diabetes.
3 Identify healthy eating guidelines for diabetes.
4 Compare basic carbohydrate counting to advanced carbohydrate counting.
5 Compose a 2000-calorie eating pattern using the carbohydrate counting method of meal planning.

6 Compare carbohydrate counting to using the Food Lists for Diabetes.
7 Describe the plate method of meal planning.
8 Determine the number of carbohydrate choices a serving of food provides by using the "Nutrition Facts" label.
9 Discuss diabetes nutrition therapy in youth and older adults.

Diabetes is one of the most costly and burdensome chronic diseases of our time and is expected to increase in prevalence due at least in part to an aging population, increasing prevalence of overweight and obesity, and growing minority populations that are at higher risk of diabetes. In 2011 to 2012, the estimated unadjusted prevalence of total diabetes using A1c or fasting plasma glucose definitions was 12.3% among American adults, with a higher prevalence among non-Hispanic black, non-Hispanic Asian, and Hispanic individuals (Menke, Casagrande, Geiss, & Cowie, 2015). An estimated 27.8% of people with diabetes have not been diagnosed (Centers for Disease Control and Prevention, 2014). Direct and indirect costs of diabetes in the United States are estimated to be $245 billion (Centers for Disease Control and Prevention, 2014). Diabetes is the seventh leading cause of death in the United States (Centers for Disease Control and Prevention, 2016).

This chapter focuses on the prevention of type 2 diabetes and nutrition therapy for type 1 and type 2 diabetes. A third type of diabetes, gestational diabetes, is presented in Chapter 11.

DIABETES

Diabetes mellitus is a heterogeneous group of metabolic disorders characterized by hyperglycemia and abnormal insulin metabolism. Absent or ineffective insulin impairs the metabolism of all three macronutrients, resulting in high blood glucose levels, increased levels of fatty acids and triglycerides in the blood, and muscle wasting (Table 19.1). Diagnostic criteria for diabetes appears in Figure 19.1.

Sustained hyperglycemia alters glucose metabolism in virtually every tissue. Damage to small vessels (microvascular) can lead to retinopathy, nephropathy, and neuropathy. Large blood vessel (macrovascular) damage increases the risk of cardiovascular disease and stroke. Other complications include impaired wound healing, gangrene, periodontal disease, and increased susceptibility to other illnesses. Intensive glucose control is associated with significantly lower rates of microvascular (retinopathy and diabetic kidney disease) and neuropathic complications in people with type 2 diabetes and in people newly diagnosed with type 1 diabetes (American Diabetes Association [ADA], 2016e).

Table 19.1	Actions of Insulin and Effects of Its Insufficiency	
Nutrient	**Action of Insulin**	**Results of Insulin Insufficiency**
Glucose	Promotes uptake of glucose into cells Promotes formation of glycogen in the liver and muscle Promotes conversion of excess glucose into triglycerides for storage	Decreases uptake of glucose into muscle and adipose Decreases glycogen formation in liver and muscle Increases glycogen breakdown in liver and muscle Increases gluconeogenesis (the formation of glucose from a noncarbohydrate source, such as amino acids or glycerol) Hyperglycemia
Protein	Promotes uptake of amino acids into tissue protein	Decreases uptake of amino acids into muscle Decreases protein synthesis Increases protein breakdown
Fat	Promotes formation of adipose from excess fat	Increases production of ketones in the liver Decreases formation of triglycerides in adipose Increases triglyceride breakdown in adipose Increases serum triglyceride and fatty acid levels

Figure 19.1 ▶
Diagnostic criteria for diabetes and prediabetes.
(Source: American Diabetes Association. [2016]. Classification and diagnosis of diabetes. Diabetes Care, *39[Suppl. 1], S13–S22.)*

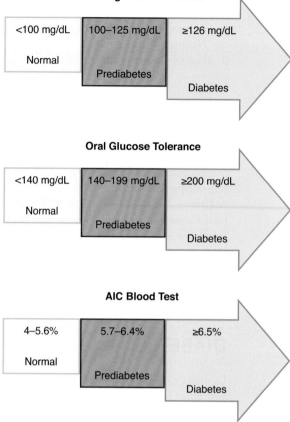

Fasting Plasma Glucose

<100 mg/dL	100–125 mg/dL	≥126 mg/dL
Normal	Prediabetes	Diabetes

Oral Glucose Tolerance

<140 mg/dL	140–199 mg/dL	≥200 mg/dL
Normal	Prediabetes	Diabetes

AIC Blood Test

4–5.6%	5.7–6.4%	≥6.5%
Normal	Prediabetes	Diabetes

Type 1 Diabetes
diabetes characterized by the absence of insulin secretion.

Polyuria
excessive urine excretion.

Polydipsia
excessive thirst.

Polyphagia
excessive appetite.

Ketoacidosis
the accumulation of ketone bodies leading to acidosis related to incomplete breakdown of fatty acids from carbohydrate deficiency or inadequate carbohydrate utilization.

Insulin Resistance
decreased cellular response to insulin.

Impaired Fasting Glucose
fasting plasma glucose levels of 100 to 125 mg/dL.

Impaired Glucose Tolerance
2-hour values in the oral glucose tolerance test of 140 to 199 mg/dL.

Hyperinsulinemia
elevated blood levels of insulin.

Type 1 Diabetes

Type 1 diabetes, formerly known as insulin-dependent diabetes mellitus, is characterized by the absence of insulin. It accounts for 5% to 10% of diabetes cases. Although type 1 can occur at any age, it is most often diagnosed before the age of 18 years. Type 1 diabetes occurs from an autoimmune response that damages or destroys pancreatic beta cells, leaving them unable to produce insulin. Interaction between genetic susceptibility and environmental factors, such as viral infection, is thought to be responsible. The classic symptoms of **polyuria**, **polydipsia**, and **polyphagia** appear abruptly. Sometimes, the first sign of the disease is **ketoacidosis**. There is no known way to prevent type 1 diabetes. All people with type 1 diabetes require exogenous insulin.

Type 2 Diabetes

Type 2 diabetes, previously referred to as non–insulin-dependent diabetes, is most often diagnosed after the age of 45 years and accounts for 90% to 95% of diagnosed cases of diabetes. Unlike type 1 diabetes, in which there is a relatively abrupt and absolute end to insulin production, type 2 diabetes is a slowly progressive disease characterized by a combination of **insulin resistance** and relative insulin deficiency. When cells do not respond to insulin as they should, the pancreas compensates by secreting higher than normal levels of insulin. **Impaired fasting glucose** and **impaired glucose tolerance** occur despite high levels of circulating insulin. Over time, chronic **hyperinsulinemia** leads to a decrease in the number of insulin receptors on the cells and a further reduction in tissue sensitivity to insulin. Insulin production progressively falls to a deficient level, and frank type 2 diabetes develops. Because hyperglycemia develops gradually in type 2 diabetes and is often not severe enough for patients to recognize any of the classic diabetes symptoms, type 2 diabetes may go

BOX 19.1 Risk Factors for Type 2 Diabetes

Testing should be considered in all adults who are overweight (BMI ≥25 kg/m² or ≥23 kg/m² in Asian Americans) and have additional risk factors:

- ≥45 years of age
- First-degree relative with diabetes
- Member of high-risk racial or ethnic group: African American, Latino/Hispanic American, Native American, Asian American, Pacific Islander
- History of gestational diabetes or giving birth to a baby weight >9 pounds
- Physical inactivity
- Hypertension
- Women with polycystic ovary syndrome
- HDL <35 mg/dL and/or triglyceride level ≥250 mg/dL

Source: American Diabetes Association. (2016). Classification and diagnosis of diabetes. *Diabetes Care, 39*(Suppl. 1), S13–S22.

Metabolic Syndrome (MetS)
a clustering of interrelated risk factors that includes hypertension, low high-density lipoprotein (HDL) cholesterol, high triglycerides levels, elevated serum glucose, and central or abdominal obesity, as indicated by waist circumference.

undiagnosed for years. Many patients will have already developed complications by the time of diagnosis (Ahmad & Crandall, 2010).

Excess weight is strongly linked to type 2 diabetes. Other risk factors are listed in Box 19.1. **Metabolic syndrome (MetS)** is a cluster of risk factors, such as central obesity, insulin resistance, dyslipidemia, and hypertension that, when combined, increases the risk of type 2 diabetes fivefold and cardiovascular disease threefold (O'Neill & O'Driscoll, 2015).

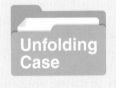

Unfolding Case

Consider Darius. He is 5 ft 10 in tall. At the time of diagnosis, he weighed 205 pounds. He wants to lose weight to get off insulin. What is his body mass index (BMI)? What risk factors does he have for type 2 diabetes? What should an initial weight loss goal be for him? Is it possible for him to manage his diabetes without insulin?

Prediabetes

Prediabetes
fasting plasma glucose of 100 to 126 mg/dL or an oral glucose tolerance test of 140 to 199 mg/dL.

Prediabetes is the period of impaired glucose metabolism that precedes the diagnosis of type 2 diabetes (see Fig. 19.1). In 2011 to 2012, the prevalence of prediabetes was 38% of the overall population (Menke et al., 2015).

Identifying and treating prediabetes is a fundamental strategy for preventing or delaying diabetes (Selph et al., 2015). Lifestyle interventions can significantly reduce the rate of diabetes onset in people at high risk for developing type 2 diabetes, namely, those with impaired fasting glucose, impaired glucose tolerance, or both (ADA, 2016h). Because of the strong link between excess weight and insulin resistance/type 2 diabetes, modest weight loss achieved through a healthy, hypocaloric eating pattern, increased physical activity, and behavior change is the primary focus of diabetes prevention (Box 19.2). A major, multicenter clinical trial called the Diabetes Prevention Program (DPP) found that in a diverse group of overweight people with impaired glucose tolerance, nutrition therapy, physical activity, and behavior change decreased the incidence of diabetes by 58% (DPP Research Group, 2002). Average weight loss among study participants was a modest 5% to 7% of initial weight. Participants also benefited from improvements in their lipid profiles, blood pressure, and markers of inflammation (Haffner et al., 2005; Ratner et al., 2005). A 10-year follow-up on the original participants showed that the lifestyle intervention group maintained a decreased risk of diabetes over time (DPP Research Group, 2009). Strategies have been observed to promote weight loss are listed in Box 19.3.

BOX 19.2 — Selected Interventions that May Prevent or Delay Type 2 Diabetes

- Intensive lifestyle intervention program that includes diet, physical activity, and behavior change to achieve a 7% loss of body weight
- Medical nutrition therapy has been shown to lower A1c.
- Increase moderate-intensity physical activity to at least 150 minutes per week.
- Consume a healthy eating pattern:
  - A Mediterranean diet rich in monounsaturated fats may lower diabetes risk.
  - Eat whole grains.
  - Eat a pattern high in fruits and vegetables that includes nuts and berries.

Source: American Diabetes Association. (2016). Prevention or delay of type 2 diabetes. *Diabetes Care, 39*(Suppl. 1), S36–S38.

Current recommendations for prediabetes screening are primarily focused on adults who are overweight or obese based on BMI until patients meet age-related screening at 45 years old (ADA, 2016c). However, a study by Mainous, Tanner, Jo, and Anton, (2016) found that in healthy weight adults aged 20 years and older, the prevalence of prediabetes was 18.5% in 2012 compared to 10.2% in 1988 to 1994. Although the reason for the increase in prevalence is unclear, researchers speculate that sedentary lifestyle could in part be responsible (Mainous et al., 2016).

DIABETES TREATMENT

Diabetes is a progressive disease that requires lifelong treatment. The cornerstones of diabetes management are education, nutrition therapy, regular physical activity, and blood glucose monitoring. Patients with type 1 diabetes also require insulin. Patients with type 2 diabetes may also need oral medication, insulin, or a combination of both. A treatment plan is created to help patients achieve metabolic goals (Box 19.4). Periodic adjustments are needed in response to disease progression or changes in health, age, or life circumstances.

Diabetes Self-Management Education (DSME)
the process of facilitating the knowledge, skill, and ability needed to self-manage diabetes.

Diabetes Self-Management Support (DSME/S)
the support needed to implement and maintain skills and behaviors needed to self-manage on an ongoing basis.

Diabetes Self-Management Education and Support

It is recommended that all people with diabetes participate in **diabetes self-management education (DSME)** and **diabetes self-management support (DSME/S)** at diagnosis and thereafter as needed to learn and sustain the knowledge, skills, and ability needed

---

BOX 19.3 — Strategies Associated with Weight Loss in Diabetes Prevention Trials

Weekly self-weighing
Eating breakfast
Restricting fast-food intake
Increasing physical activity
Reducing portion sizes
Using meal replacements (as appropriate)
Eating more "healthy" foods, such as fruits and vegetables

Source: Raynor, H., Jeffery, R., Ruggiero, A., Clark, J. M., & Delahanty, L. M. (2008). Weight loss strategies associated with BMI in overweight adults with type 2 diabetes at entry into the Look AHEAD (Action for Health in Diabetes) trial. *Diabetes Care, 31*, 1299–1304.

BOX 19.4   General Recommended Goals* from the American Diabetes Association

Diabetes Management Goals

- A1c <7%
- Blood pressure <140/80 mmHg
- LDL cholesterol <100 mg/dL
- Triglycerides <150 mg/dL
- HDL cholesterol >40 mg/dL for men, >50 mg/dL for women

*A1c, blood pressure, and cholesterol goals may be adjusted based on the individual's age, duration of diabetes, health history, and other health conditions.
Source: Evert, A., Boucher, J., Cypress, M., Dunbar, S. A., Franz, M. J., Mayer-Davis, E. J., . . . Yancy, W. S., Jr. (2013). Nutrition therapy recommendations for the management of adults with diabetes. *Diabetes Care, 36,* 3821–3842.

to manage their diabetes (Fig. 19.2) (ADA, 2016d). Examples of self-care behaviors include healthy eating, being active, monitoring glucose and eating, taking medication, problem solving, and healthy coping. Although DSME/S has been shown to reduce hospital admission and lower estimated lifetime health-care costs due to a lower risk for complications, only a very small percentage of people with newly diagnosed type 2 diabetes actually participate in such a program (Powers et al., 2015).

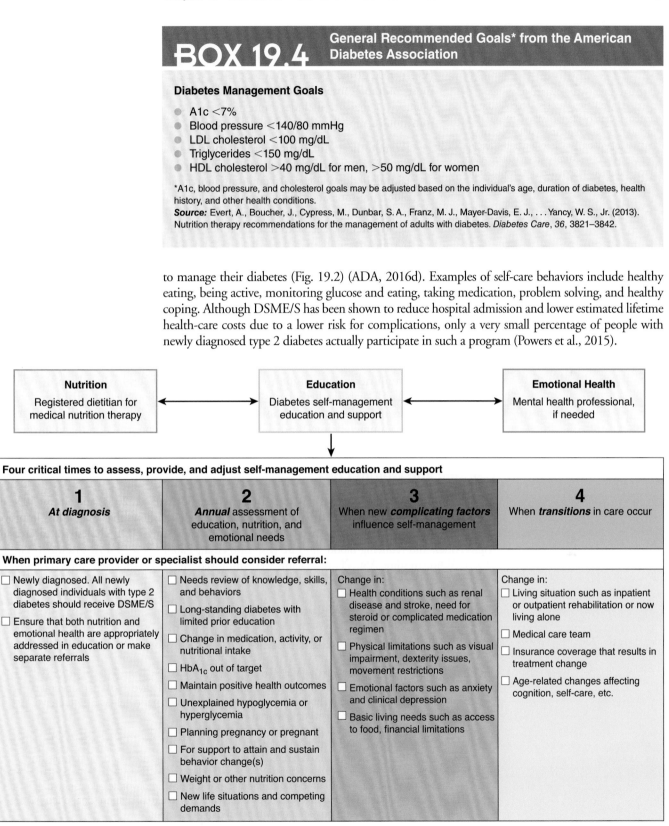

Note: Standards are also appropriate for people with other types of diabetes.

Figure 19.2 ▲ **Diabetes self-management education and support for adults with type 2 diabetes: algorithm of care.** *(Source: Powers, M. A., Bardsley, J., Cypress, M., Duker, P., Funnell, M. M., Fischl, A. H., . . . Vivian, E. [2015]. Diabetes self-management education and support in type 2 diabetes: A joint position statement of the American Diabetes Association, the American Association of Diabetes Educators, and the Academy of Nutrition and Dietetics.* Journal of the Academy of Nutrition and Dietetics, 115*[8], 1323–1334.)*

Nutrition Therapy for Diabetes

Atherosclerotic Cardiovascular Disease (ASCVD)
diseases of the cardiovascular system caused by atherosclerosis, which is the accumulation of plague within arteries. Includes acute coronary syndromes, myocardial infarction, stable or unstable angina, coronary or other arterial revascularization, stroke, transient ischemic attack, or peripheral arterial disease.

Nutrition therapy is recommended for all people with type 1 or type 2 diabetes (Evert et al., 2013). Because **atherosclerotic cardiovascular disease (ASCVD)** is the most common cause of death among adults with diabetes (Go et al., 2013), nutrition therapy for diabetes includes strategies to reduce the risk of ASCVD. The goals of nutrition therapy for adults with diabetes are to (Evert et al., 2013)

- Promote healthful eating patterns that emphasize a variety of nutrient-dense foods in the appropriate amounts to improve overall health by attaining or maintaining body weight goals; attaining individualized goals for glucose, lipids, and blood pressure; and delaying or preventing diabetes complications
- Individualize a nutrition plan based on the patients' preferences and culture, health literacy, access to healthy foods, willingness and ability to change, and barriers to change
- Preserve pleasure in eating
- Provide tools for day-to-day meal planning rather than concentrating on individual macronutrients, micronutrients, or single foods

People with diabetes generally have the same nutritional requirements as the general population and dietary recommendations to promote health and well-being in the general public—lose weight if overweight, limit saturated fat, trans fat, and added sugars, eat more fiber and less sodium—are also appropriate for people with diabetes.

An ideal macronutrient composition for all people with diabetes has not been determined nor is there a universal "diabetic diet" that is recommended for all people with diabetes (Evert et al., 2013). An individualized approach is used to accomplish the goals listed earlier. The ADA's nutrition therapy recommendations for diabetes management are presented in the following sections. Box 19.5 translates nutrition recommendations into healthy eating guidelines.

Calories and Weight Loss

More than 75% of adults with diabetes are at least overweight (Ali et al., 2013) and almost 50% are obese (Nguyen, Nguyen, Lane, & Wang, 2011). Strong evidence shows that weight loss improves A1c (Esposito et al., 2009) and lowers ASCVD risk by increasing HDL cholesterol, decreasing triglycerides, and reducing blood pressure (Esposito et al., 2009; Look AHEAD Research Group, 2013). Although some ASCVD risk factors were improved, the landmark Look AHEAD study did

BOX 19.5   Healthy Eating Guidelines for Diabetes

- Eat 3 meals a day and possibly a small evening snack.
- Spread carbohydrate choices throughout the day. Women should have 3 to 4 carbohydrate choices per meal; men should have 4 to 5 carbohydrate choices per meal. Adults can have 1 to 2 carbohydrate choices for an evening snack.
- Eat a balanced intake of a variety of nutrient-dense foods.
- Choose unprocessed foods over refined foods.
- Eat more fiber, such as from whole grains, legumes, and the skins and seeds from fruits and vegetables.
- Sugars and sweetened foods can be consumed as part of the carbohydrate allowance but should be eaten in limited amounts so as not to displace the intake of nutrient-dense foods.
- Artificially sweetened beverages are safe when used in moderation.
- Avoid sugar-sweetened beverages, canned fruit with heavy syrup, honey, molasses, and syrups.
- Choose lean protein foods. Trim visible fat. Bake, poach, steam, or boil instead of frying.
- Limit added fats and fried foods.
- Limit sodium intake to 2300 mg/day.
- Choose canola oil, olive oil, or small amounts of nuts for healthy sources of added fat.
- People who choose to drink alcohol should do so in moderation and not on an empty stomach. Beer and some mixers provide carbohydrate. Alcohol can interact with certain medications.

not show a decrease in ASCVD events among participants randomized to intensive lifestyle intervention (Look AHEAD Research Group, 2013). However, participants reaped other health benefits, such as significant weight loss, which resulted in a lower need for medication to manage glucose and ASCVD risks, less sleep apnea (Faulconbridge et al., 2012), less depression (Foster et al., 2009), and improved health-related quality of life (Williamson et al., 2009). Although a modest sustained weight loss of 5% of initial body weight may improve glucose levels, blood pressure, and/or lipids levels, a sustained weight loss of ≥7% is optimal (ADA, 2016d).

Lifestyle intervention for weight management is a three-pronged approach that includes a healthy hypocaloric eating pattern, an increase in physical activity, and lifestyle behavior changes. A hypocaloric intake may be achieved by lowering calorie intake by 500 to 700 cal/day or by choosing a calorie level within the recommended range of 1200 to 1500 cal/day diet for women and 1500 to 1800 cal/day for men (ADA, 2016d). Strategies associated with weight loss in diabetes prevention studies are listed in Box 19.3.

To achieve modest weight loss, intensive lifestyle interventions with ongoing support are recommended (ADA, 2016f). Structured programs that focus on diet, physical activity, and behavior change should be composed of ≥16 sessions over a 6-month period. Patients who achieve weight loss should enroll in a long-term (≥1 year) comprehensive weight loss maintenance program. Other options include (ADA, 2016d)

- Very-low-calorie diets (<800 cal/day) with meal replacements used for a short term may effectively achieve weight loss but must be provided by a professional in a medical care setting.
- Adjunct use of weight loss medications (see Chapter 15).
- Bariatric surgery for adults with type 2 diabetes and a BMI >35, especially if diabetes or comorbidities are difficult to control with lifestyle and medication. Bariatric surgery has been found to nearly or completely normalize blood glucose levels 2 years after surgery in 72% of patients (Sjöström et al., 2014). Bariatric surgery in severely obese patients with type 1 diabetes has been shown to produce significant and sustained weight loss and significant improvement in glycemic status and comorbid conditions (Brethauer et al., 2014). However, data are extremely limited and more research is needed.

Eating Patterns

A variety of eating patterns have been shown modestly effective in managing diabetes including Mediterranean-style, Dietary Approaches to Stop Hypertension (DASH)-style, vegan or vegetarian, low-fat, and lower carbohydrate diet (Evert et al., 2013). There is not one "ideal" pattern that all people with diabetes must follow. Total calorie intake is important regardless of the type of eating pattern selected. Patient preferences and health status should determine the type of eating pattern chosen.

Carbohydrate

Although postprandial glucose response is primarily determined by the amount of carbohydrates consumed (and the amount of available insulin), the ideal amount of carbohydrate intake for people with diabetes is unknown (Evert et al., 2013). Monitoring carbohydrate intake, such as with carbohydrate counting, and how it affects glucose response, is important for improving postprandial glucose control (Delahanty et al., 2009). Recommendations regarding the timing, amount, and consistency of carbohydrate intake are based on whether the patient manages diabetes with insulin, medication, or only diet and exercise (see "Carbohydrate Counting" section). Consistent with recommendations for the general population, nutrient-dense and high-fiber sources of carbohydrate should be chosen whenever possible over refined or processed carbohydrates with added sodium, fat, and sugar. The majority of carbohydrate calories should come from fruit, vegetables, whole grains, legumes, and low-fat milk.

Sweeteners

Substantial evidence from clinical studies demonstrates that when sucrose is **isocalorically** substituted for starch, there is no difference in glycemic control in either type 1 or type 2 diabetes (Franz et al., 2002). Sucrose and sucrose-containing foods are

Isocalorically
of the same calorie level.

not eliminated but should be substituted for other carbohydrates in the meal plan, not eaten as "extras." Many people with long-standing diabetes resist accepting this shift in thinking because sugar was once taboo. Others find the freedom to choose sweetened foods difficult not to abuse. Even though foods high in sugar do not aggravate glycemic control, they should be minimized to avoid displacing the intake of nutrient-dense foods (Evert et al., 2013). Sugar-sweetened beverages should be avoided.

Fructose consumed in fruit may result in better glycemic control compared to the same number of calories consumed from sucrose or starch (Evert et al., 2013). However, the intake of sugar-sweetened beverages containing any sugar, including high-fructose corn syrup and sucrose, should be limited or avoided to lower the risk of weight gain and a detrimental impact on serum lipid levels.

Nonnutritive and Hypocaloric Sweeteners

Nonnutritive Sweeteners
synthetically made sweeteners that do not provide calories.

Sugar Alcohols
natural sweeteners derived from monosaccharides; these are considered low-calorie sweeteners because they are incompletely absorbed. They produce a smaller rise in postprandial glucose levels and insulin secretion than sucrose.

Nonnutritive sweeteners, such as saccharin, aspartame, acesulfame potassium, and sucralose, are approved for use by the U.S. Food and Drug Administration (FDA) and may safely be used by people with diabetes. **Sugar alcohols** (sorbitol, mannitol, and xylitol) are hypocaloric sweeteners that provide fewer calories than sucrose and other natural sweeteners. They appear safe to use but may cause diarrhea when consumed in large amounts, especially in children. Although the potential benefit of using nonnutritive and hypocaloric sweeteners is a decrease in overall calorie and carbohydrate intake if they are used in place of caloric sweeteners and a compensatory increase in calories from other sources does not occur, it is not known if their use leads to weight loss (Wiebe et al., 2011).

Fiber

People with diabetes should consume as least the amount of fiber recommended for the general population, which is 14 g/1000 cal consumed, or approximately 25 g/day for women and 38 g/day for men. As with the general population, at least half of all grain choices should be whole grain. Fiber intake is associated with lower all-cause mortality in people with diabetes (Evert et al., 2013).

Glycemic Index

Glycemic Index
the incremental rise in blood glucose (above baseline) compared to that induced by a standard, usually 50 g of glucose or a white bread challenge.

Study results are mixed on whether using low **glycemic index** eating patterns improve glucose levels (Evert et al., 2013). It is difficult to draw conclusions about the value of using glycemic index because studies do not always control for the effect of fiber in foods and studies vary in how they define high and low glycemic index. Despite the lack of conclusive evidence, substituting low glycemic load foods for higher glycemic load foods may modestly improve glycemic control (Evert et al., 2013).

Fat

The ideal total fat intake for people with diabetes is not known; however, the type of fat consumed may be far more important that the total amount. With regard to specific types of fat,

- A Mediterranean-style eating pattern that is rich in monounsaturated fats may improve glucose control and blood lipids and may be an effective alternative to a low-fat, high-carbohydrate eating pattern (ADA, 2016d).
- Recommendations to eat less saturated fat and trans fat are appropriate for the general population, including people with diabetes.
- The ADA does not recommend omega-3 supplements to prevent ASCVD (Evert et al., 2013).
  - Consistent with recommendations for the general public, people with diabetes are urged to eat fish, especially fatty fish, twice a week.
- Consuming 1.6 to 3.0 g/day of **plant stanols** or **sterols** found in enriched foods may help people with diabetes and dyslipidemia lower total and low-density lipoprotein (LDL) cholesterol (Evert et al., 2013). Examples of foods that may be enriched with stanols or sterols include margarine, salad dressing, low-fat yogurt, and fruit juice.

Plant Stanols or Sterols
essential components of plant membranes that are structurally similar to cholesterol; may help lower LDL cholesterol by competing for cholesterol absorption in the gastrointestinal (GI) tract, although they themselves are poorly absorbed.

Concept Mastery Alert

A nutrition plan for a patient with nephropathy should specifically include a diet that does not exceed the individual's RDA for protein. Avoiding alcohol intake without food is good advice for everyone.

Protein

For people who do not have diabetic kidney disease, there is insufficient evidence to suggest an ideal amount of protein for optimizing glycemic control or for improving one or more ASCVD risk factors (Wheeler et al., 2012). For people with diabetic kidney disease, the Recommended Dietary Allowance (RDA) for protein (0.8 g/kg) should be maintained.

Sodium

The Institute of Medicine (2013) recommends the general adult population reduce their sodium intake to 2300 mg per day. However, it states that the available data do not support additional benefits of lowering sodium intake to <2300 mg/day for certain at-risk populations, such as people with diabetes. Sodium intake recommendations should be individualized for people with both diabetes and hypertension (Evert et al., 2013).

Alcohol

Moderate alcohol intake has minimal acute and/or long-term detrimental effects on blood glucose and may lower ASCVD risk and mortality in people with diabetes (Beulens et al., 2010). Adults with diabetes who choose to drink alcohol should limit their intake to moderate use, which is defined as one drink per day or less in women and two drinks per day or less in men. Delayed hypoglycemia is a risk, especially in people who take insulin or insulin secretagogues. Consuming alcohol with food can minimize the risk of nocturnal hypoglycemia (Evert et al., 2013).

Micronutrients and Herbal Supplements

Micronutrient supplements provide no proven benefit unless there is an underlying nutrient deficiency. There is insufficient evidence to support routine supplementation of chromium, magnesium, and vitamin D to improve glucose control in people with diabetes (Evert et al., 2013). Likewise, the use of cinnamon and other herbal supplements has not been proven to improve glucose management. Micronutrient needs should be met by consuming a varied, nutrient-dense eating pattern.

Meal Planning Approaches

A variety of meal planning approaches, such as carbohydrate counting, Food Lists for Diabetes (formerly called Exchange Lists for Meal Planning), or the plate method can be used to implement a healthy eating pattern, such as Mediterranean-style, DASH, vegetarian or vegan, low-fat, or low-carbohydrate eating patterns. The approach and eating pattern selected is based on the patient's personal and cultural preferences; literacy and numeracy; and readiness, willingness, and ability to change (Evert et al., 2013).

Carbohydrate Counting

Carbohydrate counting has become a mainstay meal planning approach; it is easier and more flexible than the more traditional exchange or food list system. In patients with type 1 diabetes, carbohydrate counting has been shown to improve quality of life, reduce BMI and waist circumference, and lower A1c (Laurenzi et al., 2011) and also to improve satisfaction with treatment (DAFNE Study Group, 2002). Carbohydrate counting is based on the underlying principle that 15 g of carbohydrates equals one carbohydrate serving or "choice." Patients may choose whatever carbohydrate sources they want as long as they adhere to their carbohydrate intake goals. Although only carbohydrates are counted, patients are encouraged to maintain a consistent intake of protein and fat because they also require insulin for metabolism, provide calories, and are essential nutrients. The two levels of carbohydrate counting are basic and advanced.

Basic Carbohydrate Counting. Basic carbohydrate counting is a structured approach with a focus on consistency in the timing and amount of carbohydrates consumed. Patients are given a meal pattern based on their calorie needs that specifies the amount of carbohydrate to be consumed at each meal and, if desired, snack. The amount of carbohydrate may be stated in grams or as the number of carbohydrate "choices" per meal based on the patient's abilities and preferences. The daily amount and timing of carbohydrate consumption remains constant, but there should be variety in the type of carbohydrates chosen. Two sample menus that count carbohydrates in an 1800-calorie meal pattern are featured in Box 19.6.

Basic carbohydrate counting is best suited for any of the following patients who (Hall, 2013)

- Want an approach that promotes weight loss. Maintaining a consistent carbohydrate intake helps, but does guarantee, a consistent calorie intake. Patients are counseled on the appropriate types and amounts of protein foods and added fats to achieve the target calorie intake and to improve blood lipid levels.
- Manage their diabetes with diet and exercise alone
- Use a split-mixed insulin regimen, such as a Humalog 72/25 twice a day that requires patients to eat at a certain time after the insulin injection to avoid hypoglycemia.
- Take a fixed dose of rapid-acting insulin with meals. Rapid-acting insulin begins to work within 10 to 20 minutes after injection; eating a predetermined amount of carbohydrates based on the onset and duration of insulin activity promotes postprandial glycemic control.

BOX 19.6 — Carbohydrate Counting: Sample 1800-Calorie Menus

Sample Menu	Carbohydrate Choices	Sample Menu	Carbohydrate Choices
Breakfast			
½ cup orange juice	1	A parfait consisting of	
1 low-fat waffle	1	1¼ cup whole strawberries	1
topped with ¾ cup blueberries	1	½ cup granola	2
1 cup nonfat milk	1	6 oz artificially sweetened	1
1 tsp light margarine		vanilla Greek yogurt	
		Coffee	
Lunch			
6-in submarine with 2 oz meat and light mayonnaise	3	Hamburger on a hamburger bun	2
1 apple	1	1 cup oven-baked French fries	1
Calorie-free soft drink		Lettuce and tomato	
		Light mayonnaise	
		1 cup nonfat milk	1
Dinner			
2 taco shells (each 5 in diameter)	1	1 cup spaghetti noodles	3
3 oz taco meat		2 meatballs	
2 cups combined lettuce, tomato, onion	1	½ cup spaghetti sauce	1
⅓ cup rice	1	Tossed salad	
1 cup cubed papaya	1	1 slice Italian bread	1
		1 tsp butter	
		Calorie-free soft drink	
Bedtime Snack			
½ cup shredded wheat	1	3 cups added popcorn	1
1 cup nonfat milk	1	Calorie-free flavored seltzer water	
Total carbohydrate choices/day	14		14

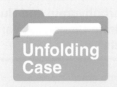

Think of Darius. He has been counseled on basic carbohydrate counting and has a meal pattern that allows him four carbohydrate choices per meal and two for a bedtime snack. His usual dinner is 4 pieces of thick crust cheese and pepperoni pizza and a sugar-free soft drink. He was shocked to learn that each piece of pizza counts as 2½ carbohydrate choices. How can Darius continue to enjoy pizza and still adhere to his meal plan?

Bolus Insulin
the rapid-acting insulin injected, such as aspart (NovoLog) and lispro (Humalog), before meals to counteract the rise in blood glucose after eating.

Insulin-to-Carbohydrate Ratio (ICR)
the number of units of rapid-acting insulin needed to handle a specific number of grams of carbohydrate consumed. An ICR of 1:15 means that 1 unit of rapid-acting insulin is needed for each 15 g of carbohydrate consumed.

Basal Insulin
the longer acting insulin injected once or twice a day, such as NHP (Humulin N, Novolin, N, Novolin NPH) and glargine (Lantus), to counteract increases in blood glucose that occur independent of food intake, such as from gluconeogenesis (formation of glucose in the liver) or hormone fluctuations.

Correction Insulin or Insulin Sensitivity Factor
the amount by which 1 unit of rapid-acting insulin will lower blood glucose as measured in mg/dL.

Advanced Carbohydrate Counting. Advanced carbohydrate counting is more flexible than basic carbohydrate counting in that it gives the patient the freedom to choose how much carbohydrate he or she wants to eat at each meal and the responsibility to calculate the corresponding insulin dose. Patients are taught how to determine their **bolus insulin** dose according to the amount of carbohydrate consumed based on a given **insulin-to-carbohydrate ratio (ICR)**. For instance, if a meal provides 45 g of carbohydrate and the individual's ICR is 1:15, the amount of bolus insulin needed is 3 units of rapid-acting insulin (45 divided by 15 = 3). Advanced carbohydrate counting is best suited to patients who

- Are willing to count the total carbohydrate grams or choices eaten in order to determine their mealtime insulin dose
- Use multiple daily insulin injections, such as **basal insulin** one to two times per day and bolus insulin at meals that is adjusted to maximize postprandial glycemic control. Patients must have basic math skills to calculate their bolus using their ICR if they do not use a pump.
- Use an insulin pump. Pumps allow basal insulin to be constantly delivered 24 hours/day to mimic pancreatic basal secretion. Pumps are programmed with the individual's ICR; the patient simply inputs the amount of carbohydrates he or she will eat, and the pump calculates and secretes the appropriate bolus dose.
- Are willing to check their blood glucose levels before and after meals. If premeal blood glucose is not within the individual's target range, **correction insulin** or **insulin sensitivity factor** is used to adjust the bolus insulin dose to compensate for the deviation. For instance, in an adult with a sensitivity factor of 40, taking 1 extra unit of rapid-acting insulin will lower the patient's blood glucose level by 40 mg/dL. If preprandial glucose is 40 mg/dL above the target range, the patient adds 1 additional unit of rapid-acting insulin to the bolus dose to correct for the higher glucose level.

Implementing Carbohydrate Counting

Patients are given a carbohydrate allowance after their total calorie and carbohydrate needs have been determined. Most people with diabetes consume about 45% of their calories from carbohydrate (Evert et al., 2013), which is within the Acceptable Macronutrient Distribution Range of 45% to 65% of total calories. Table 19.2 shows the total grams of carbohydrate and corresponding number of carbohydrate choices for various calorie level eating patterns when carbohydrates provide 45% of total calorie intake.

Patients are taught to identify sources of carbohydrates and estimate portion sizes. Patients should use the "Nutrition Facts" label for an accurate estimation of carbohydrate content (Fig. 19.3). When the "Nutrition Facts" label is not available, patients should use the serving sizes based on the Carbohydrate Choice Lists (Table 19.3).

Correctly estimating portion sizes is a crucial component of carbohydrate counting. In basic carbohydrate counting, inaccurate portion size estimates cause weight gain or loss. In advanced carbohydrate counting, inaccurate portion sizes can lead to hypo- or hyperglycemia. Food models or measuring cups can help teach appropriate portion sizes to patients. Other tactics that may help include urging patients to (Hall, 2013)

- Measure foods once per week to reinforce serving sizes and correct quantification
- Note how a portion size looks on the plate or where it comes to in their bowls or cups

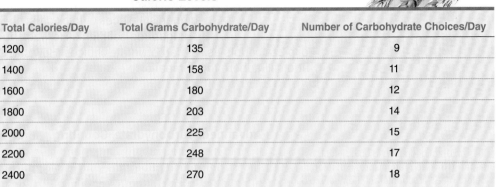

Total Calories/Day	Total Grams Carbohydrate/Day	Number of Carbohydrate Choices/Day
1200	135	9
1400	158	11
1600	180	12
1800	203	14
2000	225	15
2200	248	17
2400	270	18

Table 19.2 — Grams of Carbohydrate and Number of Carbohydrate Choices at Various Calorie Levels*

*Calculated to provide 45% of total calories from carbohydrates.

- Create a cheat sheet of the carbohydrate content of foods they usually eat
- Check the nutritional content of restaurant items online before ordering food out
- Use standard household items to approximate size. For instance, the size of a baseball is approximately 1 cup and the size of a deck of cards is approximately 3 oz.

Food Lists for Diabetes

The *Choose Your Foods: Food Lists for Diabetes* is a meal planning approach that groups foods into lists that, per serving size given, are similar in carbohydrate, protein, fat, and calories based on rounded averages (ADA & Academy of Nutrition and Dietetics, 2014). Its three major categories are carbohydrates, protein, and fats; these groupings are further divided into subgroups that form the food lists. For instance, the protein list has separate categories for lean, medium-fat, high-fat, and plant-based proteins. Any food (in the serving size specified) can be exchanged for any other within each list. A meal pattern specifies the number of servings allowed from each list for each

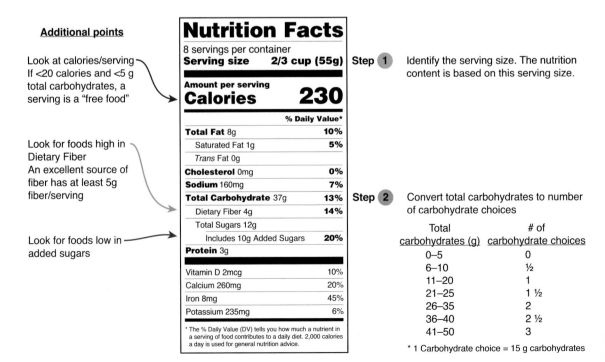

Figure 19.3 ▲ Label reading for carbohydrate counting.

Table 19.3   Carbohydrate Choice Lists

List	Representative Foods with Serving Sizes	CHO (g)	Number of Carbohydrate Choices
Starch		15	1
	Bread 1 slice white or whole-grain bread ½ English muffin, hamburger bun, or 6 in pita 1 small white, corn, or whole wheat tortilla		
	Cereals and grains ½ cup cooked cereal or grain ¾ cup unsweetened ready-to-eat cereal ⅓ cup cooked rice, pasta, or other grain		
	Starchy vegetables ½ cup mashed potatoes, corn, green peas, or yams 1 cup oven baked French-fried potatoes ½ cup marinara, pasta, or spaghetti sauce		
	Crackers and snacks 1 oz of regular potato or tortilla chips (about 13 chips) ¾ oz baked potato or pita chips (about 8 chips) 3 cups popcorn popped 1 granola or snack bar		
	Beans and lentils ½ cup cooked or canned beans, drained and rinsed ⅓ cup baked beans, canned		
Fruits		15	1
	½ cup, unsweetened canned or frozen fruit ½ cup unsweetened fruit juice		
	Fresh fruit 1 extra small banana 1 small apple ¾ cup blueberries 1 cup diced melon 1¼ cup whole strawberries		
	Dried fruit 2 tbsp raisins, cranberries, or mixed fruit		
Milk and milk substitutes	1 cup dairy milk ⅔ cup plain, light, or artificially sweetened regular or Greek yogurt	12	1
Sweets and desserts	1¼ in square unfrosted brownie 1 small frosted cupcake ½ cup fruit cobbler	15 30 45	1 2 3
Nonstarchy vegetables		5	3 servings = 1 carbohydrate choice
	½ cup cooked vegetables (fresh, canned, or frozen) such as asparagus, beets, broccoli, carrots, cauliflower, green beans, greens, mushrooms, onions, spinach, summer squash, and tomatoes 1 cup raw vegetables (excludes salad greens, which are on the Free Food List) ½ cup vegetable juice		
Free foods	Salad greens: arugula, chicory, endive, escarole, lettuce, radicchio, romaine, watercress Sugar-free gum, syrup, soft drink, or flavored water Bouillon, broth, mineral water, club soda, unsweetened cocoa powder (1 tbsp), coffee, tea, water, flavoring extracts, herbs, kelp, nonstick cooking spray, spices	<5 g	Free

Source: American Diabetes Association & Academy of Nutrition and Dietetics. (2014). *Count your carbs: Getting started.* Alexandria, VA: American Diabetes Association; Chicago, IL: Academy of Nutrition and Dietetics.

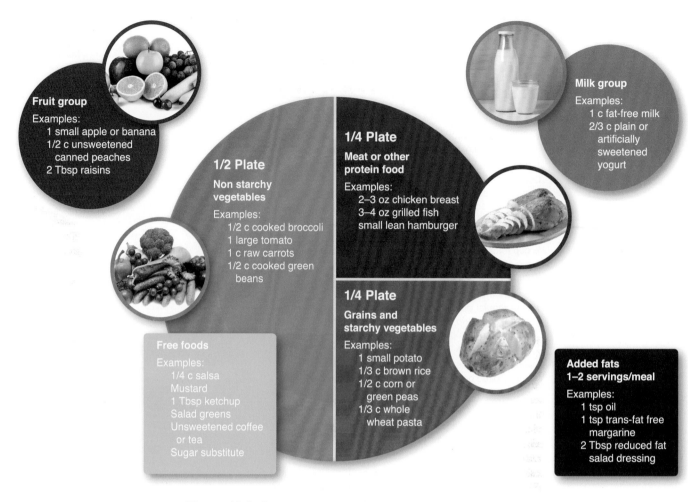

Figure 19.4 ▲ **The plate method of meal planning.**

meal and snack. As with carbohydrate counting, accurate portion sizes are vital to maintaining a consistent carbohydrate and calorie intake.

The food lists can be helpful for people who want, or need, structured meal-planning guidance and are able to understand complex details. However, the food list approach is not better than carbohydrate counting for maintaining glycemic control and is less flexible. The food lists may not be appropriate or acceptable for all age, ethnic, and cultural groups.

Plate Method for Meal Planning

The plate method for meal planning is to simply control portions and promote healthy food choices by using a dinner plate to plan meals (Fig. 19.4). This more lax approach is suited to people who have difficulty understanding health and math concepts. It may also be an effective strategy for older adults.

Nutrition Education and Counseling

People often see "diet" as the most difficult part of treatment. Learning the intricacies of eating for diabetes—what, when, and why—occurs over a continuum. Initial topics may include healthy eating guidelines (see Box 19.5), basic carbohydrate counting choice lists (see Table 19.3), and how to treat hypoglycemia (Box 19.7). More advanced nutrition topics include modifying recipes, tips for eating out (Box 19.8), and food purchasing strategies.

Often, motivation to follow a meal plan may be initially high, but commitment and diligence may dwindle when patients realize that "cheating" does not cause immediate illness. Compliance to the eating plan may improve with periodic and ongoing counseling throughout

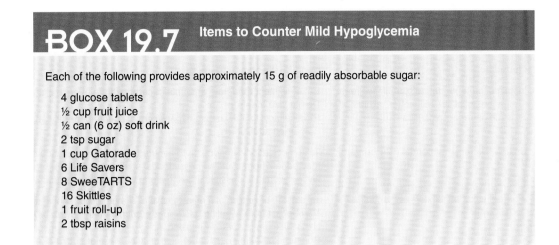

BOX 19.7 Items to Counter Mild Hypoglycemia

Each of the following provides approximately 15 g of readily absorbable sugar:

4 glucose tablets
½ cup fruit juice
½ can (6 oz) soft drink
2 tsp sugar
1 cup Gatorade
6 Life Savers
8 SweeTARTS
16 Skittles
1 fruit roll-up
2 tbsp raisins

the patient's lifetime. Periodic changes in the meal plan may be necessary to improve glycemic control, achieve lipid and blood pressure goals, manage weight, manage diabetes complications and comorbidities, and compensate for age-related changes.

Although medical nutrition therapy is the domain of the registered dietitian nutritionist, all health-care team members need to be knowledgeable in the basic principles of diabetes nutrition therapy so they can facilitate basic meal planning, dispel misconceptions, and reinforce diabetes nutrition education (Powers et al., 2015).

Diabetes Medications

People with type 1 diabetes require exogenous insulin. Most people with type 1 diabetes should be treated with multiple-dose insulin injections or continuous insulin infusion with a pump (ADA, 2016a). As stated earlier, carbohydrate intake is matched to available insulin.

In contrast, nutrition therapy and exercise are capable of controlling glucose levels for the majority of people with type 2 diabetes. However, when lifestyle changes alone do not achieve glycemic goals, metformin may be added at, or soon after, diagnosis (ADA, 2016a). Because of the progressive nature of the disease, most people with type 2 diabetes eventually require one or more oral medications, insulin, or a combination of both to manage blood glucose levels. Medication–nutrition considerations are listed in Table 19.4.

BOX 19.8 Tips for Eating Out

- Eat the same size portion you would at home. Order only what you need and want.
- Select a restaurant with a variety of choices.
- Eat slowly.
- Choose tomato juice, unsweetened fruit juice, clear broth, bouillon, consommé, or shrimp cocktail as an appetizer instead of sweetened juices, fried vegetables, or creamed or thick soups.
- Choose fresh vegetable salads and use oil and vinegar or fresh lemon instead of regular salad dressings or request that the dressing be put on the side. Avoid coleslaw and other salads with the dressing already added.
- Order plain (without gravy or sauce) roasted, baked, or broiled meat, fish and poultry instead of fried, sautéed, or breaded entrées. Avoid stews and casseroles. Request a doggie bag if the portion exceeds the meal plan allowance.
- Order steamed, boiled, or broiled vegetables.
- Choose plain, baked, mashed, boiled, or steamed potatoes; rice; or noodles.
- Select fresh fruit for dessert.
- Request a sugar substitute for coffee or tea, if desired.

Table 19.4	Recommendations for Coordinating Food Intake with Selected Medications

Medication	Food Intake Recommendations
Insulin secretagogues (e.g., sulfonylureas such as glipizide [Glucotrol]; glinides such as repaglinide [Prandin])	Eat consistent moderate amounts of carbohydrate at each meal and snack. Do not skip meals. Physical activity may cause hypoglycemia; source of readily absorbable carbohydrate should be carried at all times.
Biguanides (e.g., metformin [Glucophage])	Take medication with food or 15 minutes after eating if GI side effects persist. May benefit from avoiding gassy foods, such as cauliflower, broccoli, cabbage, legumes Hypoglycemia is possible if taking along with insulin or an insulin secretagogue.
Alpha-glucoside inhibitors (e.g., miglitol [Glyset])	Take at the beginning of a meal to have maximum effect; should not be taken when meals are missed May benefit from avoiding gassy foods, such as cauliflower, broccoli, cabbage, legumes Hypoglycemia is possible if taking along with insulin or an insulin secretagogue. Consume a source of sugar (e.g., fruit juice, regular soft drink, hard candy), not a starch, to correct hypoglycemia because drug prevents polysaccharide digestion.
Incretin mimetics (e.g., glucagon-like peptide-1 [GLP-1] analogs)	Once or twice daily injections should be preprandial. Nausea, a frequent side effect, may improve over time. Hypoglycemia is possible if taking along with insulin or an insulin secretagogue. Once weekly GLP-1s can be taken at any time during the day regardless of mealtimes.
Insulin (for either type 1 or type 2 diabetes)	Counting carbohydrates through a meal planning approach is necessary to match mealtime insulin to carbohydrate intake.
For multiple daily injections or an insulin pump	Take insulin before eating. Meals can be eaten at different times. Dose of insulin may need to be lowered to reduce the risk of hypoglycemia if physical activity occurs within 1 to 2 hours of mealtime.
For premixed insulin plan	Insulin doses and mealtimes should be consistent from day to day. Do not skip meals to reduce the risk of hypoglycemia. Physical activity may cause hypoglycemia; source of readily absorbable carbohydrate should be carried at all times.
For fixed insulin plan	Eat consistent amounts of carbohydrates each day to match set insulin dose.

Source: Evert, A., Boucher, J., Cypress, M., Dunbar, S. A., Franz, M. J., Mayer-Davis, E. J., . . . Yancy, W. S., Jr. (2013). Nutrition therapy recommendations for the management of adults with diabetes. *Diabetes Care, 36,* 3821–3842.

Physical Activity

Exercise
a specific form of physical activity that is structured and intended to improve physical fitness.

Physical Activity
all movement that increases calorie expenditure.

Exercise has been shown to improve glycemic control, lower ASCVD risk factors, contribute to weight loss, and improve well-being (ADA, 2016d). **Physical activity** may help prevent type 2 diabetes in high-risk individuals (ADA, 2016d). In people with type 2 diabetes, physical activity helps control glucose levels and may help prevent diabetes complications. It is not clear whether physical activity offers the same benefits in people with type 1 diabetes.

The ADA contends people with diabetes will benefit from following the U.S. Department of Health and Human Services (USDHHS) physical activity guidelines and therefore recommends (ADA, 2016d)

- Adults with diabetes perform at least 150 minute per week of moderate-intensity aerobic physical activity spread over at least 3 days per week with no more than 2 consecutive days without exercise.
- All adults, with or without the diagnosis of diabetes, reduce sedentary time and avoid sitting more than 90 minutes at a time.
- If not contraindicated, adults with type 2 diabetes should perform resistance training at least twice a week with each session consisting of at least one set of five or more different resistance exercises involving the large muscle groups.

To reduce the risk of hypoglycemia in people taking insulin and/or insulin secretagogues, additional carbohydrate may need to be consumed if preexercise glucose levels are <100 mg/dL, depending on whether insulin level can be lowered (e.g., with a pump or preexercise insulin dose), the time of day exercise is performed, and the intensity and duration of the activity. In people with diabetes who do not take insulin or insulin secretagogues, hypoglycemia is less likely to occur, so preventive measures are not necessary (ADA, 2016d).

ACUTE DIABETES COMPLICATIONS

Untreated or poorly controlled diabetes can lead to acute life-threatening complications related to high blood glucose concentrations. Conversely, hypoglycemia caused by overuse of medication, too little food, or too much exercise can also be life-threatening.

Diabetic Ketoacidosis

People with type 1 diabetes are susceptible to diabetic ketoacidosis (DKA), characterized by hyperglycemia (glucose levels >250 mg/dL) and ketonemia. It is caused by a severe deficiency of insulin or from physiologic stress, such as illness or infection. DKA is sometimes the presenting symptom when type 1 diabetes is diagnosed. Hyperventilation, diabetic coma, and death are possible. DKA rarely develops in people with type 2 diabetes because only very little insulin is needed to prevent ketosis. If DKA does occur in people with type 2 diabetes, infection or illness is usually to blame.

Hyperosmolar Hyperglycemic State

Hyperosmolar hyperglycemic state (HHS) is characterized by hyperglycemia (>600 mg/dL) without significant ketonemia. It occurs most commonly in people with type 2 diabetes because they have enough insulin to prevent ketosis. Dehydration and heat exposure increase the risk; illness or infection is usually the precipitating factor. Older people may be particularly vulnerable because they have a diminished sense of thirst or may be unable to replenish fluid losses due to illness or physical impairments. HHS develops relatively slowly over a period of days to weeks. The best protection against HHS is regular glucose monitoring.

Hypoglycemia

Hypoglycemia (blood glucose level <70 mg/dL) occurs from taking too much insulin or some oral medications and, inadequate food intake, delayed or skipped meals, extra physical activity, or consumption of alcohol without food. Symptoms include weakness, shakiness, dizziness, cold sweat, clammy feeling, headache, confusion, irritability, and light-headedness.

Mild hypoglycemia is treated with the "Rule of 15," which stipulates the following:

- Eat 15 g of readily absorbable carbohydrate if blood glucose is <70 mg/day (see Box 19.7). If blood glucose level is <50 mg/dL, eat 30 g of carbohydrates. Pure sugars are better than items like chocolate candy bars, which contain fat that slows the gastric emptying time and delays the rise in blood glucose.
- Wait 15 minutes. If glucose level is still <70 mg/dL, repeat the process.
- Eat a meal within an hour.

People with diabetes should carry a readily absorbable source of carbohydrate with them at all times to treat hypoglycemia. Likewise, an appropriate source of carbohydrate should be on the nightstand in case hypoglycemia develops during the night. Regular blood glucose monitoring and exercising with someone are recommended. Frequent bouts of hypoglycemia may mean the care plan needs to be revised or the client needs to be counseled to ensure better compliance.

Patients with long-standing diabetes may develop hypoglycemic unawareness. This occurs because the body no longer signals hypoglycemia. Consistent monitoring of blood glucose is especially important for people who are not cognizant of hypoglycemic symptoms.

SICK-DAY MANAGEMENT

Acute illnesses, even mild ones such as a cold or flu, can significantly raise blood glucose levels. Unless otherwise instructed by the physician, patients should maintain their normal medication schedule, monitor their blood glucose levels every 2 to 4 hours, maintain an adequate fluid intake, and continue with their normal meal plan. Softer foods such as soup, crackers, applesauce, and fruit juice may help maintain an adequate intake. If the patient cannot tolerate solids, carbohydrate targets can be met by consuming sweetened liquids, which are generally a well-tolerated source of carbohydrates and fluid. A daily intake of 150 to 200 g of carbohydrates, approximately 50 g (approximately three carbohydrate choices) every 3 to 4 hours, is recommended. Examples of items that may be best tolerated during illness are as follows (each serving specified provides approximately one carbohydrate choice [15 g of carbohydrate]):

- 6 oz regularly sweetened ginger ale
- 8 oz sports drink
- ½ cup ice cream
- ½ cup apple juice
- 1 frozen 100% juice bar
- ¼ cup sherbet or sorbet
- ½ cup gelatin
- 1 cup cream soup made with water

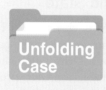

Consider Darius. He developed the flu and was advised to drink plenty of fluids; continue with his four carbohydrates per meal pattern by using regular ginger ale, fruit juice, and ice cream; and increase his monitoring of blood glucose and ketones. He is reluctant to consume regular ginger ale and ice cream because he knows sugar is bad for him. How do you respond?

Diabetes in the Hospital

Standard consistent carbohydrate meal plans are used many hospitals; these menus also typically feature heart-healthy selections that limit saturated fat, trans fat, and sodium. The previously used term "ADA diet" that reflected a specific calorie-level pattern with set percentages of carbohydrates, protein, and fat is no longer used because the ADA does not endorse any single meal plan or specified nutrient composition. Other hospital diets that are obsolete include "no concentrated sweets," "no sugar added," "low sugar," and "liberal diabetic" diets. These diets do not reflect the current nutrient recommendations for diabetes and are unnecessarily restrictive in sugar. These diets may give patients the false impression that glycemic control is achieved by limiting sugar.

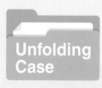

Recall Darius. He is admitted to the hospital with pneumonia and uncontrolled diabetes. He is ordered a soft diet without any carbohydrate restrictions. He is confused by the lack of restriction and announces he is no longer going to count carbohydrates because it is too confusing and difficult. What strategies are available to help Darius eat a hypocaloric meal plan to promote weight loss and manage diabetes?

LIFE CYCLE CONSIDERATIONS

Diabetes nutrition therapy can influence growth and development in children and adolescents and the quality of life in older adults. Special considerations for these groups are presented in the following sections.

Children and Adolescents

Current standards for diabetes management reflect the need to lower glucose as safely as possible (ADA, 2016b). Diabetes management in children and adolescents is complicated by the impact of growth on nutrient needs, irregular eating patterns, and erratic activity levels. Young children are unable to recognize or articulate hypoglycemia. However, hyperglycemia increases the risk of diabetes complications which may affect long-term health at an early age. For instance, youth with type 1 diabetes may have subclinical cardiovascular abnormalities within the first decade of diagnosis (ADA, 2016b). Therefore, glycemic goals are set by balancing the long-term benefits of lowering A1c against the risks of hypoglycemia and the burdens of intensive regimens (ADA, 2016b).

Failure to provide adequate calories and nutrients results in poor growth, as does poor glycemic control and inadequate insulin administration. Conversely, excessive weight gain occurs from excessive calorie intake, overtreatment of hypoglycemia, or excess insulin administration. Neither withholding food nor having a child eat when not hungry is an appropriate strategy to manage glucose levels. Rather, increased use of basal-bolus regimens, insulin pumps, frequent blood glucose monitoring, goal setting, and improved patient education in youth are associated with more children achieving blood glucose targets set by the ADA (ADA, 2016b). Advanced carbohydrate counting and intensive insulin regimens can provide flexibility for erratic eating, activity, and growth.

Although type 2 diabetes is most often diagnosed after 45 years of age, it is increasingly diagnosed in youth (Centers for Disease Control and Prevention, 2014) possibly due to the increase in pediatric obesity (Dabelea et al., 2014). Morbidity and mortality related to type 2 diabetes is greater when it is diagnosed at a young age than at the usual age of onset (Al-Saeed et al., 2016). Weight control may be key to preventing type 2 diabetes in children.

Diabetes in Later Life

There are unique considerations related to aging that affect glycemic control. Cognitive impairments, such as memory loss, impaired concentration, dementia, and depression, may preclude self-management. Physical impairments may impede exercise. Sensory impairments, such as decreased hearing, poor eyesight, and decreased senses of taste and smell, may complicate teaching and self-management. For instance, older clients who could clinically benefit from insulin may be treated instead with oral agents if poor eyesight or decreased manual dexterity precludes self-injection. Older adults may be at greater nutritional risk for a variety of reasons, including poor dentition, physical impairments that make shopping or cooking difficult, poor appetite related to lack of socialization, and an inadequate food budget. For many, a strict calorie-controlled diet may be more harmful than beneficial. Glycemic goals are based on the health of the patient, including their remaining life expectancy. For instance, suggested fasting glucose targets for older adults with diabetes are (ADA, 2016g)

- 90 to 130 mg/dL for healthy older patients with longer remaining life expectancy
- 90 to 150 mg/dL for patients with an intermediate remaining life expectancy due to multiple chronic illnesses, two or more instrumental activities of daily living (ADLs) impairments, or mild-to-moderate cognitive impairment
- 100 to 180 mg/dL for patients with very poor health and limited remaining life expectancy where benefit of stricter control is not uncertain

NURSING PROCESS

Type 2 Diabetes

Mark is 52 years old and is sedentary. His doctor monitored his fasting blood glucose and choles-terol levels for several years, urging Mark to eat better and exercise or he would eventually need medications to bring down both his glucose and cholesterol levels. Mark was unmotivated to change until he was recently diagnosed with type 2 diabetes. His mother went blind from type 2 diabetes, and he is now is convinced he must make lifestyle changes to manage his diabetes. He wants to avoid using medication. He is 5 ft 9 in tall and weighs 190 pounds.

Assessment

Medical–Psychosocial History

- Medical history and comorbidities, including hyperlipidemia, hypertension, ASCVD, renal impairments, neuropathy, and GI complaints
- Use of prescribed and over-the-counter medications
- Psychosocial and economic issues such as the living situation, cooking facilities, adequacy of food budget, education, need for food assistance, and level of family and social support
- Usual activity patterns

Anthropometric Assessment

- Height, current weight, usual weight; recent weight history
- BMI
- Waist circumference to identify abdominal obesity

Biochemical and Physical Assessment

- Hemoglobin A1c, fasting glucose levels, glucose tolerance results
- Lipid profile
- Measures of renal function, if available
- Blood pressure

Dietary Assessment

- How many meals and snacks do you usually eat in a day? Do you ever skip meals? Do you eat at regular intervals? When do you eat snacks?
- What is a typical day's intake?
- Have you ever tried to follow a diet or improve your eating habits?
- What changes can you make in your present lifestyle?
- What obstacles may prevent you from making changes?
- What changes would be difficult to make?
- What questions do you have about nutrition for diabetes?
- How is your appetite?
- Do you have any food intolerances or allergies? Do you ever have GI symptoms that affect what you eat?
- How do you feel about your weight?
- Do you have any cultural, religious, or ethnic food preferences?
- Who prepares your meals?
- Do you take vitamins, minerals, or other supplements?
- Do you use alcohol?

Diagnosis

Possible Nursing Diagnoses   Readiness for enhanced health management

Planning

Client Outcomes

Short term
The client will
- Lose 1 to 2 pounds/week
- Eat three meals plus a bedtime snack at approximately the same times every day
- Begin strategies to shift toward a nutritionally adequate, balanced, and varied diet that has
  Four carbohydrate choices at each meal and two at a bedtime snack that are composed of a
    variety of fruits, vegetables, whole grains, and low-fat or nonfat milk
  4 to 6 oz of protein/day
  Small amounts of healthy fats
  Little saturated fat and minimal trans fats

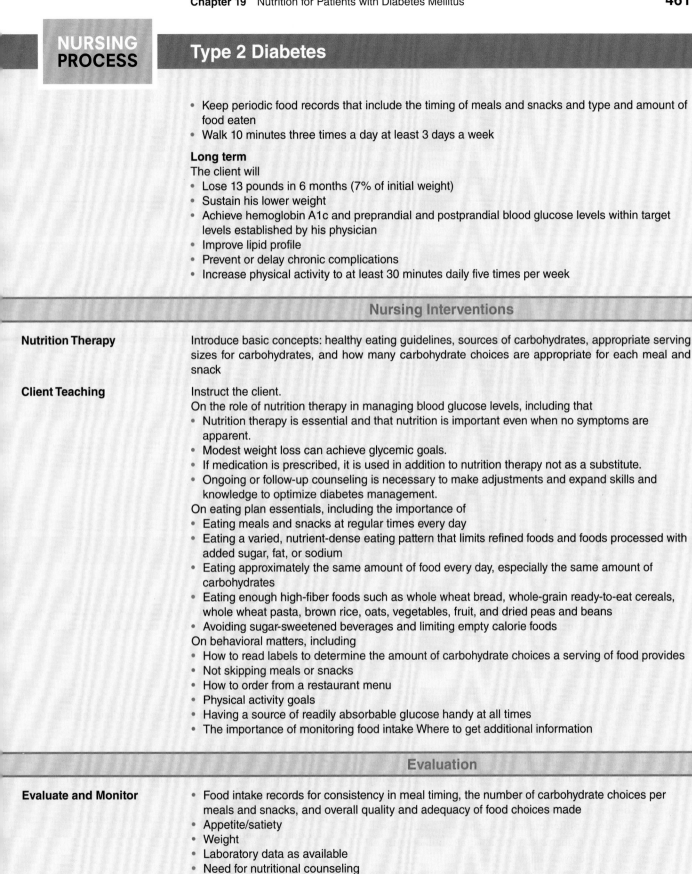

NURSING PROCESS

Type 2 Diabetes

- Keep periodic food records that include the timing of meals and snacks and type and amount of food eaten
- Walk 10 minutes three times a day at least 3 days a week

Long term
The client will
- Lose 13 pounds in 6 months (7% of initial weight)
- Sustain his lower weight
- Achieve hemoglobin A1c and preprandial and postprandial blood glucose levels within target levels established by his physician
- Improve lipid profile
- Prevent or delay chronic complications
- Increase physical activity to at least 30 minutes daily five times per week

Nursing Interventions

Nutrition Therapy

Introduce basic concepts: healthy eating guidelines, sources of carbohydrates, appropriate serving sizes for carbohydrates, and how many carbohydrate choices are appropriate for each meal and snack

Client Teaching

Instruct the client.
On the role of nutrition therapy in managing blood glucose levels, including that
- Nutrition therapy is essential and that nutrition is important even when no symptoms are apparent.
- Modest weight loss can achieve glycemic goals.
- If medication is prescribed, it is used in addition to nutrition therapy not as a substitute.
- Ongoing or follow-up counseling is necessary to make adjustments and expand skills and knowledge to optimize diabetes management.
On eating plan essentials, including the importance of
- Eating meals and snacks at regular times every day
- Eating a varied, nutrient-dense eating pattern that limits refined foods and foods processed with added sugar, fat, or sodium
- Eating approximately the same amount of food every day, especially the same amount of carbohydrates
- Eating enough high-fiber foods such as whole wheat bread, whole-grain ready-to-eat cereals, whole wheat pasta, brown rice, oats, vegetables, fruit, and dried peas and beans
- Avoiding sugar-sweetened beverages and limiting empty calorie foods
On behavioral matters, including
- How to read labels to determine the amount of carbohydrate choices a serving of food provides
- Not skipping meals or snacks
- How to order from a restaurant menu
- Physical activity goals
- Having a source of readily absorbable glucose handy at all times
- The importance of monitoring food intake Where to get additional information

Evaluation

Evaluate and Monitor

- Food intake records for consistency in meal timing, the number of carbohydrate choices per meals and snacks, and overall quality and adequacy of food choices made
- Appetite/satiety
- Weight
- Laboratory data as available
- Need for nutritional counseling
- Progress toward physical activity goals

How Do You Respond?

Are "dietetic" products like candy and cookies worth the added expense? Dietetic products are not necessarily calorie-free or specifically intended for diabetics. Foods that are labeled "dietetic" may be made without sugar, without salt, with a particular type of fat, or for special food allergies. Read the ingredient label and check with a diet counselor before adding a dietetic food to the diet—or avoid dietetic foods altogether because they are expensive and usually do not taste as good as the foods they are intended to replace.

REVIEW CASE STUDY

Keisha is a 42-year-old black female with a BMI of 29. She was recently diagnosed with diabetes and hypertension. Her mother and two sisters also have type 2 diabetes. She is the mother of three children and had gestational diabetes with her last two pregnancies. Although she knows she should exercise, she doesn't have time in her busy schedule.

The doctor gave her a 1500-calorie diet and told her if her glucose does not improve, she will have to go on medication and, possibly insulin. She has tried the "diet" but finds it too restrictive: It tells her to eat things she doesn't like (such as milk) and won't let her eat the things she loves (like sweetened tea and fast foods). She is scared of the potential for needing insulin and the complications associated with diabetes.

- What risk factors does Keisha have for type 2 diabetes?
- Is a 1500-calorie diet appropriate for her? Should it promote weight loss or maintain her current weight?
- What would you tell Keisha about weight and diabetes management?
- What would you tell her about drinking milk? What about sweetened tea and fast foods?
- What approaches would you take to improve compliance yet increase her satisfaction with eating?
- What other lifestyle changes would you propose to Keisha to manage diabetes and reduce the risk of complications?

STUDY QUESTIONS

1 Which statement indicates the patient understands nutrition recommendations regarding carbohydrate intake?
   a. "People with diabetes should avoid sugars and foods that contain sugars."
   b. "It is important to consume the proper balance of starch, sugar, and fiber at each meal."
   c. "It is important to consume the correct amount of carbohydrate at each meal and snack."
   d. "Carbohydrates must be balanced in relation to the amount of protein and fat consumed."

2 The client with type 1 diabetes asks if she can have a glass of wine with dinner on the weekends. Which of the following would be the nurse's best response?
   a. "It is better to have wine between meals than with meals so that it doesn't interfere with your normal food intake."
   b. "People with diabetes cannot have alcohol because it raises blood glucose levels very quickly."
   c. "A mixed drink would be better than wine because the mixer will help slow the absorption of the alcohol."
   d. "An occasional glass of wine with dinner will not cause any problems. Be sure to limit yourself to one serving."

3 When developing a teaching plan for a client who is taking insulin, which of the following foods would the nurse suggest the client carry with him to treat mild hypoglycemia?
   a. Crackers
   b. Peanuts
   c. Chocolate drops
   d. Life Savers

4 The best approach for monitoring carbohydrate intake is to use
   a. The food list system
   b. Carbohydrate counting
   c. The plate method
   d. The approach that best helps the individual control blood glucose levels

5 How many carbohydrate choices are provided in a serving of food that supplies 19 g of carbohydrate?
   a. 1
   b. 2
   c. 3
   d. 4

6 The nurse knows her instructions about label reading have been effective when the client verbalizes that to determine the amount of carbohydrate in a serving you must
   a. Add the grams of total carbohydrate and grams of sugars together
   b. Use only the grams of total carbohydrate
   c. Use grams of total carbohydrate after subtracting grams of dietary fiber
   d. Use only the grams of added sugars

7 What is the priority for preventing diabetes in people who are at high risk?
   a. Eat a low-carbohydrate diet.
   b. Consume a consistent amount of carbohydrate at every meal.
   c. Achieve moderate weight loss through increased activity and lowered calorie intake.
   d. Eat a low-sugar diet.

8 Which types of food provide carbohydrates? (Select all that apply.)
   a. Vegetables
   b. Fruit
   c. Milk
   d. Animal proteins

KEY CONCEPTS

- Diabetes is a group of diseases characterized by hyperglycemia. The prevalence is increasing.
- Type 1 diabetes is characterized by the lack of insulin secretion. It is usually diagnosed in children and adolescents and is related to genetic and environmental factors.
- Ninety percent to 95% of diabetes cases are type 2 diabetes. It begins with prediabetes that is characterized by insulin resistance and relative insulin deficiency. Hyperglycemia provides constant stimulation for insulin secretion, leading to hyperinsulinemia.
- Due to the strong link between excess weight and insulin resistance/type 2 diabetes, modest weight loss of 5% to 7% of body weight is the focus of diabetes prevention. However, as many as 20% of normal weight adults also have prediabetes.
- Long-term diabetes complications include damage to both small and large vessels in the body. Intensive glycemic control lowers the rates of microvascular and neuropathic complications in people with type 2 diabetes and in patients with newly diagnosed type 1 diabetes.
- DSME and support, nutrition therapy, and regular physical activity are the cornerstones of diabetes management. Many patients require oral medication, insulin, or a combination of both.
- DSME imparts the skills and knowledge necessary for patients to manage their diabetes. It is recommended for all people at the time of diabetes diagnosis. Support is ongoing and necessary in response to changes in health, age, or life circumstances. Only a small percentage of patients participate in DSME/S.
- Nutrition therapy is recommended for all people with type 1 or type 2 diabetes. The goals of nutrition therapy are to promote an overall healthy eating pattern that enables the patient to attain or maintain healthy body weight; achieve glucose, lipid, and blood pressure goals; and delay or prevent diabetes complications with an individualized meal pattern that enables the patient to enjoy eating.
- An ideal percentage of calories from carbohydrate, protein, and fat for all people with diabetes has not been identified. A universal "diabetic diet" recommended for all people with diabetes does not exist.
- A modest sustained weight loss of 5% of initial body weight may improve glucose, blood pressure, and/or lipids; however, a sustained weight loss of ≥7% is optimal.
- Lifestyle intervention for weight management is a three-pronged approach that includes a healthy hypocaloric eating pattern, an increase in physical activity, and lifestyle behavior changes. A hypocaloric intake may be achieved by lowering calorie intake by 500 to 700 cal/day or by choosing a calorie level within the recommended range of 1200 to 1500 cal/day diet for women and 1500 to 1800 cal/day for men.
- Structured lifestyle invention programs to achieve and maintain weight loss are recommended on a long-term basis. Other options for patients who do not achieve glycemic control through lifestyle modification include a very-low-calorie diet with meal replacements, obesity medication, and bariatric surgery.
- A variety of eating patterns may be effective in managing diabetes, such as Mediterranean-style, DASH-style, vegan or vegetarian, low-fat, and low carbohydrate diet. There is not one "ideal" pattern for all people with diabetes.
- The ideal amount of carbohydrate intake for people with diabetes is unknown. Recommendations regarding the timing, amount, and consistency of carbohydrate intake are based on whether the patient manages diabetes with insulin, medication, or only diet and exercise. Sources of nutrient-dense carbohydrates include whole grains, fruits, vegetables, legumes, and dairy products.
- Sugar intake is not forbidden but should be limited so as not to displace the intake of nutrient-dense foods. Sweetened beverages should be avoided.

- Nonnutritive and hypocaloric sweeteners are safe to use. It is not known whether they promote a lower calorie intake and weight loss.
- People with diabetes should eat at least as much fiber as is recommended for the general population, which is approximately 25 g/day for women and 38 g/day for men.
- Choosing carbohydrates with a low glycemic index may help manage blood glucose levels.
- The type of fat is more important than the amount of fat consumed. The amount of saturated fat, trans fat, and cholesterol recommended for the general public is also appropriate for people with diabetes. An eating pattern rich in monounsaturated fat, such a Mediterranean-style pattern, may control glucose and lipid levels better than a low-fat, high-carbohydrate pattern. Although omega-3 supplements are not recommended, people with diabetes are urged to consume at least two servings of fish, preferably fatty fish, per week.
- There is not enough evidence to suggest an ideal amount of protein for optimizing glycemic control or for improving ASCVD risk factors in people with diabetes who do not have diabetic kidney disease. The RDA for protein (0.8 g/kg) is recommended for people who have diabetic kidney disease.
- People with diabetes should limit their sodium intake to 2300 mg/day. Further sodium lowering is made on an individual basis.
- People with diabetes who choose to drink alcohol should limit their intake to one drink or less a day for women and two drinks a day or less for men. There is a risk of delayed hypoglycemia, especially in people who take insulin or insulin secretagogues.
- Micronutrient supplements are not recommended unless there is an underlying deficiency.
- The use of herbal supplements to help treat diabetes is not supported by evidence.
- Meal planning approaches include carbohydrate counting, Food Lists for Diabetes, and the plate method. Any of those approaches can be used to implement an effective eating pattern, such as the Mediterranean-style or DASH diet. Patient preference and abilities affect the approach and pattern.
- Carbohydrate counting can be basic or advanced. It is based on the concept that one carbohydrate choice provides 15 g of carbohydrate. Protein and fat are not specifically counted but should be consumed in consistent amounts daily.
- Basic carbohydrate counting stresses consistency in the timing and amount of daily carbohydrate. It is appropriate for people who do not use insulin, use a split-mixed insulin regiment, or a fixed dose of rapid-acting insulin with meals.
- Advanced carbohydrate counting allows the patient the flexibility to choose how much carbohydrate they want to eat at each meal and snack and adjust their insulin dose according to that amount and their premeal glucose level. It is appropriate for people who take multiple daily insulin injections or who use an insulin pump. Patients must be willing to quantify their food intake and check blood glucose levels before and after eating.
- The Food Lists for Diabetes, formerly called the Exchange Lists for Meal Planning, is a more complex and structured eating plan but is not superior for managing glucose levels. A meal plan specifies how many servings from each list the patient should have for every meal and snack. Any item in a list can be substituted for any other.
- The plate method uses a dinner plate to simplify meal planning. It is appropriate for people who cannot perform math calculations. It may also be suitable for older people with diabetes.
- Nutrition therapy and exercise are capable of controlling glucose levels for the majority of people with type 2 diabetes. If lifestyle changes alone do not achieve glycemic goals, oral medication and/or insulin is used. Insulin and oral medications have nutritional implications.
- All people with diabetes are urged to engage in at least 150 minutes per week of moderate physical activity and to sit less. People who use insulin may need to adjust their preexercise carbohydrate intake or insulin dose to void hypoglycemia.
- Acute diabetes complications include DKA, HHS, and hypoglycemia. Acute complications are more likely during illness. Frequent blood glucose monitoring can help avoid acute complications.
- During acute illness, people with diabetes are urged to keep their normal medication schedule, monitor their blood glucose levels closely, consume adequate fluids, and eat their usual amount of carbohydrate. Acceptable sick-day carbohydrates include sugar-sweetened carbonated beverages, fruit juice, sweetened gelatin, ice cream, and cream soups.
- Hospital diets intended for patients with diabetes were traditionally identified as "ADA diets." Because there is no one diabetic diet recommended for all people with diabetes, this term should be discontinued. Consistent carbohydrate diets or regular diets that are reviewed and corrected as needed may be used.
- Children and adolescents have a greater variation in their daily calorie needs than adults do because of their nutritional needs for growth and their more erratic activity and eating patterns. Managing diabetes is more challenging in young people.
- Older people with diabetes may need to be treated more conservatively than younger people because they are more susceptible to severe hypoglycemia, are at greater nutritional risk, and may have physical or sensory impairments that complicate self-management.

Check Your Knowledge Answer Key

1 **FALSE** Diabetes is not an inevitable consequence of pre-diabetes. Weight loss and exercise can prevent or delay diabetes and normalize blood glucose levels.

2 **FALSE** People with diabetes should consume a "normal" carbohydrate intake of 45% to 65% of total calories (within the Acceptable Macronutrient Distribution Range) just like the general population. Low-carbohydrate diets tend to be high in fat; high–saturated fat diets increase the risk of cardiovascular disease.

3 **FALSE** Modest weight loss, such as 5% to 7%, has been shown to dramatically reduce the risk of type 2 diabetes even when healthy BMI is not attained.

4 **TRUE** Alcohol is more likely to cause hypoglycemia when consumed without food rather than with food.

5 **FALSE** People with diabetes should avoid the use of fructose as an added sweetener because it causes adverse effects on serum triglycerides and LDL cholesterol but do not need to avoid natural fructose found in fruit.

6 **FALSE** People with diabetes can substitute sucrose-containing foods for other carbohydrates of equal carbohydrate content without much impact on their glucose levels. However, the intake foods with added sugar should be limited so as not to displace the intake of nutrient-dense foods.

7 **FALSE** Hypoglycemia is a risk with insulin and certain oral medications but not with all medications, so the use of snacks should be tailored to the individual's insulin and/or medication regimen. People with type 2 diabetes who are controlled by diet alone do not need snacks, and snacks may be counterproductive in people trying to lose weight.

8 **FALSE** People who practice carbohydrate counting cannot ignore protein and fat intake because they also are metabolized by insulin and provide calories and nutrients. A carbohydrate counting meal pattern should specify the appropriate intake of protein (4–8 oz/day depending on total calorie needs) and small amounts of healthy fats.

9 **FALSE** Although a chocolate candy bar does provide ample sugar, it also provides substantial amounts of fat that delay the absorption of sugar. The best choice for treating mild hypoglycemia is readily absorbable pure sugars, such as glucose tablets, fruit juice, soft drinks, or Life Savers.

10 **TRUE** People with diabetes should limit their intake of saturated fat and trans fat because their risk of ASCVD is very high.

Student Resources on thePoint®
For additional learning materials, activate the code in the front of this book at
http://thePoint.lww.com/activate

Websites

American Diabetes Association at www.diabetes.org
Joslin Diabetes Center at www.joslin.org
National Institute of Diabetes and Digestive and Kidney Diseases at www.niddk.nih.gov

References

Ahmad, L., & Crandall, J. (2010). Type 2 diabetes prevention: A review. *Clinical Diabetes, 28,* 53–59.

Ali, M., Bullard, K., Saaddine, J., Cowie, C. C., Imperatore, G., & Gregg, E. W. (2013). Achievement of goals in U.S. diabetes care, 1999–2010. *The New England Journal of Medicine, 368,* 1613–1624.

Al-Saeed, A., Constantino, M., Molyneaux, M., D'Souza, M., Limacher-Gisler, F., Luo, C., . . . Wong, J. (2016). An inverse relationship between age of type 2 diabetes onset and complication risk and mortality: The impact of you-onset type 2 diabetes. *Diabetes Care, 39,* 823–829.

American Diabetes Association. (2016a). Approaches to glycemic treatment. *Diabetes Care, 39*(Suppl. 1), S52–S59.

American Diabetes Association. (2016b). Children and adolescents. *Diabetes Care, 39*(Suppl. 1), S86–S93.

American Diabetes Association. (2016c). Classification and diagnosis of diabetes. *Diabetes Care, 39*(Suppl. 1), S13–S22.

American Diabetes Association. (2016d). Foundations of care and comprehensive medical evaluation. *Diabetes Care, 39*(Suppl. 1), S23–S35.

American Diabetes Association. (2016e). Glycemic targets. *Diabetes Care, 39*(Suppl 1), S39–S46.

American Diabetes Association. (2016f). Obesity management for the treatment of type 2 diabetes. *Diabetes Care, 39*(Suppl. 1), S47–S51.

American Diabetes Association. (2016g). Older adults. *Diabetes Care, 39*(Suppl. 1), S81–S85.

American Diabetes Association. (2016h). Prevention or delay of type 2 diabetes. *Diabetes Care, 39*(Suppl. 1), S36–S38.

American Diabetes Association & Academy of Nutrition and Dietetics. (2014). *Choose your foods: Food lists for diabetes.* Alexandria, VA: American Diabetes Association; Chicago, IL: Academy of Nutrition and Dietetics.

Beulens, J., Algra, A., Soedamah-Muthu, S., Visseren, F. L., Grobbee, D. E., & van der Graaf, Y. (2010). Alcohol consumption and risk of recurrent cardiovascular events and mortality in patients with clinically manifest vascular disease and diabetes mellitus: The Second Manifestations of ARTerial (SMART) disease study. *Atherosclerosis, 212,* 281–286.

Brethauer, S., Aminian, A., Rosenthal, R., Kirwan, J. P., Kashyap, S. R., & Schauer, P. R. (2014). Bariatric surgery improves the metabolic profile of morbidly obese patients with type 1 diabetes. *Diabetes Care, 37*(3), e51–e52.

Centers for Disease Control and Prevention. (2014). National Diabetes Statistics Report: Estimates of diabetes and its burden in the United States, 2014. Available at http://www.cdc.gov/diabetes/pubs/statsreport14/national-diabetes-report-web.pdf. Accessed on 7/18/16.

Centers for Disease Control and Prevention. (2016). Leading causes of death. Available at http://www.cdc.gov/nchs/fastats/leading-causes-of-death.htm. Accessed on 3/2/16.

Dabelea, D., Mayer-Davis, E., Saydah, S., Imperatore, G., Linder, B., Divers, J., . . . Hamman, R. F. (2014). Prevalence of type 1 and type 2 diabetes among children and adolescents from 2001 to 2009. *JAMA, 311*, 1778–1786.

DAFNE Study Group. (2002). Training in flexible, intensive insulin management to enable dietary freedom in people with type 2 diabetes: Dose adjustment for normal eating (DAFNE) randomised controlled trial. *BMJ, 325*, 746–749.

Delahanty, L., Nathan, D., Lachin, J., Hu, F. B., Cleary, P. A., Ziegler, G. K., . . . Wexler, D. J. (2009). Association of diet with glycated hemoglobin during intensive treatment of type 1 diabetes in the Diabetes Control and Complications Trial. *The American Journal of Clinical Nutrition, 89*, 518–524.

Diabetes Prevention Program Research Group. (2002). Reduction in the evidence of type 2 diabetes with lifestyle intervention or metformin. *The New England Journal of Medicine, 346*, 393–403.

Diabetes Prevention Program Research Group. (2009). 10-Year follow-up of diabetes incidence and weight loss in the Diabetes Prevention Program outcomes study. *Lancet, 374*, 1677–1686.

Esposito, K., Maiorino, M., Ciotola, M., Di Palo, C., Scognamiglio, P., Gicchino, M., . . . Giugliano, D. (2009). Effects of a Mediterranean-style diet on the need for antihyperglycemic drug therapy in patients with newly diagnosed type diabetes: A randomized trial. *Annals of Internal Medicine, 151*, 306–314.

Evert, A., Boucher, J., Cypress, M., Dunbar, S. A., Franz, M. J., Mayer-Davis, E. J., . . . Yancy, W. S., Jr. (2013). Nutrition therapy recommendations for the management of adults with diabetes. *Diabetes Care, 36*, 3821–3842.

Faulconbridge, L., Wadden, T., Rubin, R., Wing, R. R., Walkup, M. P., Fabricatore, A. N., . . . Ewing, L. J. (2012). One-year changes in symptoms of depression and weight in overweight/obese individuals with type 2 diabetes in the Look AHEAD study. *Obesity (Silver Spring), 20*, 783–793.

Foster, G., Borradaile, K., Sanders, M., Millman, R., Zammit, G., Newman, A. B., . . . Kuna, S. T. (2009). A randomized study on the effect of weight loss on obstructive sleep apnea among obese patients with type 2 diabetes: The Sleep AHEAD study. *Archives of Internal Medicine, 169*, 1619–1626.

Franz, M., Bantle, J., Beebe, C., Brunzell, J. D., Chiasson, J. L., Garg, A., . . . Wheeler, M. (2002). Evidence-based nutrition principles and recommendations for the treatment and prevention of diabetes and related complications. *Diabetes Care, 25*, 148–198.

Go, A., Mozaffarian, D., Roger, V., Benjamin, E. J., Berry, J. D., Borden, W. B., . . . Turner, M. B. (2013). Executive summary: Heart disease and stroke statistics—2013 update: A report from the American Heart Association. *Circulation, 127*, 143–152.

Haffner, S., Temprosa, M., Crandall, J., Fowler, S., Goldberg, R., Horton, E., . . . Barrett-Connor. (2005). Intensive lifestyle intervention or metformin on inflammation and coagulation in participants with impaired glucose tolerance. *Diabetes, 54*, 1566–1572.

Hall, M. (2013). Understanding advanced carbohydrate counting—a useful tool for some patients to improve blood glucose control. *Today's Dietitian, 15*, 40.

Institute of Medicine. (2013). Sodium intake in populations: Assessment of evidence. Available at http://www.nationalacademies.org/hmd/Reports/2013/Sodium-Intake-in-Populations-Assessment-of-Evidence.aspx. Accessed on 8/18/16.

Laurenzi, A., Bolla, A., Panigoni, G., Doria, V., Uccellatore, A., Peretti, E., . . . Scavini, M. (2011). Effects of carbohydrate counting on glucose control and quality of life over 24 weeks in adults patients with type 1 diabetes on continuous subcutaneous insulin infusion: A randomized, prospective clinical trial (GIOCAR). *Diabetes Care, 34*, 823–827.

Look AHEAD Research Group. (2013). Cardiovascular effects of intensive lifestyle intervention in type 2 diabetes. *The New England Journal of Medicine, 369*, 145–154.

Mainous, A., Tanner, R., Jo, A., & Anton, S. (2016). Prevalence of prediabetes and abdominal obesity among healthy-weight adults: 18-Year trend. *Annals of Family Medicine, 14*, 304–310.

Menke, A., Casagrande, S., Geiss, L., & Cowie, C. (2015). Prevalence of and trends in diabetes among adults in the United States, 1988-2012. *JAMA, 314*, 1021–1029.

Nguyen, N., Nguyen, X., Lane, J., & Wang, P. (2011). Relationship between obesity and diabetes in a US adult population: Findings from the National Health and Nutrition Examination Survey, 1999-2006. *Obesity Surgery, 21*, 351–355.

O'Neill, S., & O'Driscoll, L. (2015). Metabolic syndrome: A closer look at the growing epidemic and its associated pathologies. *Obesity Reviews, 16*, 1–12. doi:10.1111/obr.12229

Powers, M., Bardsley, J., Cypress, M., Duker, P., Funnell, M. M., Fischl, A. H., . . . Vivian, E. (2015). Diabetes self-management education and support in type 2 diabetes: A joint position statement of the American Diabetes Association, the American Association of Diabetes Educators, and the Academy of Nutrition and Dietetics. *Journal of the Academy of Nutrition and Dietetics, 115*, 1323–1334.

Ratner, R., Goldberg, R., Haffner, S., Marcovina, S., Orchard, T., Fowler, S., & Temprosa, M. (2005). Impact of intensive lifestyle and metformin therapy on cardiovascular disease risk factors in the Diabetes Prevention Program. *Diabetes Care, 28*, 888–894.

Selph, S., Dana, T., Blazina, I., Bougatsos, C., Patel, H., & Chou, R. (2015). Screening for type 2 diabetes mellitus: A systematic review for the U.S. Preventive Services Task Force. *Annals of Internal Medicine, 162*, 765–776.

Sjöström, L., Peltonen, M., Jacobson, P., Ahlin, S., Andersson-Assarsson, J., Anveden, Å., . . . Carlsson, L. M. (2014). Association of bariatric surgery with long-term remission of type 2 diabetes and with microvascular and macrovascular complications. *JAMA, 311*, 2297–2304.

Wheeler, M., Dunbar, S., Jaacks, L., Karmally, W., Mayer-Davis, E. J., Wylie-Rosett, J., & Yancy, W. S., Jr. (2012). Macronutrients, food groups, and eating patterns in the management of diabetes: A systematic review of the literature, 2010. *Diabetes Care, 35*, 434–445.

Wiebe, N., Padwal, R., Field, C., Marks, S., Jacobs, R., & Tonelli, M. (2011). A systematic review on the effect of sweeteners on glycemic response and clinically relevant outcomes. *BMC Medicine, 9*, 123.

Williamson, D., Rejeski, J., Lang, W., Van Dorsten, B., Fabricatore, A. N., & Toledo, K. (2009). Impact of a weight management program on health-related quality of life in overweight adults with type 2 diabetes. *Archives of Internal Medicine, 169*, 163–171.

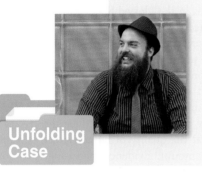

Unfolding Case

Jacob Holzhausen

Jacob is 49 years old and wants to eat healthier and lose weight. He is 6 ft 1 in tall, weighs 298 pounds, and does not exercise. His physician advised him to get down to 250 pounds and told him to follow a 2000-calorie diet. He has prediabetes, hypertension, and hypercholesterolemia. He lives alone and doesn't cook. Instead, he normally eats fast food meals. He admits to being a heavy beer drinker.

Check Your Knowledge

True	False		
☐	☐	1	Of all seven metrics that define cardiovascular health, the one most in need of improvement among American adults is diet.
☐	☐	2	The Dietary Approaches to Stop Hypertension (DASH) diet lowers blood pressure primarily because it is low in sodium.
☐	☐	3	For cardiovascular disease (CVD) risk reduction, it is more effective to focus on single nutrients (e.g., fat or sodium) than the whole eating pattern.
☐	☐	4	High triglyceride levels are a component of metabolic syndrome (MetS) but are not considered to be directly atherogenic but rather a biomarker of CVD.
☐	☐	5	A traditional Mediterranean diet is a low-fat diet.
☐	☐	6	Foods with components that provide cardiometabolic benefits include fish and nuts.
☐	☐	7	Trans fats increase low-density lipoprotein cholesterol (LDL-C) and therefore risk of CVD.
☐	☐	8	Alcohol has both positive and negative effects on heart health.
☐	☐	9	Only people with blood pressure greater than 120/80 mmHg can benefit from lowering their sodium intake.
☐	☐	10	The need to restrict sodium intake in patients with heart failure is clearly established.

Learning Objectives

Upon completion of this chapter, you will be able to

1 List the metrics that define cardiovascular health.
2 Discuss the metrics that define an optimal healthy diet score for a 2000-calorie intake.
3 Summarize the characteristics of a Dietary Approaches to Stop Hypertension (DASH) diet.
4 Compare the DASH diet with the traditional Mediterranean diet.
5 Plan a 2000-calorie DASH eating plan menu.

6 Name foods associated with cardiometabolic benefits.
7 Name foods associated with cardiometabolic risks.
8 Counsel a client on ways to lower sodium intake.

Cardiovascular disease (CVD) refers to heart and blood vessel conditions such as coronary heart disease (CHD), stroke, hypertension, and heart failure. Although mortality from CVD has been declining over the last few decades in the United States and many Western industrialized countries, it remains the leading cause of death in United States and worldwide (Mozaffarian et al., 2015). CVD is responsible for nearly 1 out of 3 deaths in the United States and more deaths than from all forms of cancer combined (Mozaffarian et al., 2015). Poor diet quality affects several major cardiovascular risk factors, including blood pressure, serum lipid levels, insulin resistance, and weight.

The relationship between diet and CVD has been a major focus of health research for almost half a century (Mente, de Koning, Shannon, & Anand, 2009). For decades, Americans were urged to follow a low-fat diet to reduce the risk of CVD. It is now known that the quality of fat consumed is more important than the total amount. Evidence increasingly supports the shift away from focusing on single nutrients (e.g., fat) to promoting healthy dietary patterns (e.g., a Dietary Approaches to Stop Hypertension-style or Mediterranean-style pattern).

This chapter discusses cardiovascular health and various CVD risks, dietary strategies for the risk reduction, and nutrition therapy for established CVD and heart failure.

Quick Bite **Estimated prevalence of CVD among American adults**

High blood pressure: 80 million
CHD: 15.5 million
Myocardial infarction (MI): 7.6 million
Chest pain: 8.2 million
Heart failure: 5.7 million
Stroke (all types): 6.6 million

Source: Mozaffarian, D., Benjamin, E., Go, A., Arnett, D. K., Blaha, M. J., Cushman, M., . . . Turner, M. B. (2015). Heart disease and stroke statistics—2016 update: A report from the American Heart Association. *Circulation, 133*, e38–e360. doi:10.1161/cir.0000000000000350

CARDIOVASCULAR HEALTH

The 2020 goal of the American Heart Association is "to improve the cardiovascular health of all Americans by 20% while reducing deaths from CVD and stroke by 20%" (Lloyd-Jones et al., 2010). The new concept of cardiovascular health is defined according to seven metrics: smoking, body mass index (BMI), physical activity, diet quality, total cholesterol level, blood pressure, and fasting plasma glucose level (Table 20.1). It is estimated that 80% of CVD can be prevented by not smoking; eating healthily; being physically active; maintaining a healthy weight; and controlling hypertension, diabetes, and high lipid levels (Mozaffarian et al., 2015).

A scoring system is used to rate cardiovascular health as ideal, intermediate, or poor for each metric and overall. Table 20.1 shows the percentage of American adults who meet the criteria for each metric. Americans score as "ideal" most often in the category of "not currently a smoker" (77.8%) and least often in consuming a healthy eating pattern, such as a DASH-type pattern (1.5%) (Mozaffarian et al., 2015). Poor diet quality, overweight/obesity, hypertension, hypercholesterolemia, and metabolic syndrome are presented in the following sections.

Diet Quality

Of all seven metrics that define cardiovascular health, healthy diet pattern has the worst compliance scores with only 1.5% of adults achieving an ideal score (>80 out of 100 points) (Mozaffarian et al., 2015). An "ideal diet" is described as a calorie-appropriate DASH-type eating plan characterized by five primary and three secondary features as listed in Table 20.1. Comparing 2011 to 2012 scores for the five primary healthy diet metrics to the previous period in 2009 to 2010, American adults (Mozaffarian et al., 2015)

- Did not show overall improvement in ideal adherence. However, more adults achieved intermediate adherence (a score of 40%–79%) and fewer had poor adherence (a score of <40%)
- Improved most in increasing whole grain intake and reducing consumption of sugar sweetened beverages
- Had a small, nonsignificant increase in fruit and vegetable intake
- Showed virtually no improvement in fish and sodium intake

Table 20.1	Definition of Ideal Cardiovascular Health Metrics and the Percentage of Adults 20 Years and Older Who Meet the Criteria for Ideal in Each Metric	

Ideal Health Factors	Percentage of Adults Who Achieve Ideal Metric
Total cholesterol <200 mg/dL	46.6
Blood pressure <120 mmHg or <80 mmHg	42.2
Not currently a smoker	77.8
Fasting plasma glucose <100 mg/dL	53.0
Ideal Health Behaviors	
Physically active ≥150 minutes/week at moderate to vigorous intensity or ≥75 minutes/week at vigorous intensity	44.0
BMI <25 kg/m²	31.3
A DASH-type pattern that meets four to five of these goals	1.5
≥4.5 cups/day fruits and vegetables	17.2
≥2 servings fish/week	21.2
<1500 mg/day sodium	3.1
<36 oz/week sugar sweetened beverages	66.0
Three or more 1-oz servings whole grains/day	12.0
Secondary diet metrics	
≥4 servings/week nuts/legumes/seeds	42.0
<2 servings/week processed meats	62.1
<7% total calories from saturated fat	25.9

BMI, body mass index; DASH, Dietary Approaches to Stop Hypertension.
Sources: Lloyd-Jones, D., Hong, Y., Labarthe, D., Mozaffarian, D., Appel, L. J., Van Horn, L., . . . Rosamond, W. D. (2010). Defining and setting national goals for cardio-vascular health promotion and disease reduction: The American Heart Association's Strategic Impact Goal through 2020 and beyond. *Circulation, 121*, 586–613 and Mozaffarian, D., Benjamin, E., Go, A., Arnett, D. K., Blaha, M. J., Cushman, M., . . . Turner, M. B. (2015). Heart disease and stroke statistics—2016 update: A report from the American Heart Association. *Circulation, 133*, e38–e360. doi:10.1161/cir.0000000000000350

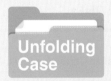

Recall Jacob. A diet history reveals that his typical first meal of the day is two egg-and-sausage breakfast sandwiches along with coffee, cream, and sugar. Lunch is two peanut butter and jelly sandwiches on white bread with chips and soda. Dinner is a submarine sandwich, pizza, or tacos. During the evening he eats chips and salsa while drinking three to four beers. How does his usual intake compare to the ideal diet metrics? What specific suggestions would you make to improve his usual intake?

Saturated Fat or Fatty Acids
fatty acids in which all the carbon atoms are bonded to as many hydrogen atoms as they can hold, so no double bonds exist between carbon atoms; animal fats (meat and dairy), coconut oil, palm oil, and palm kernel oil are the biggest sources.

Trans Fats
fatty acids with hydrogen atoms on opposite sides of the double bond. Most trans fats in the diet come from partially hydrogenated fats.

Eating Pattern Recommendations

Current dietary recommendations for the primary or secondary prevention of CVD focus on eating patterns, not individual nutrients, that inherently reflect nutrient targets, such as reducing intakes of sodium, added sugars, **saturated fat or fatty acids**, and **trans fat** and increasing intakes of potassium and fiber. Foods with a positive impact on cardiometabolic factors (Table 20.2) are emphasized, and those with a negative impact (Table 20.3) are avoided.

For "healthy" people, the DASH- and Mediterranean-style eating patterns may help prevent hypertension, CHD, stroke, type 2 diabetes, and obesity if calories are appropriate. For people who are not "healthy" (e.g., those who are being

Table 20.2   Foods Associated with Cardiometabolic Benefits

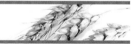

Food	Components Implicated in Benefits	Possible Cardiometabolic Benefits
Fruits and vegetables	Antioxidant vitamins, potassium, magnesium, fiber, phytochemicals	Improvements in blood pressure, lipid levels, insulin resistance, weight control Lower incidence of CHD Lower incidence of stroke (fruit) Benefits are not replicated with equivalent amounts of mineral or fiber supplements.
Whole grains	B vitamins, vitamin E, fiber, folate, minerals, phytochemicals, polyunsaturated fatty acids	Improvements in glucose-insulin homeostasis; may reduce inflammation and promote weight loss Whole-grain oats decrease LDL cholesterol without lowering HDL-C Higher fiber content contributes to the lower incidence of CHD, diabetes, and possibly stroke from whole grains; the effect of whole grains is not replicated from equivalent amounts of supplemental fiber bran, or isolated micronutrients.
Fish	Specific proteins, unsaturated fats, vitamin D, selenium, omega-3 fatty acids	In human trials, fish oil lowers triglyceride levels, systolic and diastolic blood pressure, and resting heart rate. May reduce inflammation and limit platelet aggregation Lower incidence of CHD, ischemic stroke, cardiac death
Nuts	Unsaturated fatty acids, vegetable proteins, fiber, folate, minerals, antioxidants, phytochemicals	Lower total cholesterol, LDL cholesterol, and postprandial hyperglycemia from high-carbohydrate meals When added to weight loss diets, weight loss is either unchanged or greater. Lower incidence of CHD
Dairy products	It is not known which constituents of dairy products offer cardiometabolic benefits; possibly specific fatty acids, proteins, vitamins, minerals, and other nutrients	May improve satiety and weight loss May contribute to improvements in blood pressure, lipid levels, and insulin resistance regardless of changes in weight Lower risk of stroke and diabetes
Vegetable oils	Polyunsaturated fatty acids (PUFAs), monounsaturated fatty acids, plant-derived omega-3 fatty acids	Improvements in blood lipids and lipoproteins and lower CVD events when PUFAs replace saturated fatty acids Monounsaturated fats from vegetable oils (e.g., olive oil) may lower CVD risk.
Legumes	Micronutrients, phytochemicals, fiber	Nutrient package may reduce cardiometabolic risk.

CHD, chronic heart disease; LDL, low-density lipoprotein; HDL-C, high-density lipoprotein; CVD, cardiovascular disease.
Source: Mozaffarian, D., Appel, L., & Van Horn, L. (2011). Components of a cardioprotective diet: New insights. *Circulation, 123*, 2870–2891.

Table 20.3   Foods Associated with Cardiometabolic Risks

Food	Components Implicated in Adverse Effects	Possible Cardiometabolic Risks
Foods and fats containing partially hydrogenated vegetable oils, such as commercially baked products and stick margarine	Trans fatty acids	Strongest link to CHD risk of all types of fat
Red and processed meats such as bacon, sausage, hot dogs	Heme iron, saturated fatty acids, dietary cholesterol; sodium and preservatives (in processed meats)	Consumption of processed meats associated with higher incidence of CHD and diabetes mellitus Red meat and processed meat may increase risk of CHD when they are eaten in place of poultry, fish, and plant proteins.
Sugar-sweetened beverages, sweets, and grain-based desserts and bakery foods	Sugars, refined grains	Sugar-sweetened beverages are linked to obesity; lack of satiety from liquid sugar may contribute to positive calorie balance. Sugar-sweetened beverages may displace the intake of more healthful beverages. High sugar-sweetened beverage consumption associated with higher incidence of diabetes, MetS, and possibly CHD Refined carbohydrates are devoid of beneficial nutrients and may displace more healthful foods.

CHD, chronic heart disease; MetS, metabolic syndrome.
Source: Mozaffarian, D., Appel, L., & Van Horn, L. (2011). Components of a cardioprotective diet: New insights. *Circulation, 123*, 2870–2891.

treated for CHD, hypertension, or diabetes or have had an MI or stroke), these eating patterns and lifestyle changes are an integral part of management. With attention to cultural considerations, as appropriate (Box 20.1), these eating pattern and lifestyle recommendations come close to being "one size fits all." Tips for choosing "ideal" eating pattern are summarized in Box 20.2.

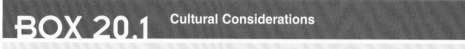

BOX 20.1 Cultural Considerations

For all cultural groups, emphasize the positive aspects of their eating styles and suggest ways to lower saturated fat and sodium content of traditional foods.

African American Tradition

Traditional soul foods tend to be high in saturated fat and sodium. On the positive side, there is a heavy emphasis on vegetables and complex carbohydrates.
   Suggested changes in cooking techniques include

- Using nonstick skillets sprayed with cooking spray when pan-frying eggs, fish, and vegetables
- Using small amounts of liquid smoke flavoring in place of bacon, salt pork, or ham
- Using more seasonings, such as onion, garlic, and pepper, in place of some of the salt
- Using turkey ham or turkey sausage in place of bacon
- Using "lite" or sugar-free syrups

Mexican American Tradition

The traditional diet is primarily vegetarian with a heavy emphasis on fruits, vegetables, rice, and dried peas and beans. Processed foods are used infrequently.
   Cooking techniques rely on frying and stewing with liberal amounts of oil or lard. An alternative is to sauté or stew with small amounts of canola or olive oil. High-fat meats and lard are commonly used. Using less meat, choosing lower fat varieties, trimming visible fat, and substituting oil for lard are heart healthy alternatives.

Chinese American Tradition

Traditional Chinese cooking relies heavily on vegetables and rice with plants providing the majority of calories. Meat is used more as a condiment than an entrée. Cooking techniques tend to preserve nutrients. Sauces add little fat.
   Sodium intake is high related to heavy use of soy sauce, monosodium glutamate (MSG), and salted pickles. Reduced-sodium soy sauce is available, but it is still high in sodium. Because of the difficulty in eliminating the use of soy sauce, a more practical approach is to gradually use less.

Native American/Alaska Native Traditions

Widely diverse eating styles make useful generalizations difficult.
   In general,

- Encourage traditional cooking methods such as baking, roasting, boiling, and broiling.
- Encourage the use of traditional meats, such as fish, deer, and caribou.
- Remove fat from canned meats.
- Use vegetable oil for frying instead of lard or shortening.

Jewish Tradition

Many traditional foods are high in sodium such as *kosher* meats (salt is used in the koshering process), herring, lox, pickles, canned chicken broth or soups, and delicatessen meats (e.g., corned beef, pickled tongue, pastrami).
   Pareve (neutral) nondairy creamers are often used as a dairy substitute in meals containing meat, but they are high in saturated fat. Encourage light and fat-free versions.
   Encourage methods to lower fat in traditional recipes such as

- Baking instead of frying potato pancakes
- Limiting the amount of schmaltz (chicken fat) used in cooking
- Using reduced-fat or fat-free cream cheese on bagels
- Using low-fat or nonfat cottage cheese, sour cream, and yogurt in kugels and blintzes

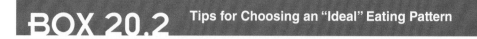

BOX 20.2   Tips for Choosing an "Ideal" Eating Pattern

Replace foods high in saturated fat with foods that provide unsaturated fats.

- Avoid fatty meats.
- Avoid processed meat.
- Choose lean meats and poultry and remove skin from poultry before eating.
- Use liquid oils such as canola, olive, and soybean in place of solid fats such as butter, stick margarine, shortening, and lard.

Choose low-fat dairy products.

- Enjoy low fat or non-fat milk, yogurt, and cheese.

Choose whole grains.

- Replace white enriched breads and cereals with whole grains, such as whole wheat, oats, barley, corn, popcorn, brown rice, wild rice, buckwheat, triticale, bulgur, millet, quinoa, and sorghum.

Eat more fruits and vegetables.

- Eat a variety of fresh, frozen, and canned fruits and vegetables without added sugars, salt, or high-calorie sauces.
- Eat occasional meatless meals that feature legumes, tofu, or vegetables.
- Snack on fresh or dried fruits, fresh vegetables with "healthy" dip, or frozen fruit bars.

Eat more fish.

- Eat oily fish, such as mackerel, salmon, herring, lake trout, tuna, and white fish, at least twice a week.

Avoid added fats, added sugars, and sodium.

- Read "Nutrition Facts" labels.
- Limit high-calorie bakery products—they usually contain white flour, added sugars, and saturated and trans fats.
- Avoid sugar-sweetened beverages.
- Prepare foods from "scratch" instead of purchasing convenience foods and mixes, which tend to be high in sodium.
- Use herbs and spices, lemon juice, and flavored vinegars to flavor vegetables and other foods.

The Dietary Approaches to Stop Hypertension Diet

Dietary Approaches to Stop Hypertension (DASH) was a multicenter feeding study funded by the National Heart, Lung, and Blood Institute (Appel et al., 1997) that set out to test whether eating whole "real" foods rather than individual nutrients would lower blood pressure as a result of some combination of nutrients, interactions among individual nutrients, or other food factors (Appel et al., 1997). The results clearly showed that eating a diet high in fruit, vegetables, and low-fat dairy products; moderate in whole grains, poultry, fish, and nuts; and low in fat, red meat, sweets, and sugar-sweetened beverages substantially lowers both systolic and diastolic blood pressures as well as low-density lipoprotein cholesterol (LDL-C). Reductions in blood pressure were similar in men and women and similar in magnitude to the effects seen with drug monotherapy for mild hypertension. In people who have type 2 diabetes, the DASH diet has been shown to improve numerous cardiac risk factors, including waist circumference, systolic and diastolic blood pressure, fasting blood glucose, hemoglobin A1c, triglyceride levels, LDL-C, high-density lipoprotein cholesterol (HDL-C), and total cholesterol (Azadbakht et al., 2011).

The DASH diet is a healthy eating pattern appropriate for all people, unless contraindicated. Table 20.4 lists food group serving recommendations for various calorie levels. The DASH diet is frequently featured in lay publications. U.S. News & World Report ranks the DASH diet as the best overall "diet" (as in eating plan, not weight loss diet) out of 38 diets evaluated and the best diet for healthy eating (Haupt, 2016).

The original DASH eating plan was rich in potassium, magnesium, and calcium, as well as fiber and protein; low in total fat, saturated fat, and cholesterol; and protein content was slightly increased. It is likely that several aspects of the diet, not just one nutrient or food, lowered blood

Table 20.4	The Dietary Approaches to Stop Hypertension Eating Plan at Various Calorie Levels				

Food Group and Representative Serving Sizes	Servings Per Day			Examples of Foods	Significance to the DASH Eating Pattern
	1600 Calories	2000 Calories	2600 Calories		
Grain 1 slice bread; ½ cup cooked rice, pasta, or cereal; 1 oz ready to eat cereal	6	6–8	10–11	Whole grains are recommended for most grain servings, such as whole wheat bread, whole-grain cereals, whole wheat pasta, and brown rice	Provide calories and fiber
Vegetables 1 cup raw leafy vegetable ½ cup cut-up raw or cooked vegetable ½ cup vegetable juice	3–4	4–5	5–6	All fresh, plain frozen, and low-sodium canned vegetables Use preparation methods to retain the fiber content, such as leaving skins on potatoes	Provide potassium, magnesium, and fiber
Fruits 1 medium fruit ¼ cup dried fruit ½ cup fresh, frozen, or canned fruit ½ cup fruit juice	4	4–5	5–6	All; eat skins and seeds for fiber whenever possible Whole fruits are better choices than fruit juice.	Provide potassium, magnesium, and fiber
Fat-free or low-fat milk and milk products 1 cup milk or yogurt 1½ oz natural cheese	2–3	2–3	3	Fat-free or low-fat milk; fat-free, low-fat, or reduced-fat cheese; fat-free or low-fat regular or frozen yogurt	Provide calcium, magnesium, potassium, and protein
Lean meats, poultry, and fish 1 oz lean meat, poultry, or fish 1 egg	3–4 or less	6 or less	6 or less	Choose only lean meats; broil, roast, or poach meats; trim away visible fat Limit egg yolks to 4 per week	Provide protein and magnesium
Nuts, seeds, and legumes ⅓ cup or 1½ oz nuts 2 tbsp peanut butter 2 tbsp or ½ oz seeds ½ cup cooked legumes	3–4 per week	4–5 per week	1	Any unsalted nuts and seeds Any dried peas and beans (drain and rinse canned varieties)	Provide calories, magnesium, protein, and fiber
Fats and oils 1 tsp soft margarine 1 tsp oil 1 tbsp mayonnaise 2 tbsp salad dressing	2	2–3	3	Soft trans fat-free margarines in tubs or spray form Vegetable oils such as canola, olive, corn, and safflower oils Low-fat mayonnaise Light salad dressing	DASH diet provided 27% of calories from fat including fat in food and fat added to foods.
Sweets and added sugars 1 tbsp sugar 1 tbsp jelly or jam ½ cup sorbet and ices	3 or less per week	5 or less per week	Less than 2	Sweets that are low in fat such as sorbets, ices, fruit bars, angel food cake, fig bars, gelatin, hard candy, maple syrup	DASH diet is low in sugar.
Maximum sodium limit	2300 mg/day	2300 mg/day	2300 mg/day		

Source: National Heart, Lung, and Blood Institute. (2015). *In brief: Your guide to lowering your blood pressure with DASH.* Available at https://www.nhlbi.nih.gov/files/docs/public/heart/dash_brief.pdf. Accessed on 8/7/16.

pressure (Appel et al., 2006). Especially noteworthy is that the decrease in blood pressure occurred without lowering sodium intake and without lowering calories to produce weight loss.

A second study, DASH-sodium, was designed to test whether limiting sodium on a DASH diet would yield even better results (Sacks et al., 2001). The results showed the following:

- Lowering sodium with either the control diet or DASH diet lowers blood pressure; the lower the sodium intake, the lower the blood pressure.
- At each sodium level, blood pressure was lower on the DASH diet than on the control diet.

Table 20.5	2000-Calorie Dietary Approaches to Stop Hypertension Menus at Two Sodium Levels		
2300-mg Sodium Menu	**Sodium (mg)**	**Substitutions to ↓ Sodium to 1500 mg**	**Sodium (mg)**
Breakfast		The same as the 2400-mg sodium menu except	
¾ cup wheat flakes cereal	199	2 cups puffed wheat cereal	1
1 slice whole wheat bread	149		149
1 medium banana	1		1
1 cup nonfat milk	126		126
1 cup orange juice	5		5
1 tsp soft margarine	51	1 tsp soft margarine, unsalted	1
Lunch			
Beef sandwich			
2 oz ham, low sodium	101	2 oz beef, eye of round	35
1 tbsp Dijon mustard	360	1 tbsp low-fat mayonnaise	101
2 slices cheddar cheese, reduced fat	260	2 slices Swiss cheese, natural	109
1 sesame roll	319		319
1 large leaf romaine lettuce	1		1
2 slices tomato	22		22
1 cup low-fat, low-sodium potato salad	12		12
1 medium orange	0		0
Dinner			
3 oz cod with lemon juice	90		90
½ cup brown rice	5		5
½ cup cooked spinach	88		88
1 small corn bread muffin	363	1 small dinner roll	146
1 tsp soft margarine	51	1 tsp soft margarine, unsalted	1
Snacks			
1 cup fruit yogurt, fat free, no added sugar	107		107
½ cup dried fruit	6		6
2 large graham cracker rectangles	156		156
1 tbsp peanut butter, reduced fat	101	1 tbsp peanut butter, unsalted	3
Total sodium (mg)	**2228**		**1539**

- The greatest reduction in blood pressure occurred at 1500 mg of sodium.
- The greatest blood pressure reductions occurred in blacks; middle-aged and older people; and people with hypertension, diabetes, or chronic kidney disease.

Table 20.5 shows two 2000-calorie DASH menus, one with 2300 mg of sodium and the other at 1500 mg. Given that more than 75% of the sodium in a typical American diet comes from processed foods, it is difficult for people who regularly consume processed, prepackaged, and restaurant foods to lower their sodium intake (Box 20.3). Breads and rolls, cold cuts and cured meats, pizza, soup, sandwiches, and poultry are identified as the top six sources of sodium in a typical American eating pattern (American Heart Association, n.d.). Compliance to a lower sodium intake may improve by gradually lowering intake. Tips to lower sodium intake appear in Box 20.4.

BOX 20.3 The Effect of Food Processing on Sodium Content

Food Groups	Sodium (mg)
Whole and other grains and grain products*	
Cooked cereal, rice, pasta, unsalted, ½ cup	0–5
Ready-to-eat cereal, 1 cup	0–360
Bread, 1 slice	110–175
Vegetables	
Fresh or frozen, cooked without salt, ½ cup	1–70
Canned or frozen with sauce, ½ cup	140–460
Tomato juice, canned, ½ cup	330
Fruit	
Fresh, frozen, canned, ½ cup	0–5
Low-fat or fat-free milk and milk products	
Milk, 1 cup	107
Yogurt, 1 cup	175
Natural cheeses, 1½ oz	110–450
Processed cheeses, 2 oz	600
Nuts, seeds, and legumes	
Peanuts, salted, ½ cup	120
Peanuts, unsalted, ½ cup	0–5
Beans, cooked from dried or frozen, without salt, ½ cup	0–5
Beans, canned, ½ cup	400
Lean meats, fish, and poultry	
Fresh meat, fish, poultry, 3 oz	30–90
Tuna canned, water pack, no salt added, 3 oz	35–45
Tuna canned, water pack, 3 oz	230–350
Ham, lean, roasted, 3 oz	1020
Convenience and Fast Foods	**Sodium (mg)**
1 packet dry onion soup mix	3132
1 tsp salt	2325
1 fast-food single cheeseburger with condiments and bacon	1314
One 6-in, fast-food tuna salad sub	1293
1 large fast-food taco	1233
2 fast-food pancakes with syrup	1104
1 cup canned macaroni and cheese	1061
1 fast-food beef chimichanga	910

*Whole grains are recommended for most grain servings.

Since the DASH-sodium trial, studies have tested whether a lower carbohydrate DASH diet would yield similar or better results than the original DASH diet. The OmniHeart (Optimal Macronutrient Intake Trial to Prevent Heart Disease) randomized trial replaced some of the carbohydrate in the original DASH diet with either protein, half of which was from plant sources, or **unsaturated fat or fatty acids**, predominately **monounsaturated fat or monounsaturated fatty acids** (Appel et al., 2005). Results showed that both the protein and unsaturated fat DASH diets significantly lowered blood pressure in all participants, including those with hypertension. Although the effect on specific lipoprotein levels differed between the two modifications, the estimated CHD risk was similar on both diets and lower than that of the original DASH diet. Adherence to the modified DASH diets was also high. The take away message is that compared to the typical American eating pattern, a DASH pattern—original, lower in sodium, or lower in carbohydrates—provides major health benefits. These findings highlight the importance of specific food choices in the DASH pattern (e.g., the high fruit, vegetable, dairy content and low content of red meat and sweets) rather than the macronutrient composition (Mozaffarian, Appel, & Van Horn, 2011).

Unsaturated Fat or Fatty Acids
fatty acids in which one or more double bonds exist between carbon atoms. A fatty acid with one double bond is classified as a monounsaturated fat. Polyunsaturated fats have two or more double bonds between carbon atoms.

Monounsaturated Fat or Monounsaturated Fatty Acids
fatty acids that have only one double bond between two carbon atoms; olive oil, canola oil, and poultry are rich sources.

BOX 20.4 Tips to Lower Sodium Intake

In General

- Eat more meals at home. Cook in batches and freeze for use on busy days.
- Avoid or limit convenience foods, such as boxes mixes, frozen dinners, and canned goods.
- Compare labels to find items lowest in sodium.
- Don't add salt when cooking.

Grains

- Find lower sodium varieties by comparing labels.
- Cook rice and pasta without adding salt.
- Eat cereals without added salt, such as oatmeal, shredded wheat, and puffed whole-grain cereal.
- Avoid instant flavored rice, pasta, and cereal mixes.

Vegetables

- Eat more fresh or frozen vegetables without salt added.
- Rinse canned vegetables before using.
- Switch to pasta sauce without added salt or dilute regular bottled pasta sauce with equal parts of no-salt-added tomato sauce.
- Substitute fresh vegetables for pickles and other pickled foods.

Fruits

- Fresh, frozen, and canned fruits are salt-free; enjoy.

Milk and Milk Products

- Use cheese sparingly, especially processed cheeses.

Protein Foods

- Choose fresh poultry, fish, and lean meat instead of canned, smoked, deli, or other processed varieties.
- Limit frozen dinners.

- Limit cured meat intake, such as sausages and hot dogs. Compare labels to find lower sodium varieties.
- Limit imitation crab and lobster products.
- Limit soy substitutes, such as imitation ground beef or chicken.
- Use no-salt-added nut butters.

Fats and Oils

- Use homemade vinegar and oil dressings instead of bottled salad dressings.

Miscellaneous

- Use herbs and spices instead of salt to season foods.
- Replace garlic and onion salts with garlic and onion powders.
- Use reduced-salt or no-salt-added condiments such as ketchup, soy sauce, and mayonnaise.
- Use no-salt-added broth to make soup instead of using canned soup.

When Eating Out

- Request that food not be salted, if possible.
- Choose fruit juice instead of soup for an appetizer.
- Use oil and vinegar or fresh lemon instead of regular salad dressing.
- Choose foods that are grilled, baked, or roasted.
- Order plain meat and vegetables without gravy or sauce, or order them "on the side" and use sparingly.
- Choose plain baked potatoes and season sparingly with sour cream, butter, or pepper.
- Select fresh fruit for dessert. If the client is going to splurge, ice cream or sherbet is a better choice than pie, cake, cookies, or other desserts.
- Avoid fast-food restaurant meals, which usually are high in sodium. If you have to go, order a child-sized meal.
- Order sandwiches without mayonnaise, sauces, or condiments; load with lettuce, tomato, and onion.

Mediterranean-Style Eating Pattern

Arguably, the healthiest and best-studied eating pattern is a Mediterranean-style pattern (Fig. 20.1). Although there is not a uniform definition of a Mediterranean-style diet, it is characterized by a high intake of olive oil, fruits, nuts, vegetables, and cereals; moderate intake of fish and poultry; low intake of dairy products, red meat, processed meats, and sweets; and wine in moderation, consumed with meals (Estruch et al., 2013). Generally, a Mediterranean-style eating pattern is moderate in total fat (32%–35% of total calories), relatively low in saturated fat (9%–10% of total calories), high in fiber (27–37 g/day), and high in unsaturated fats (Eckel et al., 2014). Adherence to the diet can be easily achieved because it is a palatable eating pattern (Lopez-Garcia et al., 2014).

The benefits of a Mediterranean diet may be due to the synergy among various nutrients and foods (Jacobs, Gross, & Tapsell, 2009). Observational studies have attributed cardiovascular benefits to the Mediterranean diet (Mente et al., 2009), olive oil (Buckland et al., 2012), and nuts (Afshin, Micha, Khatibzadeh, & Mozaffarian, 2014). The eating pattern, and to a lesser degree its individual components, lowers CVD risk by improving blood pressure, lipid levels, insulin resistance, BMI, and waist circumference and through its anti-inflammatory and antioxidant effects (Widmer, Flammer, Lerman, & Leman, 2015). A large primary prevention trial in Spain among people at high risk for CVD compared a low-fat diet to a Mediterranean-style diet supplemented

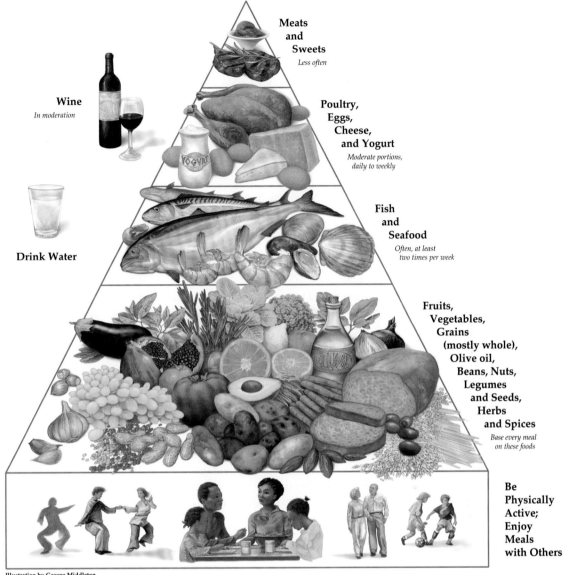

FIGURE 20.1 ▲ Mediterranean diet pyramid. *(© 2009 Oldways Preservation and Exchange Trust, www.oldwayspt.org)*

with either extra virgin oil or nuts (Box 20.5) (Estruch et al., 2013). The study was actually halted early when it became overwhelmingly evident that those assigned to the Mediterranean diet had a significant decrease in the risk of stroke, MI, and cardiovascular deaths (Estruch et al., 2013). This landmark study is one of the largest randomized trials on the primary prevention of CVD and places the Mediterranean diet in the forefront of CVD prevention (Widmer et al., 2015).

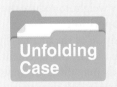

Unfolding Case

Think of Jacob. Is 2000 calories an appropriate weight loss diet for a male? What factors should be considered when deciding whether Jacob should be counseled to adhere to a DASH diet or a Mediterranean-style eating pattern? Can either pattern be adjusted to the appropriate calorie level? Jacob says he prefers a Mediterranean-style pattern because it includes wine, which he will drink in place of beer. What does Jacob need to know about alcohol and his CVD risks?

BOX 20.5 | Food Options for Mediterranean-Diet Study Participants

Foods recommended

- ≥3 servings/day of fresh fruit
- ≥2 servings/day of vegetables
- ≥3 servings/week of fish or seafood, especially fatty fish
- ≥3 servings/week legumes
- White meats in place of red meat
- ≥7 glasses/week of wine with meals for habitual drinkers

Plus:

- ≥4 tbsp olive oil/day (polyphenol-rich extra-virgin olive oil, not ordinary refined variety) for participants in the Mediterranean diet plus olive oil group
- ≥3 servings/week of nuts for participants in the Mediterranean diet plus nuts group. Participants were advised to eat 1 oz of nuts daily: 15 g of walnuts, 7.5 g of almonds, and 7.5 g of hazelnuts

Foods discouraged

- Soda (<1 drink/day)
- Commercial bakery products, sweets, pastries (<3 servings/week)
- Spreadable fats (<1 serving/day)
- Red and processed meats (<1 serving/day)

Source: Estruch, R., Ros, E., Salas-Salvadó, J., Covas, M. I., Corella, D., Arós, F., ... Martínez-González, M. A. (2013). Primary prevention of cardiovascular disease with a Mediterranean diet. *The New England Journal of Medicine, 368,* 1279–1290.

Dietary Supplements

There is a lack of convincing evidence to support the use of supplements to lower CVD risk. Results of the Physician's Health Study II showed that taking a daily multivitamin did not reduce major cardiovascular events, MI, stroke, or CVD mortality in male physicians after more than a decade of treatment and follow-up (Sesso et al., 2012). Certain supplements, including beta-carotene, calcium, and vitamin E, can even be harmful (Mozaffarian, Appel, et al., 2011).

Fish oil supplements of 1 to 2 g/day have shown CVD benefits in some studies but not in others (Mozaffarian et al., 2015). A meta-analysis of all randomized controlled trials showed a significant decrease in cardiac mortality but no significant effects on other CVD end points (Mozaffarian et al., 2015).

Overweight and Obesity

An ideal weight for cardiovascular health is set at BMI <25 kg/m^2; only 31.3% of American adults met that criterion in 2011 to 2012 (Mozaffarian et al., 2015). Overweight and obesity are major risk factors for CVD, including CHD, stroke, heart failure, and arrhythmias, because they raise LDL-C levels, decrease insulin sensitivity, increase blood pressure, and lower HDL-C. In a study of people who have carotid atherosclerosis, weight loss diets induced a significant reversal of atherosclerosis, which appears to be related to decreases in systolic blood pressure (Shai et al., 2010). Attaining and maintaining healthy weight to reduce the risk of CVD are appropriate goals throughout the lifecycle in the general population.

Although the macronutrient composition of the diet has little effect on weight loss, the quality of foods consumed may be a factor in weight management. Emerging evidence suggests that even when calorie value is the same, foods may differ in how likely they are to promote weight gain (Mozaffarian et al., 2015). High glycemic carbohydrates such as potatoes, white bread, white rice, low-fiber breakfast cereals, sweets/desserts, sugar-sweetened beverages, and red and processed meats are linked to weight gain. Note that these are foods that Americans are advised to limit. Conversely, nuts, whole grains, fruits, vegetables, legumes, fish, and yogurt—foods that are integral to a healthy eating pattern—are associated with weight loss over time (Mozaffarian, Hao, Rimm, Willett, & Hu, 2011; J. Smith et al., 2015). See Chapter 15 for more on overweight and obesity.

Hypertension

Hypertension is a major risk factor for stroke, CHD, heart failure, and kidney disease. It is arbitrarily defined as sustained elevated blood pressure greater than or equal to 140/90 mmHg. The definition is considered arbitrary, not absolute, because problems associated with high blood pressure increase progressively throughout the range of usual blood pressure starting at around 115/75 mmHg (Appel et al., 2011). African American adults have the highest prevalence of hypertension in the world at 44.9% of men and 46.1% of women. Compared to non-blacks, blacks develop hypertension earlier in life, have much higher average blood pressures, and have higher rates of hypertension-related complications, especially fatal stroke and end-stage kidney disease (Mozaffarian et al., 2015). Compared with other modifiable risk factors, high blood pressure is the leading cause of death in women and the second leading cause of death in men behind smoking (Mozaffarian et al., 2015).

In addition to overweight and obesity, nutrition-related risk factors for hypertension include

- *Salt sensitivity.* One definition of salt sensitivity is a change in blood pressure of 5% to 10% or at least 5 mmHg in response to a change in salt intake (Sullivan, 1991). Independent of blood pressure, salt sensitivity is a risk for cardiovascular and other diseases, even in salt-sensitive people who are normotensive (Felder, White, Williams, & Jose, 2013). There are no lab tests for salt sensitivity, and accurate testing is not easily or inexpensively performed.
- *High salt intake.* Lowering sodium intake to lower blood pressure is a recommendation in almost every country that has issued guidelines for preventing and treating CVD (Whelton et al., 2012). There is strong and consistent clinical trial evidence that lowering sodium intake lowers blood pressure in adults with hypertension and prehypertension, men and women, African Americans and non-African American adults, and in older and younger adults (Eckel et al., 2014). Observational data suggest that lower sodium intake is associated with lower risk of cardiovascular events in people with and without hypertension. The American Heart Association guideline on lifestyle management to reduce cardiovascular risk recommends that adults who would benefit from blood pressure lowering should consume no more than 2400 mg/day of sodium but that greater lowering to 1500 mg/day can result in a greater decrease in blood pressure (Eckel et al., 2014). In addition, even if those targets are not achieved, lowering sodium intake by at least 1000 mg/day lowers blood pressure. Despite the recommendation, controversy exists over what is an optimal sodium intake for people with or without high blood pressure (Graudal, Jürgens, Baslund, & Alderman, 2014).
- *Alcohol.* Although alcohol has the beneficial effect of raising HDL-C, chronic alcohol consumption (>3 drinks/day) is associated with an increased incidence of hypertension and CVD (Sesso, Cook, Buring, Manson, & Gaziano, 2008). If people choose to drink, alcohol intake should be limited to two drinks or less per day for men and one drink or less per day for women.
- *Low intake of potassium.* A meta-analysis of randomized controlled trials shows that potassium lowers blood pressure, with stronger effects in people who have hypertension and when sodium intake is high (Binia, Jaeger, Hu, Singh, & Zimmermann, 2015). A high potassium intake is associated with a decrease in blood pressure, stroke, and CVD risk (Aaron & Sanders, 2013).

Dietary interventions known to lower blood pressure include weight loss if overweight or obese, a decrease in sodium and alcohol intake, and adoption of the DASH eating plan. The DASH diet has been shown to prevent hypertension in people who are normotensive or prehypertensive; eliminate the need for medication in people with stage 1 hypertension; and lower blood pressure and reduce the dose of medication needed in people whose blood pressure is controlled with medication (Appel et al., 2006).

Hypercholesterolemia

Hypercholesterolemia is the cause of atherosclerosis, the underlying process responsible for most clinical atherosclerotic cardiovascular disease (ASCVD) events, such as MI, ischemic stroke, or

Table 20.6   Classification of Cholesterol

Total Cholesterol	
<200 mg/dL	Desirable
200–239 mg/dL	Borderline high
≥240 mg/dL	High
LDL Cholesterol	
<100 mg/dL	Optimal (ideal)
100–129 mg/dL	Near optimal/above optimal
130–159 mg/dL	Borderline high
160–189 mg/dL	High
≥190 mg/dL	Very high
HDL Cholesterol	
<40 mg/dL men	Risk factor for heart disease and stroke
<50 mg/dL women	Risk factor for heart disease and stroke
≥60 mg/dL	High; provides some protection against heart disease

LDL, low-density lipoprotein; HDL, high-density lipoprotein.
Source: Adult Treatment Panel. (2001). Clinical guidelines for cholesterol testing and management. The National Cholesterol Education Program, a division of the National Heart, Lung, Blood Institute. Available at www.nhlbi.nih.gov/guidelines /cholesterol/dskref.htm. Accessed on 8/7/16.

Non-HDL-C
non-HDL-C = total cholesterol − HDL-C. Includes atherogenic lipoproteins such as LDL-C, intermediate density lipoproteins, very-low-density lipoproteins (VLDL), VLDL remnants, chylomicron remnants, and lipoprotein (a). Non-HDL-C may be a stronger predictor of ASCVD morbidity and mortality than LDL-C.

Atherogenic Lipoproteins
lipoproteins that cause atherosclerosis and ASCVD, namely, non-HDL-C.

renal failure (Jacobson et al., 2014). Total cholesterol is a measure several lipoproteins, including LDL-C, HDL-C (Table 20.6), and **non-HDL-C** lipoproteins (Table 20.7). LDL-C and non-HDL-C are **atherogenic lipoproteins**; HDL-C levels are strongly inversely correlated with the incidence of CHD (Di Angelantonio et al., 2009). Because these lipoproteins have different effects on health, total cholesterol is less meaningful than non-HDL-C levels or the ratio of total cholesterol to HDL-C (Virani et al., 2012). Triglycerides are another form of lipid in the blood.

Low-Density Lipoprotein Cholesterol

Atherosclerosis is a progressive systemic disease process characterized by the buildup of fatty plaques that can develop in the large and small arteries that supply blood to

Table 20.7   Classification of Non-High-Density Lipoprotein Cholesterol (Non-HDL-C)* Levels

Non-HDL-C	Classification
<130	Desirable
130–159	Above desirable
160–189	Borderline high
190–219	High
≥220	Very high

*non-HDL-C = total cholesterol − HDL-C.
Source: Jacobson, T., Ito, M., Maki, K., Orringer, C. E., Bays, H. E., Jones, P. H., . . . Brown, W. V. (2014). National Lipid Association recommendations for patient-centered management of dyslipidemia: Part 1—executive summary. *Journal of Clinical Lipidology, 8,* 473–488.

the heart, brain, kidneys, and extremities. Atherosclerosis often begins early in life and progresses asymptomatically for decades before resulting in a clinical ASCVD event (Jacobson et al., 2014).

Lowering of LDL-C is the gold standard of atherosclerosis prevention (Whayne, 2011). Large-scale randomized controlled trials have shown that drug therapies, particularly statins, effectively lower atherogenic cholesterol and reduce ASCVD morbidity and mortality (Jacobson et al., 2014). Lifestyle interventions may be the sole treatment initially in patients at low or moderate risk before drug therapy is instituted (Jacobson et al., 2014). In high-risk patients, lifestyle interventions and drug therapy may be started concurrently. Lifestyle interventions can improve lipid levels, weight status, blood pressure, and insulin resistance (Jacobson et al., 2014).

Dietary factors that may raise LDL-C include, saturated fat, trans fats, and an excessive calorie intake (Jacobson et al., 2014). Reducing saturated fat intake lowers both LDL-C and HDL-C but has a greater impact on LDL-C. Although the general consensus from epidemiologic studies is that there is a correlation between saturated fat and CHD (Mente et al., 2009), the source of saturated fat may also affect its effect on risk: A higher intake of saturated fat in dairy products may be associated with lower CVD risk, whereas a higher intake of saturated fat in meat may increase CVD risk (de Oliveira Otto et al., 2012). Likewise, it may be that the effects of saturated fatty acids are modified by which foods or nutrients are increased or decreased in ex-

> **Isocaloric**
> having similar or the same calorie value.

change for saturated fatty acids. For instance, **isocaloric** replacement of saturated fats with carbohydrates has been shown to increase the risk of coronary events (Jakobsen et al., 2009), whereas replacing saturated fat with unsaturated fat and replacing trans fat with monounsaturated fat has been shown to be inversely associated with CVD (Guasch-Ferré et al., 2015). What is known is that eating patterns that reduce CVD risk include foods high in unsaturated fat, such as vegetable oils, nuts, and fish, and limit the intake of red meat (saturated fat) and trans fats.

Dietary recommendations for lowering LDL-C include following a DASH-type dietary pattern, lowering saturated fat intake to 5% to 6% of total calories, and reducing the percentage of calories from trans fat (Eckel et al., 2014). The most favorable impact on lipid profiles is seen when saturated fat is replaced by polyunsaturated fats, followed by monounsaturated fatty acids, then carbohydrates, preferably in the form of whole, not refined grains (Eckel et al., 2014). Weight loss is recommended for people who are overweight or obese. Additional dietary strategies, such as using plant sterols/stanols and soluble fiber, may be considered.

High-Density Lipoprotein Cholesterol

HDL-C is believed to reduce the risk of atherosclerosis by moving cholesterol from peripheral tissues back to the liver and possibly through other mechanisms, such as anti-inflammatory and antithrombotic effects (Duffy & Rader, 2009). The level of HDL-C is an important risk indicator; however, low HDL-C is not recommended as a target of therapy per se (Jacobson et al., 2014). Lifestyle interventions to lower atherogenic cholesterol, namely, regular physical activity, weight loss, and smoking cessation, increase HDL-C.

Triglycerides

According to the American Heart Association, triglycerides are not directly atherogenic but are an important biomarker of CVD risk because they are associated with other atherogenic particles

> **Omega-3 Fatty Acids**
> polyunsaturated fatty acids in which the first double bond is three carbon atoms away from the methyl (CH_3) end of the carbon chain. Eicosapentaenoic acid (EPA) and docosahexaenoic acid (DHA), commonly referred to as fish oils, are omega-3 fatty acids found in oily fish.

(Miller et al., 2011). High triglycerides are not a target of therapy until they are very high ($\geq$500 mg/dL and especially if $\geq$1000 mg/dL); triglyceride lowering at that point is to reduce the risk of pancreatitis. When triglycerides are 200 to 499 mg/dL, the target of therapy is to lower LDL-C (Jacobson et al., 2014). Triglyceride levels can decrease 20% to 50% as a result of healthy lifestyle changes, such as weight loss, limiting carbohydrates, eliminating trans fats, restricting fructose and saturated fatty acids, choosing a Mediterranean diet, and consuming **omega-3 fatty acids** from fish oil (Miller et al., 2011). Alcohol is also avoided.

Metabolic Syndrome

Metabolic syndrome (MetS), a multicomponent risk factor for both ASCVD and type 2 diabetes, is considered a worldwide epidemic (Alberti et al., 2009). It consists of a cluster of metabolic

Table 20.8	Diagnostic Criteria for Metabolic Syndrome
Risk Factor	**Defining Level**
Metabolic syndrome is confirmed by the presence of any three of the following five risks:	
Central obesity Men Women	>40-in waist >35-in waist Or population- and country-specific definitions, especially Asians and non-Europeans who have predominantly lived outside the United States
Elevated triglycerides	≥150 mg/dL, or taking medication for high triglyceride levels
Low HDL-C Men Women	<40 mg/dL in men <50 mg/dL in women Or taking medication for low HDL-C
Elevated blood pressure	≥130 mmHg systolic blood pressure ≥85 mmHg diastolic blood pressure Or taking medication for hypertension or taking antihypertensive medication with a history of hypertension
Elevated fasting glucose	≥100 mg/dL or taking medication to control blood sugar level

HDL-C, high-density lipoprotein cholesterol.
Source: Alberti, K., Eckel, R., Grundy, S., Zimmet, P. Z., Cleeman, J. I., Donato, K. A., . . . Smith, S. C., Jr. (2009). Harmonizing the metabolic syndrome: A joint interim statement of the International Diabetes Federation Task Force on Epidemiology and Prevention; National Heart, Lung, and Blood Institute: American Heart Association; World Heart Federation: International Atherosclerosis Society; and International Association for the Study of Obesity. *Circulation, 120*, 1640–1645.

abnormalities, namely, elevated triglycerides, low HDL-C, high blood pressure, high fasting blood glucose levels, and central obesity (Alberti et al., 2009). Although there is disagreement over the diagnostic criteria used to define MetS, three abnormal findings out of five qualify a person for MetS (Table 20.8). Of all possible combinations of three of the five risk factors, the combination of central obesity, elevated blood pressure, and hyperglycemia confer the greatest risk for ASCVD (Franco et al., 2009). It is estimated that 13.3% to 44% of excess CVD mortality in the United States is due to MetS or MetS-related existing CVD (Mozaffarain et al., 2015).

A review of 13 randomized controlled trials indicated that lifestyle interventions are more effective than drug treatment in reversing MetS (Dunkley et al., 2012); reversing MetS prevents its progression to CVD and type 2 diabetes. Weight loss via improvements in eating patterns and physical activity can improve all of the clinical markers (Bassi et al., 2014). A Mediterranean-style diet may improve central obesity, plasma glucose, blood pressure, and levels of HDL-C and triglycerides (Kastorini et al., 2011).

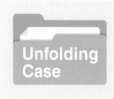

Consider Jacob. Does he meet the criteria for having MetS? Does his diet contribute to his risk of MetS? What should be Jacob's highest dietary priority? How would you respond when he asks if he can use meal replacements for two meals a day so he doesn't have to think about what to eat?

CARDIOVASCULAR DISEASES

Nutrition therapy for CHD and heart failure are presented in the following sections.

Coronary Heart Disease

CHD accounts for more than half of all CVD events in American adults under the age of 75 years (Mozaffarian et al., 2015). Improvements in the prevalence of certain risk factors, such as smoking, total cholesterol levels, systolic blood pressure, and physical activity contribute to the decrease in the death rate from CHD seen over the last several decades (Ford et al., 2007). However, increases in BMI and diabetes mellitus prevalence have, in part, offset some of those favorable improvements (Mozaffarian et al., 2015).

Most atherosclerotic plaques are unstable; blood clots that form after these plaques rupture are responsible for causing ischemia (e.g., MI or stroke) and tissue damage. Because atherosclerosis is a systemic process, older patients with CHD often also have peripheral arterial disease and cerebrovascular disease that may impair ability to function and quality of life (Fleg et al., 2013). CHD-related complications, including heart failure and heart rhythm disorders, are a major cause of chronic disability, loss of independence, and impaired quality of life.

Although statins are the most effective strategy to lower LDL-C to prevent recurrent ASCVD events, lifestyle modifications, including regular physical activity and weight management are fundamental (Fleg et al., 2013). The Lyon Diet Heart Study, a secondary prevention trial in patients with recent MI, showed rates of CHD events and death were reduced for up to 4 years after an initial event in those assigned a Mediterranean diet (de Lorgeril et al., 1999). Likewise, Lopez-Garcia et al. (2014) found an inverse relationship between adherence to a Mediterranean-style eating pattern and all-cause mortality in men and women with CVD, showing that a healthy diet can still be beneficial at an advanced stage of the atherosclerotic process. For secondary prevention in people with established coronary and other atherosclerotic vascular disease, the American Heart Association and American College of Cardiology Foundation recommend saturated fat intake be limited to <7% of total calories, trans fatty acids to <1% of total calories, and cholesterol to <200 mg/day (S. Smith et al., 2011)—nutrient targets that can be met with a Mediterranean-style diet (Tuttle et al., 2008).

Studies using daily supplements of 1 g of omega-3 fatty acids for MI survivors have yielded mixed results. A recent trial showed 4 g/day of Lovaza, a prescription omega-3 fatty acid supplement, taken within a month of hospitalization for an MI and continuing for 6 months, led to less fibrosis of the heart muscle in the area of the MI and less blood left in the left ventricle after the heart muscle fully contracted (Heydari et al., 2016). This amount of omega-3 fatty acids is therapeutic and cannot be obtained by eating the recommended two servings per week of fish. More research is needed to determine the usefulness of omega-3 supplements for MI survivors.

Heart Failure

Heart failure (HF) is a complex syndrome characterized by specific symptoms—particularly dyspnea, fatigue, and fluid retention—that result from any structural or functional impairment of ejection of blood (Yancy et al., 2013). An estimated 5.7 million American adults ≥20 years of age have HF (Mozaffarian et al., 2015). Findings from the Physicians Health Study indicate that lifetime risk of HF is reduced by healthy lifestyle factors, such as normal weight, not smoking, regular physical activity, moderate alcohol intake, eating breakfast cereals, and consuming fruits and vegetables (Djousse, Driver, & Gaziano, 2009). Advances in treatment options have led to improvements in outcomes over the past decade; however, the 1-year mortality rate remains high at 29.6% (Chen, Normand, Wang, & Krumholz, 2011).

Cachexia
a wasting syndrome characterized by loss of lean tissue, muscle mass, and bone mass.

Malnutrition among patients with advanced HF, known as cardiac **cachexia**, may occur from decreased sensation of hunger, diet restrictions, fatigue, malabsorption related to gastrointestinal edema, shortness of breath, nausea, or anxiety. Sarcopenia, characterized by progressive and generalized loss of skeletal muscle mass and strength, can also be common in patients with HF (Someya, Wakabayashi, Hayashi, Akiyama, & Kimura, 2016). A high-calorie, high-protein intake with adequate levels of micronutrients is indicated for HF patients with cachexia and/or sarcopenia. Calorie and protein density are important to maximize intake. Supplements of the omega-3 fatty acid EPA may improve cardiac function and long-term prognosis of chronic HF patients with dyslipidemia (Kohashi et al., 2014). If enteral feedings are necessary, a concentrated formula is used to limit fluid intake.

An association has been demonstrated between HF and micronutrient status, particularly deficiencies in vitamins A, C, D, E, thiamin, other B vitamins, selenium, zinc, and copper (McKeag, McKinley, Woodside, Harbinson, & McKeown, 2012). Micronutrient deficiencies may occur from poor intake, inflammation, oxidative stress, and increased urinary losses secondary to drug therapy (McKeag et al., 2012). Although observational studies suggest a relationship between HF and altered micronutrient intake and status, research is limited, and more studies are needed to determine whether micronutrient supplements are appropriate.

Nutrition Therapy for Heart Failure

Sodium restriction for HF is widely used and highly debated

- The Heart Failure Society of America recommends that sodium be limited to between 2000 and 3000 mg/day for patients with the clinical syndrome of HF and to less than 2000 mg/day for people in moderate to severe HF (Box 20.6) (Lindenfeld et al., 2010).

BOX 20.6   Low-Sodium Eating Pattern

A low-sodium eating pattern usually limits sodium intake to 1500 to 2000 mg/day.

General Guidelines

- Read "Nutrition Facts" labels; choose foods that provide 140 mg of sodium or less per serving. Foods that provide more than 300 mg sodium per serving may be too high in sodium to be included in a low-sodium pattern.
- Avoid processed and prepared foods and beverages high in sodium; use fresh, frozen, and canned low-sodium products.
- Do not use salt in cooking or at the table.
- Recommended foods include

  Breads that provide <80 mg sodium per slice; many ready-to-eat cereals, cooked cereals, pasta, rice, quinoa, and other starches cooked without salt
  Fresh and frozen vegetables; low-sodium or sodium-free canned vegetables and soups
  Fresh and canned fruit; dried fruit
  Low-fat and nonfat milk and yogurt; small amounts of low-fat natural cheese; cream cheese; low-sodium cottage cheese
  Fresh and frozen meats and fish; low-sodium canned tuna, dried peas and beans, eggs, edamame, unsalted nuts or peanut butter
  Angel food cake, granola bars, unsalted pretzels or popcorn, vanilla wafers, frozen fruit bars
  Tub or liquid margarine; vegetable oils

Patient Teaching

Provide general information:

- Reducing sodium intake will help the body rid itself of excess fluid and help lower high blood pressure.
- Sodium appears in the diet in the form of salt and, to some degree, in almost all foods and beverages. Most unprocessed, unsalted foods are low in sodium. The majority of the sodium in a typical American diet comes from processed foods. Sodium-containing compounds are used extensively as preservatives (sodium propionate, sodium sulfite, and sodium benzoate), leavening agents (sodium bicarbonate,

baking soda, and baking powder), and flavor enhancers (e.g., salt, MSG) and are found in foods that may not taste salty.
- Salt substitutes replace sodium with potassium or other minerals. "Low-sodium" salt substitutes are not sodium free and may contain half as much sodium as regular table salt. Use neither type without a physician's approval.
- The preference for salty taste eventually will decrease.
- When an occasional food containing 300 mg or more per serving is eaten, balance it out with low-sodium foods the rest of the day.
- Try to make low-sodium choices while dining out (see Box 20.4).

Teach the client food preparation techniques to minimize sodium intake:

- Prepare foods from "scratch" whenever possible.
- Experiment with sodium-free seasonings, such as herbs, spices, lemon juice, vinegar, and wine. Fresh ingredients are more flavorful than dried ones.
- Try a commercial "salt alternative" for sodium-free flavor enhancement.
- Consult a low-sodium cookbook or online low-sodium recipes.

Teach the client how to read labels:

- Salt, MSG, baking soda, and baking powder contain significant amounts of sodium. Other sodium compounds such as sodium nitrite, benzoate of soda, sodium saccharin, and sodium propionate add less sodium to the diet.
- Sodium labeling terms are reliable:
  - "Sodium-free" and "salt-free" foods provide <5 mg sodium/serving.
  - "Very low sodium" provides <35 mg sodium/serving.
  - "Low sodium" provides <140 mg sodium/serving.
- A variety of low- and reduced-sodium products are available, such as bread and bread products, cereal, crackers, cakes, cookies, pastries, soups, bouillon, canned vegetables, tomato products, meats, entrées, processed meats, hard and soft cheeses, condiments, nuts and peanut butter, butter, margarine, salad dressings, and snack foods. The difference in flavor between some low-sodium products and their high-sodium counterparts is barely noticeable; others taste flat and may need to have herbs or spices added.

- The European Society of Cardiology 2012 guidelines on HF cite salt restriction as an area in need of clinical research. No recommendation is made due to insufficient evidence on its effectiveness and safety of restricting sodium (McMurray et al., 2012).
- The American College of Cardiology Foundation/American Heart Association HF management guidelines state that sodium restriction is reasonable for patients with symptomatic HF but does not suggest intake targets (Yancy et al., 2013).

Despite the theoretical basis for limiting sodium intake, sodium restriction is not well supported by current evidence (Yancy et al., 2013). An observational study by Doukky et al. (2016) found that sodium restriction (<2500 mg/day) in symptomatic patients with chronic HF was associated with higher risk of death or HF hospitalization. Furthermore, sodium restriction was not associated with improved quality of life, physical functioning, 6-minute walk distance, or symptoms. However, a randomized controlled trial by Colin-Ramirez et al. (2015) found that a sodium intake of ≤1500 mg/day resulted in improvements in quality of life and B-type natriuretic peptide, a biomarker of volume overload and surrogate prognostic marker in HF. Randomized clinical trials are needed to determine the optimal sodium intake for HF.

Other diet modifications are made as appropriate, such as

- A fluid restriction of less than 2 L/day may be considered for patients with severe hyponatremia (serum sodium <130 mEq/L) and for all patients with fluid retention that is difficult to control despite high doses of diuretic medication and sodium restriction.
- Appropriate nutrition therapy if comorbidities exist, such as diabetes, renal disease, or hyperlipidemia
- Protein fortification because patients with HF have protein needs higher than normal (1.12 g/kg not the Recommended Dietary Allowance of 0.8 g/kg), even when they are not malnourished (Nutrition Care Manual, 2016). Patients who are malnourished require more.
- Small, frequent meals to limit gastric distention and pressure on the heart
- Soft, easy-to-chew foods for patient with fatigue
- Oral nutrition supplements for additional protein and calories for patients with weight loss or muscle wasting (cardiac cachexia)
- Potassium and thiamin supplements, as needed, to compensate for losses in patients on diuretics

NURSING PROCESS

Heart Failure

Mrs. Gigante is a 79-year-old widow admitted with moderate to severe HF, with a long-standing history of hypertension and one previous MI. She lives alone. She relies heavily on convenience foods, such as canned and packaged soups, frozen dinners, canned pasta, and tuna fish sandwiches, because she is too tired to cook. She appears frail and has significant lower extremity edema. Her physician has ordered a low-sodium diet.

Assessment

Medical–Psychosocial History

- Medical history and comorbidities including diabetes, hypertension, MI, alcohol abuse, and other CHD risk factors
- Use of medications that affect nutrition, such as diuretics, antihypertensives, antidiabetics, and lipid-lowering medications; adherence to prescribed drug therapy
- Complaints including activity intolerance, fatigue, and shortness of breath
- Behaviors suggesting restlessness, anxiety, or confusion
- Psychosocial and economic issues, such as living situation, cooking facilities, financial status, education, and eligibility for the Meals on Wheels program
- Understanding of the relationship between sodium, fluid accumulation, and symptoms of congestive HF
- Motivation to change eating style

NURSING PROCESS	**Heart Failure**

Anthropometric Assessment	• Height, weight; body mass index (BMI) • Recent weight history, especially rapid weight gain
Biochemical and Physical Assessment	• Blood pressure • Measure of edema • Laboratory values related to comorbidities, such as total cholesterol, LDL, HDL, and triglyceride levels • Serum osmolality, serum sodium • Intake and output • Lung sounds for crackles • Respirations for breathing effort
Dietary Assessment	• How many meals and snacks do you usually eat? • What is your usual 24-hour food intake like? • What cooking methods do you use to prepare your food? • How is your appetite? • Do you feel full quickly after you start to eat? • Have you ever been advised to follow a certain kind of diet in the past? If so, how did you change your eating habits? • Do you watch the kind of fats you eat? • Do you try to limit your intake of salt? • How many glasses of fluid do you drink in a day? • Do you have health impairments that affect your ability to shop, cook, or eat? • Do you have any cultural, religious, or ethnic influences on your food preferences or eating habits? • Do you take any vitamins, minerals, and nutritional supplements? If so, what are the reasons? • Do you use alcohol or caffeine?

Diagnosis

Possible Nursing Diagnoses	Excess fluid volume related to fluid retention as evidenced by 3+ peripheral edema

Planning

Client Outcomes	The client will • Attain and maintain normal fluid balance • Consume a varied and nutritious diet with adequate calories to attain healthy body weight • Limit sodium intake • Explain how and why sodium is limited in her diet

Nursing Interventions

Nutrition Therapy	• Provide a 2-g sodium diet as ordered. • Provide five to six small meals to limit gastric distention and pressure on the heart. • Monitor input and output for need for fluid restriction.

NURSING PROCESS

Heart Failure

Client Teaching

Instruct the client
On the roles of sodium, fluid, and medication in managing HF
On the availability of a Meals on Wheels–type program. Explain that Meals on Wheels can provide her with the appropriate diet after discharge to ensure that she gets the proper foods even on days when she feels short of breath or too tired to cook. (Notify the discharge planner that the client may be a candidate for Meals on Wheels.)
On eating plan essentials, such as
- Eliminating the use of salt in cooking and at the table
- Using low-sodium canned foods when available
- Avoiding processed foods; choosing plain wholesome foods
- Increasing intake of high-potassium foods
- Avoiding alcohol
- Adhering to fluid restriction if appropriate
On behavioral matters, including the following:
- How to read labels to identify and avoid foods that provide more than 300 mg sodium per serving
- Trying for a gradual reduction in sodium intake, which may be easier to comply with than an abrupt withdrawal of sodium. Because the preference for salt gradually diminishes when intake is limited, following a low-sodium diet tends to get easier with time.
- Timing meals and snacks to avoid shortness of breath and fatigue
- Identifying physical activity goals, if applicable and appropriate

Evaluation

Evaluate and Monitor

- Monitor weight daily for rapid weight gain.
- Monitor edema and other signs and symptoms of fluid retention.
- Assess tolerance to small meals.
- Determine need for additional diet counseling.

How Do You Respond?

I do everything right and still my LDL cholesterol is sky high. Why? People with a genetic form of hypercholesterolemia generally have an LDL of 190 mg/dL or higher. For them, diet will not effectively lower LDL to acceptable levels. Still, a healthy eating pattern, regular physical activity, and weight loss are important—maybe even more important than for other people—because of the potential beneficial effects on other risks, such as blood pressure and insulin sensitivity.

Why should I eat less sodium if my blood pressure is normal? Even for people who are normotensive, lowering sodium intake will blunt the rise in blood pressure that occurs with aging (Appel et al., 2011). In addition to its effect on blood pressure, a high sodium intake also increases the risk of fibrosis in the heart, kidneys, and arteries; kidney damage, gastric cancer, and possibly osteoporosis by increasing the excretion of calcium. Reducing sodium intake is considered an important public health effort to prevent CVD, stroke, and kidney disease (Appel et al., 2011).

REVIEW CASE STUDY

Matt is 34 years old. His BMI is 28 and has steadily increased over the last few years when he accepted a position with his company that requires frequent travel. It is hard for him to exercise, and he eats out often. He is a "steak and potatoes" kind of guy who wouldn't dream of eating lunch or dinner without meat as the centerpiece of the meal. At his most recent annual employee physical, Matt's total cholesterol level was 245 mg/dL, his HDL level was 50, fasting glucose level was 92, and his blood pressure was 154/85 mmHg. His father died of a heart attack at age 49 years. Matt feels doomed by genetics and is resistant to going on medication because of the potential side effects. He is willing to try to change his diet and lifestyle but is skeptical that it will help.

- What risks does Matt have for heart disease?
- Knowing that he is willing to change his diet and lifestyle, what additional information would you ask of Matt before devising a teaching plan?
- What diet recommendations would you prioritize in helping Matt initiate a healthy eating pattern? What suggestions could you offer him to help him meet these recommendations?
- How would you respond to Matt's skepticism that lifestyle factors will probably not lower his risk of heart disease?

STUDY QUESTIONS

1 Which statement indicates the patient understands the instruction about a DASH-style diet?
   a. "The most important thing about a DASH diet is to eat less cholesterol. No egg yolks for me."
   b. "I need to eat more fruits, vegetables, and whole grains."
   c. "As long as I don't add salt to my food while cooking or at the table, I will be able to achieve a low-sodium diet."
   d. "I had given up sugar-sweetened soft drinks but now I am going to go back to drinking them because they are allowed on my diet."

2 The client asks if he can continue using butter on his DASH-style healthy diet. Which of the following would be the nurse's best response?
   a. "No, butter does not fit into a heart healthy diet."
   b. "Butter is not limited in a heart healthy diet because most people only use small amounts."
   c. "You can use small amounts of butter if you are willing to compromise on other foods, such as switching to fat-free salad dressing."
   d. "You can use small amounts of butter if you give up meat entirely."

3 When developing a teaching plan for a client on a low-sodium diet, which of the following foods would the nurse advise the client to limit?
   a. Processed cheese
   b. Canned fruit
   c. Eggs
   d. Milk

4 The nurse knows that instructions for a Mediterranean-style eating pattern have been effective when the client expresses a need to eat more
   a. Fish and nuts
   b. Lean red and deli meats
   c. Milk and cheese
   d. Italian bread and white pasta

5 Which of the following recommendations would be most appropriate to limit trans fats?
   a. Avoid red meats.
   b. Avoid egg yolks and shellfish.
   c. Avoid corn oil.
   d. Avoid commercially made baked goods and stick margarines containing partially hydrogenated vegetable oils.

6 A client asks how to alter a diet to lower high triglyceride levels. Which of the following is the nurse's best response?
   a. "Alcohol lowers triglycerides, but don't drink more than 2 drinks daily."
   b. "Eliminate egg yolks and butter."
   c. "Eat less sodium by avoiding processed foods and don't salt your food at the table."
   d. "Eat a Mediterranean-style eating pattern."

7 The client understands that losing weight will lower her risk for CVD. What does the client need to know about weight loss diets?
   a. For overall health, it doesn't matter what kind of diet you choose.
   b. A very-low-carbohydrate diet is best because it promotes quick weight loss and foods that provide carbohydrates are detrimental to cardiovascular health.
   c. The appropriate calorie level DASH diet can promote weight loss while providing adequate amounts of food components that have cardiometabolic benefits.
   d. Low-fat diets are the best for cardiovascular health because it is beneficial to eat less of all types of fat in the diet.

8 The number of servings of fish recommended is
   a. 2 per month
   b. 1 per week
   c. 2 per week
   d. 3 to 4 per week

KEY CONCEPTS

- The American Heart Association defines cardiovascular health with seven metrics, one of which is a healthy diet. A healthy diet is defined as a calorie-appropriate DASH-style diet that emphasizes fruits, vegetables, whole grains, fish, and nuts, legumes, and seeds and limits sodium, sugar sweetened beverages, processed meats, and saturated fat.

- Diet quality is the cardiovascular health metric most in need of improvement. Although American adults are consuming fewer sugar sweetened beverages and processed meats, they need to eat more whole grains, fruits, and vegetables.

- Dietary recommendations to prevent or treat CVD focus on eating patterns, not single nutrients. Nutrient targets, such as reducing intakes of sodium, added sugars, saturated fat, and trans fat and increasing intakes of potassium and fiber, are achieved within the context of a healthy eating pattern.

- The DASH diet is high in fruit, vegetables, low-fat dairy products, whole grains, poultry, fish, and nuts; and low in fat, red meat, sweets, and sugar-sweetened beverages. It substantially lowers both systolic and diastolic blood pressures and LDL-C.

- A Mediterranean-style diet is generally high in olive oil, fruits, nuts, vegetables, and cereals; moderate in fish and poultry; low in dairy products, red meat, processed meats, and sweets; and moderate in wine, which is consumed with meals. It has been shown to lower CVD risk by improving blood pressure, lipid levels, insulin resistance, BMI, and waist circumference and through its anti-inflammatory and antioxidant effects.

- With the exception of fish oil supplements, supplements have not been shown to reduce cardiac risks, and some may even increase risk.

- Overweight and obesity are major risk factors for CVD, including CHD, stroke, HF, and arrhythmias because they raise LDL-C levels, decrease insulin sensitivity, increase blood pressure, and lower HDL-C.

- Weight loss, a decrease in sodium and alcohol intake, and adoption of the DASH eating plan are dietary strategies that lower blood pressure. The DASH diet has been shown to prevent hypertension in people who are normotensive or prehypertensive, eliminate the need for medication in people with stage 1 hypertension, and to lower blood pressure and reduce the dose of medication needed in people whose blood pressure is controlled with medication.

- People who choose to drink alcohol should limit their intake to 2 drinks per day (males) or 1 drink per day (females).

- Alcohol not only has positive health benefits, such as raising HDL-C and reducing platelet aggregation, but it also raises blood pressure and other health risks.

- Hypercholesterolemia is the cause of atherosclerosis, the underlying process responsible for most clinical ASCVD events, such as MI, ischemic stroke, or renal failure. LDL-C and non-HDL-C are atherogenic; HDL-C is protective against ASCVD.

- Lowering LDL-C may decrease the risk of ASCVD. Dietary recommendations for lowering LCL-cholesterol include following a DASH type dietary pattern, reducing saturated fat intake to 5% to 6% of total calories, and reducing the percentage of calories from trans fat. Saturated fat should be replaced by polyunsaturated fats or monounsaturated fatty acids for the most favorable impact on lipid levels.

- Lifestyle interventions that lower LDL-C, such as regular physical activity, weight loss, and smoking cessation, increase HDL-C.

- High triglycerides are a biomarker for CVD risk, not independently atherogenic. Nutrition interventions to lower triglycerides include weight loss, reducing carbohydrate intake, eliminating trans fats, lowering saturated fat and fructose intake, and eating omega-3 fatty acids from fish. Alcohol is restricted. A Mediterranean-style eating pattern is recommended.

- MetS is a risk factor for CVD and type 2 diabetes. Diagnosis is made when three of the following are present: hypertension, high triglycerides, low HDL-C, central obesity, and elevated fasting glucose. A Mediterranean-style eating pattern is recommended.

- Lifestyle modifications, including regular physical activity and weight management are fundamental to treating existing CHD. To reduce the risk of a second CVD event, the American Heart Association recommends saturated fat intake be limited to <7% of total calories, trans fatty acids to <1% of total calories, and cholesterol to <200 mg/day. These nutrient targets can be met with a Mediterranean-style diet.

- Lifetime risk of HF may be lowered by healthy lifestyle factors, such as normal weight, not smoking, regular physical activity, moderate alcohol intake, eating breakfast cereals, and consuming fruits and vegetables. The use of a sodium-restricted diet to treat HF is controversial. Other possible diet modifications include a fluid restriction, a high-protein, high calorie intake, small frequent meals, and a soft diet.

Check Your Knowledge Answer Key

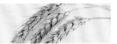

1 **TRUE** Of all seven metrics that define cardiovascular health—smoking, physical activity, diet quality, body weight, total cholesterol level, glucose level, and blood pressure—diet quality is the one most in need of improvement. Only 1.5% of adults have an eating pattern that qualifies as ideal.

2 **FALSE** The original DASH diet study was not lower in sodium. It is speculated that one of the factors that make the DASH diet effective in lowering blood pressure is its high content of potassium, magnesium, and calcium from fruit, vegetables, nuts, and dairy.

3 FALSE It is believed that to reduce the risk of CVD focus should be on the whole eating pattern rather than individual nutrients. The DASH diet and Mediterranean-style diet are associated with decreased risk of CVD.

4 TRUE High triglyceride levels are a component of MetS but are not considered to be directly atherogenic. However, they are an important biomarker of CVD risk.

5 FALSE A traditional Mediterranean diet is not a low-fat diet, but it is low in animal fat, which means it is low in saturated fat and cholesterol. Its relatively high fat content, mostly in the form of monounsaturated fats, comes from olives and olive oil.

6 TRUE Foods with components that provide cardiometabolic benefits include fish and nuts as well as fruits, vegetables, whole grains, vegetable oils, dairy products, and legumes.

7 TRUE Trans fats increase LDL-C and therefore increase the risk of CVD.

8 TRUE Alcohol increases HDL-C, lowers systemic inflammation, and reduces platelet aggregation. However, high intakes increase blood pressure and triglyceride levels and are associated with liver damage, physical abuse, and vehicular and work accidents.

9 FALSE All Americans, whether normotensive or hypertensive, are urged to lower their sodium intake to lower blood pressure.

10 FALSE A low-sodium diet for HF is based on expert consensus, not randomized study evidence. The theoretical basis is that lowering sodium lowers fluid retention; however, some studies suggest that lowering sodium actually worsens fluid retention.

Student Resources on thePoint

For additional learning materials, activate the code in the front of this book at
http://thePoint.lww.com/activate

Websites

American Heart Association at www.americanheart.org
Heart and Stroke Foundation of Canada at www.hsf.ca
Mediterranean Diet Pyramid at www.oldways.org
National Heart, Lung and Blood Institute at www.nhlbi.nih.gov; to estimate your risk of heart disease, go to http://cvdrisk.nhlbi.nih.gov/

References

Aaron, K., & Sanders, P. (2013). Role of dietary salt and potassium intake in cardiovascular health and disease: A review of the evidence. *Mayo Clinic Proceedings, 88,* 987–995. doi:10.1016/j.mayocp.2013.06.005

Afshin, A., Micha, R., Khatibzadeh, S., & Mozaffarian, D. (2014). Consumption of nuts and legumes and risk of incident ischemic heart disease, stroke, and diabetes: A systematic review and meta-analysis. *The American Journal of Clinical Nutrition, 100,* 278–288.

Alberti, K., Eckel, R., Grundy, S., Zimmet, P. Z., Cleeman, J. I., Donato, K. A., . . . Smith, S. C., Jr. (2009). Harmonizing the metabolic syndrome: A joint interim statement of the International Diabetes Federation Task Force on Epidemiology and Prevention; National Heart, Lung, and Blood Institute: American Heart Association; World Heart Federation: International Atherosclerosis Society; and International Association for the Study of Obesity. *Circulation, 120,* 1640–1645.

American Heart Association. (n.d.). *Sodium breakup.* Available at http://sodiumbreakup.heart.org/sodium-411/sources-of-sodium/. Accessed 8/1/16.

Appel, L. J., Brands, M. W., Daniels, S. R., Karanja, N., Elmer, P. J., & Sacks, F. M. (2006). Dietary approaches to prevent and treat hypertension: A scientific statement from the American Heart Association. *Hypertension, 47,* 296–308.

Appel, L. J., Frohlich, E., Hall, J., Pearson, T. A., Sacco, R. L., Seals, D. R., . . . Van Horn, L. V. (2011). The importance of population-wide sodium reduction as a means to prevent cardiovascular disease and stroke. *Circulation, 123,* 1138–1143.

Appel, L. J., Moore, T., Obarzanek, E., Vollmer, W. M., Svetkey, L. P., Sacks, F. M., . . . Karanja, N. (1997). A clinical trial of the effects of dietary patterns on blood pressure. *The New England Journal of Medicine, 336,* 1117–1124.

Appel, L. J., Sacks, F., Carey, V., Obarzanek, E., Swain, J. F., Miller, E. R., III, . . . Bishop, L. M. (2005). Effects of protein, monounsaturated fat, and carbohydrate intake on blood pressure and serum lipids: Results of the OmniHeart randomized trial. *JAMA, 294,* 2455–2464.

Azadbakht, L., Fard, N., Karimi, M., Baghaei, M. H., Surkan, P. J., Rahimi, M., . . . Willett, W. C. (2011). Effects of the Dietary Approaches to Stop Hypertension (DASH) eating plan on cardiovascular risks among type 2 diabetic patients: A randomized crossover clinical trial. *Diabetes Care, 34,* 55–57.

Bassi, N., Karagodin, I., Wang, S., Vassallo, P., Priyanath, A., Massaro, E., & Stone, N. J. (2014). Lifestyle modification for metabolic syndrome: A systematic review. *The American Journal of Medicine, 12,* 1242.e1–1242.e10.

Binia, A., Jaeger, J., Hu, Y., Singh, A., & Zimmermann, D. (2015). Daily potassium intake and sodium-to-potassium ratio in the reduction of blood pressure: A meta-analysis of randomized controlled trials. *Journal of Hypertension, 33,* 1509–1520.

Buckland, G., Travier, N., Barricarte, A., Ardanaz, E., Moreno-Iribas, C., Sánchez, M. J., . . . Gonzalez, C. A. (2012). Olive oil intake and CHD in the European Prospective Investigation into Cancer and Nutrition Spanish cohort. *The British Journal of Nutrition, 108,* 2075–2082.

Chen, J., Normand, S., Wang, Y., & Krumholz, H. (2011). National and regional trends in heart failure hospitalization and mortality rates for Medicare beneficiaries, 1998-2008. *JAMA, 306,* 1669–1678.

Colin-Ramirez, E., McAlister, F., Zheng, Y., Sharma, S., Armstrong, P. W., & Ezekowitz, J. A. (2015). The long-term effects of dietary sodium restriction on clinical outcomes in patients with heart failure. The SODIUM-HF (Study of Dietary Intervention Under 100 mmol in Heart Failure): A pilot study. *American Heart Journal, 169,* 274–281.

de Lorgeril, M., Salen, P., Martin, J., Monjaud, I., Delaye, J., & Mamelle, N. (1999). Mediterranean diet, traditional risk factors, and the rate of cardiovascular complications after myocardial infarction: Final report of the Lyon Diet Heart Study. *Circulation, 99,* 779–785.

de Oliveira Otto, M., Moazffarian, D., Kromhout, D., Bertoni, A. G., Sibley, C. T., Jacobs, D. R., Jr., & Nettleton, J. A. (2012). Dietary intake of saturated fat by food source and incident cardiovascular disease: The Multi-Ethnic Study of Atherosclerosis. *The American Journal of Clinical Nutrition, 96,* 397–404.

Di Angelantonio, E., Sarwar, N., Perry, P., Kaptoge, S., Ray, K. K., Thompson, A., . . . Danesh, J. (2009). Major lipids, apolipoproteins, and risk of vascular disease. *JAMA, 302,* 1993–2000.

Djousse, L., Driver, J., & Gaziano, M. (2009). Relation between modifiable lifestyle factors and lifetime risk of heart failure. *JAMA, 302,* 394–400.

Doukky, R., Avery, E., Mangla, A., Collado, F. M., Ibrahim, Z., Poulin, M. F., . . . Powell, L. H. (2016). Impact of dietary sodium restriction on heart failure outcomes. *JACC. Heart Failure, 4,* 24–35.

Duffy, D., & Rader, D. (2009). Update on strategies to increase HDL quantity and function. *Nature Reviews. Cardiology, 6,* 455–463.

Dunkley, A., Charles, K., Gray, L., Camosso-Stefinovic, J., Davies, M. J., & Khunti, K. (2012). Effectiveness of interventions for reducing diabetes and cardiovascular disease risk in people with metabolic syndrome: Systematic review and mixed treatment comparison meta-analysis. *Diabetes, Obesity and Metabolism, 14,* 616–625.

Eckel, R., Jakicic, J., Ard, J., de Jesus, J. M., Houston Miller, N., Hubbard, V. S., . . . Yanovski, S. Z. (2014). 2013 AHA/ACC guideline on lifestyle management to reduce cardiovascular risk: A report of the American College of Cardiology/American Heart Association Task Force on practice guidelines. *Journal of the American College of Cardiology, 63,* 2960–2984. doi:10.1016/j.jacc.2013.11.003

Estruch, R., Ros, E., Salas-Salvadó, J., Covas, M. I., Corella, D., Arós, F., . . . Martínez-González, M. A. (2013). Primary prevention of cardiovascular disease with a Mediterranean diet. *The New England Journal of Medicine, 368,* 1279–1290.

Felder, R., White, M., Williams, S., & Jose, P. (2013). Diagnostic tools for hypertension and salt sensitivity testing. *Current Opinion in Nephrology and Hypertension, 22,* 65–76.

Fleg, J., Forman, D., Berra, K., Bittner, V., Blumenthal, J. A., Chen, M. A., . . . Zieman, S. J. (2013). Secondary prevention of atherosclerotic cardiovascular disease in older adults: A scientific statement from the American Heart Association. *Circulation, 128,* 2422–2446.

Ford, E., Ajani, U., Croft, J., Critchley, J. A., Labarthe, D. R., Kottke, T. E., . . . Capewell, S. (2007). Explaining the decrease in U.S. deaths from coronary disease, 1980–2000. *The New England Journal of Medicine, 356,* 2388–2398.

Franco, O., Massaro, J., Civil, J., Cobain, M. R., O'Malley, B., & D'Agostino, R. B., Sr. (2009). Trajectories of entering the metabolic syndrome: The Framingham Heart Study. *Circulation, 120,* 1943–1950.

Graudal, N., Jürgens, G., Baslund, B., & Alderman, M. (2014). Compared with usual sodium intake, low- and excessive-sodium diets are associated with increased mortality: A meta-analysis. *American Journal of Hypertension, 27,* 1129–1137.

Guasch-Ferré, M., Babio, N., Martínez-González, M. A. M., Corella, D., Ros, E., Martín-Peláez, S., . . . Salas-Salvadó, J. (2015). Dietary fat intake and risk of cardiovascular disease and all-cause mortality in a population at high risk of cardiovascular disease. *The American Journal of Clinical Nutrition, 102,* 1563–1573.

Haupt, A. (2016). *What is the "best diet" for you?* Available at http://health.usnews.com/health-news/health-wellness/articles/2016-01-05/what-is-the-best-diet-for-you. Accessed on 7/29/16.

Heydari, B., Abdullah, S., Pottala, J., Shah, R., Abbasi, S., Mandry, D., . . . Kwong, R. Y. (2016). Effect of omega-3 acid ethyl esters on left ventricular remodeling after acute myocardial infarction. *Circulation, 134,* 378–391.

Jacobs, D., Gross, M., & Tapsell, L. (2009). Food synergy: An operational concept for understanding nutrition. *The American Journal of Clinical Nutrition, 89,* 1543S–1548S.

Jacobson, T., Ito, M., Maki, K., Orringer, C. E., Bays, H. E., Jones, P. H., . . . Brown, W. V. (2014). National Lipid Association recommendations for patient-centered management of dyslipidemia: Part 1— executive summary. *Journal of Clinical Lipidology, 8,* 473–488.

Jakobsen, M., O'Reilly, E., Heitmann, B., Pereira, M. A., Bälter, K., Fraser, G. E., . . . Ascherio, A. (2009). Major types of dietary fat and risk of coronary heart disease: A pooled analysis of 11 cohort studies. *The American Journal of Clinical Nutrition, 89,* 1425–1432.

Kastorini, C., Milionis, H., Ioannidi, A., Kalantzi, K., Nikolaou, V., Vemmos, K. N. . . . Panagiotakos, D. B. (2011). Adherence to the Mediterranean diet in relation to acute coronary syndrome or stroke nonfatal events: A comparative analysis of a case/case-control study. *American Heart Journal, 162,* 717–724.

Kohashi, D., Nakagoni, A., Saiki, Y., Morisawa, T., Kosugi, M., Kusama, Y., . . . Shimizu, W. (2014). Effects of eicosapentaenoic acid on the levels of inflammatory markers, cardiac function and long-term prognosis in chronic heart failure patients with dyslipidemia. *Journal of Atherosclerosis and Thrombosis, 21,* 712–729.

Lindenfeld, J. J., Albert, N., Boehmer, J., Collins, S. P., Ezekowitz, J. A., Givertz, M. M., . . . Walsh, M. N. (2010). HFSA 2010 comprehensive heart failure practice guideline. *Journal of Cardiac Failure, 16,* 475–539.

Lloyd-Jones, D., Hong, Y., Labarthe, D., Mozaffarian, D., Appel, L. J., Van Horn, L., . . . Rosamond, W. D. (2010). Defining and setting national goals for cardiovascular health promotion and disease reduction: The American Heart Association's Strategic Impact Goal through 2020 and beyond. *Circulation, 121,* 586–613.

Lopez-Garcia, E., Rodriguez-Artalejo, F., Li, T., Fung, T. T., Li, S., Willett, W. C., . . . Hu, F. B. (2014). The Mediterranean-style dietary pattern and mortality among men and women with cardiovascular disease. *The American Journal of Clinical Nutrition, 99,* 172–180.

McKeag, N., McKinley, M., Woodside, J., Harbinson, M. T., & McKeown, P. P. (2012). The role of micronutrients in heart failure. *Journal of the Academy of Nutrition and Dietetics, 112,* 870–886.

McMurray, J. J., Adamopoulos, S., Anker, S. D., Auricchio, A., Böhm, M., Dickstein, K., . . . Ponikowski, P. (2012). ESC guidelines for the diagnosis and treatment of acute and chronic heart failure 2012: The Task Force for the Diagnosis and Treatment of Acute and Chronic Heart Failure 2012 of the European Society of Cardiology. Developed in collaboration with the Heart Failure Association (HFA) of the ESC. *European Journal of Heart Failure, 14,* 803–869.

Mente, A., de Koning, L., Shannon, H., & Anand, S. (2009). A systematic review of the evidence supporting a causal link between dietary factors and coronary heart disease. *Archives of Internal Medicine, 169,* 659–669.

Miller, M., Stone, N., Ballantyne, C., Bittner, V., Criqui, M. H., Ginsberg, H. N., . . . Pennathur, S. (2011). Triglycerides and cardiovascular disease: A scientific statement from the American Heart Association. *Circulation, 123,* 2292–2333.

Mozaffarian, D., Appel, L., & Van Horn, L. (2011). Components of a cardioprotective diet: New insights. *Circulation, 123,* 2870–2891.

Mozaffarian, D., Benjamin, E., Go, A., Arnett, D. K., Blaha, M. J., Cushman, M., . . . Turner, M. B. (2015). Heart disease and stroke statistics—2016 update: A report from the American Heart Association. *Circulation, 133*, e38–e360. doi:10.1161/cir.0000000000000350

Mozaffarian, D., Hao, T., Rimm, E., Willett, W. C., & Hu, F. B. (2011). Changes in diet and lifestyle and long-term weight gain in women and men. *The New England Journal of Medicine, 364*, 2392–2404.

Nutrition Care Manual. (2016). *Heart failure. Nutrition prescription.* Available at http://www.nutritioncaremanual.org. Accessed on 8/3/16.

Sacks, F., Svetkey, L., Vollmer, W., Appel, L. J., Bray, G. A., Harsha, D., . . . Lin, P. H. (2001). Effects on blood pressure of reduced dietary sodium and the Dietary Approaches to Stop Hypertension (DASH) diet. *The New England Journal of Medicine, 344*, 3–10.

Sesso, H., Christen, W., Bubes, V., Smith, J. P., MacFadyen, J., Schvartz, M., . . . Gaziano, J. M. (2012). Multivitamins in the prevention of cardiovascular disease in men. The Physicians' Health Study II randomized controlled trial. *JAMA, 308*, 1751–1760.

Sesso, H., Cook, N., Buring, J., Manson, J. E., & Gaziano, J. M. (2008). Alcohol consumption and the risk of hypertension in women and men. *Hypertension, 51*, 1080–1087.

Shai, I., Spence, J., Schwarzfuchs, D., Henkin, Y., Parraga, G., Rudich, A., . . . Stampfer, M. J. (2010). Dietary intervention to reverse carotid atherosclerosis. *Circulation, 121*, 1200–1208.

Smith, J., Hou, T., Ludwig, D., Rimm, E. B., Willett, W., Hu, F. B., & Mozaffarian, D. (2015). Changes in intake of protein foods, carbohydrate amount and quality, and long-term weight change: Results from 3 prospective cohorts. *The American Journal of Clinical Nutrition, 101*, 1216–1224.

Smith, S., Benjamin, E., Bonow, R., Braun, L. T., Creager, M. A., Franklin, B. A., . . . Taubert, K. A. (2011). ANA/ACCF secondary prevention and risk reduction therapy for patients with coronary and other atherosclerotic vascular disease: 2011 Update: A guideline from the American Heart Association and American College of Cardiology Foundation endorsed by the World Heart Federation and the Preven-tive Cardiovascular Nurses Association. *Journal of the American College of Cardiology, 58*, 2432–2446.

Someya, R., Wakabayashi, H., Hayashi, K., Akiyama, E., & Kimura, K. (2016). Rehabilitation nutrition for acute heart failure on inotropes with malnutrition, sarcopenia, and cachexia: A case report. *Journal of the Academy of Nutrition and Dietetics, 116*, 765–767.

Sullivan, J. (1991). Salt sensitivity. Definition, conception, methodology, and long-term issues. *Hypertension, 17*(1 Suppl.), I61–I68.

Tuttle, K., Shuler, L., Packard, D., Milton, J. E., Daratha, K. B., Bibus, D. M., & Short, R. A. (2008). Comparison of low-fat versus Mediterranean-style dietary intervention after first myocardial infarction (from the Heart Institute of Spokane Diet Intervention and Evaluation Trial). *The American Journal of Cardiology, 101*, 1523–1530.

Virani, S., Wang, D., Woodard, L., Chitwood, S. S., Landrum, C. R., Zieve, F. J., . . . Petersen, L. A. (2012). Non-high-density lipoprotein cholesterol reporting and goal attainment in primary care. *Journal of Clinical Lipidology, 6*, 545–552.

Whayne, T. (2011). Atherosclerosis: Current status of prevention and treatment. *The International Journal of Angiology, 20*, 213–222.

Whelton, P., Appel, L., Sacco, R., Anderson, C. A., Antman, E. M., Campbell, .N., . . . Van Horn, L. V. (2012). Sodium, blood pressure, and cardiovascular disease: Further evidence supporting the American Heart Association sodium reduction recommendations. *Circulation, 126*, 2880–2889.

Widmer, R., Flammer, A., Lerman, L., & Leman, A. (2015). The Mediterranean diet, its components, and cardiovascular disease. *The American Journal of Medicine, 128*, 229–238.

Yancy, C., Jessup, M., Bozkurt, B., Butler, J., Casey, D. E., Drazner, M. H., . . . Wilkoff, B. L. (2013). 2013 ACCF/AHA guideline for the management of heart failure: Executive summary: A report of the American College of Cardiology Foundation/American Heart Association Task Force of practice guidelines. *Circulation, 128*, 1810–1852.

Chapter 21

Nutrition for Patients with Kidney Disorders

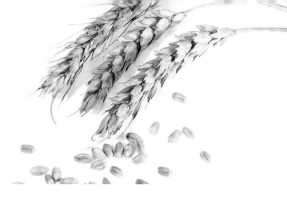

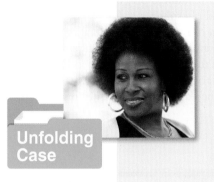

Unfolding Case

Sonja Fern

Sonja is 46 years old, is 6 ft 1 in tall, and weighs 218 pounds. She has intentionally lost 25 pounds in the last month after donating one of her kidneys. She was extremely moved by the significance of being healthy enough to help a friend through organ donation and recognizes that she must proactively protect her remaining kidney to preserve her own health. She had borderline hypertension before the surgery, is a previous heavy smoker, but has no other medical history. She has adopted a lacto-ovo vegetarian eating pattern and occasionally eats fish.

Check Your Knowledge

True	False		
☐	☐	1	A Dietary Approaches to Stop Hypertension (DASH) diet may help prevent chronic kidney disease.
☐	☐	2	Foods high in protein tend to be high in phosphorus.
☐	☐	3	Milk is the best source of protein for people with chronic kidney disease.
☐	☐	4	All people with chronic kidney disease need to limit their potassium intake.
☐	☐	5	People with chronic renal disease tend to have accelerated atherosclerosis and may benefit from eating a heart-healthy diet.
☐	☐	6	Dialysis increases protein requirements.
☐	☐	7	People receiving peritoneal dialysis absorb calories from the dialysate.
☐	☐	8	People with nephrotic syndrome need to eat a high-protein diet to compensate for urinary protein losses.
☐	☐	9	People with calcium oxalate renal stones should avoid calcium.
☐	☐	10	Increasing fluid intake is recommended to decrease the risk of recurrent kidney stone formation.

Learning Objectives

Upon completion of this chapter, you will be able to

1 Explain general nutrition recommendations for nephrotic syndrome.
2 Discuss nutrition and lifestyle interventions that may help prevent chronic kidney disease (CKD).
3 Describe the impact CKD has on nutritional status and requirements.
4 Compare nutrition guidelines for predialysis to those for patients on dialysis.
5 Explain nutrition guidelines for posttransplant patients.
6 Give examples of the challenges in providing adequate nutrition to people with acute kidney injury.
7 Describe dietary recommendations for various types of kidney stones.

Nitrogenous Wastes
wastes produced from nitrogen—namely, ammonia, urea, uric acid, and creatinine.

Renin
an enzyme secreted by the kidneys that activates the precursor of angiotensin, a hormone involved in blood pressure regulation.

Erythropoietin
a hormone secreted by the kidneys that stimulates the bone marrow to produce red blood cells.

The kidneys perform many vital functions. They maintain normal blood volume and composition by reabsorbing needed nutrients and excreting wastes through urine; urinary excretion is the primary method by which the body rids itself of excess water, **nitrogenous wastes** from protein metabolism, electrolytes, sulfates, organic acids, toxic substances, and drugs. The kidneys help to regulate acid–base balance by secreting hydrogen ions to increase pH and excreting bicarbonate to lower pH. The kidneys are involved in blood pressure regulation through the action of **renin** and in red blood cell production through the action of **erythropoietin**. Because vitamin D is converted to its active form in the kidneys, the kidneys play an important role in maintaining normal metabolism of calcium and phosphorus.

Impaired kidney function can cause widespread alterations in metabolism, bone health, fluid balance, nutritional status, and nutrition requirements. Kidney disease is the ninth leading cause of death in the United States (Centers for Disease Control and Prevention [CDC], 2016). Kidney diseases vary in severity, chronicity, and etiology. Nutrition therapy for nephrotic syndrome, chronic kidney disease, acute kidney injury, and urolithiasis is presented in the following text.

NEPHROTIC SYNDROME

Nephrotic Syndrome
a collection of symptoms that occurs when increased capillary permeability in the glomeruli allows serum proteins to leak into the urine.

Hypoalbuminemia
low blood levels of albumin, the most abundant plasma protein.

Hyperlipidemia
abnormally high level of lipids in the blood, such as low-density lipoprotein cholesterol and triglycerides.

Nephrotic syndrome refers to a collection of symptoms caused by alterations in the kidney's glomerular basement membrane that result in large urinary losses of albumin and other plasma proteins. It can arise from any kidney disease that damages the glomeruli, such as diabetes, autoimmune diseases (e.g., lupus, IgA nephropathy), infection, and certain chemicals.

Hypoalbuminemia, hyperlipidemia, and edema are major features of **nephrotic syndrome**. The majority of the urinary protein excreted is albumin; **hypoalbuminemia** leads to edema related to altered oncotic pressure. **Hyperlipidemia** increases the risk of cardiovascular disease (CVD) and progressive renal damage. Possible complications related to the loss of other plasma proteins include anemia (loss of transferrin), increased risk of infection (loss of immunoglobulins), vitamin D deficiency (loss of vitamin D–binding protein), and increased blood clotting (loss of anti–blood clotting proteins). Protein-calorie malnutrition may develop. In some cases, treating the underlying disorder corrects nephrotic syndrome. In others, especially diabetes, nephrotic syndrome may be the beginning of CKD.

Nutrition Therapy for Nephrotic Syndrome

The goals of nutrition therapy are to help control edema, replace nutrients lost in the urine, protect kidney function, reduce the risk of atherosclerosis, and maintain good nutritional status (Kalista-Richards, 2011). Although nephrotic syndrome is characterized by increased urinary losses of plasma proteins, a high-protein diet is contraindicated because it exacerbates urinary protein losses, promoting further kidney damage. Usually restrictions of saturated fat, trans fat, and cholesterol are recommended to control lipid levels; however, nutrition therapy may not be effective for dyslipidemia associated with nephrotic syndrome and pharmacology is generally needed. General nutrition recommendations for nephrotic syndrome are summarized in Box 21.1.

BOX 21.1   **General Nutrition Recommendations for Nephrotic Syndrome**

- Restrict sodium to 2 g/day to help control edema and blood pressure (Cadnapaphornchai, Tkachenko, Shehekochikhin, & Schrier, 2014).
- Restrict fluid only in patients with hyponatremia.
- Limit protein to 0.8 g/kg/day (the RDA) to 1.0 g/kg/day (Cadnapaphornchai et al., 2014), with at least half of the protein from high biologic value (HBV) sources, such as meat, fish, poultry, milk, eggs, and soy (Kalista-Richards, 2011). Provide adequate calories to spare protein and maintain weight.
- Provide supplemental vitamin D when vitamin D deficiency is diagnosed.

Table 21.1	Glomerular Filtration Rate (GFR) Categories in Chronic Kidney Disease (CKD)		
CKD Stage	**GFR Category**	**GFR Range (mL/min/1.73 m^2)**	**Description of Kidney Function**
1	G1	≥90	Normal or high
2	G2	60–89	Mildly decreased
3	G3a	45–59	Mildly to moderately decreased
3	G3b	30–44	Moderately to severely decreased
4	G4	15–29	Severely decreased
5	G5	<15	Kidney failure

Source: Kidney Disease: Improving Global Outcomes CKD Work Group. (2013). KDIGO 2012 clinical practice guideline for the evaluation and management of chronic kidney disease. *Kidney International*, *3*, 1–150.

CHRONIC KIDNEY DISEASE

Chronic Kidney Disease (CKD)
a decrease in kidney function defined as an estimated GFR <60 mL/min/1.73 m^2 and/or evidence of kidney damage, including persistent albuminuria, defined as >30 mg of urine albumin per gram of urine creatinine.

Glomerular Filtration Rate (GFR)
the rate at which the kidneys form filtrate estimated from the amount of creatinine excreted per 24 hours. Normal GFR is about 120 to 130 mL/min.

Estimated Glomerular Filtration Rate (eGFR)
determined through an equation that takes into account serum creatinine level, age, gender, and race. Used interchangeably with the term glomerular filtration rate (GFR).

Chronic kidney disease (CKD) is a general term for heterogeneous abnormalities of kidney structure or function, present for more than 3 months, with implications for health (Kidney Disease: Improving Global Outcomes [KDIGO] CKD Work Group, 2013). Classification of CKD is based on cause, **glomerular filtration rate (GFR)** category (Table 21.1), and persistent albuminuria category (Table 21.2). **Estimated glomerular filtration rate (eGFR)** and albuminuria are used to assess the risk of CKD progression, the suggested frequency of medical monitoring, and when referral to a nephrologist is recommended (KDIGO CKD Work Group, 2013).

CKD is associated with significant morbidity and increased risk of death from any cause (Johnson et al., 2013). CVD risk increases with only mild kidney impairment and rises as the disease progresses (McMahon et al., 2013). It accounts for more than 50% of deaths in patients with CKD (Briasoulis & Bakris, 2013). CKD patients are 16 to 40 times more likely to die than reach end-stage renal disease (ESRD) (CDC, 2014).

Inflammation—and inflammatory conditions—play an important role in CKD (Mas et al., 2015). Diabetes and hypertension are the leading causes of CKD, accounting for 72% of new cases in the United States in 2011 (CDC, 2014). Other risk factors for CKD include CVD, obesity, advancing age, and a family history of CKD. Individuals of African American, Native American, or Hispanic ethnicities are at increased risk for CKD (Qaseem, Hopkins, Sweet, Starkey, & Shekelle, 2013).

Table 21.2	Albuminuria Categories in Chronic Kidney Disease Based on Albumin-to-Creatinine Ratio	
Persistent Albuminuria Category	**Albumin-to-Creatinine Ratio**	**Description**
A1	<30 mg/g or <3 mg/mmol	Normal to mildly increased
A2	30–300 mg/g or 3–30 mg/mmol	Moderately increased (compared to young adult level)
A3	>300 mg/g or >30 mg/mmol	Severely increased (including nephrotic syndrome)

Source: Kidney Disease: Improving Global Outcomes CKD Work Group. (2013). KDIGO 2012 clinical practice guideline for the evaluation and management of chronic kidney disease. *Kidney International*, *3*, 1–150.

Symptoms and Complications of Chronic Kidney Disease

CKD symptoms may take months to 10 years or more to develop. If present, early symptoms of CKD are nonspecific, such as anorexia, fatigue, malaise, headache, dry skin, nausea, and unintentional weight loss. Hypertension may occur at any stage, either as the cause or a result of the disease (Aoun, Cochran, & Pavlinac, 2014). As kidney function deteriorates, complications increase in frequency and severity; however, complications can occur at any stage and can lead to death before CKD progresses to ESRD. Complications may arise from diminishing kidney function, CVD, or from treatments. Complications are interrelated and multifactorial, and the disruption to homeostasis is profound (Box 21.2).

Protein-Energy Wasting

Protein-Energy Wasting (PEW)
a state of lean body mass wasting and depletion of fat mass which is a strong risk factor for adverse outcomes and death related to CKD. Also called uremic malnutrition.

Protein-energy wasting (PEW) naturally develops as CKD progresses and is an inherent feature of advanced disease (Carrero et al., 2013). Potential causes of PEW include inadequate intake related to anorexia and/or dietary restrictions, increased nutrient losses, inflammation, hypercatabolism caused by comorbidities, and metabolic derangements such as metabolic acidosis, insulin resistance, or increased glucocorticoid activity (Kovesdy, Kopple, & Kalantar-Zadeh, 2013). Although low-protein diets can alleviate uremic symptoms and possibly delay the progression of CKD, the concern is that they may increase the risk of PEW.

Undernutrition is a strong predictor of adverse outcomes; however, it is not clear whether correcting undernutrition improves clinical outcomes. The ideal amount of protein for PEW is not known (Kovesdy et al., 2013). Protein supplements (e.g., HBV proteins or specially formulated essential amino acids or keto acid/EAA supplements) may improve markers of PEW but additional benefits have not been proven (Kovesdy et al., 2013). Adequate calories, prevention or correction of metabolic acidosis and inflammation, and the use of specially formulated protein supplements are strategies that may improve PEW. Enteral or parenteral nutrition or initiation of dialysis may be considered if poor nutritional status continues (Kovesdy et al., 2013).

Suggestions to Help Maintain Kidney Health

Primary prevention is the most effective way to reduce the personal and public health burden of CKD because often by the time biochemical evidence of CKD appears there is irreversible fibrosis within the kidney that eliminates the possibility of a "cure" (Johnson et al., 2013). However, dietary guidelines for the prevention of CKD have not been established. Nutrition and lifestyle behaviors recommended to prevent CVD, such as to increase physical activity, not smoke, and attain/maintain healthy weight, may also reduce the risk of CKD given their shared risk factors.

BOX 21.2 Complications of Chronic Kidney Disease

- Malnutrition which may impair immunity, wound healing, and GI function
- Protein-energy wasting (PEW) with loss of muscle mass and calorie reserves
- Fluid retention as evidenced by increased blood pressure, weight gain, edema, shortness of breath, and lung crackles
- Uremic syndrome, characterized by anemia, bone disease, hormonal imbalances, bleeding impairment, impaired immunity, fatigue, decreased mental acuity, muscle twitches, cramps, anorexia, unpleasant nausea, vomiting, diarrhea, itchy skin, and gastritis, related to the retention of nitrogenous wastes in the blood
- Metabolic acidosis because the kidneys are unable to excrete hydrogen ions produced through normal metabolic processes. Metabolic acidosis may cause bone and muscle mass loss,

negative nitrogen balance, increased protein catabolism, and decreased protein synthesis.
- Anemia related to impaired synthesis of erythropoietin; GI absorption of iron is also impaired, and iron intake may be inadequate.
- Chronic kidney disease mineral and bone disorder (CKD-MBD) related to abnormalities in calcium, phosphorus, parathyroid hormone, and/or vitamin D metabolism; bone abnormalities; and calcification of other vascular or other soft tissue
- Impaired synthesis of renin contributes to hypertension.
- Metabolism is altered from impaired inactivation of certain peptide hormones, such as insulin, parathyroid hormone, and glucagon.
- Accelerated atherosclerosis increases the risk of coronary heart disease, myocardial infarction, and further renal damage.

A recent prospective cohort study has found that participants who consumed an eating pattern similar to the Dietary Approaches to Stop Hypertension (DASH) diet had a lower risk for kidney disease independent of demographic characteristics, kidney disease risk factors, and baseline kidney function (Rebholz et al., 2016). The DASH diet is high in fruits, vegetables, whole grains, nuts and legumes, and low-fat dairy products and low in red and processed meats, sugar-sweetened beverages, and sweets (see Chapter 20). Benefits may be attributed to its effect on lowering blood pressure and reducing inflammation. In addition, researchers specifically found that high intakes of nuts, legumes, and low-fat dairy products were associated with a lower risk for kidney disease, whereas high red and processed meat intake was associated with a higher kidney disease risk.

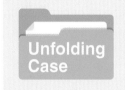

Think of Sonja. What is her body mass index (BMI)? What risk factors for CKD did she have or currently has? What interventions would you suggest to help her maintain kidney health? Is a lacto-ovo eating pattern adequate and appropriate?

Suggestions to help maintain kidney health are listed in Box 21.3 (Johnson et al., 2013). Controlling risk factors for CKD, especially blood pressure and glucose levels, are the focus of nutrition therapy for early stages of kidney impairment.

Control Blood Pressure

CKD impairs urinary excretion of sodium, which in turn raises blood pressure, which increases the risk of CVD. Sodium restriction has been shown to reduce blood pressure as well as **proteinuria**

Proteinuria
protein in the urine; also known as albuminuria.

and albuminuria, which are strong predictors of CKD progression and CVD events (McMahon et al., 2013). A high sodium intake has also been reported to impair the ability of angiotensin-converting enzyme inhibitors (ACEIs) to suppress the progression of CKD (Mitch & Remuzzi, 2016).

The Institute of Medicine (2013) recently suggested a range of 1500 to 2300 mg sodium per day for the general population, including people with diabetes, CKD, or CVD. However, the report also stated that at the lower end of that range (1500 mg), people with diabetes, CKD, or CVD have been shown to have a potentially higher risk of adverse effects, especially in patients who also have heart failure. Patients who achieve an intake of 2300 mg/day should be assessed whether further sodium lowering is appropriate.

Other interventions that improve blood pressure include the DASH diet, regular physical activity, weight loss, and limiting alcohol intake.

BOX 21.3 Suggestions to Help Maintain Kidney Health

- Limit sodium to 2300 mg or less to help control blood pressure.
- Manage diabetes, if appropriate.
- Avoid excessive protein. A reasonable intake range is 0.8 to 1.0 g/kg/day.
- Eat more fruits and vegetables (e.g., adding 2–4 cups fruits and vegetables to the usual intake), which may lower blood pressure. Goraya, Simoni, Jo, and Wesson (2012) found a high fruit and vegetable intake (e.g., a DASH-style eating pattern) significantly improves urinary markers of kidney damage in patients with GFR category 2.
- A Mediterranean-style eating pattern may improve dyslipidemia.
- Increasing fiber intake may reduce inflammation.
- Attain and maintain healthy weight.
- Engage in regular physical activity.
- Stop smoking.

Source: Johnson, D., Atai, E., Chan, M., Phoon, R. K., Scott, C., Toussaint, N. D., . . . Wiggins, K. J. (2013). KHA-CARI guideline: Early chronic kidney disease: Detection, prevention and management. *Nephrology, 18*, 340–350.

> **Unfolding Case**
>
> **Consider Sonja.** A diet history revealed she uses soy protein–based entrees, which she recently realized are high in sodium. Her typical pattern also includes one serving of yogurt per day, vegetables, fruit, and occasionally whole wheat bread. She dislikes milk and gave up sugar-sweetened beverages. She drinks two "large" glasses of wine 3 to 4 days/week and admitted a weakness for white bread and potatoes. When she is stressed, she goes to the vending machine and buys two candy bars and hides them in her clothes so her coworkers won't know she is eating. How does her intake compare to a DASH-style pattern? What are the positive features of her current pattern? Is her alcohol intake considered moderate? What options would you suggest in place of high-sodium soy entrees?

Manage Diabetes

Control of blood glucose may reduce the risk of CVD and help delay the progression of CKD (National Kidney Disease Education Program [NKDEP], 2015) (see Chapter 19). Intensive diabetes treatment early in the course of type 1 diabetes has been shown to provide long-lasting benefits on the course of kidney disease that persist at least 18 years after the initial intervention (DCCT/EDIC Research Group, 2014). An A1c goal of approximately 7% is recommended to reduce the risk of CVD, slow the progression of albuminuria, and reduce the loss of kidney function (DCCT/EDIC Research Group, 2014).

A large international study of people with type 2 diabetes found that an eating pattern rich in fruits and vegetables and moderate in alcohol was associated with a decreased risk of developing CKD and slower progression of early kidney disease (Dunkler et al., 2013). Researchers speculate that the benefits of a healthy diet, such as the DASH diet, may be attributed to a slower progression of atherosclerosis and reduced inflammation. Interestingly, neither a low-protein nor a low-sodium diet decreased the incidence and progression of CKD in this high-risk population of people with type 2 diabetes. However, it is reasonable to advise people with type 2 diabetes and vascular disease to avoid excesses of protein and sodium within the context of a healthy eating pattern to lower their risk for CKD.

Nutrition Therapy for Glomerular Filtration Rate Categories 3 to 5 Without Dialysis

Although diet is important in preventing or delaying CKD progression and managing symptoms, the majority of evidence supporting nutrition therapy interventions is based on low-level evidence or isolated randomized clinical trials (Ash, Campbell, Bogard, & Millichamp, 2014). Nutrition therapy recommendations vary among experts, the level of existing kidney function, and comorbidities. Control of blood pressure and glucose levels remain crucial strategies as kidney disease progresses; therefore, sodium restriction and a healthy eating pattern, such as a DASH diet, are stressed. Dietary modifications are individualized according complications and laboratory values (Table 21.3). Additional points are summarized in the following sections.

Protein

Protein restriction has been recommended for more than 50 years as a strategy to delay the progression of CKD (Mandayam & Mitch, 2006). Limiting protein intake may reduce albuminuria and improve blood glucose control, hyperlipidemia, blood pressure, renal bone disease, and metabolic acidosis (NKDEP, 2015). However, because CKD patients are at risk for PEW, the diet must provide sufficient protein to meet needs and prevent loss of protein mass.

Although it is agreed upon that excesses and deficiencies of protein should be avoided, the ideal intake of protein in patients with CKD is not known. Recommendations vary among guideline sources, the stage of CKD, and comorbidities. For predialysis CKD patients who do

Table 21.3 Predialysis (Glomerular Filtration Rate Categories 3–5) Nutrition Guidelines

Nutrient	Nutrition Intervention	Selection Details
Protein	Avoid excessive protein intake. For people with diabetes: 0.8–1.0 g/kg/day For people who do not have diabetes: 0.6–0.8 (0.6 g/kg/day may be more beneficial but is difficult to achieve) Avoiding excessive protein also reduces intake of phosphorus and metabolic acid.	Eat small portions of meat, fish, poultry, eggs, dairy, legumes, and nuts. Spread sources of protein over the day. Choose at least 50% high biologic value proteins (meat, fish, poultry, milk, yogurt, soy) to potentially slow CKD progression, especially in people with diabetes.
Sodium	Limit to 2300 mg/day or less	Choose fresh or plain frozen vegetables over canned and fresh meat over processed meat. Avoid convenience items such as canned or dried soups, bottled salad dressings, and frozen dinners. Use herbs and spices as alternatives to salt to season food. Read "Nutrition Facts" labels and compare brands to choose lower sodium items.
Fat	Limit saturated fat and trans fat; choose unsaturated fats, including sources of omega-3 fatty acids.	Use oils and products made with oil instead of solid fats. Choose fish and poultry over red meats. Buy lean cuts of meat and drain fat when possible.
Potassium	Limit potassium when serum value is 5 mEq/L or higher.	Read "Nutrition Facts" label to compare potassium content of similar products (potassium must appear on the label by 7/26/18). Protein foods (meat, fish, poultry, beans, dairy, nuts) provide potassium. Choose refined grains over whole grain breads and cereals. The potassium content of fruits and vegetables varies (see Table 21.5). The potassium content of most vegetables can be leached by soaking sliced vegetables in water overnight, draining the water, and then boiling them in fresh water. Avoid salt substitutes that contain potassium. Limit foods that contain potassium chloride on the ingredient list; it may be used in place of salt in some packaged foods. For people with diabetes, use apple, grape, or cranberry juice instead of orange juice for hypoglycemia.
Phosphorus	Restriction may not be necessary until CKD is advanced; recommended level of restriction has not been determined.	Phosphorus intake is decreased when protein (meat, fish, poultry, dairy, legumes, nuts) intake is restricted. To lower intake even more, limit foods with phosphorus additives (e.g., "phos" identified on the ingredient list). Some food manufacturers post nutrition information that includes phosphorus content on their websites.
Calcium	Calcium recommendations have not yet been established.	Phosphate binders that contain calcium contribute to total daily intake. Dairy products provide calcium, phosphorus, protein, and potassium, so they may not be the best calcium source for people with CKD.

Source: National Kidney Disease Education Program. (2015). *Chronic kidney disease and diet: Assessment, management, and treatment. Treating CKD patients who are not on dialysis*. Available at https://www.niddk.nih.gov/health-information/health-communication-programs/nkdep/a-z/Documents/ckd-diet-assess-manage-treat-508.pdf. Accessed on 8/30/16.

not have diabetes, protein intake may be limited to 0.6 to 0.8 g/kg/day (Aoun et al., 2014). For people with diabetic kidney disease, protein allowance may be slightly higher at 0.8 to 1.0 g/kg/day (NKDEP, 2015), based on studies that show this level of protein stabilizes or reduces albuminuria, slows the deterioration of GFR, and may possibly prevent kidney failure (Burrowes, 2008).

In international settings where keto acid analogs are available, a very-low-protein diet (0.3–0.5 g/kg/day) with supplements of keto acid analogs may be considered for adults with CKD who do not have diabetes and are not on dialysis (Aoun et al., 2014). Compared to a conventional low-protein diet, very-low-protein diets supplemented with keto analogs have been shown to slow the rate of decline in kidney function in patients with GFR categories 4 to 5 and significantly improve quality of life (Garneata & Mircescu, 2013). Crucial to the success of this type of regimen is a high level of motivation in the patient, intensive education and support, and ongoing nutrition counseling.

Calories

Adequate calories are needed to ensure that dietary protein is used for repair rather than being metabolized as a source of energy. Although obesity has been linked to a higher risk of CKD (Kopple & Feroze, 2011), higher body mass has been associated with lower mortality in stage 5 kidney failure (Kalantar-Zadeh et al., 2012). Generally, 25 to 35 cal/kg/day are recommended depending on goal weight.

Fat

Although clinical trials testing the effectiveness of heart-healthy diets in CKD patients are lacking, CKD patients are advised to limit their intake of saturated fat, trans fat, and cholesterol. Unsaturated fats, such as fatty fish, avocados, olive oil, nuts, and seeds, are an important source of heart-healthy calories.

Potassium

Patients with CKD are at risk of hyperkalemia due to reduced urinary excretion. Other contributing factors include metabolic acidosis, catabolism, and the use of ACEIs or angiotensin receptor blockers (ARBs) to control blood pressure. Although hyperkalemia can occur in stages 3 to 4, it is more typically seen in stage 5 kidney failure. For all CKD stages, potassium allowance is based on the individual's serum potassium levels.

A typical low potassium diet provides 2 g/day. To lower the potassium content in tuberous vegetables (e.g., turnip, taro, potato), patients are advised to peel, cut into small pieces to increase the surface area, and boil in a large amount of water to leach potassium. By July 26, 2018, food manufacturers are required to list potassium on the revised "Nutrition Facts" label for the first time since the inception of the "Nutrition Facts" label. That change will help patients make informed food purchases because taste does not reflect potassium content as it often does with sodium content. Patients are advised to avoid potassium-based salt substitutes.

Phosphorus and Calcium

As kidney function deteriorates, the conversion of vitamin D to its active form is impaired, leading to alterations in the metabolism of calcium, phosphorus, and magnesium. CKD progression leads to a gradual decline in phosphorus excretion, resulting in hyperphosphatemia, bone demineralization, and bone pain. Hyperphosphatemia, hypocalcemia, and low levels of active vitamin D stimulate parathyroid hormone (PTH) secretion, creating secondary hyperparathyroidism that further aggravates loss of bone mass and increases the risk that damaging deposits of calcium and phosphorus will form in the kidneys and other soft tissues such as the eyes, skin, heart, lungs, and blood vessels. Hyperphosphatemia plays a crucial role in the development of CKD-mineral and bone disorder (MBD) and increases the risk of CVD events and mortality in patients with CKD (Mitch & Remuzzi, 2016).

A phosphate-restricted diet (e.g., 800–1000 mg/day) and phosphate binders, along with vitamin D and supplemental calcium, are used to treat and prevent secondary hyperparathyroidism, renal bone disease, and soft tissue calcification. Animal proteins are rich in phosphates, therefore restricting protein reduces phosphorus intake. However, low-phosphorus diets can be challenging to achieve because inorganic phosphate additives are widely used as food preservatives, and they are better absorbed than naturally occurring phosphorus in foods. In addition, "Nutrition Facts" labels are not required to list phosphorus content. Because serum phosphate levels are difficult to control through dietary restriction alone, phosphate binders may be prescribed with meals and snacks to impair phosphorus absorption.

Dietary calcium recommendations have not been established (NKDEP, 2015). Milk products, a rich source of calcium, are generally restricted because they are also sources of protein and phosphorus. Calcium-based phosphate binders contribute to total calcium intake. Supplements of vitamin D increase the risk for hypercalcemia.

Quick Bite Foods high in phosphorus

Meat, fish, poultry
Dairy products
Bran cereals and oatmeal
Nuts
Legumes
Colas
Frozen, convenience, and prepackaged foods with phosphorus-based additives or preservatives

Vitamin and Mineral Supplementation

There is little certainty about the vitamin needs of people with CKD (Steiber & Kopple, 2011) and wide variations exist in the use of vitamin and mineral supplements. In general,

- Vitamin intake may be inadequate secondary to anorexia or dietary restrictions. For instance, intakes of riboflavin and vitamin B_{12} may be inadequate in patients on a low-protein diet (0.6 g/kg/day) because protein foods are sources of both of these vitamins.
- Certain medications may interfere with vitamin metabolism, particularly of vitamin B_6.
- Vitamin deficiencies are common in people with advanced kidney disease who do not take supplements yet in advanced CKD, certain vitamins may accumulate due to impaired excretion (Steiber & Kopple, 2011).Generally, a renal-specific multivitamin, with higher amounts of water-soluble vitamins is prescribed. Data do not support routine supplementation with niacin and vitamins A, E, and K (NKDEP, 2015).
- The need for vitamin D is determined on an individual basis.
- Intravenous (IV) iron supplementation, in conjunction with erythropoietin, is more effective in improving iron status than oral iron supplements (Beto, Ramirez, & Bansal, 2014).

Nutrition Therapy During Dialysis

Patients undergoing dialysis are at considerable increased risk of morbidity and mortality related to persistent inflammation, malnutrition, and metabolic abnormalities (Huang, Lindholm, Stenvinkel, & Carrero, 2013). The goal of nutrition therapy is to match dietary intake with renal replacement therapy (RRT) while preventing nutrition deficiencies (Beto et al., 2014). The diet is complex and dynamic. The nutrient recommendations are used as a guideline; the patient's actual needs are based on individual assessment. Table 21.4 outlines nutrition recommendations for patients undergoing dialysis. Additional points are summarized in the following sections.

Table 21.4 — Recommended Nutrition Guidelines for Adults on Dialysis or After Transplantation

Nutrient	CKD Stage 5 with RRT (Kidney Failure)	Posttransplantation (Guided by CKD Stage/Category of Kidney Function)
Protein	1.1–1.5 g/kg of BW/day (HD with at least 50% HBV to achieve/maintain adequate serum albumin levels in conjunction with sufficient protein-sparing calorie intake)	0.8–1.0 g/kg of BW/day with 50% HBV
Energy	25–35 kcal/kg of BW/day to achieve or maintain goal body weight; include estimated caloric absorption from PD fluid as applicable	25–35 kcal/kg of BW/day to achieve or maintain goal body weight
Fat	Focus on type of fat and carbohydrate to manage dyslipidemia, if present.	Focus on type of fat and carbohydrate to reduce cardiovascular risk or manage immunosuppressant medication adverse effects (e.g., dyslipidemia, glucose intolerance).
Saturated fat	Reduce and substitute saturated fat sources with healthier fat sources.	Reduce and substitute saturated fat sources with healthier fat sources.
Sodium	2.0–3.0 g/day (HD) to control interdialytic fluid gain; 2.0–4.0 g/day (PD) to control hydration status	General population recommendation of ≤2.4 g/day
Potassium	2.0–4.0 g/day or 40 mg/kg of BW/day in HD or individualized in PD to achieve normal serum levels	No restriction unless hyperkalemia is present and then individualized
Calcium	2 g elemental/day from dietary and medication sources	Individualized to kidney function
Phosphorus	800–1000 mg/day to achieve goal serum level of 3.5–5.5 mg/dL* or below; coordinate with oral phosphate binder prescription	Individualized to stage of kidney function
Fiber	Same as general population; 25–35 g/day	Same as general population; 25–35 g/day
Fluid	1000 mL/day (+ urine output if present) in HD; greater in PD individualized to fluid status	No restriction; matched to urine output if appropriate

RRT, renal replacement therapy; CKD, chronic kidney disease; HD, hemodialysis; HBV, high biologic value; BW, body weight; PD, peritoneal dialysis.
*To convert mg/dL phosphorus to mmol/L, multiply mg/dL by 0.323. To convert mmol/L phosphorus to mg/dL, multiply mmol/L by 3.10. Phosphorus of 3.10 mg/dL = 1.00 mmol/L.
Sources: Beto, J. A., Ramirez, W. E., & Bansal, V. K. (2014). Medical nutrition therapy in adults with chronic kidney disease: Integrating evidence and consensus into practice for the generalist registered dietitian nutritionist. *Journal of the Academy of Nutrition and Dietetics, 114*(7), 1077–1087; and Information from this table is available online at www.adjrnl.org.

Protein

The protein allowance for patients treated with dialysis is increased by approximately 50% or more above the Recommended Dietary Allowance (RDA) to account for the loss of serum proteins and amino acids in the **dialysate**. Achieving a higher protein intake within the confines of other restrictions, especially phosphorus restriction, can be challenging. Box 21.4 illustrates a menu at two different protein levels.

Calories

Calorie recommendations do not change from predialysis to dialysis. However, people who undergo peritoneal dialysis absorb a significant amount of calories daily through the dextrose in the dialysate, which needs to be considered. Dialysate calories can be estimated by a mathematical formula that takes into account several factors, including the number of exchanges and the dextrose concentration of the exchanges (Pace, Tootell, & Mahony, 2013). A feeling of fullness may occur from dwelling dialysate and impair intake. Smaller, more frequent meals and eating during or after draining may improve intake (Pace et al., 2013).

BOX 21.4 Sample Chronic Kidney Disease Menus: for Predialysis and While on Hemodialysis

Menus appropriate for a 165 pound/75 kg man

Sample CKD predialysis menu providing 50 g protein (0.7 g protein/kg)	**Sample CKD menu for hemodialysis, providing 97 g protein (1.3 g protein/kg)**
Breakfast	
½ cup apricot nectar	½ cup apricot nectar
1 English muffin	1 English muffin
At least 1 tbsp trans fat–free margarine	1 tbsp trans fat–free margarine
Jelly	2 eggs fried in trans fat–free margarine
Coffee	Jelly
Sugar	1 cup coffee
Nondairy creamer	Sugar
	Nondairy creamer
Lunch	
Sandwich made with	Sandwich made with
2 oz turkey	4 oz turkey
2 slices whole wheat bread	2 slices whole wheat bread
Salad dressing	Salad dressing
Lettuce and 1 slice tomato	Lettuce and 1 slice tomato
1 small apple	1 small apple
½ cup low-fat milk	½ cup low-fat milk
Snack	
2 fruit roll-ups	
Dinner	
2 oz grilled salmon	5 oz grilled salmon
½ cup unsalted rice with margarine	½ cup unsalted rice with margarine
½ cup carrots with margarine	½ cup carrots
Lettuce, onions, cucumbers, green salad with olive oil and vinegar dressing	Lettuce, onions, cucumbers, green pepper salad with olive oil and vinegar dressing
⅛ blueberry pie	⅛ blueberry pie
Ginger ale	1 cup ginger ale
Snacks	
Carbonated beverages*	
Marshmallows, gumdrops, hard candy	Marshmallows, gumdrops, hard candy

CKD, chronic kidney disease.
*As allowed, depending on fluid needs.

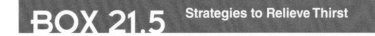

BOX 21.5 Strategies to Relieve Thirst

- Use ice or popsicles within the fluid allowance—very cold things are better at relieving thirst.
- Suck on hard candy or mints.
- Chew gum.
- Rinse your mouth without swallowing using refrigerated water.
- Rinse your mouth occasionally with refrigerated mouthwash.
- Suck on a lemon wedge.
- Eat bread with applesauce or jelly with margarine.
- Control blood glucose levels, as appropriate.
- Try frozen low-potassium fruit, such as grapes.
- Use small glasses instead of large ones.
- Apply petroleum jelly to the lips.

Phosphorus

When dialysis begins and protein allowance increases, phosphorus intake correspondingly increases, yet the recommendation is to limit intake to 800 to 1000 mg. People who adhere to a low-phosphorus diet are at risk of consuming an inadequate protein diet, which can lead to malnutrition and PEW. A study by Shinaberger et al. (2008) concluded that the risk of controlling serum phosphorus by restricting dietary protein may outweigh the benefit of controlling phosphorus and may lead to greater mortality, especially in patients on maintenance hemodialysis. Phosphate binders, which decrease gastrointestinal (GI) absorption of phosphorus and promote fecal excretion, allow for a higher protein (and phosphorus) intake. Phosphate binders, which must be taken with all meals and snacks, are necessary to control serum phosphorus levels for the majority of patients.

Fluid

For people on hemodialysis, fluid allowance equals the volume of any urine produced plus 1000 mL. Fluid intake is monitored by weight gain: Anuric hemodialysis patients should not gain more than approximately 2 pounds/day between treatments. For many patients on hemodialysis, limiting fluid intake is the biggest challenge. Teaching clients *why* the fluid restriction is important is only half the battle; teaching them *how* to control their intake and thirst is vital. Strategies to relieve thirst are listed in Box 21.5. Peritoneal dialysis patients usually have fewer problems with fluid retention.

Guidelines for Chronic Kidney Disease Meals

The diet for CKD is challenging; modifications can be numerous, extensive, and lifelong, and changes are frequent. It is a difficult task to design a meal plan that balances what the individual needs with what the individual can tolerate and will accept. Box 21.6 lists strategies that may help promote dietary adherence.

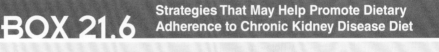

BOX 21.6 Strategies That May Help Promote Dietary Adherence to Chronic Kidney Disease Diet

- Provide positive messages about what to eat rather than emphasizing food restrictions.
- Encourage social support from family and friends.
- Foster the patient's perception as successfully adhering to the plan. People who are more confident in their ability to adhere to the eating plan make better choices.
- Provide feedback on self-monitoring and laboratory data. Correlation of records with laboratory data enables the client to see cause and effect, reinforces the importance of nutrition therapy, and opens the door for problem solving.
- For patients who must restrict their intake of protein, encourage the use of low-protein breads, cereals, cookies, and pastas. Acceptability varies greatly among low-protein products, so if a client does not like one brand, it does not mean he or she will not like another.

Patients who are taught how to restrict their protein intake must also learn how to replace protein calories with protein-free foods. The taste and texture of protein-free foods, which may also be low in phosphorus and sodium, are often unacceptable to patients. Patients may find protein-free pasta much more palatable than protein-free bread (D'Alessandro et al., 2013). Intense nutrition counseling may also improve patient adherence to a low-protein diet (Paes-Barreto et al., 2013).

Food lists, with the number of daily servings permitted from each list specified, may be used to help patients implement their prescribed diet (Table 21.5). An individualized meal plan corresponds as closely as possible to the patient's food preferences and habits. Portion sizes are specified to help ensure relative consistency in nutrient intake. The composition and complexity of the meal plan differs with the type of treatment used (e.g., predialysis, hemodialysis, or peritoneal dialysis). For instance, people not receiving dialysis may not need to limit their intake of potassium and would be free to choose among low-, medium-, and high-potassium fruits and vegetables, whereas people undergoing hemodialysis may need to limit their intake of fruits and vegetables to those that are low in potassium. Guidelines for implementing nutrition therapy recommendations for CKD are featured in Box 21.7.

Kidney Transplantation

Kidney transplantation is a treatment option for people with kidney failure. Posttransplant nutrition guidelines are summarized in Table 21.4. As with all major surgeries, the immediate postoperative diet is high in protein and adequate in calories to promote healing; nutrient needs gradually decrease after the initial postoperative period. During the first 1 to 3 months posttransplant, the need for protein may be 1.3 to 2.0 g/kg of **dry weight** (Pace et al., 2013). Most dietary parameters are removed when the new kidney functions normally, although side effects from immunosuppressant drugs may require some dietary modifications. A lifelong commitment to a calorie-appropriate, heart-healthy eating pattern, such as a Mediterranean-style eating pattern is important to decrease the risk of obesity, hypertension, diabetes, and hyperlipidemia and to maximize bone density.

Dry weight
the lowest body weight safety achieved after dialysis without precipitating symptoms of low blood pressure.

BOX 21.7   Guidelines for Implementing Nutrition Therapy for Chronic Kidney Disease

- Initially weigh or measure portion sizes and, thereafter, periodically spot-check portion sizes for accuracy because either too little or too much protein in the diet can cause uremic symptoms to return.
- Be sure to eat a good breakfast if appetite decreases as the day progresses, which may occur secondary to uremia.
- Limit meat intake to less than 5 to 6 oz/day for most men and less than 4 oz/day for most women. Think of meat as a side dish, not the main entrée.
- Spread protein allowance over the whole day instead of saving it all for one meal.
- Limit dairy products, including milk, yogurt, ice cream, and frozen yogurt, to ½ cup/day. Nondairy creamers are a low-phosphorus alternative, but they can be high in saturated fat.
- Limit cheese to 1 oz hard cheese per day or ⅓ cup cottage cheese per day.
- Limit high-phosphorus foods to one serving or less per day. High-phosphorus foods include beer, chocolate, cola, nuts, peanut butter, dried peas and beans, bran, bran cereals, and some whole grains.
- Do not add salt during cooking or at the table. Avoid processed foods, regular canned vegetables, convenience foods, and seasonings that contain salt (e.g., onion salt, lemon pepper, monosodium glutamate [MSG]).
- Eat heart healthy by choosing lean meats, fatty meats, nonfat milk and dairy products, trans fat–free margarines, and canola and olive oils.
- Try highly seasoned or strongly flavored foods if uremia has caused a change in the sense of taste.
- Eat a consistent intake of carbohydrate with regularly timed meals to control blood glucose levels, if appropriate.
- Seek physician approval before using any vitamin, mineral, or supplement.

| Table 21.5 | Food Lists for Chronic Kidney Disease with Meal Plan Allowances* | | | | | | |

Food List/Representative Foods and Serving Sizes	Approximations/Averages per Serving						
	Calories	Protein (g)	Carbohydrates (g)	Fat (g)	Sodium (mg)	Potassium (mg)	Phosphorus (mg)
Protein Choices							
Meat, Poultry, and Fish _____ servings allowed per day 1 serving = 1 oz beef, fish, lamb, pork, veal, poultry	75	7	0	5	65	115	70
Meat Alternatives _____ servings allowed per day 1 serving = 1 oz cheese, 1 large egg, 1 oz unsalted nuts, 2 tbsp peanut butter, ¼ cup tofu	90	7	5	5–10	100	100	120
Legumes _____ servings allowed per day 1 serving = ⅓ cup black beans, black-eyed peas, kidney beans, garbanzo beans, lentils, hummus	90	6	15	≤1	<10	250	100
Protein Foods with Higher Amounts of Sodium and Phosphorus _____ servings allowed per day 1 serving = 4 slices bacon, ¼ cup canned salted tuna or sardines, 1 oz processed cheese, 1 oz deli meats, 2 oz hot dogs, 1–2 oz soy burgers	75–250	7	0–5	10	≥200	50–150	100–300
Dairy Choices							
Dairy Foods _____ servings allowed per day 1 serving = 1 cup low-fat or nonfat milk, 1 cup low-fat plain or sugar-free yogurt	120	8	12	5	≥120	≥350	≥220
Dairy Foods with Higher Amounts of Calories, Carbohydrates, and Fat _____ servings allowed per day 1 serving = 1 cup eggnog, 1 cup ice cream, 1 cup whole milk, 1 cup regular sweetened and/or frozen yogurt	Varies; higher than dairy foods	Varies; higher than dairy foods	≥15	≥10	Varies; higher than dairy foods	Varies; higher than dairy foods	Varies; higher than dairy foods
Dairy Alternatives _____ servings allowed per day 1 serving = ½ cup almond milk, rice milk, soy milk	75	1	2–12	7	40	60	60
Bread, Cereal, and Grain Choices							
Bread, Cereal, and Grain Foods _____ servings allowed per day 1 serving = 1 slice bread, ½ cup cooked cereal, 4 unsalted crackers, ⅓ cup cooked pasta, ⅓ cup rice, one 6-in flour tortilla	80	2	15	4	150	50	30

(continued)

Table 21.5 — Food Lists for Chronic Kidney Disease with Meal Plan Allowances* (continued)

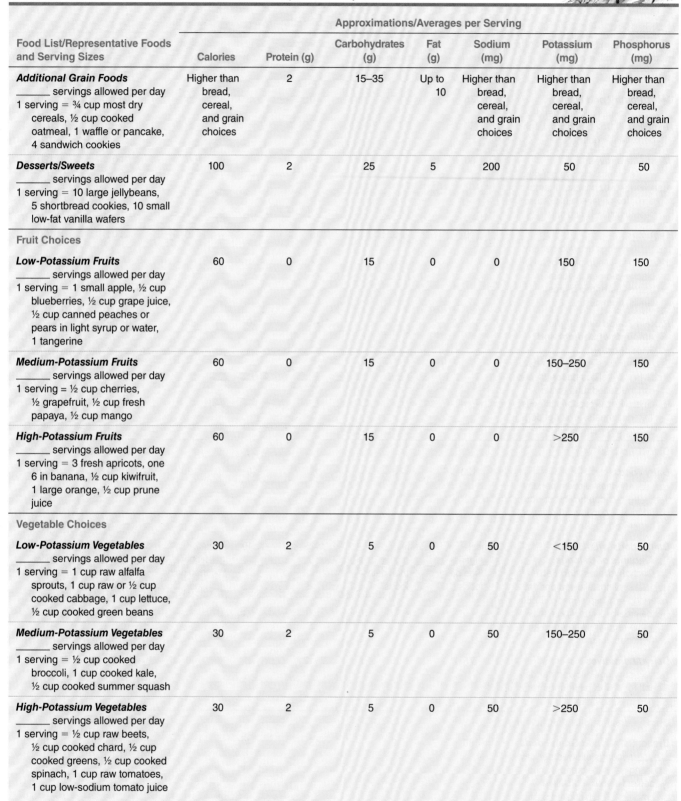

Food List/Representative Foods and Serving Sizes	Calories	Protein (g)	Carbohydrates (g)	Fat (g)	Sodium (mg)	Potassium (mg)	Phosphorus (mg)
Additional Grain Foods _____ servings allowed per day 1 serving = ¾ cup most dry cereals, ½ cup cooked oatmeal, 1 waffle or pancake, 4 sandwich cookies	Higher than bread, cereal, and grain choices	2	15–35	Up to 10	Higher than bread, cereal, and grain choices	Higher than bread, cereal, and grain choices	Higher than bread, cereal, and grain choices
Desserts/Sweets _____ servings allowed per day 1 serving = 10 large jellybeans, 5 shortbread cookies, 10 small low-fat vanilla wafers	100	2	25	5	200	50	50
Fruit Choices							
Low-Potassium Fruits _____ servings allowed per day 1 serving = 1 small apple, ½ cup blueberries, ½ cup grape juice, ½ cup canned peaches or pears in light syrup or water, 1 tangerine	60	0	15	0	0	150	150
Medium-Potassium Fruits _____ servings allowed per day 1 serving = ½ cup cherries, ½ grapefruit, ½ cup fresh papaya, ½ cup mango	60	0	15	0	0	150–250	150
High-Potassium Fruits _____ servings allowed per day 1 serving = 3 fresh apricots, one 6 in banana, ½ cup kiwifruit, 1 large orange, ½ cup prune juice	60	0	15	0	0	>250	150
Vegetable Choices							
Low-Potassium Vegetables _____ servings allowed per day 1 serving = 1 cup raw alfalfa sprouts, 1 cup raw or ½ cup cooked cabbage, 1 cup lettuce, ½ cup cooked green beans	30	2	5	0	50	<150	50
Medium-Potassium Vegetables _____ servings allowed per day 1 serving = ½ cup cooked broccoli, 1 cup cooked kale, ½ cup cooked summer squash	30	2	5	0	50	150–250	50
High-Potassium Vegetables _____ servings allowed per day 1 serving = ½ cup raw beets, ½ cup cooked chard, ½ cup cooked greens, ½ cup cooked spinach, 1 cup raw tomatoes, 1 cup low-sodium tomato juice	30	2	5	0	50	>250	50

Table 21.5	Food Lists for Chronic Kidney Disease with Meal Plan Allowances* (continued)						
Food List/Representative Foods and Serving Sizes	Approximations/Averages per Serving						
	Calories	Protein (g)	Carbohydrates (g)	Fat (g)	Sodium (mg)	Potassium (mg)	Phosphorus (mg)
Fat Choices							
Healthier, Unsaturated Fats _____ servings allowed per day 1 serving = 1 tsp trans fat–free margarine, 1 tbsp trans fat–free margarine spread, 1 tsp canola, corn, olive, soybean, or peanut oil	100	0	4	5	≥55	10	5
Saturated Fats (Limit Use) 1 tsp bacon fat, 1 tsp butter, 2 tbsp half-and-half, 1 tbsp cream cheese, 2 tbsp powdered cream substitute, 1 tbsp whipped cream, 1 tsp lard							
Fluid Choices _____ servings allowed per day Includes coffee, diet soft drinks, tea, water, soup, broth, sugar-free gelatin	Amounts vary. Requires careful label reading						

*The patient's daily allowance for each subgroup would be specified based on the individual nutrition prescription.
Source: Academy of Nutrition and Dietetics. (n.d.). *Diabetes and chronic kidney disease stages 1-4: Nutrition guidelines*. Available at https://www.nutritioncaremanual .org/vault/2440/web/files/CKD-DiabetesNutritionTherapy.pdf. Accessed on 8/14/16.

ACUTE KIDNEY INJURY

Acute kidney injury (AKI) is characterized by a sudden decrease (up to 48 hours) in kidney function. Common life-threatening complications include volume overload, hyperkalemia, acidosis, and uremia. AKI seldom exists as an isolated organ failure but rather is often a complication of sepsis, critical illness, burns, cardiac surgery, trauma, and multiple-organ failure. The mortality rate for AKI diagnosed in intensive care unit (ICU) patients is up to 50%, with infection, cardiorespiratory complications, and CVD the three main leading causes of death (Li, Tang, Zhang, & Wu, 2012). Primary treatment goals are to correct fluid overload, severe acidosis, hyperkalemia, and hematologic abnormalities.

PEW may affect up to 40% of AKI patients in the ICU and represents a major negative prognostic factor (Fiaccadori, Regolisti, & Maggiore, 2013). The pathogenesis of PEW in AKI is complex and involves many factors including a systemic inflammatory response, loss of kidney homeostatic function, insulin resistance, and oxidative stress (Fiaccadori et al., 2013). Dialysis contributes to nutrient losses.

Nutrition Therapy for Acute Kidney Injury

The goals of nutrition therapy are to prevent PEW, reestablish appropriate immune function, reduce mortality, and diminish the inflammatory response and oxidative stress (McCarthy & Phipps, 2014). The metabolic derangements that occur in hypercatabolic patients with AKI, such as accelerated protein breakdown, increased energy expenditure, and alterations in carbohydrate, protein, and fat metabolism, make it difficult to achieve nutrition goals. Conversely, overfeeding, such as from failing to account for the calorie content of RRT solutions, may increase the risk of hyperglycemia, liver disease, electrolyte disorders, and fluid overload (Fiaccadori et al., 2013). Individualized assessment and monitoring are necessary to avoid both under- and overfeeding.

Nutrition support in the form of enteral and/or parenteral nutrition is often required for AKI patients, even though it is not known if nutrition support positively affects patient outcomes (Fiaccadori et al., 2013). The optimal intake of calories and nutrients for AKI has not been determined. For instance, nutrition guidelines frequently suggest 25 to 35 cal/kg/day even though the evidence supporting such recommendations is weak and based on small or very small single-center studies (Bellomo et al., 2014). Clinicians rely on best practice recommendations and institutional protocols due to the lack of evidence-based nutrition therapy recommendations to improve mortality and outcomes (McCarthy & Phipps, 2014).

Nutrition therapy is affected by the underlying disease process, preexisting comorbidities, and current complications (McClave et al., 2016). Although the evidence base is limited, a group of U.S. experts in AKI and critical care nephrology agree with the following international recommendations that pertain to nutrition (Palevsky et al., 2013)

- Enteral nutrition is the preferred route for delivering nutrition.
- Total calorie intake should be 20 to 30 cal/kg/day in patients with any stage of AKI.
- Provide 0.8 to 1.0 g protein/kg/day to noncatabolic patients who do not need dialysis, 1.0 to 1.5 g/kg/day in patients with AKI on RRT, and up to a maximum of 1.7 g/kg/day in patients on continuous renal replacement therapy (CRRT) and in hypercatabolic patients.
- Protein restriction should not be used as a strategy to prevent or delay initiation of RRT.

Standard enteral formulas are recommended, although a specialty formula designed for renal failure may be considered in patients who develop significant electrolyte abnormalities (McClave et al., 2016). If calorie targets are not met within 3 to 5 days, parenteral nutrition may be used as a complement to EN to achieve adequate calorie intake, especially in patients receiving RRT (McClave et al., 2016; Singer et al., 2011).

In patients who are not given dialysis, intakes of potassium, magnesium, phosphorus, and calcium are adjusted according to serum concentrations. Because deficiencies of certain vitamins and minerals may occur over time with RRT, single nutrients or renal multivitamin preparations may be prescribed.

KIDNEY STONES

Kidney stones form when insoluble crystals precipitate out of urine. They vary in size from sand-like "gravel" to large, branching stones, and although they form most often in the kidney, they can occur anywhere in the urinary system.

Risks for kidney stone formation include dehydration or low urine volume, urinary tract obstruction, gout, chronic inflammation of the bowel, and intestinal bypass or ostomy surgery. Serum electrolytes, calcium, and creatinine may suggest underlying medical conditions. Assessment of urine pH and the composition of the stone may help direct preventive measures (Pearle et al., 2014). Prospective data from cohort studies indicate obesity, weight gain, and other characteristics related to metabolic syndrome increase the risk of kidney stone formation (Taylor, Stampfer, & Curhan, 2005), which may explain the increasing prevalence of kidney stones since 1994 (Scales, Smith, Hanley, & Saigal, 2012).

Dietary Risk Factors for Kidney Stones

Dietary factors can affect the risk of developing most types of stones, although diet is not always involved.

Fluid

A low fluid intake concentrates the urine, increasing the likelihood of chemicals precipitating out to form kidney stones—regardless of the composition of the stone.

Oxalate
a salt of oxalic acid. Oxalate has no known function in the body and is normally excreted in urine. Excess oxalate can bind with calcium in the urine to form calcium oxalate kidney stones.

Hyperoxaluria
elevated levels of oxalate in the urine.

Oxalate

Approximately 80% of kidney stones contain calcium and most calcium stones are composed of primarily of calcium **oxalate** (Noori et al., 2014). **Hyperoxaluria** can be caused by genetic disorders, chronic bowel inflammation, or a high-oxalate intake. Typically, patients with hyperoxaluria are advised to drink more fluids, consume adequate calcium, and avoid oxalate-rich foods (Box 21.8), despite the lack of substantial data supporting the recommendation to limit oxalate (Noori et al., 2014).

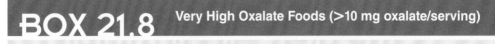

BOX 21.8 Very High Oxalate Foods (>10 mg oxalate/serving)

- Fruits: avocado, dates, grapefruit, kiwi, orange, raspberries, canned pineapple
- Vegetables: beets, navy beans, okra, rhubarb, spinach, yams, turnips, kale
- Grains: brown rice, bulgur, grits, cornmeal, pancakes, bran cereals
- Nuts: almonds, cashews, peanuts
- Miscellaneous: hot chocolate, potato chips, peanut butter

Source: Harvard School of Public Health at https://regepi.bwh.harvard.edu/health/Oxalate/files/Oxalate%20Content%20 of%20Foods.xls.

Calcium

Because dietary calcium favorably binds with dietary oxalate in the intestines to form an insoluble compound that the body cannot absorb, an adequate calcium intake helps reduce the risk of calcium oxalate stones.

Protein

High intakes of animal protein may increase the risk of kidney stones by increasing urinary excretion of calcium, oxalate, and uric acid and reducing urinary pH (Seiner, Ebert, Nicolay, & Hesse, 2003).

Sodium

A high sodium intake promotes urinary calcium excretion by decreasing calcium reabsorption by the kidney (Nouvenne et al., 2010).

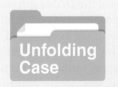

Recall Sonja. An increase in her stress level has caused her to give up on her lacto-ovo vegetarian eating pattern. Her blood pressure is increasing, and her weight loss has stalled. To make matters worse, she recently went to an ambulatory care center with excruciating back pain and was diagnosed with kidney stones, which she passed hours after receiving IV fluids. She is worried she will have more kidney stones that may eventually damage her only kidney. What would you tell her about reducing her risk of stone recurrence? What should her nutritional priorities be to maintain kidney health? What other lifestyle interventions would you recommend?

Nutrition Therapy for Kidney Stones

Although dietary changes can reduce the risk of stone formation, it is important to first determine whether an individual's eating pattern plays a causative role; if nutrition is not a cause, it cannot be a cure (Penniston, 2015). Table 21.6 lists dietary recommendations for the medical management of kidney stones.

A well-accepted strategy for reducing the recurrence of stones is to increase fluid intake (Ferraro, Taylor, Gambaro, & Curhan, 2013). Although there is not a definite threshold for urine volume and increased risk of stone formation, an accepted goal is to drink enough fluid to produce at least 2.5 L of urine daily (Pearle et al., 2014).

Studies suggest not all fluids have the same impact on the risk of kidney stone formation. Sugar-sweetened soda and punch have been found to increase the risk of stone formation, whereas coffee, tea, beer, wine, and orange juice are associated with a lower risk (Ferraro et al., 2013). In prospective cohort studies, caffeine intake was found to be independently associated with a lower risk of incident kidney stones (Ferraro, Taylor, Gambaro, & Curhan, 2014).

An individual's eating pattern may also influence risk of kidney stone formation. In a randomized controlled trial, the DASH diet, despite its high oxalate content, decreased the risk of stone formation by 35% compared to a 14% risk reduction in participants who followed the low-oxalate

Table 21.6   Dietary Recommendations for Kidney Stones

Type of stone	Possible Diet Modifications
All types of stones	Ensure adequate fluid intake to achieve ≥2.5 L urine daily. Limiting sugar-sweetened beverages may help reduce risk.
Calcium stones with high urinary calcium	Limit sodium to ≤2300 mg/day. Consume 1000–1200 mg calcium/day from food and beverages; avoid calcium supplements.
Calcium oxalate stones with high urinary oxalate	Limit oxalate-rich foods (see Box 21.8). Consume 1000–1200 mg calcium from food and beverages primarily with meals to bind oxalate. Avoid vitamin C supplements and other over the counter supplements.
Calcium stones with low urinary citrate	Increase fruit and vegetable intake if acid load of eating pattern contributes to low urinary citrate. Limit nondairy animal protein to decrease potential renal acid load of eating pattern.
Calcium stones or uric acid stones with high urinary uric acid	No relevant studies refute or confirm diet to manage high urinary uric acid in uric acid or calcium stone formers. Patients may benefit from limiting high and moderately high purine foods. Increase fruit and vegetable intake to increase alkalinity of eating pattern. Limit intake of nondairy animal protein to decrease the acid load of the eating pattern and increase urine pH.
Cystine stones	Increase fluid to produce a urine volume of ≥4 L. Limit sodium to ≤2300 mg/day. All animal proteins contain cystine and methionine, which is metabolized to cysteine; limiting animal proteins may be prudent.

Source: Pearle, M., Goldfarb, D., Assimos, D., Curhan, G., Denu-Ciocca, C. J., Matlaga, B. R., . . . White, J. R. (2014). Medical management of kidney stones: AUA guideline. *Journal of Urology, 192,* 316–324. doi:10.1016/j.juro.2014.05.006

diet (Noori et al., 2014). The effectiveness of the DASH diet may be due to its high-content fruits, vegetables, and dairy products, which provide ample calcium, magnesium, and potassium. The result is more calcium to bind with oxalate in the intestine and a favorable increase in urinary pH. A normal calcium intake (1200 mg/day) from food and beverages consumed primarily with meals is recommended to decrease the risk of stone formation (Pearle et al., 2014). The study data do not support the common practice of restricting dietary oxalate (a single component), particularly if that means a lower intake of fruits, vegetables, and whole grains (a healthy eating pattern).

NURSING PROCESS

Chronic Kidney Disease

Carlos is 66 years old and has had type 2 diabetes for 20 years. He is 5 ft 7 in tall and weighs 172 pounds. His hemoglobin A1c is 8.2; he takes insulin twice a day. He has a history of hypertension and mild anemia and complains of sudden weight gain and "swelling." His blood urea nitrogen (BUN) and creatinine have been steadily increasing over the last several years, and his GFR is currently 63. During his last appointment, the doctor told Carlos to watch his sugar intake and avoid salt. At this visit, Carlos' chief complaint is that he does not have an appetite anymore; he attributes his change in taste to not salting his food. The doctor has asked you to talk to Carlos about his diet.

Assessment

Medical–Psychosocial History

- Medical history including cardiovascular disease, hypertension, diabetes, and renal disease
- Medications that affect nutrition such as diuretics, insulin, and lipid-lowering medications
- Physical complaints such as fatigue, taste changes, anorexia, nausea, vomiting, diarrhea, muscular twitches, and muscle cramps
- Psychosocial and economic issues such as living situation, cooking facilities, financial status, employment, and education
- Understanding of the relationship between diet and renal function
- Motivation to change eating style

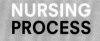

Chronic Kidney Disease

Anthropometric Assessment	• Current height, weight, and BMI • Recent weight history

Biochemical and Physical Assessment	• Blood values of
	  • BUN and creatinine
	  • Sodium, potassium, and other electrolytes
	  • Phosphorus and calcium
	  • Glucose
	  • Lipid profile
	  • Hemoglobin and hematocrit
	• eGFR
	• Urinalysis for volume, urea, protein, etc.
	• Blood pressure

Dietary Assessment	• What kind of nutrition counseling have you had in the past? • How many meals and snacks do you usually eat? • What is a typical day's intake for you? • Do you follow a diet for diabetes? What gives you the most difficulty? • How is your appetite? • Do you have any food allergies or intolerances? • Do you have any feeding issues, such as difficulty chewing or swallowing? • What kind of protein do you eat most often? What is a typical serving size? Is it spread out over the day? • Do you drink milk and, if so, how much per day? • How successful were you "watching your protein and avoiding salt"? • How often do you eat high-sodium foods, such as cold cuts, bacon, frankfurters, smoked meats, sausage, canned meats, chipped or corned beef, buttermilk, cheese, crackers, canned soups and vegetables, convenience products, pickles, and condiments? • Do you use a salt substitute? • Do you regularly eat fruits and vegetables? How many servings of each do you consume in an average day? • How much fluid do you drink daily? What is your favorite beverage? • Do you have any cultural, religious, and ethnic food preferences? • Do you use vitamins, minerals, or nutritional supplements? If so, what, how much, and why do you use them? • Do you drink alcohol? • How often do you eat out?

Diagnosis

Possible Nursing Diagnosis	Imbalanced nutrition: eating less than the body needs related to anorexia, taste changes, dietary restrictions

Planning

Client Outcomes	The client will • Consume adequate calories to prevent weight loss • Attain and maintain adequate nutritional status • Experience improved appetite • Practice self-management strategies especially self-monitoring sodium intake • Achieve normal or near-normal electrolyte levels • Maintain adequate glucose control • Achieve and maintain normal blood pressure • Maintain normal urinary output • Describe the rationale and principles of nutrition therapy for CKD and implement appropriate dietary changes • Prevent further kidney damage

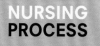

NURSING PROCESS: Chronic Kidney Disease

Nursing Interventions

Nutrition Therapy　Provide a 2000-calorie carbohydrate-controlled diet with 2300 mg sodium, as ordered.

Client Teaching　Instruct the client on
1. The role of nutrition therapy in the treatment of CKD
2. Eating plan essentials including
   - Maintaining a consistent carbohydrate intake that is adequate in calories
   - Limiting high-sodium foods, not adding salt during cooking or at the table
   - Using sodium-free seasonings and salt alternatives to improve the flavor of food
3. Behavioral matters including
   - How to weigh and measure foods to ensure accurate portion sizes
   - Weighing oneself at approximately the same time every day with the same scale while wearing the same amount of clothing. Unexpected weight gain or loss should be reported to the physician.
4. That heart-healthy cookbooks and cookbooks for diabetes may help increase variety and interest in eating
5. Changing eating attitudes
   - Learn to view the diet as an integral component of treatment and a means of life support
   - Adhering to the diet can improve the quality of life and decrease the workload on the kidneys

Evaluation

Evaluate and Monitor
- Monitor weight.
- Monitor lab values, blood glucose, blood pressure, and urine output.
- Monitor appetite.
- Evaluate food records, if available.
- Provide periodic feedback and reinforcement.

How Do You Respond?

Does cranberry juice prevent urinary tract infections? Cranberry has been found to be effective against urinary tract infections by preventing bacteria from adhering to the lining of the urinary tract, thereby promoting their excretion. However, the effects are transitory, so regular, perhaps more than twice daily, intake is necessary. Clients who are prone to urinary tract infections and like cranberry juice should be encouraged to consume it regularly. Cranberry juice appears more effective than cranberry capsules or tablets (Wang et al., 2012).

Are omega-3 fish oil supplements beneficial for people on hemodialysis?
A cornerstone study of the benefits of n-3 fatty acids in hemodialysis patients found that 4 g/day of fish oil supplements was associated with improved graft patency, lower rates of thrombosis, and fewer graft failures (Lok et al., 2012). Clinical studies generally show that n-3 supplements also have the potential to lower inflammatory markers in hemodialysis patients (Hung et al., 2015; Tayyebi-Khosroshahi et al., 2012), and that long-term supplementation has the potential to limit low-grade inflammation that exacerbates the progression of CKD (Mas et al., 2015). Furthermore, in the general population, n-3 fatty acids are associated with improvements in CVD risk factors, such as blood pressure and triglyceride levels (Mori, 2014). Until all the evidence is in, CKD patients—with or without RRT—should be encouraged to eat more fatty fish for their cardioprotective benefits, such as improvements in blood pressure, triglyceride levels, blood clotting, and inflammation (Mori, 2014).

REVIEW CASE STUDY

Dorothea is a 72-year-old black woman who is 5 ft 5 in tall and weighs 149 pounds. She has coronary heart disease and a long-standing history of hypertension with progressive loss of kidney function. She recently started receiving hemodialysis and is gaining about 4 pounds/day between treatments. She has convinced herself that because she is on dialysis, she can eat and drink whatever she wants and "the machine will take care of it."

Yesterday, she ate the following as shown on the right:

- What risk factors does Dorothea have for CKD?
- Based on her age, weight, and use of hemodialysis, what should the composition of her diet be (e.g., number of calories, grams of protein, grams of sodium)?
- Why is she gaining 4 pounds/day between treatments? What is a more reasonable goal? What would you suggest she do to achieve the goal?
- Evaluate her protein intake and recommend changes she could make to achieve her protein goals.
- What foods is she eating that are not heart healthy? What substitutions would you recommend?

- Evaluate her sodium intake and recommend changes she could make to limit her sodium intake.
- What foods is she eating that are high in potassium? What alternatives would you suggest?
- What would you tell Dorothea about the use of dialysis and her theory about eating anything she wants?
- Which is the lesser risk: getting enough calories and protein by eating non-heart-healthy foods or adhering to the sodium and other restrictions but not getting enough calories and protein?

Breakfast: Grits with cheese; bacon; biscuit with butter; coffee

Lunch: Hamburger on bun with ketchup and mustard; potato chips; banana; sweetened tea

Dinner: Fried chicken; macaroni and cheese; collard greens; pound cake; sweetened tea

STUDY QUESTIONS

1 Which statement indicates the patient needs further instruction about diet for nephrotic syndrome?
a. "I know I need to eat a high-protein diet to replace the protein lost in urine."
b. "I need to limit my intake of saturated fat and cholesterol."
c. "I should not use salt in cooking or at the table and avoid foods high in sodium such as processed foods, fast foods, convenience foods, condiments, and canned meat and vegetables."
d. "I am going to try substituting soy protein for animal sources of protein because it may be better for me."

2 A client with predialysis CKD asks if it is okay that she saves all her meat allowance for her evening meal. Which of the following would be the nurse's best response?
a. "You cannot have any meat on a predialysis diet."
b. "It doesn't matter when you eat your meat allowance, so if you prefer to save it all for dinner, that is fine."
c. "If you want to eat your meat allowance all at one time, it would be better to eat it for breakfast so that your body has all day to metabolize it."
d. "It is best if you spread your meat allowance out over the whole day."

3 When developing a teaching plan for a client who must restrict potassium, which fruits and vegetables would the nurse suggest?
a. Grapefruit, tomatoes, and beets
b. Kiwifruit, kale, and tomatoes
c. Apple, blueberries, and green beans
d. Apricots, broccoli, and spinach

4 The nurse knows her instructions about preventing future calcium oxalate stones have been effective when the client verbalizes he should
a. Avoid milk, cheese, and other sources of calcium
b. Take megadoses of vitamin C
c. Consume a normal amount of dietary calcium spread out over the course of the day
d. Eat a high-protein diet

5 How do the protein recommendations for those with CKD without diabetes differ from those who have diabetes?
a. Protein is more restricted for people who do not have diabetes.
b. Protein is more restricted for people who have diabetes.
c. The protein recommendations do not differ for people with diabetes or without diabetes.
d. There are no specific protein recommendations for people with diabetes because carbohydrates and fat are the priority concerns.

6 A client on hemodialysis asks if she can use popsicles to help relieve her thirst. Which of the following is the nurses' best response?

  a. "That's a great idea as long as you deduct the equivalent amount of fluid from your total daily fluid allowance."

  b. "Popsicles are empty calories. You are better off drinking just plain water."

  c. Popsicles are great at relieving thirst, and because they are solid, they do not count as fluid, so you can eat them as desired."

  d. "Hot things are better at relieving thirst than cold things. Try small amounts of hot tea or coffee to relieve your thirst."

7 One of the factors that influence protein allowance during AKI is the individual's

  a. Level of activity

  b. Degree of catabolism

  c. Blood pressure

  d. Serum albumin concentration

8 The client asks if she will need to follow a diet after she recovers from her kidney transplant. Which of the following is the nurse's best response?

  a. "You will always have to limit protein and phosphorus intake to help preserve the health of the new kidney."

  b. "After recovery, all restrictions are lifted and you can eat anything you want."

  c. "You may need to modify some aspects of your diet because of side effects from the medications you will be taking, and you should continue to eat a heart-healthy diet to decrease the risks of diabetes, hypertension, heart disease, and obesity."

  d. "All the restrictions you followed before dialysis will resume after you recover from the transplant."

KEY CONCEPTS

- Loss of renal function profoundly affects metabolism, nutritional status, and nutritional requirements. The nutrients most affected are protein, calcium, phosphorus, vitamin D, fluid, sodium, and potassium.

- People with nephrotic syndrome lose protein, mostly albumin, in the urine. Hypoalbuminemia and hyperlipidemia are other characteristics. Protein intake should be limited to 0.8 to 1.0 g/kg/day, an amount consistent with the RDA for protein, to minimize protein loss in the urine. Sodium intake is limited to control edema; a fluid restriction is usually not necessary.

- Primary prevention efforts are crucial because by the time biochemical evidence of CKD appears, there may be irreversible fibrosis within the kidney that eliminates the possibility of a "cure."

- Nutrition and lifestyle behaviors recommended to prevent CVD, such as to increase physical activity, not smoke, and attain/maintain healthy weight, may also reduce the risk of CKD. The DASH diet has been found to reduce the risk of kidney damage.

- Controlling blood pressure and managing diabetes may slow the progression of CKD. Reducing sodium intake, losing weight, eating a DASH-style eating pattern, avoiding excess alcohol intake, and regular physical activity help control blood pressure.

- Diet modifications for CKD are complex, unpalatable, and frequently adjusted according to the client's laboratory values and symptoms.

- Avoiding excess protein and limiting sodium are the cornerstones of nutrition therapy for categories 3 to 5 CKD. Managing blood pressure and blood glucose levels remains crucial. A heart-healthy diet is recommended because the risk of CVD is high in patients with CKD.

- There is a narrow margin of error regarding protein intake: Too little protein contributes to PEW, whereas too much exacerbates nitrogenous waste retention. Adequate calories are vital whenever protein intake is restricted to ensure that the protein consumed will be used for specific protein functions, not for energy requirements.

- Usually, as renal function deteriorates, potassium and phosphorus intakes may be restricted.

- In patients with CKD, calcium metabolism is impaired because of faulty vitamin D metabolism, impaired intestinal absorption, and hyperphosphatemia. A high-calcium intake from food is not achievable when phosphorus is restricted.

- When dialysis is instituted, a high-protein intake is recommended to compensate for protein lost through the dialysate. Calories need to be adequate to spare protein.

- People on hemodialysis generally have more severe restrictions in sodium and fluid than people on peritoneal dialysis.

- Clients who experience renal transplantation may need to alter their diets to lessen the side effects of immunosuppressant therapy. They should commit to a lifestyle of healthy eating to reduce the risk of diabetes, hypertension, obesity, and heart disease.

- AKI represents an even greater nutritional challenge than CKD. Protein, sodium, potassium, phosphorus, and fluid are adjusted according to laboratory data, use of RRT, renal function, and degree of catabolism.

- Consuming adequate fluid is a strategy to prevent recurrence of kidney stones regardless of the type of stone. Patients with a history of calcium oxalate kidney stones should avoid megadoses of vitamin C and eat a normal calcium intake spread out over the day. A DASH diet may be even more effective than lowering oxalate intake because its emphasis on fruits, vegetables, and dairy products provides ample calcium to bind with oxalate and raises urinary pH.

Check Your Knowledge Answer Key

1 **TRUE** A DASH-style diet has been found to reduce the risk of kidney disease independent of demographic characteristics, kidney disease risk factors, and baseline kidney function. Its benefits may be attributed to improving blood pressure and inflammation.

2 **TRUE** Foods high in protein tend to be high in phosphorus. Other high-phosphorus foods include cola, chocolate, beer, bran, and bran cereal.

3 **FALSE** Although milk is an excellent source of HBV protein, it is high in phosphorus and thus can only be consumed in limited amounts (½ cup/day).

4 **FALSE** Although patients with CKD are at risk for hyperkalemia due to decreased potassium excretion, metabolic acidosis, and certain medications, hyperkalemia is usually not seen until CKD is advanced.

5 **TRUE** People with chronic renal disease are at high risk for CVD and may benefit from eating a heart-healthy diet, such as a DASH diet or Mediterranean-style eating pattern.

6 **TRUE** The requirement for protein increases for people on dialysis to account for the loss of serum proteins and amino acids in the dialysate. Protein requirement may increase 50% to 100% above the RDA.

7 **TRUE** People receiving peritoneal dialysis may absorb 100 to 200 g of glucose from the dialysate, which is 340 to 680 calories.

8 **FALSE** Despite urinary losses of plasma proteins, a high-protein diet is contraindicated for people with nephrotic syndrome because it exacerbates urinary protein losses, which promotes further kidney damage.

9 **FALSE** Most people with hypercalciuria should consume a normal calcium intake. Restricting calcium intake does not decrease the risk of calcium stones because it increases urinary oxalate concentration.

10 **TRUE** Increasing fluid intake is a recommended strategy to prevent recurrence of any type of kidney stone. Fluid dilutes the urine to lower the risk of stone formation.

Student Resources on thePoint®
For additional learning materials, activate the code in the front of this book at
http://thePoint.lww.com/activate

Websites

American Association of Kidney Patients at www.aakp.org

American Kidney Fund at www.kidneyfund.org

National Institute of Diabetes and Digestive and Kidney Diseases at www.niddk.nih.gov

National Kidney and Urologic Diseases Information Clearinghouse (NKUDIC) at http://kidney.niddk.nih.gov

National Kidney Disease Education Program (NKDEP) at www.nkdep.nih.gov/professionals/index.htm

National Kidney Foundation at www.kidney.org

Oxalosis and Hyperoxaluria Foundation at www.ohf.org

References

Aoun, A., Cochran, C., & Pavlinac, J. (2014). *Chronic kidney disease toolkit.* Chicago IL: Academy of Nutrition and Dietetics.

Ash, S., Campbell, K., Bogard, J., & Millichamp, A. (2014). Nutrition prescription to achieve positive outcomes in chronic kidney disease: A systematic review. *Nutrients, 6*(1), 416–451.

Bellomo, R., Cass, A., Cole, L., Finfer, S., Gallagher, M., Lee, J., . . . Scheinkestel, C. (2014). Calorie intake and patient outcomes in severe acute kidney injury: Findings from the Randomized Evaluation of Normal vs. Augmented Level of Replacement Therapy (RENAL) study trial. *Critical Care, 18,* R45. doi:10.1186/cc13767

Beto, J., Ramirez, W., & Bansal, V. (2014). Medical nutrition therapy in adults with chronic kidney disease: Integrating evidence and consensus into practice for the generalist registered dietitian nutritionist. *Journal of the Academy of Nutrition and Dietetics, 114,* 1077–1087.

Briasoulis, A., & Bakris, G. (2013). Chronic kidney disease as a coronary artery disease equivalent. *Current Cardiology Reports, 15,* 340.

Burrowes, J. (2008). New recommendations for the management of diabetic kidney disease. *Nutrition Today, 43,* 65–69.

Cadnapaphornchai, M., Tkachenko, O., Shehekochikhin, D., & Schrier, R. (2014). The nephrotic syndrome: Pathogenesis and treatment of edema formation and secondary complications. *Pediatric Nephrology, 29,* 1159–1167.

Carrero, J., Stenvinkel, P., Cuppari, L., Ikizler, T. A., Kalantar-Zadeh, K., Kaysen, G., . . . Franch, H. A. (2013). Etiology of the protein-energy wasting syndrome in chronic kidney disease: A consensus statement from the International Society of Renal Nutrition and Metabolism (ISRNM). *Journal of Renal Nutrition, 23,* 77–90.

Centers for Disease Control and Prevention. (2014). *National chronic kidney disease fact sheet, 2014.* Available at http://www.cdc.gov/diabetes/pubs/pdf/kidney_Factsheet.pdf. Accessed on 8/9/16.

Centers for Disease Control and Prevention. (2016). *Leading causes of death.* Available at http://www.cdc.gov/nchs/fastats/leading-causes-of-death.htm. Accessed on 8/9/16.

D'Alessandro, C., Rossi, A., Innocenti, M., Ricchiuti, G., Bozzoli, L., Sbragia, G., . . . Cupisti, A. (2013). Dietary protein restriction for renal patients: Don't forget protein-free foods. *Journal of Renal Nutrition, 23,* 367–371.

DCCT/EDIC Research Group. (2014). Effect of intensive diabetes treatment of albuminuria in type 1 diabetes: Long-term follow-up of the Diabetes Control and Complications Trial and Epidemiology of Diabetes Interventions and Complications study. *Lancet. Diabetes & Endocrinology, 2,* 793–800.

Dunkler, D., Dehghan, M., Teo, K., Heinze, G., Gao, P., Kohl, M., . . . Oberbauer, R. (2013). Diet and kidney disease in high-risk individuals with type 2 diabetes mellitus. *JAMA Internal Medicine, 173,* 1682–1692.

Ferraro, P., Taylor, E., Gambaro, G., & Curhan, G. (2013). Soda and other beverages and the risk of kidney stones. *Clinical Journal of the American Society of Nephrology, 8,* 1389–1395.

Ferraro, P., Taylor, E., Gambaro, G., & Curhan, G. (2014). Caffeine intake and the risk of kidney stones. *The American Journal of Clinical Nutrition, 100,* 1596–1603.

Fiaccadori, E., Regolisti, G., & Maggiore, U. (2013). Specialized nutritional support interventions in critically ill patients on renal replacement therapy. *Current Opinion in Clinical Nutrition and Metabolic Care, 16,* 217–224. doi:10.1097/MCO.0b013e32835c20b0

Garneata, L., & Mircescu, G. (2013). Effect of low-protein diet supplemented with keto acids on progression of chronic kidney disease. *Journal of Renal Nutrition, 23,* 210–213.

Goraya, N., Simoni, J., Jo, C., & Wesson, D. (2012). Dietary acid reduction with fruits and vegetables or bicarbonate attenuates kidney injury in patients with a moderately reduced glomerular filtration rate due to hypertensive nephropathy. *Kidney International, 81,* 86–93.

Huang, X., Lindholm, B., Stenvinkel, P., & Carrero, J. (2013). Dietary fat modification in patients with chronic kidney disease: n-3 fatty acids and beyond. *Journal of Nephrology, 26,* 960–974.

Hung, A., Booker, C., Ellis, C., Siew, E. D., Graves, A. J., Shintani, A., . . . Himmelfarb, J. (2015). Omega-3 fatty acids inhibit the up-regulation of endothelial chemokines in maintenance hemodialysis patients. *Nephrology, Dialysis, Transplantation, 30,* 266–274.

Institute of Medicine. (2013). *Sodium intake in populations: Assessment of evidence.* Available at http://www.nap.edu/catalog/18311/sodium-intake-in-populations-assessment-of-evidence. Accessed on 8/18/16.

Johnson, D., Atai, E., Chan, M., Phoon, R. K., Scott, C., Toussaint, N. D., . . . Wiggins, K. J. (2013). KHA-CARI guideline: Early chronic kidney disease: Detection, prevention and management. *Nephrology, 18,* 340–350.

Kalantar-Zadeh, K., Streja, E., Molnar, E., Lukowsky, L. R., Krishnan, M., Kovesdy, C. P., & Greenland, S. (2012). Mortality prediction by surrogates of body composition: An examination of the obesity paradox in hemodialysis patients using composite ranking score analysis. *American Journal of Epidemiology, 175,* 793–803.

Kalista-Richards, M. (2011). The kidney: Medical nutrition therapy—yesterday and today. *Nutrition in Clinical Practice, 26,* 143–150.

Kidney Disease: Improving Global Outcomes CKD Work Group. (2013). KDIGO 2012 clinical practice guideline for the evaluation and management of chronic kidney disease. *Kidney International, 3,* 1–150.

Kopple, J., & Feroze, U. (2011). The effect of obesity on chronic kidney disease. *Journal of Renal Nutrition, 21,* 66–71.

Kovesdy, C., Kopple, J., & Kalantar-Zadeh, K. (2013). Management of protein-energy wasting in non-dialysis-dependent chronic kidney disease: Reconciling low protein intake with nutritional therapy. *The American Journal of Clinical Nutrition, 97,* 1163–1177. doi:10.3945/ajcn.112.036418

Li, Y., Tang, X., Zhang, J., & Wu, T. (2012). Nutrition support for acute kidney injury. *Cochrane Database of Systematic Reviews, (8),* CD005426.

Lok, C., Moist, L., Hemmelgarn, B., Tonelli, M., Vazquez, M. A., Dorval, M., . . . Stanley, K. (2012). Effect of fish oil supplementation on graft patency and cardiovascular events among patients with new synthetic arteriovenous hemodialysis grafts: A randomized controlled trial. *JAMA, 307,* 1809–1816.

Mandayam, S., & Mitch, W. (2006). Dietary protein restriction benefits patients with chronic kidney disease. *Nephrology, 11,* 53–57.

Mas, E., Barden, A., Burke, V., Beilin, L. J., Watts, G. F., Huang, R. C., . . . Mori, T. A. (2015). A randomized controlled trial of the effects of n-3 fatty acids on resolvins in chronic kidney disease. *Clinical Nutrition, 35,* 331–336. doi:10.1016/j.clnu.2015.04.004

McCarthy, M., & Phipps, S. (2014). Special nutrition challenges: Current approach to acute kidney injury. *Nutrition in Clinical Practice, 29,* 56–62.

McClave, S., Taylor, B., Martindale, R., Warren, M. M., Johnson, D. R., Braunschweig, C., . . . Compher, C. (2016). Guidelines for the provision and assessment of nutrition support therapy in the adult critically ill patient: Society of Critical Care Medicine (SCCM) and American Society for Parenteral and Enteral Nutrition (ASPEN). *Journal of Parenteral and Enteral Nutrition, 40,* 159–211.

McMahon, E., Bauer, J., Hawley, C., Isbel, N. M., Stowasser, M., Johnson, D. W., & Campbell, K. L. (2013). A randomized trial of dietary sodium restriction in CKD. *Journal of the American Society of Nephrology, 24,* 2096–2103.

Mitch, W., & Remuzzi, G. (2016). Diets for patients with chronic kidney disease, should we reconsider? *BMC Nephrology, 17,* 80. doi:10.1186/s12882-016-0283-x

Mori, T. (2014). Dietary n-3 PUFA and CVD: A review of the evidence. *The Proceedings of the Nutrition Society, 73,* 57–64.

National Kidney Disease Education Program. (2015). *Chronic kidney disease and diet: Assessment, management, and treatment. Treating CKD patients who are not on dialysis.* Available at https://www.niddk.nih.gov/health-information/health-communication-programs/nkdep/a-z/Documents/ckd-diet-assess-manage-treat-508.pdf. Accessed on 8/30/16.

Noori, N., Honarkar, E., Goldfarb, D., Kalantar-Zadeh, K., Taheri, M., Shakhssalim, N., . . . Basiri, A. (2014). Urinary lithogenic risk profile in recurrent stone formers with hyperoxaluria: A randomized controlled trial comparing DASH (Dietary Approaches to Stop Hypertension)-style and low-oxalate diets. *American Journal of Kidney Diseases, 63,* 456–463.

Nouvenne, A., Meschi, T., Prati, B., Guerra, A., Allegri, F., Vezzoli, G., . . . Borghi, L. (2010). Effects of a low-salt diet on idiopathic hypercalciuria in calcium-oxalate stone formers: A 3-mo randomized controlled trial. *The American Journal of Clinical Nutrition, 91,* 565–570.

Pace, R., Tootell, F., & Mahony, L. (2013). Nutritional consequences and benefits of alternatives to in-center hemodialysis. *Renal Nutrition Forum, 32*(2), 1–7.

Paes-Barreto, J., Silva, M., Qureshi, A., Bregman, R., Cervante, V. F., Carrero, J. J., & Avesani, C. M. (2013). Can renal nutrition education improve adherence to a low-protein diet in patients with stages 3 to 5 chronic kidney disease. *Journal of Renal Nutrition, 23,* 164–171.

Palevsky, P., Liu, K., Brophy, P., Chawla, L. S., Parikh, C. R., Thakar, C. V., . . . Weisbord, S. D. (2013). KDOQI US commentary on the 2012 KDIGO clinical practice guideline for acute kidney injury. *American Journal of Kidney Diseases, 61,* 649–672.

Pearle, M., Goldfarb, D., Assimos, D., Curhan, G., Denu-Ciocca, C. J., Matlaga, B. R., . . . White, J. R. (2014). Medical management of kidney stones: AUA guideline. *Journal of Urology, 192,* 316–324. doi.org/10.1016/j.juro.2014.05.006

Penniston, K. (2015). The nutrition consult for recurrent stone formers. *Current Urology Reports, 16*, 47. doi:10.1007/s11934-015-0518-6

Qaseem, A., Hopkins, R., Jr., Sweet, D., Starkey, M., & Shekelle, P. (2013). Screening, monitoring, and treatment of stage 1 to 3 chronic kidney disease: A clinical practice guideline from the American College of Physicians. *Annals of Internal Medicine, 159*, 835–847.

Rebholz, C., Crews, D., Grams, M., Steffen, L. M., Levey, A. S., Miller, E. R., III, . . . Coresh, J. (2016). DASH (Dietary Approaches to Stop Hypertension) diet and risk of subsequent kidney disease. *American Journal of Kidney Diseases, 68*, 853–861. doi:10.1053/j.ajkd.2016.05.019

Scales, C., Jr., Smith, A., Hanley, J. M., & Saigal, C. (2012). Prevalence of kidney stones in the United States. *European Urology, 62*, 160–165.

Seiner, R., Ebert, D., Nicolay, C., & Hesse, A. (2003). Dietary risk factors for hyperoxaluria in calcium oxalate stone formers. *Kidney International, 63*, 1037–1043.

Shinaberger, C., Greenland, S., Kopple, J., Van Wyck, D., Mehrotra, R., Kovesdy, C. P., & Kalantar-Zadeh, K. (2008). Is controlling phosphorus by decreasing dietary protein intake beneficial or harmful in persons with chronic kidney disease? *American Journal of Clinical Nutrition, 88*, 1511–1518.

Singer, P., Anbar, R., Cohen, J., Shapiro, H., Shalita-Chesner, M., Lev, S., . . . Madar, Z. (2011). The Tight Calorie Control Study (TICACOS): A prospective, randomized, controlled pilot study of nutritional support in critically ill patients. *Intensive Care Medicine, 37*, 601–619.

Steiber, A., & Kopple, J. (2011). Vitamin status and needs for people with stages 3–5 chronic kidney disease. *Journal of Renal Nutrition, 21*, 355–368.

Taylor, E., Stampfer, M., & Curhan, G. (2005). Obesity, weight gain, and the risk of kidney stones. *JAMA, 293*, 455–462.

Tayyebi-Khosroshahi, H., Houshyar, J., Dehgan-Hesari, R., Alikhah, H., Vatankhah, A. M., Safaeian, A. R., & Zonouz, N. R. (2012). Effect of treatment with omega-3 fatty acids on C-reactive protein and tumor necrosis factor-alfa in hemodialysis patients. *Saudi Journal of Kidney Diseases and Transplantation, 23*, 500–506.

Wang, C., Fang, C., Chen, N., Liu, S. S., Yu, P. H., Wu, T. Y., . . . Chen, S. C. (2012). Cranberry-containing products for prevention of urinary tract infections in susceptible populations: A systematic review and meta-analysis of randomized controlled trials. *Archives of Internal Medicine, 172*, 988–996.

Chapter 22

Nutrition for Patients with Cancer or HIV/AIDS

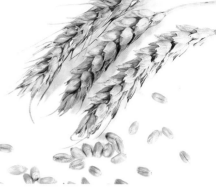

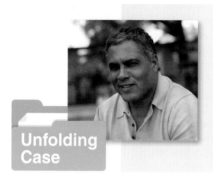

Unfolding Case

Patrick Hannon

Patrick is 50 years old, is 6 ft tall, and considers himself healthy. His normal adult weight is 258 pounds. He is a "meat-and-potatoes" kind of guy and admits to being sedentary. His wife convinced him to have a routine colonoscopy—since it is recommended at age 50 years—which lead to a diagnosis of stage III colon cancer. He had a partial colectomy and lymph node removal. He is undergoing adjuvant chemotherapy.

Check Your Knowledge

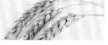

True	False		
☐	☐	1	Obesity increases the risk of several types of cancer.
☐	☐	2	Weight loss is an indicator of poor prognosis in people with cancer.
☐	☐	3	Clients who are adequately nourished may be better able to withstand the effects of cancer treatment.
☐	☐	4	Cachexia is directly related to the amount of calories consumed.
☐	☐	5	The appetite of clients with anorexia tends to improve as the day progresses.
☐	☐	6	Cancer survivors are urged to follow nutrition guidelines to reduce the risk of cancer in the future.
☐	☐	7	Many cancer patients treated with chemotherapy report a metallic taste alteration.
☐	☐	8	Clients with HIV who are experiencing malabsorption always have diarrhea.
☐	☐	9	Clients with HIV/AIDS may have problems with appetite and intake similar to those of cancer clients.
☐	☐	10	Nutritional counseling of clients with HIV/AIDS should include how to avoid foodborne illnesses.

Learning Objectives

Upon completion of this chapter, you will be able to

1 Evaluate a person's usual diet according to dietary guidelines to reduce the risk of cancer.
2 Summarize how cancer and cancer therapies affect nutritional status.
3 Give examples of ways to modify the diet to alleviate side effects of anorexia, nausea, fatigue, taste changes, mouth sores, dry mouth, and diarrhea.
4 Discuss ways to increase a client's calorie and protein intake.
5 Explain how HIV/AIDS affects nutritional status.
6 List food safety practices.
7 Teach a person living with HIV/AIDS guidelines for a healthy eating pattern.

Cancer and HIV/AIDS can cause devastating weight loss and malnutrition. Although nutrition therapy cannot cure either disease, it has the potential to maximize the effectiveness of drug therapy, alleviate the side effects of the disease and its treatments, and improve overall quality of life.

CANCER

Cancer is a group name for more than 100 different types of malignancies characterized by the uncontrolled growth of cells. Individual cancers differ in where they develop, how quickly they grow, the type of treatment they respond to, and how much they affect nutritional status. Cancer is currently the second leading cause of death in the United States (S. Murphy, Kochanek, Xu, & Arias, 2015) but is expected to surpass heart disease as the leading cause of death in the next few years (Siegel, Miller, & Jemal, 2015).

The relationship between nutrition and cancer is multifaceted:

- Analysis of global research indicates that approximately a third of cancers are preventable through lifestyle modification, namely, consuming a healthy eating pattern, maintaining healthy weight, and engaging in regular physical activity (American Institute for Cancer Research [AICR], n.d.-a). An eating pattern that provides a variety of fruits and vegetables, whole grains, and fish or poultry or is lower in red and processed meats is associated with a lower risk of developing certain cancers or dying from cancer (Kushi et al., 2012).
- The local effects of tumors, particularly those of the gastrointestinal (GI) tract, can impede eating, such as dysphagia related to head and neck cancers.
- Depending on the type of cancer and stage of diagnosis, cancer can alter metabolism and physiology, such as by causing glucose intolerance, insulin resistance, increased lipolysis, and increased whole-body protein turnover. Such changes affect requirements for macro- and micronutrients (Rock et al., 2012).
- Anorexia may be present in 15% to 25% of cancer patients at the time of diagnosis and is virtually a universal side effect in patients with widespread metastatic disease (National Cancer Institute [NCI], 2016). It may occur from a variety of factors, such as pain, depression/anxiety, early satiety, fatigue, nausea, loss of taste, sore mouth, dry mouth, thick saliva, or esophagitis. Anorexia can lead to weight loss, malnutrition, cachexia, and poor prognosis.
- Cancer treatments can alter nutrient intake, absorption, or need. Although some effects may be relatively short term, such as the increased need for protein and calories to heal from surgery, others may be more long lasting, such as chronic dysphagia that may persist for years after treatment for head and neck cancer is completed.
- Adequate nutrition during the course of cancer treatment may improve tolerance to treatment, enhance immune function, aid in recovery, and maximize quality of life.
- Because cancer survivors are at a significantly higher risk for developing second primary cancers, cancer prevention strategies (e.g., a healthy eating pattern, healthy weight, regular physical activity) are important after treatment is completed (Rock et al., 2012).
- For people living with advanced cancer, diet modifications and some physical activity may improve quality of life and enhance well-being (Rock et al., 2012).

Nutrition in Cancer Prevention

Tobacco cessation is inarguably the leading behavioral strategy for reducing the risk of cancer. For nontobacco users, the most important modifiable determinants of cancer risk are body weight, dietary choices, and levels of physical activity (Kushi et al., 2012). Cancer prevention guidelines to maintain healthy body weight, increase physical activity, consume a healthy eating pattern, and avoid excessive alcohol intake (Table 22.1) are also associated with a lower risk of cardiovascular disease (CVD) and diabetes (Ford et al., 2009). Adhering to guidelines to reduce the risk of cancer has been shown to reduce the risk of dying from cancer, CVD, and all causes combined (McCullough et al., 2011). All people, including cancer survivors, are urged to adopt healthy lifestyle behaviors to reduce the risk of cancer and other chronic diseases.

Table 22.1 Summary of American Cancer Society Guidelines on Nutrition and Physical Activity for Cancer Prevention

Guideline	Rationale
Achieve and maintain a healthy weight throughout life. • Be as lean as possible throughout life without being underweight. • Avoid excess weight gain at all ages. For those who are currently overweight or obese, losing even a small amount of weight has health benefits and is a good place to start. • Engage in regular physical activity and limit consumption of high-calorie foods and beverages as key strategies for maintaining a healthy weight.	Some of the strongest links to cancer risk are excess body weight. There is convincing evidence that overweight and obesity increase the risk of 11 cancers including bowel, breast (postmenopausal), prostate (advanced cancer), pancreatic, endometrial, kidney, liver, gallbladder, esophageal (adenocarcinoma), ovarian, and stomach cancers (AICR, 2016). Body fatness may also be associated with an increased risk of non-Hodgkin lymphoma and multiple myeloma (Kushi et al., 2012). There are a few possible mechanisms by which body fatness may increase cancer risk including increasing hormones that promote cancer cell growth; promoting insulin resistance and hyperinsulinism, which increases the risk of certain cancers; altering endogenous growth factors; altering immune system functioning; or promoting low levels of chronic inflammation, which can promote cancer cell growth and development (de Pergola & Silvestris, 2013).
Adopt a physically active lifestyle. • Adults should engage in at least 150 minutes of moderate-intensity or 75 minutes of vigorous-intensity activity each week, or an equivalent combination, preferably spread throughout the week. • Children and adolescents should engage in at least 1 hour of moderate- or vigorous-intensity activity each day, with vigorous-intensity activity occurring at least 3 days each week. • Limit sedentary behavior such as sitting, lying down, watching television, or other forms of screen-based entertainment. • Doing some physical activity above usual activities, no matter what one's level of activity, can have many health benefits.	Epidemiologic evidence suggests physical active people have a lower risk of certain cancers than sedentary people (NCI, 2016). Physical activity may lower the risk of cancers of the breast, colon, and endometrium and advanced prostate cancer and may possibly lower the risk of pancreatic cancer (Kushi et al., 2012). Physical activity may help decrease cancer risk through its impact on sex hormones, insulin, prostaglandins, and immunity. Physical activity provides an added benefit of helping avoid excess body weight. Although the optimal intensity, duration, and frequency of physical activity needed to reduce the risk of cancer are not known, it is likely that activity in amounts higher than recommended may provide greater cancer risk reduction (Kushi et al., 2012). Evidence suggests that sitting time, independent of physical activity level, may contribute to the risk of various types of cancer. The health benefits of physical activity accumulate over a lifetime.
Consume a healthy diet, with an emphasis on plant foods. • Choose foods and beverages in amounts that help achieve and maintain a healthy weight. • Limit consumption of processed meat and red meat. • Eat at least 2.5 cups of vegetables and fruits each day. • Choose whole grains instead of refined grain products.	Assessing the impact of overall intake on cancer risk encompasses determining which foods may be protective and which may increase risk. Lifelong eating patterns may be important but cannot be detected by relatively short-term, randomized clinical trials (NCI, 2016). Convincing evidence links the intake of red and processed meats to colorectal cancer (World Cancer Research Fund/AICR, 2011). Of dietary factors that may be protective against cancer risk, fruits and nonstarchy vegetables show the greatest consistency and are associated with "probably decreased risk of certain cancers" (NCI, 2016). Observational studies suggest a strong inverse relationship between whole-grain intake and GI cancers, certain hormone-related cancers, and pancreatic cancer (Jonnalagadda et al., 2011).
If you drink alcoholic beverages, limit consumption. • Drink no more than one drink per day for women or two drinks per day for men.	Strong evidence links alcohol to cancer of the mouth, pharynx, and larynx, esophagus, liver, colon/rectum, and breast (AIRC, n.d.-b).

Source: Kushi, L., Doyle, C., McCullough, M., Rock, C. L., Demark-Wahnefried, W., Bandera, E. V., . . . Thun, M. (2012). American Cancer Society guidelines on nutrition and physical activity for cancer prevention. *CA: A Cancer Journal for Clinicians, 62,* 30–67.

The focus of nutrition guidelines has shifted away from single nutrients or food groups and toward eating patterns because of the complex mixtures and interactions between food components. Reedy et al. (2014) found that people who adhered closest to any of the four healthy eating patterns studied, including the Mediterranean-style and DASH eating patterns, had a 12% to 28% decreased risk of all-cause, CVD, and cancer mortality. Results did not show that any single component of the eating patterns was largely responsible for the outcome but suggest whole grains, vegetables, fruit, and plant-based proteins are beneficial. Trichopoulou, Lagiou, Kuper, and Tichopoulos (2000) estimate that up to 25% of colorectal cancer; 15% of breast cancer; and 10% of prostate, pancreas, and endometrial cancers could be prevented if populations of Western countries adopt a traditional Mediterranean-style eating pattern. Protective benefits of a Mediterranean-style eating pattern may be due to its emphasis on plant foods and olive oil and its relatively low intake of red meat, processed meat, and sweets (Giacosa et al., 2013).

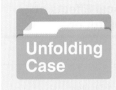

Unfolding Case

Think of Patrick. What lifestyle factors may have increased his risk for cancer? Is it appropriate for him to adopt healthy lifestyle behaviors while he is undergoing chemotherapy?

Currently, there is insufficient evidence to support the use of multivitamin and mineral supplements or single vitamins or minerals for cancer prevention (Fortmann, Burda, Senger, Lin, & Whitlock, 2013). Antioxidants, such as beta-carotene, vitamin C, and vitamin E have been theorized to have a preventive role in cancer; however, studies have not confirmed benefit and have even demonstrated an increased risk from consuming these nutrients through supplements. For instance, studies have shown increases in lung cancer risk in smokers and former smokers taking beta-carotene supplements (Gallicchio et al., 2008) and increases in prostate cancer risk in men taking vitamin E supplements (Klein et al., 2011). In the Women's Antioxidant Cardiovascular Study, total cancer incidence was not lowered in women taking supplements of vitamin C, vitamin E, or beta-carotene when compared to a placebo (Lin et al., 2009). Other nutrients of interest include vitamin D and omega-3 fatty acids, both of which are currently being studied for their effect on cancer risk in a large scale randomized trial (Manson et al., 2012).

The Impact of Cancer on Nutrition

Nutrition is affected in multiple ways by cancer and its treatment, some of which are listed in Box 22.1. Malnutrition is a common problem in patients with cancer and is associated with increased morbidity and mortality and decreased quality of life (NCI, 2016). Depending on the site of the cancer, 15% to 69% of patients with upper GI cancer have already experienced significant weight loss, defined as a loss of at least 10% of body weight in 6 months at the time of diagnosis (Silvers, Savva, Huggins, Truby, & Haines, 2014). Weight loss is an indicator of poor prognosis in people with cancer. Local tumor effects and metabolic changes contribute to the risk of malnutrition and weight loss.

Local Tumor Effects

Local tumor effects occur when the tumor impinges on surrounding tissue, impairing its ability to function. The effects vary with the site and size of the tumor and are most likely to affect nutrition when the GI tract is involved (Table 22.2). GI obstruction can cause anorexia, dysphagia, early satiety, nausea, vomiting, pain, or diarrhea, leading to weight loss and malnutrition.

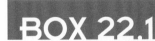

BOX 22.1   Cancer-Related Nutrition Impact Symptoms

- Unintended weight loss
- Loss of lean body mass and muscle strength
- Fatigue
- Impaired wound healing
- Altered immune system functioning
- Altered glucose metabolism
- Impaired quality of life
- Depression
- Reduced response to treatment, increased treatment toxicities, treatment delays
- Increased hospitalization or length of stay

Source: Thompson, K., Elliott, L., Fuchs-Tarlovsky, V., Levin, R. M., Voss, A. C., & Piemonte, T. (2016). Oncology evidence-based nutrition practice guidelines for adults. *Journal of the Academy of Nutrition and Dietetics*. doi:10.1016/j .and.2016.05.010

Table 22.2	Potential Local Effects of Cancer on Nutrition	

Site	Potential Effects
Brain/CNS	Eating disabilities Chewing and swallowing difficulties
Head and neck	Difficulty in chewing and swallowing
Esophagus	Dysphagia related to obstruction Gastroesophageal reflux disease
Stomach	Early satiety, nausea, vomiting Impaired motility Obstruction, which may necessitate tube feeding or TPN
Bowel	Maldigestion and malabsorption Obstruction, which may necessitate tube feeding or TPN
Liver	Watery diarrhea related to an increase in serotonin, histamines, and other substances
Pancreas	Maldigestion and malabsorption Diabetes

CNS, central nervous system.

Metabolic Changes and Cachexia

Tumor-induced weight loss occurs frequently in patients with solid tumors of the lung, pancreas, and upper GI tract (NCI, 2016). Tumor cells can produce proinflammatory and procachectic factors that stimulate inflammation and the breakdown of body protein and fat. The body responds with inflammatory and endocrine changes. The interplay between tumor and host leads to a systemic inflammatory response. The catabolic state is characterized by insulin resistance, decreased muscle protein synthesis, increased body protein turnover, and accelerated fat breakdown.

The cascade of metabolic changes resulting from the effects of the tumor, the body's response, and the host–tumor interaction can lead to cancer cachexia, an advanced protein calorie malnutrition characterized by involuntary weight loss, muscle wasting, and decreased quality of life (Donohoe, Ryan, & Reynolds, 2011). States of cachexia in cancer are (Thompson et al., 2016)

Cachexia
a wasting syndrome associated with cancer characterized by progressive loss of body weight, fat, and lean body mass.

- Precachexia, characterized by loss of appetite and altered glucose intolerance. Precachexia may precede substantial involuntary weight loss (e.g., up to 5% of weight). Factors that influence its variable progression include cancer type, cancer stage, systemic inflammation, inadequate food intake, and lack of response to anticancer therapy.
- Cachexia, a multifactorial syndrome characterized by ongoing loss of skeletal muscle mass (with or without loss of fat mass) that leads to progressive functional impairment. Major features include negative protein and calorie balance. Any patient who has experienced unintentional weight loss is considered at risk for cachexia. Cachexia cannot be treated with nutrition therapy alone because although anorexia is frequently present, abnormal metabolism and inflammation are contributing factors.
- Refractory cachexia, which may result from very advanced cancer or a rapidly progressive cancer that is unresponsive to anticancer therapy. This stage is actively catabolic and efforts to manage weight loss are no longer possible or appropriate. Life expectancy is less than 3 months.

Management of cachexia is a complex challenge. Early interventions to prevent weight loss in precachexia or cachexia are more likely to be effective than interventions that are delayed (Thompson et al., 2016). Medications to control side effects of cancer and its treatment, such as nausea, diarrhea, constipation, dry mouth, and pain, may help prevent weight loss. Medications to stimulate appetite and promote weight gain may be used, depending on the patient's wishes, medical condition, and life expectancy (Table 22.3). Nutrition therapy aimed at preserving lean muscle mass and fat stores may improve quality of life and affect overall survival (NCI, 2016).

Table 22.3 Drugs Commonly Used for Anorexia-Cachexia Syndrome

Drug Category	Common Drugs Used	Comments
Progestational agents	Megestrol acetate, medroxyprogesterone	Promotes weight gain, but weight gain is primarily fat/water weight, not lean body tissue
Glucocorticoids	Prednisolone, dexamethasone, methylprednisolone	Stimulates appetite; studies show positive but short-term effects on appetite and quality of life but minimal or no effect on weight gain; risks limit suitability for long-term use
Cannabinoids	Dronabinol	Inconsistent evidence of effectiveness; has not shown superior benefit in promoting weight gain and appetite
Antihistamines	Cyproheptadine	Not well studied in cancer patients. Sedation effect may limit usefulness.
Antidepressants/antipsychotics	Mirtazapine, olanzapine	Clinical data supporting routine use in cancer patients is lacking.
Anti-inflammatory agents	Thalidomide, pentoxifylline, melatonin, omega-3 fatty acids (EPA)	All have been shown to decrease tumor necrosis factor-alpha; mixed results regarding weight gain and appetite stimulation
Anabolic agents	Oxandrolone, nandrolone decanoate, fluoxymesterone	Limited reports of successful appetite stimulation in cancer patients

Source: National Cancer Institute. (2016). *Nutrition in cancer care (PDQ)—health professional version.* Available at http://www.cancer.gov/about-cancer/treatment/side-effects/appetite-loss/nutrition-hp-pdq. Accessed on 9/3/16.

The Impact of Cancer Treatments

Cancer treatments include surgery, chemotherapy, radiation, immunotherapy, hemopoietic and stem cell transplantation, or a combination of therapies. Each treatment modality can contribute to progressive nutritional deterioration related to localized or systemic side effects that interfere with intake, increase nutrient losses, or alter metabolism. Comorbidities may complicate treatment and nutritional status. The success of treatment is influenced by the patient's ability to tolerate therapy, which is affected by nutritional status. Patients who undergo aggressive cancer treatment typically need aggressive nutrition management (NCI, 2016).

Nutrition therapy, used as an adjuvant to effective cancer therapy, helps to sustain the client through adverse side effects and may reduce morbidity and mortality. Adequate calories and protein help prevent catabolism and loss of **lean body mass**. Oral nutrition supplements are commonly used. Enteral nutrition initiated before treatment begins, especially in patients treated for head and neck cancers, and may help prevent significant weight loss. Conversely, inadequate nutrition can contribute to the incidence and severity of treatment side effects and increase the risk of infection, thereby reducing the chance for survival (Vigano, Watanabe, & Bruera, 1994).

Lean Body Mass
the weight of the body minus the weight of fat.

Surgery

Surgery is often the primary treatment for cancer. People who are malnourished prior to surgery are at higher risk of postoperative morbidity and mortality. If time allows, nutritional deficiencies are corrected before surgery and may require the use of oral nutrition supplements, enteral or parenteral nutrition, and/or use of medications to stimulate appetite.

Postsurgical nutritional requirements increase for protein, calories, vitamin C, B vitamins, and iron to replenish losses and promote healing. Physiologic or mechanical barriers to good nutrition can occur depending on the type of surgery, with the greatest likelihood of complications arising from GI surgeries. Table 22.4 outlines potential side effects and complications incurred for various types of surgery.

Chemotherapy

Given alone or in combination, chemotherapy drugs damage the reproductive ability of both malignant and normal cells, especially rapidly dividing cells such as well-nourished cancer cells and normal cells of the GI tract, respiratory system, bone marrow, skin, and gonadal tissue. Cyclic administration of multiple drugs is given in maximum-tolerated doses.

Table 22.4   Potential Complications of Surgery

Type	Potential Complications
Head and neck resection	Impaired ability to speak, chew, salivate, swallow, smell, taste, and/or see Tube-feeding dependency Negative impact on nutritional status can be profound
Esophagectomy or esophageal resection	Early satiety Regurgitation Fistula formation Stenosis Vagotomy → decreased stomach motility, decreased gastric acid production, diarrhea, steatorrhea
Gastric resection	Dumping syndrome: crampy diarrhea that develops quickly after eating, accompanied by flushing, dizziness, weakness, pain, distention, and vomiting Hypoglycemia Esophagitis Decreased gastric motility Fat malabsorption and diarrhea Deficiencies in iron, calcium, and fat-soluble vitamins Vitamin B_{12} malabsorption related to lack of intrinsic factor
Intestinal resection	Malnutrition related to generalized malabsorption Fluid and electrolyte imbalance Diarrhea Increased risk of renal oxalate stone formation Metabolic acidosis
Massive bowel resection	Steatorrhea Malnutrition related to severe generalized malabsorption Metabolic acidosis Dehydration
Ileostomy or colostomy	Fluid and electrolyte imbalance
Pancreatic resection	Generalized malabsorption Diabetes mellitus

The side effects of chemotherapy vary with the type of drug or combination of drugs used, dose, rate of excretion, duration of treatment, and individual tolerance. Chemotherapy side effects are systemic and, therefore, potentially more numerous than the localized effects seen with surgery or radiation. The most commonly experienced nutrition-related side effects are anorexia, taste alterations, early satiety, nausea, vomiting, mucositis/esophagitis, diarrhea, and constipation (NCI, 2016). Side effects increase the risk of malnutrition and weight loss, which may prolong recovery time between treatments. When subsequent chemotherapy treatments are delayed, successful treatment outcome is potentially threatened.

Radiation

Radiation causes cell death; particles of radioactive energy break chemical bonds, disrupting reproductive ability. Although radiation injures all rapidly dividing cells, it is most lethal for the poorly differentiated and rapidly proliferating cells of cancer tissue. Recovery from sublethal doses of radiation occurs in the interval between the first dose and subsequent doses. Normal tissue appears to recover more quickly from radiation damage than does cancerous tissue.

The type and intensity of radiation side effects depend on the type of radiation used, the site, the volume of tissue irradiated, the dose of radiation, the duration of therapy, and individual tolerance. Patients most at risk for nutrition-related side effects are those who have cancers of the head and neck, lungs, esophagus, cervix, uterus, colon, rectum, and pancreas (Table 22.5). Side effects usually develop around the second or third week of treatment and then diminish 2 or 3 weeks after radiation therapy is completed. Some side effects may be chronic.

Table 22.5	**Potential Complications of Radiation**
Area	**Potential Complications**
Head and neck	Altered or loss of taste (mouth blindness) Xerostomia (dry mouth) Thick salivary secretions Difficulty swallowing and chewing Loss of teeth Mucositis Stomatitis
Lower neck and midchest	Acute: esophagitis with dysphagia Delayed: fibrosis, esophageal stricture, dysphagia Nausea Edema
Abdomen and pelvis	Acute or chronic bowel damage can cause diarrhea, nausea, vomiting, enteritis, and malabsorption Bowel constriction, obstruction, or fistula formation Chronic blood loss from intestine and bladder Pelvic radiation can cause increased urinary frequency, urgency, and dysuria
Central nervous system	Nausea Dysgeusia

Immunotherapy

Immunotherapy seeks to enhance the body's immune system to help control cancer. The most common side effects include fever, which increases protein and calorie requirements, and nausea, vomiting, diarrhea, anorexia, and fatigue. Actual side effects depend on the type of immunotherapy used. Left untreated, symptoms can cause gradual or drastic weight loss, which can lead to malnutrition and complicated or delayed recovery.

Hemopoietic and Peripheral Blood Stem Cell Transplantation

Hemopoietic and stem cell transplants are preceded by high-dose chemotherapy and possibly total-body irradiation to suppress immune function and destroy cancer cells. Numerous nutritional side effects may arise from these treatments and immunosuppressant medications, which are given before and after the procedure. Anorexia, taste alterations, nausea, vomiting, dry mouth, thick saliva, mucositis, stomatitis, and esophagitis may occur. Intestinal damage may cause severe diarrhea, malabsorption, and weight changes.

Parenteral nutrition may be needed for 1 to 2 months after bone marrow transplantation to ensure an adequate intake. When an oral diet resumes, a liquid diet restricted in lactose, fiber, and fat is given to minimize malabsorption and improve tolerance. Solid foods are gradually reintroduced. **Neutropenia** leaves the patient susceptible to infection, so precautionary measures must be taken to prevent foodborne illness (Box 22.2); however, a **neutropenic diet** is generally not necessary, although facility protocols differ. A high-protein, high-calcium diet may be needed to counter the negative nitrogen and calcium balances caused by immunosuppressant medications.

Neutropenia
abnormally low number of neutrophils in the blood, which increases the risk of infection.

Neutropenic Diet
a diet intended to protect people with low neutrophil counts from bacteria and other organisms in some food and drinks. Eliminates fresh fruits, vegetables, raw nuts, yogurt, and other products with live active cultures.

Nutrition Therapy During Cancer Treatment

A "typical" cancer patient does not exist. Whereas some patients present with weight loss and malnutrition at the time of cancer diagnosis, others are asymptomatic, and a substantial proportion are overweight or obese (Barrera & Demark-Wahnefried, 2009). The course of treatment may be aggressive or palliative; it may include surgery, chemotherapy, radiation, or a combination of treatments. The effect on nutritional status and intake may be mild or dramatic. Virtually all cancer patients could benefit from a nutrition consult with a dietitian to create a nutrition care plan and meal plan (NCI, 2016).

BOX 22.2	Strategies to Reduce the Risk of Foodborne Illness

- Wash hands before and after handling food and eating and after using the restroom.
- Cook all meat, fish, and poultry to the well-done stage.
- Refrigerate foods immediately after purchase.
- Avoid cross-contamination by using separate cutting boards and work surfaces for raw meats and poultry; keep work surfaces clean.
- Wash fruits and vegetables thoroughly in clean water.
- Thaw food in the refrigerator, never at room temperature.
- If the microwave is used to thaw frozen meat, cook the meat immediately after it is defrosted.
- Refrigerate leftovers immediately after eating; thoroughly reheat before eating.
- Discard leftovers after 24 hours.
- Keep hot foods >140°F and cold foods <40°F.
- Use expiration dates on food packaging to discard foods that may be unsafe to eat.
- Avoid salad bars and buffets when eating out.
- Avoid:
  - Raw or undercooked meat and poultry
  - Raw or undercooked fish, such as sushi, ceviche, or refrigerated smoked fish
  - Unpasteurized milk
  - Soft cheeses made from unpasteurized milk such as feta, brie, camembert, Queso fresco
  - Foods that contain raw or undercooked eggs, such as homemade Caesar salad dressing, raw cookie dough, and eggnog
  - Raw sprouts (alfalfa, bean, and others), unwashed fresh vegetables, and any moldy or damaged fruits and vegetables
  - Hot dogs, deli meats, and luncheon meats that have not been reheated
  - Unpasteurized, refrigerated pates or meat spreads

Quick Bite Selected high-calorie, high-protein oral nutrition supplements

	Calories (per ~240 mL)	Protein (g/~240 mL)
Boost	240	10
Boost Compact	240/125 mL	10 g/125 mL
Boost High-Protein	240	15
Boost Plus	360	14
Carnation Breakfast Essentials (powder mix made with 8 oz fat-free milk)	220	13
Carnation Breakfast Essentials	240	10
Carnation Breakfast Essentials High Protein	220	15
Ensure Original	220	9
Ensure Plus	350	13
Ensure Enlive	350	20
Ensure High Protein	160	16

The goals of nutrition therapy are to

- Manage weight. For normal-weight and underweight patients, the goal is to prevent weight loss. Preventing weight gain is appropriate for those who are overweight or obese; have certain hormonal cancers, such as prostate or breast cancer; and are treated with long-term, high-dose steroid therapy.
- Maintain lean body mass, muscle strength, and functional capacity
- Minimize nutrition-related side effects and complications. For instance, IJpma, Renken, ter Horst, and Reyners (2015) found 9.7% to 78% of participants with various cancers, chemotherapy treatments, and treatment phases reported a metallic taste. Although it is not known what the consequences are of metallic taste due to limited research, it may likely reduce intake, weight, and quality of life.
- Prevent or reverse nutrient deficiencies. Food sources of nutrients are preferred over nutrient supplements.
- Maximize quality of life: improve tolerance to treatment, improve immunocompetence, and promote wound healing.

Calories and Protein

Throughout all phases of cancer care, an adequate intake of calories and protein are essential for maintaining optimal nutritional status. Consuming enough calories to prevent weight loss is especially important for patients at risk for unintentional weight loss, such as those who are already malnourished or those whose anti-cancer treatments affect the GI tract (Rock et al., 2012). Unfortunately, evidence is limited to support any given formula to estimate calorie and protein needs. Generally, calorie needs range from 25 to 30 cal/kg for nonambulatory or sedentary adults to 35 cal/kg or more for hypermetabolic or severely stressed patients. Protein needs range from 1.0 for normal maintenance to 2.5 g/kg for patients with protein wasting.

Promoting an Oral Intake

An oral intake is the preferred route for feeding patients. The challenge may be to simply get patients to eat enough to avoid weight loss. Strategies that may help promote intake are to

- Modify the diet as needed in response to side effects or complications (Box 22.3)
- Provide small, frequent snacks throughout the day rather than three large meals. Smaller feedings are less overwhelming, especially in patients with anorexia.
- Increase the calorie and protein density of foods offered to improve overall intake without increasing the volume of food needed (Box 22.4).
- Provide high-protein, high-calorie oral nutrition supplements to augment or replace solid foods when intake is inadequate. This may be the easiest and most consistent way to achieve a high-calorie, high-protein intake.
- Encourage light physical activity such as walking
- Provide appetite stimulants as ordered (see Table 22.3)

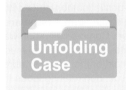

Recall Patrick. He is experiencing anorexia, nausea, vomiting, and mouth sores from chemotherapy and now weighs 236 pounds. What percentage of his usual weight has he lost? Is that significant? What strategies would you suggest he try to maintain an adequate oral intake?

Fish Oil

The Academy of Nutrition and Dietetics makes a strong and imperative recommendation that when interventions are unsuccessful in enabling a patient to achieve an adequate intake and loss of weight and lean body mass continues, the use of eicosapentaenoic acid (EPA) via dietary supplements (e.g., pills, capsules) or via enriched oral nutrition supplements should be considered (Thompson et al., 2016). Dietary supplements containing fish oil have been shown to cause statistically significant preservation of weight or an increase in weight in patients with a variety of cancers (Bonatto et al., 2012; Finocchiaro et al., 2012) and to increase lean body mass (LBM) and functional status (Fearon et al., 2006). Likewise, oral nutrition supplements enriched with EPA have been found to promote statistically significant weight gain or preservation of weight and increase LBM in patients with various cancers (van der Meij et al., 2010; Weed et al., 2011).

Enteral and Parenteral Nutrition Support

For both physiologic and psychological reasons, an oral diet is preferred whenever possible. When oral intake is inadequate or contraindicated, enteral or parenteral nutrition can provide supplemental or complete nutrition. A client may be a candidate for nutrition support if one or more of the following criteria are met (NCI, 2016):

- Weight of less than 80% of ideal or a recent unintentional weight loss of more than 10% of usual weight
- Malabsorption of nutrients related to disease, short bowel syndrome, or cancer treatments
- Fistulas or draining abscesses
- Inability to eat or drink for more than 5 days
- Moderate or high nutritional risk as determined by nutritional screening or assessment
- Client or caregiver demonstrate competency in nutrition support for discharge planning

BOX 22.3   Guidelines for Managing Side Effects or Complications that Affect Nutrition

Anorexia

- Plan a daily menu in advance.
- Overeat during "good" days.
- Eat a high-protein, high-calorie, nutrient-dense breakfast if appetite is best in the morning.
- Eat a small high-calorie meals every 2 hours.
- Seek help preparing meals.
- Add extra protein and calories to food.
- Eat nutrient-dense foods first.
- Limit liquids with meals to avoid early satiety and bloating at mealtime.
- Use nutrition supplements (instant breakfast mixes, milk shakes, commercial supplements) in place of meals when appetite deteriorates or the client is too tired to eat.
- Make eating a pleasant experience by eating in a bright, cheerful environment, playing soft music, and enjoying the company of friends or family.
- Avoid strong food odors if they contribute to anorexia. Cook outdoors on a grill, serve cold foods rather than hot foods, or use takeout meals that do not need to be prepared at home. In the hospital, the tray cover should be removed before the tray is placed in front of the client so that food odors can dissipate.
- Try different foods.
- Perform frequent mouth care to reduce aftertastes.

Nausea

- Rinse mouth before and after eating.
- Eat frequently. Some people feel better by keeping a small amount of food in the stomach at all times.
- Slowly sip fluids throughout the day.
- Drink ginger ale or ginger tea.
- Eat foods served cold, such as chicken salad instead of hot baked chicken or deli roast beef instead of pot roast.
- Eat high-carbohydrate, low-fat, easy-to-digest foods such as toast, crackers, pretzels, yogurt, sherbet, cooked cereal, soft or canned fruits, watermelon, bananas, fruit juices, and angel food cake.
- Avoid fatty, greasy, fried, spicy, or foods with a strong odor.
- Sit up for 1 hour after eating.
- Keep track of and avoid foods that cause nausea.
- Avoid eating 1–2 hours before chemotherapy or radiotherapy.
- Take antiemetics as prescribed even when symptoms are absent.

Fatigue

- Eat a hearty breakfast because fatigue may worsen as the day progresses.
- Engage in regular exercise if possible.
- Consume easy-to-eat foods that can be prepared with a minimal amount of effort, such as frozen dinners, takeout foods, sandwiches, instant breakfast mixes and liquid formulas, cheese and crackers, peanut butter on crackers, yogurt, and pudding.
- If weight loss isn't a problem, avoid overeating for energy. Excess weight worsens fatigue.
- Enlist the help of friends and family to provide meals.

Taste Changes

- Eat cold or frozen foods.
- Use sugar-free lemon drops, gum, or mints to counter a metallic or bitter taste in the mouth.
- Brush your teeth or rinse with a mouthwash before eating.
- Eat small frequent meals.
- Use plastic utensils if food has a metallic taste.
- Drink tart juice before eating, such as cranberry or orange juice, to mask a metallic taste.
- Experiment with tart foods such as pickles, vinegar, or relishes to help overcome metallic taste.
- Eat meat with something sweet, such as pork with applesauce or turkey with cranberry sauce.
- Substitute poultry, eggs, cheese, and mild fish for beef and pork if they have a "bad," "rotten," or "fecal" taste.
- Avoid foods that are offensive; stick to those that taste good.
- Try new foods, such as lemon yogurt in place of strawberry.

Sore Mouth (Stomatitis)

- Practice good oral hygiene (thorough cleaning with a soft-bristle toothbrush or cotton swabs plus frequent mouth rinses with normal saline and water or baking soda and water). Commercial mouthwashes containing alcohol may irritate and burn the oral mucosa.
- Eat cold or room temperature foods.
- Eat soft, nonirritating foods that are easy to chew and swallow, such as bananas, applesauce, watermelon, canned fruit, cottage cheese, yogurt, mashed potatoes, macaroni and cheese, puddings, milk shakes, oral nutrition supplements, scrambled eggs, oatmeal, and other cooked cereals.
- Add gravy, broth, or sauces to increase the fluid content of foods, as appropriate.
- Cook food until soft and tender
- Cut food into small pieces.
- Numb the mouth with frozen bananas, ice chips, ice cream, or popsicles.
- Avoid spices, acidic foods, coarse foods, salty foods, alcohol, and smoking that can aggravate an already irritated oral mucosa.
- Consume high-calorie, high-protein drinks in place of traditional meals.
- Use a straw to drink liquids.
- Avoid wearing ill-fitting dentures.
- Glutamine swishes may reduce the duration and severity of mucositis.

Xerostomia (Dry Mouth)

- Use an alcohol-free mouth rinse before eating.
- Drink fluids with meals and all day long.
- Eat moist foods softened with gravies or sauces. Casseroles and stews are easier to eat than baked or roasted meats.
- Avoid dry, coarse foods and very spicy or salty foods.
- Avoid foods that stick to the roof of the mouth such as peanut butter.
- Avoid sugary food and beverages that promote dental decay.
- Drink high-calorie, high-protein liquids between meals.
- Stimulate saliva production with citrus fruits if tolerated, such as lemons, oranges, limes, and grapefruit.

BOX 22.3 — Guidelines for Managing Side Effects or Complications that Affect Nutrition (continued)

- Consume frozen desserts, such as ice cream and frozen yogurt.
- Eating papaya may help break up "ropy" saliva.
- Use ice chips and sugar-free hard candies and gum between meals to relieve dryness.
- Use a straw to drink liquids.
- Apply a moisturizer to the lips to help prevent drying.
- Brush after every meal and snack.
- Avoid tobacco and alcohol because they dry the mouth.

Diarrhea

- Replace fluid and electrolytes with broth, soups, sports drinks, and canned fruit.
- Drink at least 1 cup of liquid after each loose bowel movement.
- Limit caffeine, hot or cold liquids, and high-fat foods because they aggravate diarrhea.
- Avoid gassy foods and liquids such as dried peas and beans, cruciferous vegetables, carbonated beverages, and chewing gum.

- Try foods high in pectin and other soluble fibers to slow transit time, such as oatmeal, cooked carrots, bananas, peeled apples, and applesauce.
- Avoid sugar-free candy or gum containing sorbitol because it can contribute to osmotic diarrhea.
- Unless tolerance to lactose has been confirmed, limit or avoid milk.

Constipation

- Increase fiber gradually by eating more fruits, vegetables, and legumes. Replace refined grains with and whole grain bread and cereals.
- Consume 2 tbsp wheat bran, which can be sprinkled on cooked or ready to eat cereal, salad, applesauce, or yogurt. After 3 days, increase by 1 tbsp daily until constipation is resolved. Bran intake should not exceed 6 tbsp/day.
- Eat dried fruit, such as raisins, dates, or prunes.
- Eat high-fiber foods throughout the day.
- Drink 8–10 cups of fluid/day.
- Take walks and exercise regularly.

BOX 22.4 — Ways to Increase the Protein and Calorie Density of Foods

To Increase Protein and Calories

- Add skim milk powder to milk to make double-strength milk; chill well before serving.
- Use double-strength milk on hot or cold cereals and in scrambled eggs, soups, gravies, casseroles, milk shakes, and milk-based desserts.
- Substitute whole milk for water in recipes.
- Add grated cheese to soups, casseroles, vegetable dishes, rice, and noodles.
- Use peanut butter as a spread on slices of apple, banana, pear, crackers, or waffles; use as a filling for celery.
- Add finely chopped, hard-cooked eggs to sauces; add cream to soups and casseroles.
- Choose desserts made with eggs or milk such as sponge cake, angel food cake, custard, and puddings.
- Dip meat, poultry, and fish in eggs or milk and coat with bread or cereal crumbs before baking, broiling, or pan frying.
- Use yogurt, especially Greek yogurt, as a topping for fruit, plain cakes, or other desserts; use in gravies and dips.

To Increase Calories

- Mix cream cheese with butter and spread on hot bread and rolls.
- Whenever possible, add butter to hot foods: breads, pancakes, waffles, soups, vegetables, potatoes, cooked cereal, rice, and pasta.
- Substitute mayonnaise for salad dressing in salads, eggs, casseroles, and sandwiches.
- Add dried fruit, nuts, or granola to desserts and cereal.
- Use whipped cream on pies, fruit pudding, gelatin, ice cream, and other desserts and in coffee, tea, and hot chocolate.
- Use marshmallows in hot chocolate, on fruits, and in desserts.
- Top baked potatoes, vegetables, and fruits with sour cream.
- Snack frequently on nuts, dried fruit, candy, buttered popcorn, cheese, granola, and ice cream.
- Use honey on toast, cereal, and fruit and in coffee and tea.

Enteral Nutrition

Enteral nutrition (EN) is indicated for patients who are unable meet their nutritional requirements orally and have a functional GI tract. For instance, patients undergoing chemoradiation to the head and neck or esophagus often have tumor-related weight loss and cachexia before treatment even begins. In this population, the early use of percutaneous endoscopic gastrostomy (PEG) tube feedings has been found to decrease weight loss, at least in some patients, preventing them from developing cachexia (Arends et al., 2006). Other indications include cancers of the stomach, intestine, or pancreas and severe complications or side effects from chemotherapy and/or radiation that are jeopardizing the treatment plan of a malnourished patient (NCI, 2016). For more on EN, including potential benefits and contraindications (see Chapter 14).

Disease-specific enteral formulas, enriched with specific nutrients, may enhance nutrition support for cancer patients. Studies have shown increased benefits among various cancer patients who have received enteral formulas enriched with EPA (R. Murphy et al., 2011; van der Meij et al., 2012), formulas that have a high ratio of fat to carbohydrate plus added n-3 fatty acids (Fietkau et al., 2013), formulas enriched with arginine (Buijs et al., 2010), and formulas enriched with glutamine (NCI, 2016). More research is needed to evaluate benefits and possible disadvantages of these nutrients.

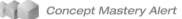

Concept Mastery Alert

Arginine-enriched formulas have been shown to be beneficial when patients with head and neck cancer are malnourished. Patients with gastrointestinal cancer have been shown to benefit from glutamine-enriched formulas.

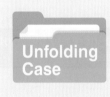

Unfolding Case

Recall Patrick. His weight loss continues and he is having difficulty staying hydrated due to mouth sores and vomiting. Are there additional diet modifications you would recommend that may enable him to consume adequate fluids and calories? Is he a candidate for EN? What are the potential risks and benefits?

Parenteral Nutrition

Parenteral nutrition (PN) can be a lifesaving therapy because it can deliver nutrients to patients who have a nonfunctional GI tract, such as those with obstruction, intractable nausea and/or vomiting, short bowel syndrome, or ileus (NCI, 2016). Other indications include severe diarrhea or malabsorption, severe mucositis or esophagitis, high-output GI fistula that cannot be bypassed by enteral intubation, and severe preoperative malnutrition. PN increases the risk of serious infectious, metabolic, and mechanical complications and should not be used for less than 5 days or in patients with poor prognosis not warranting aggressive nutritional support (NCI, 2016). Artificial nutrition, such as EN and PN, has not been shown to improve outcomes in terminally ill patients (McClave et al., 2016).

Nutrition in Palliative Care

The goals of nutrition intervention during palliative care are to establish and maintain a sense of well-being and enhance quality of life (Rock et al., 2012). Not all advanced cancer patients are malnourished or underweight. Dietary choices can help relieve cancer symptoms of treatment side effects. Eating is encouraged as a source of pleasure, not as an adjunct to treatment, and the patient's preferences are more important than the nutritional quality of the foods consumed. Box 22.5 lists supportive measures for nutrition in palliative care.

Nutrition for Cancer Survivors

Cancer survivors are urged to follow nutrition and physical activity guidelines for cancer prevention—namely, maintain a healthy weight, be physically active, and eat a mostly plant-based

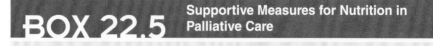

BOX 22.5 Supportive Measures for Nutrition in Palliative Care

- Control unpleasant side effects, such as pain, constipation, nausea, vomiting, and heartburn, with medication.
- Respect the client's wishes regarding the level of nutritional support desired.
- Provide adequate mouth care to control dryness and thirst.
- Respect the client's personal tastes and preferences.
- Ensure a pleasant eating environment and serve attractive food.
- Serve food of appropriate textures.
- Use a team approach that includes physician, dietitian, and nurse.

diet (Box 22.6). Convincing evidence shows that obesity is associated with an increased risk of breast cancer recurrence (Protani, Coory, & Martin, 2010) and emerging evidence suggests obesity also increases the recurrence of other cancers (Amling, 2004). Likewise, data from observational studies of colorectal cancer survivors indicate that people who report a healthy eating pattern (high in fruits, vegetables, whole grains, and low-fat dairy products) have improved overall survival and lower rates of colorectal recurrence and mortality than those who consume a typical Western eating pattern (Meyerhardt et al., 2007). Although scientific evidence supporting nutrition guidelines for cancer survivors is currently limited (Robien, Denmark-Wahnefried, & Rock, 2011), a healthy lifestyle may reduce cancer recurrence as well as the risk of other chronic diseases.

Dietary Supplements

Although routine vitamin and mineral supplements have previously been recommended during and after treatment as an "insurance policy" for obtaining adequate nutrients, this practice has come under scrutiny as more evidence suggests supplements may not be helpful or may increase the risk of mortality (Rock et al., 2012). For instance, supplements were found to increase the number of colorectal cancers in participants receiving folic acid in the Aspirin/Folate Polyp Prevention Study (Cole et al., 2007). Both the American Cancer Society and the American Institute for Cancer Research recommend that cancer survivors obtain nutrients from food, not supplements. Supplements should be considered only if there is biochemical or clinical evidence of nutrient deficiency or if it is determined that nutrient intakes are consistently lower than two-thirds of recommended intake levels (Rock et al., 2012).

BOX 22.6 Guidelines for Cancer Survivors: Recommendations to Reduce Cancer Risk

1. Be as lean as possible without becoming underweight.
2. Be physically active for at least 30 minutes every day.
3. Avoid sugary drinks and limit consumption of energy-dense foods (particularly processed foods high in added sugar, low in fiber or high in fat).
4. Eat more of a variety of vegetables, fruits, whole grains, and legumes such as beans.
5. Limit consumption of red meats (such as beef, pork, and lamb) and avoid processed meats.
6. If consumed at all, limit alcoholic drinks to two for men and one for women a day.
7. Limit consumption of salty foods and foods processed with salt (sodium).
8. Do not rely on supplements to protect against cancer.
9. Do not smoke or chew tobacco.

Source: American Institute for Cancer Research. (2016). *AICR's guidelines for cancer survivors.* Available at http://www.aicr.org/patients-survivors/aicrs-guidelines-for-cancer.html. Accessed on 9/8/16.

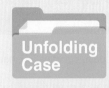

Consider Patrick. He completed the recommended course of chemotherapy and will be closely followed to ensure the treatment was effective. He has high anxiety and fear that the cancer will return and wants to do everything he can to reduce the risk. What would you say to Patrick to help manage his fear? What weight, intake, and exercise goals would you recommend Patrick set?

HIV AND AIDS

HIV is a chronic infectious disease that attacks the immune system, specifically CD4 cells. The stages of HIV are

- Acute infection, which occurs within 2 to 4 weeks of HIV infection and may last for a few weeks. Symptoms are flu-like.
- Clinical latency, which may also be called asymptomatic HIV infection or chronic HIV infection. During this period, symptoms may be absent. Without combination antiretroviral therapy, this period may last a decade. People who begin antiretroviral therapy soon after diagnosis may remain in this stage for decades. Clinical latency progresses to AIDS when **viral load** increases, CD4 cell count drops, and symptoms develop.
- AIDS is diagnosed when CD4 cell count is ≤200 cells/mm or if certain opportunistic illnesses develop. Symptoms include chills, fever, weakness, and weight loss. Life expectancy is approximately 3 years. Untreated HIV leads to AIDS in most people.

Viral Load
the level of virus or viral markers measured in the blood.

Antiretroviral Therapy (ART)
a combination of ART medications that are typically used to control and reduce viral load.

Since the introduction of combination **antiretroviral therapy (ART)** in the mid-1990s, morbidity and mortality from HIV has dramatically declined (Montaner et al., 2014). Life expectancy of HIV-infected adults receiving ART is nearing that of the general population (Rodger et al., 2013) and chronic and age-related conditions are becoming increasingly prevalent as the population receiving ART lives longer (Thompson-Paul et al., 2015). In fact, AIDS is the cause of death in less than one-quarter of deaths among HIV-infected people, whereas up to half are due to noninfectious causes such as CVD, non–AIDS-related cancers, and kidney disease (Weber et al., 2013).

Nutrition Consequences

Any infection challenges nutritional status, and the chronicity of HIV infection intensifies the challenge. Inflammatory, hormonal, and immune responses can increase metabolic rate and nutrient requirements, promote loss of lean body tissue, cause anorexia, and alter nutrient storage and availability. Infections in the intestines can lead to diarrhea, malabsorption of nutrients, blood loss, and damage to the intestinal lining. Opportunistic infections and cancers often result in weight loss. Severe infection increases the risk of malnutrition. ART medications have multiple adverse side effects that may affect overall intake, metabolism, or nutrient utilization. People who are malnourished at the time of diagnosis may be at higher risk for disease progression related to malnutrition-related immune suppression (Dong, 2016).

HIV-Associated Weight Loss and Wasting

Widespread use of ART has significantly improved morbidity and mortality related to HIV infection and dramatically reduced the incidence of wasting (Erlandson et al., 2016).

However, the initial loss of weight or lean body mass due to HIV replication may not be fully restored after ART begins. A high incidence of wasting continues to be a problem in some Americans, especially in adults who use drugs and have food insecurity, have high viral loads, or have low incomes (Keithley & Swanson, 2013). HIV-associated wasting reflects a loss of both fat and lean tissue and is defined as any one of the following (Guaraldi, Chiara, Zona, & Bagni, 2012; Wanke et al., 2000):

- Unintentional weight loss of 10% body weight in 1 year
- Unintentional weight loss of 5% body weight in 6 months
- Body mass index (BMI) <20

Cytokines
a group name for more than 100 different proteins involved in immune responses; they are also critical for normal growth and development. Prolonged production of proinflammatory cytokines promotes hypercatabolism (hyper = excessive; catabolism = breaking down phase of metabolism).

Like cancer cachexia, the etiology of HIV-associated wasting is multifactorial and not completely understood. Wasting is likely mediated in part by inflammatory changes, such as excessive production of **cytokines** that increase calorie expenditure and protein breakdown (Melchior et al., 1991). Inadequate calorie intake may be a primary contributor (Mulligan & Schambelan, 2003). Diarrhea and malabsorption of nutrients decrease nutrient availability. Wasting has been associated with accelerated disease progression, diminished strength, and muscle fatigue and weakness. Severe wasting increases the risk of death.

Impaired Intake

Inadequate food intake may occur from

- Anorexia related to depression, fatigue, pain, anxiety, or as a side effect of medication
- Oral infections that cause pain, dysphagia, or altered taste
- Respiratory infections that cause shortness of breath and chest pain
- Medication side effects, such as nausea, vomiting, food aversions, or diarrhea
- Food insecurity and low income

Gastrointestinal Complications

Infections in the esophagus, stomach, or small intestines can significantly affect nutrient intake, digestion, or absorption. Bacterial overgrowth can occur from the use of medications to control infections caused by viruses, parasites, or fungi and may cause GI discomfort, vomiting, diarrhea, and malabsorption. Because malabsorption can occur in the absence of diarrhea, malabsorption cannot be excluded on the basis of normal bowel patterns alone. Most ART have GI side effects, such as anorexia, nausea, and diarrhea.

HIV-Associated Lipodystrophy

Lipodystrophy
also called fat redistribution syndrome; a condition characterized by changes in body shape and metabolism. Characteristics may occur separately or in combination.

Exposure to ART is associated with a significant risk of adverse metabolic effects, including **lipodystrophy**, insulin resistance, hyperlipidemia, and an increase cardiovascular morbidity in patients with HIV (Deshpande, Toshniwal, Joshi, & Jani, 2016). Patients with HIV lipodystrophy develop fat redistribution, which is characterized by peripheral fat wasting with loss of subcutaneous fat in the face, arms, legs, and buttocks and accumulation of fat in the back of the neck and trunk; however, some patients have only fat gain, some only fat loss, and some have both. Metabolic disturbances of HIV lipodystrophy include insulin resistance, and hyperlipidemia, which increase the risk of diabetes and atherosclerotic CVD. Although HIV lipodystrophy is associated with ART, its exact etiology is unclear (Deshpande et al., 2016). Emotional distress caused by the significant changes in body shape and social stigmatization may cause some patients to decrease or stop their ARTs because they are implicated in its cause.

Cardiovascular Disease Risk

The risk of myocardial infarction may be increased by 50% in HIV-infected people compared to uninfected people, likely due to HIV infection, ART, and comorbid disease (Freiberg et al., 2013). Although the mechanism by which HIV infection increases the risk of MI is not known,

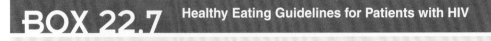

BOX 22.7   Healthy Eating Guidelines for Patients with HIV

- Eat a calorie appropriate eating pattern rich in whole grains, vegetables, fruits with lean sources of protein such as skinless poultry, lean cuts of beef and pork, and legumes.
- Choose low fat or nonfat milk and dairy products.
- Eat fish and seafood for healthy omega-3 fats.
- Eat healthy fats in moderation, such as oils, seeds, nuts, nut butters, and avocados.
- Eat some carbohydrate, protein, and fat at each meal and snack.
- Drink adequate fluids.
- Practice food safety guidelines.
- Limit solid fats such as butter, margarine, and shortenings and foods made with solid fats.
- Limit sweetened beverages and high fat desserts such as cookies, cakes, and ice cream.
- Limit salt intake to 2300 mg/day.
- Manage side effects or symptoms that affect nutrition, such as anorexia, nausea, vomiting, and diarrhea.

inflammation, CD4 cell count depletion, altered coagulation, and endothelial dysfunction may be factors. As noted earlier, ART is associated with lipodystrophy, which is linked to insulin resistance, diabetes, dyslipidemia, and increased risk of atherosclerosis. Results from the Strategies for Management of Antiretroviral Therapy study suggest that the virus plays a larger role than ART in MI risk (El-Sadr et al., 2006).

Nutrition Therapy for HIV/AIDS

There is not a one-size-fits-all diet for HIV/AIDS nor are there unanimously agreed upon recommendations for calories or nutrients despite the universal goals of maintaining body weight and lean body mass. An individualized assessment identifies the patient's needs based on weight, laboratory values, body composition, and clinical data. A healthy eating pattern of appropriate calories is the general approach (Box 22.7). Ideally, nutrition therapy begins soon after diagnosis because the effectiveness of nutrition therapy may be limited once the client is ill enough to need hospital care.

Weight Management

For patients with weight loss or wasting, a high-calorie, high-protein diet is recommended. As in the case of cancer, oral nutrition supplements are frequently used because they tend to leave the stomach quickly, are easy to consume, and provide significant quantities of calories and protein. Small frequent feedings (e.g., six to nine times daily) are encouraged.

Although weight loss and wasting are associated with HIV, weight gain and overweight and obesity are becoming increasingly prevalent (Lakey, Yang, Yancy, Chow, & Hicks, 2013). A study by Tate et al. (2012) in the Southern United States found that the prevalence of overweight or obesity in HIV-infected study participants was 45% before ART was initiated and increased to 56% after 2 years of ART. In the general population, obesity is associated with increased risk of chronic diseases, such as diabetes and CVD; HIV-infection likely exacerbates the risk of these conditions in obese patients. Moderate weight loss may be recommended for overweight or obese HIV-infected patients.

Protein

In theory, protein need may increase in response to opportunistic infections; however, no studies have confirmed that increasing protein is beneficial during opportunistic infections (Dong, 2016). There is no evidence to indicate protein need increases in HIV-infected adults nor is there evidence to suggest that protein need does not increase (Raiten, Mulligan, Papathakis, & Wanke, 2011).

Fat

When initiated at the time ART is started, a heart-healthy eating pattern low in saturated fat, trans fat, and cholesterol with increased monounsaturated fats, polyunsaturated fats, and fiber has been shown to prevent dyslipidemia in HIV-infected people (Lazzaretti, Kuhmmer, Sprinz, Polanczyk, & Ribeiro, 2012). The diet also prevented some of the weight gain and fat distribution of lipodystrophy syndrome, most likely because calorie intake was also reduced. For patients who have hyperlipidemia, a heart-healthy eating pattern such as a Mediterranean-style diet is recommended. Several studies in patients with HIV and hypertriglyceridemia have found fish oil helps lower triglycerides (Dong, 2016).

Vitamins and Minerals

Observational studies suggest a high prevalence of serum micronutrient deficiencies among people with HIV and that poor intake or low serum levels of some vitamins and minerals are associated with faster HIV disease progression and mortality (World Health Organization [WHO], 2003). Nutrient deficiencies may occur from poor intake, malabsorption, infections, or diet–medication interactions. In general, dietary intake of micronutrients at RDA amounts is a reasonable recommendation for people with clinically stable disease (Forrester & Sztam, 2011). In some people infected with HIV, short-term, high-dose multiple micronutrient supplementation may be beneficial, depending on the patient's nutritional status and immune status and the presence of coinfections (Forrester & Sztam, 2011). A meta-analysis by Carter et al. (2015) found micronutrient supplementation significantly and substantially slowed the progression of HIV in adults not on ART and that it may reduce mortality. Evidence suggests potential harm from higher doses of selected micronutrients, especially of vitamin A and zinc in some populations (Raiten et al., 2011).

Manage Symptoms

Clients with HIV/AIDS may experience problems with appetite and intake similar to those of cancer clients. Diet modifications recommended for side effects or complications of cancer are also appropriate for people infected with HIV (see Box 22.3).

Enteral and Parenteral Nutrition Support

Clients who are unable to consume an adequate oral intake may require EN for supplemental or complete nutrition. The same guidelines for use apply in HIV as in other populations, with extra attention to ensure sanitary conditions. PN is reserved for clients whose GI tract is nonfunctional. Hydrolyzed formulas consumed orally may be just as effective as PN in preventing weight loss in patients with severe malabsorption—with none of the risk associated with PN.

Food and Drug Interactions

Due to food–drug interactions, medication schedules and food restrictions are both complex and strict. Some drug combinations that must be taken three or more times a day have significant adverse GI side effects such as nausea, vomiting, and diarrhea. Lipodystrophy and peripheral neuropathy may be long-term effects. The bioavailability of some medications depends on the medication being taken with food (Table 22.6). A study by Kalichman et al. (2015) showed that greater alcohol use, not believing medications are necessary, and being prescribed an ART regimen that requires the simultaneous intake of food significantly predicted poor ART adherence in patients with food insecurity. Access to food must be assessed when ART is being prescribed.

Food Safety

Because HIV-infected patients have compromised immune systems, steps should be taken to reduce the risk of foodborne illness. Food safety strategies are listed in Box 22.2 (see Chapter 9 for more on foodborne illness).

Table 22.6	Single HIV/AIDS Medications and Timing of Food Intake		
Generic Name (Brand Name)	Take with Food	Take on Empty Stomach	No Food Restrictions
Nucleoside reverse transcriptase inhibitors (NRTIs)			
Abacavir (Ziagen)			✓
Didanosine (Videx)		✓	
Emtricitabine (Emtriva)			✓
Lamivudine (Epivir)			✓
Stavudine (Zerit)			✓
Tenofovir (Viread)			✓
Zidovudine (Retrovir)			✓
Nonnucleoside reverse transcriptase inhibitors (NNRTIs)			
Efavirenz (Sustiva)		✓ May take with a light low-fat snack. Fat increases absorption and may increase the risk of adverse effects.	
Etravirine (Intelence)	✓		
Nevirapine (Viramune)			✓
Rilpivirine (Endurant)	✓		
Protease inhibitors			
Atazanavir (Reyataz)	✓		
Darunavir (Prezista)	✓		
Fosamprenavir (Lexiva)			✓
Indinavir (Crixivan)		✓ If unboosted, take 1 hour before or 2 hours after a meal.	
Nelfinavir (Viracept)	✓		
Ritonavir (Norvir)	✓		
Saquinavir (Invirase)	✓ Take within 2 hours after a meal.		
Tipranavir (Aptivus)			✓ Taking with food may improve tolerance.
Fusion inhibitors			
Enfuvirtide (Fuzeon)			✓
Entry inhibitors			
Maraviroc (Selzentry)			✓
Integrase inhibitors			
Dolutegravir (Tivicay)			✓
Elvitegravir (Vitekta)	✓		✓
Raltegravir (Isentress)			✓
Pharmacokinetic enhancers			
Cobicistat (Tybost)	✓		

Sources: AIDSinfo. (2016). *HIV treatment: FDA-approved HIV medicines*. Available at https://aidsinfo.nih.gov/education-materials /fact-sheets/21/58/fda-approved-hiv-medicines. Accessed on 9/11/16; U.S. Department of Veterans Affairs. (2016). *ARVs: Food requirements*. Available at http://www.hiv.va.gov/provider/manual-primary-care/food-supplements-table1.asp?backto=provider /manual-primary-care/food-supplements&backtext=Back%20to%20Food%20and%20Supplements%20Chapter. Accessed on 9/11/16.

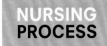
NURSING PROCESS

Cancer

Karen is a 59-year-old former smoker who now calls herself a "health nut." She was recently diagnosed with lung cancer. She had surgery to remove her right lung and is receiving chemotherapy for cancerous "spots" on the left lung and stomach. She has lost 28 pounds and complains of nausea, vomiting, and a bad taste in her mouth. Because she has followed a healthy diet to prevent cancer for years, she is reluctant to now change her eating habits and eat more protein, fat, and calories. Right now, she is eating mostly fruit, sherbet, and skim milk.

Assessment

Medical–Psychosocial History	• Medical history such as diabetes, heart disease, or hypertension • Types of drugs the client is receiving through chemotherapy; other prescribed medications that affect nutrition • Physician's goals and plan of treatment • Pattern of nausea and vomiting • Client's understanding of increased nutritional needs related to cancer and cancer therapies • Willingness to change her attitudes toward food and nutrition • Psychosocial and economic issues such as financial status, employment, and outside support system • Usual activity patterns
Anthropometric Assessment	• Height, current weight, usual weight • Rate of weight loss; percentage of usual body weight loss • BMI
Biochemical and Physical Assessment	• Laboratory data: prealbumin, serum electrolytes, any abnormal values • Nitrogen balance study, if available • General appearance/evidence of muscle wasting
Dietary Assessment	• How many daily meals and snacks are you eating? • What is a typical day's intake for you? • How is your appetite? When is your appetite the best? • What do you do to alleviate nausea? • How has your sense of taste changed? What do you do to cope with the changes? • Do you have any food allergies or intolerances? • Do you have any cultural, religious, or ethnic food preferences? • Do you use vitamins, minerals, or nutrition supplements? • Do you use liquid formulas, such as instant breakfast mixes or commercial products? • How much liquid do you consume in a day? • Do you use alcohol?

Diagnosis

Possible Nursing Diagnoses	• Imbalanced nutrition: eating less than the body requires related to nausea, vomiting, and taste changes secondary to cancer/cancer therapy as evidenced by 28-pound weight loss

NURSING PROCESS   Cancer

Planning

Client Outcomes

The client will
- Eat six to eight times daily
- Add to the protein and calorie density of foods she eats
- Drink at least 16 oz of a high-calorie, high-protein supplement daily
- Switch from skim milk to whole milk, as tolerated
- Verbalize interventions she will try to help alleviate nausea and taste alterations
- Verbalize the importance of consuming adequate protein and calories and the role of fat in providing calories
- Maintain present weight until chemotherapy is completed

Nursing Interventions

Nutrition Therapy

Provide regular diet as ordered with high-protein, high-calorie, in-between meal supplements.

Client Teaching

Instruct the client
- That an adequate nutritional status reduces the side effects of treatment, may make cancer cells more receptive to treatment, and may improve quality of life; poor nutritional status may potentiate chemotherapeutic drug toxicity.
- That a preventive eating style is no longer appropriate; consuming adequate protein and calories (even fat calories) is the major priority.

Instruct the client on eating plan essentials, including
- Protein sources the client may tolerate despite nausea and taste changes such as eggs, cheese, mild fish, nuts, dried peas and beans, milk shakes, eggnogs, puddings, ice cream, instant breakfast mixes, and commercial supplements
- How to increase the protein and calorie density of foods eaten (see Box 22.4)
- To eat small, frequent "meals" to help maximize intake but to avoid eating 12 hours before chemotherapy
- To drink ample fluids 1–2 days before and after chemotherapy to enhance excretion of the drugs and to decrease the risk of renal toxicity

Instruct the client on interventions to minimize nausea, such as
- Eating foods served cold or at room temperature
- Eating high-carbohydrate, low-fat foods such as toast, crackers, yogurt, sherbet, cooked cereal, soft or canned fruits, watermelon, bananas, fruit juices, and angel food cake
- Avoiding fatty, greasy, fried, and strongly seasoned foods

Instruct the client on behavior to help maximize intake, including
- Viewing food as a medicine, rather than a social pleasure, that must be "taken" even when the desire to eat is lacking
- Keeping track of and avoiding foods that cause nausea
- Taking antiemetics as prescribed even when symptoms are absent
- Sucking on sugarless hard candy during chemotherapy and using plastic utensils and dishes to mitigate the "bad taste" in her mouth
- Avoiding anything that tastes unpleasant

Evaluation

Evaluate and Monitor

- Monitor weight.
- Monitor food intake records.
- Monitor management of side effects; suggest additional interventions as needed.

How Do You Respond?

Why do cancer prevention guidelines suggest red meat intake be limited? The World Cancer Research Fund International Continuous Update Project report found convincing evidence that red meat and processed meats increase the risk of colorectal cancer (World Cancer Research Fund/AICR, 2011). Studies suggest up to 18 oz/week of red meat can be safely consumed without significantly increasing cancer risk. However, cancer risk starts to increase when even small amounts of processed meats are eaten daily. The risk may be related to substances that occur naturally in red meat (e.g., heme) and substances that are produced when red meat is processed (e.g., nitrites that can become carcinogenic compounds) or cooked (e.g., heterocyclic amines formed at high heat). Other hypotheses are that processed meats are high in fat, contributing to an excess calorie intake and an increase in bile acids and that people who have a high red meat intake tend to eat less plant-based foods and thus miss out on their cancer-protective substances. Although more research is needed to fully explain the relationship between red and processed meats and cancer, it is prudent to limit red meat to less than 18 oz/week and eat very little, if any, processed meats.

Doesn't canola oil cause cancer? The rumor that canola oil causes cancer stems from the fact that canola is derived from rapeseed. Rapeseed is naturally high in erucic acid, a fatty acid shown to be harmful to animals. However, in the 1970s, traditional plant breeding methods led to the creation of a low–erucic acid rapeseed, which is used to make canola oil. There are no human health risks associated with canola oil.

REVIEW CASE STUDY

Steve is a 39-year-old male who has been HIV positive for 6 years. His waistline is expanding, and he blames that for his recent onset of heartburn. Based on a physical examination and insulin resistance, his doctor diagnosed lipodystrophy syndrome. Steve is 6 ft tall and weighs 190 pounds. His weight has been stable for the last several years, although he feels "fatter." He is on ART but is thinking of discontinuing the medication if it is the cause of his change in shape. He is willing to exercise but wants maximum benefit from minimum effort. He is also willing to change his eating habits but relies heavily on eating out. A typical day's intake is shown on the right:

- Evaluate Steve's current weight. Would you recommend weight loss?
- How does Steve's weight affect heartburn and insulin resistance?
- How does his usual intake affect heartburn and insulin resistance?
- What are Steve's nutrition-related problems? What nutrition therapy recommendations would you make?
- What would you tell Steve about exercise?
- What criteria would you monitor to evaluate the effectiveness of nutrition therapy?

Breakfast: A fast-food egg, bacon, and cheese sandwich on an English muffin; hash browns; large black coffee
Lunch: Double hamburger; french fries; cola
Dinner: Grilled steak; baked potato with sour cream; water
Snacks: Chips

STUDY QUESTIONS

1 The nurse knows her instructions about healthy eating to reduce the risk of cancer have been understood when the client states
   a. "If I follow those healthy eating guidelines, I will not get cancer."
   b. "To reduce the risk of cancer, I have to eat a vegetarian diet."
   c. "There is not enough known about diet and cancer to make informed choices about what to eat to reduce the risk of cancer."
   d. "A mostly plant-based diet may reduce the risk of cancer."

2 The nurse knows her instructions on how to reduce the risk of foodborne illness have been understood when the client states
   a. "It is okay to thaw food at room temperature as long as I cook it immediately after it is defrosted."
   b. "Leftovers are not safe to eat."
   c. "Fruits and vegetables do not need to be washed if I peel them or eat them after they are cooked."
   d. "All meat, fish, and poultry should be cooked to the well-done stage."

3 Which of the following strategies would the nurse suggest
to help the client increase the protein density of his diet?
a. Top baked potatoes with sour cream
b. Mix cream cheese with butter and spread on hot bread
c. Substitute milk for water in recipes
d. Add whipped cream to coffee

4 Which of the following meals would be most appropriate
for a patient who has nausea?
a. Cottage cheese and fresh fruit plate
b. Fried chicken and coleslaw
c. Pot roast and roasted potatoes with gravy
d. Spaghetti with marinara sauce and salad

5 The client asks what foods she can eat for protein because
meat tastes "rotten" to her. Which of the following would
be the nurse's best response?
a. Cheese omelet, cold chicken sandwich, shrimp salad
b. Vegetable soup, pulled-pork sandwich, meatloaf with gravy
c. Spaghetti with meatballs, tacos, peanut butter and jelly
sandwich
d. Hot dogs, hamburgers, vegetable pizza

6 A client asks if it is okay to drink nutrition supplements in
place of eating solid food because it seems to be the only
thing she tolerates. Which of the following is the nurse's
best response?
a. "Nutrition formulas are okay to use as a supplement in
your diet, but they do not provide enough nutrition to
use them in place of a meal."

b. "Nutrition formulas are rich in nutrients and can be used
in place of meals if they are what you are able to tolerate
best."
c. "It is fine to rely on nutrition supplements but vary the
brand to ensure you are getting adequate nutrition."
d. "Nutrition supplements generally are too high in calories
and protein to use in place of meals."

7 Which statement indicates the client with HIV needs further instruction about healthy eating?
a. "Eating fat increases my chances of getting fat around
my middle, so I am trying to choose all nonfat or low-fat
food."
b. "Because I have HIV, it is too late for healthy eating to
be beneficial."
c. "Protein is the most important nutrient, so I am eating
extra red meat at every meal."
d. "Unsaturated fats in olive oil, canola oil, nuts, and avocado are healthiest. I am eating more of them and less of
solid fats."

8 When should nutrition become part of the care plan for a
client with HIV?
a. Soon after diagnosis
b. When the client begins to lose weight
c. After an acute episode of illness
d. When weight loss is more than 5% of initial weight

KEY CONCEPTS

- Cancer is a group name for different diseases that differ in
their impact on nutrition.
- As many as a third of cancers may be related to lifestyle
behaviors. Eating a plant-based eating pattern, being physically active, and avoiding excess weight may reduce the risk
of cancer.
- Tumors in the GI tract are more likely than other tumors to
produce local effects that affect nutrition.
- Cancer may alter metabolism by causing glucose intolerance and insulin resistance, increasing energy expenditure,
increasing protein catabolism, increasing fat catabolism,
and increasing the use of fat for energy.
- Anorexia, a common problem in people with cancer, may
lead to weight loss and malnutrition. Pain, depression/
anxiety, early satiety, taste changes, fatigue, and nausea caused
by cancer or its treatment may be contributing factors.
- Cancer cachexia is a progressive wasting syndrome characterized by preferential loss of lean body mass. Altered metabolism and anorexia are involved. The severity of cachexia
is not directly related to calorie intake or tumor weight.
- Nutrition therapy may help sustain the client through adverse side effects of cancer treatments and may reduce morbidity and mortality.

- Requirements for protein, calories, vitamin C, B vitamins,
and iron increase after surgery to replenish losses and promote healing. Compared to other surgeries, GI surgeries
have the greatest chance of affecting nutrition.
- Unlike surgery and radiation, chemotherapy produces systemic side effects. Anorexia, nausea and vomiting, taste alterations, sore mouth or throat, diarrhea, early satiety, and
constipation are the most common nutrition-related side
effects of chemotherapy.
- Nutrition-related side effects from radiation are most likely
to occur in people who have cancers of the head and neck,
lungs, esophagus, cervix, uterus, colon, rectum, and pancreas.
- People who have bone marrow transplantation may need
total parenteral nutrition (TPN) for 1 to 2 months or longer
after the procedure.
- The goal of nutrition therapy for people being treated for
cancer is to prevent weight loss (even in overweight patients) and maintain lean body mass. Avoiding unintentional weight gain is a goal for people who are overweight
or obese at the time of diagnosis and in those with certain
hormonal cancers, such as breast and prostate cancers.
- There are no validated parameters for determining the nutrition needs of patients with cancer. Generally, a high-calorie,

high-protein diet with small frequent meals is recommended for patients who are underweight or losing weight. The diet is modified to alleviate nutrition-related side effects.

- Increasing the calorie and protein densities of the diet is generally more acceptable than increasing the volume of food served.
- An oral diet is used whenever possible. EN and PN are options in specific situations.
- Malnutrition may speed the progression from HIV disease to AIDS.
- The cause of HIV-associated wasting is multifactorial. Impaired intake and altered metabolism may be at least partially responsible.

- The exact nutritional requirements of patients infected with HIV are not known. Calories should be appropriate to attain and maintain healthy weight. There are no data to support an increased need for protein. A heart-healthy eating plan may help control lipodystrophy syndrome and reduce the risk of CVD.
- Patients with HIV may experience side effects similar to those of people with cancer. Diet modifications can help alleviate side effects to promote an adequate intake.
- Drugs used for HIV/AIDS may interact with certain foods. Complex and strict dietary restrictions may be necessary to maximize drug effectiveness.
- Patients with HIV should practice food sanitation and safety to decrease the risk of foodborne illness.

Check Your Knowledge Answer Key

1 **TRUE** Convincing evidence links obesity with several types of cancer, such as pancreatic, kidney, and postmenopausal breast.
2 **TRUE** Weight loss is an indicator of poor prognosis in cancer patients.
3 **TRUE** Clients who are adequately nourished are better able to withstand the effects of cancer treatments.
4 **FALSE** Although anorexia can contribute to the development of cachexia, neither the incidence nor the severity of cachexia can be related directly to calorie intake.
5 **FALSE** The cancer patient's appetite is generally better in the morning and tends to deteriorate as the day progresses.
6 **TRUE** Cancer survivors are urged to follow nutrition guidelines to reduce the risk of cancer in the future.

7 **TRUE** Many cancer patients treated with chemotherapy report a metallic taste alteration.
8 **FALSE** Diarrhea does not necessarily accompany malabsorption caused by HIV infection. Malabsorption cannot be ruled out on the basis of bowel movements alone.
9 **TRUE** Patients with HIV/AIDS may experience problems related to appetite and intake similar to those of cancer patients.
10 **TRUE** The risk of foodborne infections in patients with HIV/AIDS can be reduced by educating them on food and water safety such as the importance of refrigerating foods, washing fruit and vegetables, and cooking meats thoroughly.

Student Resources on thePoint®
For additional learning materials, activate the code in the front of this book at
http://thePoint.lww.com/activate

Websites

Websites related to cancer
American Cancer Society at www.cancer.org
American Institute for Cancer Research at www.aicr.org
National Cancer Institute at www.cancer.gov
National Center for Complementary and Alternative Medicine (NCCAM) at www.nccam.nih.gov
Oncology Nursing Society at www.ons.org

Websites related to HIV/AIDS
AIDSinfo (A Service of the U.S. Department of Health and Human Services) at www.aidsinfo.nih.gov
Center for HIV Information from the University of California San Francisco School of Medicine at www.hivinsite.org
Health Resources and Services Administration (HRSA) HIV/AIDS Services at http://hab.hrsa.gov

References

American Institute for Cancer Research. (n.d.-a). *AICR annual report 2014/2015*. Available at http://www.aicr.org/assets/docs/pdf/financial/aicr-annual-report-2014-2015.pdf?_ga=1.22292411.1043066767.1471888558. Accessed on 12/8/16.

American Institute for Cancer Research. (n.d.-b). *The facts about alcohol*. Available at http://www.aicr.org/assets/docs/pdf/fact-sheets/facts-about-alcohol.pdf?_ga=1.219400089.1043066767.1471888558. Accessed on 12/8/16.

American Institute for Cancer Research. (2016). *What you need to know about obesity and cancer*. Available at http://www.aicr.org/learnmore-about-cancer/infographics/infographic-obesity-and-cancer.html. Accessed on 12/8/16.

Amling, C. (2004). The association between obesity and the progression of prostate and renal cell carcinoma. *Urologic Oncology, 22,* 478–484.

Arends, J., Bodoky, G., Bozzetti, F., Fearon, K., Muscaritoli, M., Selga, G., . . . Zander, A. (2006). ESPEN guidelines on enteral nutrition: Non-surgical oncology. *Clinical Nutrition, 25*, 245–259.

Barrera, S., & Demark-Wahnefried, W. (2009). Nutrition during and after cancer therapy. *Oncology, 23*(2 Suppl.), 15–21.

Bonatto, S., Oliveira, H., Nunes, E., Pequito, D., Iagher, F., Coelho, I., . . . Fernandes, L. C. (2012). Fish oil supplementation improves neutrophil function during cancer chemotherapy. *Lipids, 47*, 383–389.

Buijs, N., van Bokhorst-de van der Schueren, M., Langius, A., Leemans, C. R., Kuik, D. J., Vermeulen, M. A., & van Leeuwen, P. A. (2010). Perioperative arginine-supplemented nutrition in malnourished patients with head and neck cancer improves long-term survival. *The American Journal of Clinical Nutrition, 92*, 1151–1156.

Carter, G., Indyk, D., Johnson, M., Andreae, M., Suslov, K., Busani, S., . . . Sacks, H. S. (2015). Micronutrients in HIV: A Bayesian meta-analysis. *PLoS One, 10*(4), e0120113. doi:10.1371/journal.pone.0120113

Cole, B., Baron, J., Sandler, R., Haile, R. W., Ahnen, D. J., Bresalier, R. S., . . . Greenberg, E. R. (2007). Folic acid for the prevention of colorectal adenomas: A randomized clinical trial. *JAMA, 297*, 2351–2359.

de Pergola, G., & Silvestris, F. (2013). Obesity as a major risk factor for cancer. *Journal of Obesity, 2013*, 291546. doi:10.1155/2013/291546

Deshpande, A., Toshniwal, H., Joshi, S., & Jani, R. (2016). A prospective, multicentre, open-label single-arm exploratory study to evaluate efficacy and safety of Saroglitazar on hypertriglyceridemia in HIV associated lipodystrophy. *PLoS One, 11*(1), e0146222. doi:10.1371/journal.pone.0146222

Dong, K. (2016). HIV/AIDS. *In Academy of Nutrition and Dietetics Nutrition Care Manual*. Available at https://www.nutritioncaremanual.org/topic.cfm?ncm_category_id=1&lv1=20149&ncm_toc_id=20149&ncm_heading=&. Accessed on 9/6/16.

Donohoe, C., Ryan, A., & Reynolds, J. (2011). Cancer cachexia: Mechanisms and clinical implications. *Gastroenterology Research and Practice, 2011*, 601434.

El-Sadr, W., Lundgren, J., Neaton, J., Gordin, F., Abrams, D., Arduino, R. C., . . . Rappoport, C. (2006). CD4+ count-guided interruption of antiretroviral treatment. *The New England Journal of Medicine, 355*, 2283–2296.

Erlandson, K., Li, X., Abraham, A., Margolick J. B., Lake, J. E., Palella, F. J., Jr., . . . Brown, T. T. (2016). Long-term impact of HIV wasting on physical function. *AIDS, 30*, 445–454.

Fearon, K., Barber, M., Moses, A., Ahmedzai, S. H., Taylor, G. S., Tisdale, M. J., & Murray, G. D. (2006). Double-blind, placebo-controlled, randomized study of eicosapentaenoic acid diester in patients with cancer cachexia. *Journal of Clinical Oncology, 24*, 3401–3407.

Fietkau, R., Lewitzki, V., Kuhnt, T., Hölscher, T., Hess, C. F., Berger, B., . . . Lubgan, D. (2013). A disease-specific enteral nutrition formula improves nutritional status and functional performance in patients with head and neck and esophageal cancer undergoing chemoradiotherapy: Results of a randomized, controlled, multicenter trial. *Cancer, 119*, 3343–3353.

Finocchiaro, C., Segre, O., Fadda, M., Monge, T., Scigliano, M., Schena, M., . . . Canuto, R. A. (2012). Effect of n-3 fatty acids on patients with advanced lunch cancer: A double-blind, placebo-controlled study. *The British Journal of Nutrition, 108*, 327–333.

Ford, E., Bergmann, M., Kröger, J., Schienkiewitz, A., Weikert, C., & Boeing, H. (2009). Healthy living is the best revenge: Findings from the European Prospective Investigation into Cancer and Nutrition-Potsdam study. *Archives of Internal Medicine, 169*, 1355–1362.

Forrester, J., & Sztam, K. (2011). Micronutrients in HIV/AIDS: Is there evidence to change the WHO 2003 recommendations? *American Journal of Clinical Nutrition, 94*(Suppl.), 1683S–1689S.

Fortmann, S., Burda, B., Senger, C., Lin, J. S., & Whitlock, E. P. (2013). Vitamin and mineral supplements in the primary prevention of cardiovascular disease and cancer: An updated systematic evidence review for the U.S. Preventive Services Task Force. *Annals of Internal Medicine, 159*, 824–834.

Freiberg, M., Chang, C. C., Kuller, L., Skanderson, M., Lowy, E., Kraemer, K. L., . . . Justice, A. C. (2013). HIV infection and the risk of acute myocardial infarction. *JAMA Internal Medicine, 173*, 614–622.

Gallicchio, L., Boyd, K., Matanoski, G., Tao, X. G., Chen, L., Lam, T. K., Shiels, M., . . . Alberg, A. J. (2008). Carotenoids and the risk of developing lung cancer: A systematic review. *The American Journal of Clinical Nutrition, 88*, 372–383.

Giacosa, A., Barale, R., Bavaresco, L., Gatenby, P., Gerbi, V., Janssens, J., . . . Rondanelli. (2013). Cancer prevention in Europe: The Mediterranean diet as a protective choice. *European Journal of Cancer Prevention*. doi:10.1097/CEJ.0b013e328354d2d7

Guaraldi, G., Chiara, S., Zona, S., & Bagni, B. (2012). Anthropometry in the assessment of HIV-related lipodystrophy. In V. Preedy (Ed.), *Handbook of anthropometry: Physical measures of human form in health and disease* (pp. 2459–2471). New York, NY: Springer Science and Business Media.

IJpma, I., Renken, R., ter Horst, G., & Reyners, A. K. (2015). Metallic taste in cancer patients treated with chemotherapy. *Cancer Treatment Reviews, 41*, 179–186

Jonnalagadda, S., Harnack, L., Lui, R., McKeown, N., Seal, C., Liu, S., & Fahey, G. C. (2011). Putting the whole grain puzzle together: Health benefits associated with whole grains—summary of American Society for Nutrition 2010 Satellite Symposium. *The Journal of Nutrition, 141*, 1011S–1022S.

Kalichman, S., Washington, C., Grebler, T., Hoyt, G., Welles, B., Kegler, C., . . . Cherry, C. (2015). Medication adherence and health outcomes of people with HIV who are food insecure and prescribed antiretrovirals that should be taken with food. *Infectious Diseases and Therapy*. doi:10.1007/s40121-015-0056-y

Keithley, J., & Swanson, B. (2013). HIV-associated wasting. *The Journal of the Association of Nurses in AIDS Care, 24*(1 Suppl.), S103–S111.

Klein, E. A., Thompson, I. M., Jr., Tangen, C. M., Crowley, J. J., Lucia, M. S., Goodman, P. J., . . . Baker, L. H. (2011). Vitamin E and the risk of prostate cancer: The Selenium and Vitamin E Cancer Prevention Trial (SELECT). *JAMA, 306*, 1549–1556.

Kushi, L., Doyle, C., McCullough, M., Rock, C. L., Demark-Wahnefried, W., Bandera, E. V., . . . Thun, M. (2012). American Cancer Society guidelines on nutrition and physical activity for cancer prevention. *CA: A Cancer Journal for Clinicians, 62*, 30–67.

Lakey, W., Yang, L. Y., Yancy, W., Chow, S. C., & Hicks, C. (2013). Short communication: From wasting to obesity: Initial antiretroviral therapy and weight gain in HIV-infected persons. *AIDS Research and Human Retroviruses, 29*(3). doi:10.1089/aid.2012.0234

Lazzaretti, R., Kuhmmer, R., Sprinz, E., Polanczyk, C. A., & Ribeiro, J. P. (2012). Dietary intervention prevents dyslipidemia associated with highly active antiretroviral therapy in human immunodeficiency virus type 1-infected individuals. *Journal of the American College of Cardiology, 59*, 979–988.

Lin, J., Cook, N., Albert, C., Zaharris, E., Gaziano, J. M., Van Denburgh, M., . . . Manson, J. E. (2009). Vitamins C and E and beta carotene supplementation and cancer risk: A randomized controlled trial. *Journal of the National Cancer Institute, 101*, 14–23.

Manson, J., Bassuk, S., Lee, I., Cook, N. R., Albert, M. A., Gordon, D., . . . Buring, J. E. (2012). The VITamin D and OmegA-3 TriaL (VITAL): Rationale and design of a large randomized controlled trial of vitamin D and marine omega-3 fatty acid supplements for the primary prevention of cancer and cardiovascular disease. *Contemporary Clinical Trials, 33*, 159–171.

McClave, S., Taylor, B., Martindale, R., Warren, M. M., Johnson, D. R., Braunschweig, C., . . . Compher, C. (2016). Guidelines for the provision and assessment of nutrition support therapy in the adult critically ill patients: Society of Critical Care Medicine (SCCM) and American Society for Parenteral and Enteral Nutrition (A.S.P.E.N.). *Journal of Parenteral and Enteral Nutrition, 40,* 159–211.

McCullough, M., Patel, V., Kushi, L., Patel, R., Willett, W. C., Doyle, C., . . . Gapstur, S. M. (2011). Following cancer prevention guidelines reduces risk of cancer, cardiovascular disease, and all-cause mortality. *Cancer Epidemiology, Biomarkers & Prevention, 20,* 1089–1097.

Melchior, J., Salmon, D., Rigaud, D., Leport, C., Bouvet, E., Detruchis, P., . . . Apfelbaum, M. (1991). Resting energy expenditure is increased in stable, malnourished HIV-infected patients. *The American Journal of Clinical Nutrition, 53,* 437–441.

Meyerhardt, J., Niedzwiecki, D., Hollis, D., Saltz, L. B., Hu, F. B., Mayer, R. J., . . . Fuchs, C. S. (2007). Association of dietary patterns with cancer recurrence and survival in patients with stage III colon cancer. *JAMA, 298,* 754–764.

Montaner, J., Lima, V., Harrigan, P., Lourenço, L., Yip, B., Nosyk, B., . . . Kendall, P. (2014). Expansion of HAART coverage is associated with sustained decreases in HIV/AIDS morbidity, mortality and HIV transmission: The "HIV Treatment as Prevention" experience in a Canadian setting. *PLoS One, 9*(2), e87872. doi:10.1371/journal.pone.0087872

Mulligan, K., & Schambelan, M. (2003). *HIV-associated wasting.* Available at http://hivinsite.ucsf.edu/InSite?page=kb-04-01-08. Accessed on 9/6/16.

Murphy, R., Mourtzakis, M., Chu, Q., Baracos, V. E., Reiman, T., & Mazurak, V. C. (2011). Nutritional intervention with fish oil provides a benefit over standard of care for weight and skeletal muscle mass in patients with nonsmall cell lung cancer receiving chemotherapy. *Cancer, 117,* 1775–1782.

Murphy, S., Kochanek, K., Xu, J., & Arias, E. (2015). *Mortality in the United States, 2014* (NCHS Data Brief, No. 229). Hyattsville, MD: National Center for Health Statistics. Available at http://www.cdc.gov/nchs/data/databriefs/db229.pdf. Accessed on 9/2/16.

National Cancer Institute. (2016). *Nutrition in cancer care (PDQ)— health professional version.* Available at http://www.cancer.gov/about-cancer/treatment/side-effects/appetite-loss/nutrition-hp-pdq. Accessed on 9/3/16.

Protani, M., Coory, M., & Martin, J. (2010). Effect of obesity on survival of women with breast cancer: Systematic review and meta-analysis. *Breast Cancer Research and Treatment, 123,* 627–635.

Raiten, D., Mulligan, K., Papathakis, P., & Wanke, C. (2011). Executive summary: Nutritional care of HIV-infected adolescents and adults, including pregnant and lactating women: What do we know, what can we do, and where do we go from here? *American Journal of Clinical Nutrition, 94*(Suppl.), 1667S–1676S.

Reedy, J., Krebs-Smith, S., Miller, P., Liese, A. D., Kahle, L. L., Park, Y., & Subar, A. F. (2014). High diet quality is associated with decreased risk of all-cause, cardiovascular disease, and cancer mortality among older adults. *The Journal of Nutrition, 144,* 881–889.

Robien, K., Denmark-Wahnefried, W., & Rock, C. L. (2011). Evidence-based nutrition guidelines for cancer survivors: Current guidelines, knowledge gaps, and future research directions. *Journal of the American Dietetic Association, 111,* 368–375.

Rock, C., Doyle, C., Denmark-Wahnefried, W., Meyerhardt, J., Courneya, K. S., Schwartz, A. L., . . . Gansler, T. (2012). Nutrition and physical activity guidelines for cancer survivors. *CA: A Cancer Journal for Clinicians, 62,* 232–274.

Rodger, A., Lodwick, R., Schechter, N., Deeks, S., Amin, J., Gilson, R., . . . Phillips, A. (2013). Mortality in well controlled HIV in the continuous antiretroviral therapy arms of the SMART and ESPRIT trials compared with the general population. *AIDS, 27,* 973–979.

Siegel, R., Miller, K., & Jemal, A. (2015). Cancer statistics, 2015. *CA: A Cancer Journal for Clinicians, 65,* 5–29.

Silvers, M., Savva, J., Huggins, C., Truby, H., & Haines, T. (2014). Potential benefits of early nutritional intervention in adults with upper gastrointestinal cancer: A pilot randomized trial. *Supportive Care in Cancer, 22,* 3035–3044.

Tate, T., Willig, A., Willing, J., Raper, J. L, Moneyham, L., Kempf, M. C., . . . Mugavero, M. J. (2012). HIV infection and obesity: Where did all the wasting go? *Antiviral Therapy, 17,* 1281–1289.

Thompson, K., Elliott, L., Fuchs-Tarlovsky, V., Levin, R. M., Voss, A. C., & Piemonte, T. (2016). Oncology evidence-based nutrition practice guidelines for adults. *Journal of the Academy of Nutrition and Dietetics.* Advance online publication. doi:10.1016/j.and.2016.05.010

Thompson-Paul, A., Wei, S., Mattson, C., Robertson, M., Hernandez-Romieu, A. C., Bell, T. K., & Skarbinski, J. (2015). Obesity among HIV-infected adults receiving medical care in the United States: Data from the cross-sectional medical monitoring project and National Health and Nutrition Examination Survey. *Medicine (Baltimore), 94*(27), e1081. doi:10.1098/MD.0000000000001081

Trichopoulou, A., Lagiou, P., Kuper, H., & Tichopoulos, D. (2000). Cancer and Mediterranean dietary traditions. *Cancer Epidemiology, Biomarkers & Prevention, 9,* 869–873.

van der Meij, B., Langius, J., Smit, E., Spreeuwenberg, M. D., von Blomberg, B. M., Heijboer, A. C., . . . van Leeuwen, P. A. (2010). Oral nutritional supplements containing (n-3) polyunsaturated fatty acids affect the nutritional status of patients with stage III non-small cell lung cancer during multimodality treatment. *The Journal of Nutrition, 140,* 1774–1780.

van der Meij, B., Langius, J., Spreeuwenberg, M., Slootmaker, S. M., Paul, M. A., Smit, E. F., & van Leeuwen, P. A. (2012). Oral nutritional supplements containing n-3 polyunsaturated fatty acids affect quality of life and functional status in lung cancer patients during multimodality treatments: An RCT. *European Journal of Clinical Nutrition, 66,* 399–404.

Vigano, A., Watanabe, S., & Bruera, E. (1994). Anorexia and cachexia in advanced cancer patients. *Cancer Surveillance, 21,* 99–115.

Wanke, C., Silva, M., Knox, A., Forrester, J., Speigelman, D., & Gorbach, S. L. (2000). Weight loss and wasting remain common complications in individuals infected with human immunodeficiency virus in the era of high active antiretroviral therapy. *Clinical Infectious Diseases, 31,* 803–805.

Weber, R., Ruppik, M., Richenbach, M., Spoerri, A., Furrer, H., Battegay, M., . . . Ledergerber, B. (2013). Decreasing mortality and changing patterns of causes of death in the Swiss HIV Cohort Study. *HIV Medicine, 14,* 195–207.

Weed, H., Ferguson, M., Gaff, R., Hustead, D. S., Nelson, J. L., & Voss, A. C. (2011). Lean body mass gain in patients with head and neck squamous cell cancer treated perioperatively with a protein- and energy-dense nutritional supplement containing eicosapentaenoic acid. *Head Neck, 33,* 1027–1033.

World Cancer Research Fund/American Institute for Cancer Research. (2011). *Continuous update project report: Food, nutrition, physical activity, and the prevention of colorectal cancer 2011.* Available at http://www.aicr.org/continuous-update-project/reports/Colorectal-Cancer-2011-Report.pdf. Accessed on 12/8/16.

World Health Organization. (2003). *Nutrient requirements for people living with HIV/AIDS: Report of a technical consultation.* Available at www.who.int/nutrition/publications/Content_nutrient_requirements.pdf. Accessed on 9/8/16.

Dietary Reference Intakes (DRIs): Recommended Dietary Allowances and Adequate Intakes, Total Water and Macronutrients

Dietary Reference Intakes (DRIs): Recommended Dietary Allowances and Adequate Intakes, Total Water and Macronutrients. Food and Nutrition Board, Institute of Medicine, National Academies

Life Stage Group	Total Water[a] (L/d)	Carbohydrate (g/d)	Total Fiber (g/d)	Fat (g/d)	Linoleic Acid (g/d)	α-Linolenic Acid (g/d)	Protein[b] (g/d)
Infants							
0–6 mo	0.7*	60*	ND	31*	4.4*	0.5*	9.1*
7–12 mo	0.8*	95*	ND	30*	4.6*	0.5*	11.0+
Children							
1–3 y	1.3*	**130**	19*	ND[c]	7*	0.7*	**13**
4–8 y	1.7*	**130**	25*	ND	10*	0.9*	**19**
Males							
9–13 y	2.4*	**130**	31*	ND	12*	1.2*	**34**
14–18 y	3.3*	**130**	38*	ND	16*	1.6*	**52**
19–30 y	3.7*	**130**	38*	ND	17*	1.6*	**56**
31–50 y	3.7*	**130**	38*	ND	17*	1.6*	**56**
51–70 y	3.7*	**130**	30*	ND	14*	1.6*	**56**
>70 y	3.7*	**130**	30*	ND	14*	1.6*	**56**
Females							
9–13 y	2.1*	**130**	26*	ND	10*	1.0*	**34**
14–18 y	2.3*	**130**	26*	ND	11*	1.1*	**46**
19–30 y	2.7*	**130**	25*	ND	12*	1.1*	**46**
31–50 y	2.7*	**130**	25*	ND	12*	1.1*	**46**
51–70 y	2.7*	**130**	21*	ND	11*	1.1*	**46**
>70 y	2.7*	**130**	21*	ND	11*	1.1*	**46**
Pregnancy							
14–18 y	3.0*	**175**	28*	ND	13*	1.4*	**71**
19–30 y	3.0*	**175**	28*	ND	13*	1.4*	**71**
31–50 y	3.0*	**175**	28*	ND	13*	1.4*	**71**
Lactation							
14–18 y	3.8*	**210**	29*	ND	13*	1.3*	**71**
19–30 y	3.8*	**210**	29*	ND	13*	1.3*	**71**
31–50 y	3.8*	**210**	29*	ND	13*	1.3*	**71**

Note: This table (taken from the DRI reports, see www.nap.edu) presents Recommended Dietary Allowances (RDA) in **bold type** or Adequate Intakes (AI) in ordinary type followed by an asterisk (*). An RDA is the average daily dietary intake level sufficient to meet the nutrient requirements of nearly all (97–98 percent) healthy individuals in a group. It is calculated from an Estimated Average Requirement (EAR). If sufficient scientific evidence is not available to establish an EAR, and thus calculate an RDA, an AI is usually developed. For healthy breastfed infants, the AI is the mean intake. The AI for other life stage and gender groups is believed to cover the needs of all healthy individuals in the group, but lack of data or uncertainty in the data prevent being able to specify with confidence the percentage of individuals covered by this intake.

[a]Total water includes all water contained in food, beverages, and drinking water.
[b]Based on g protein per kg of body weight for the reference body weight, e.g., for adults 0.8 g/kg body weight for the reference body weight.
[c]Not determined.

Sources: *Dietary Reference Intakes for Energy, Carbohydrate, Fiber, Fat, Fatty Acids, Cholesterol, Protein, and Amino Acids* (2002/2005); *Dietary Reference Intakes for Water, Potassium, Sodium, Chloride, and Sulfate* (2005). These reports may be accessed via http://www.nap.edu.
Reprinted with permission from the National Academies Press, Copyright 2005, National Academy of Sciences.

Dietary Reference Intakes (DRIs): Recommended Dietary Allowances and Adequate Intakes, Vitamins

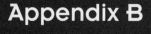

Appendix B begins on page 546.

Dietary Reference Intakes (DRIs): Recommended Dietary Allowances and Adequate Intakes, Elements

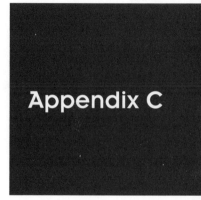

Appendix C is on page 548.

Dietary Reference Intakes (DRIs): Recommended Dietary Allowances and Adequate Intakes, Vitamins. Food and Nutrition Board, Institute of Medicine, National Academies

Life Stage Group	Vitamin A (μg/d)[a]	Vitamin C (mg/d)	Vitamin D (μg/d)[b,c]	Vitamin E (mg/d)[d]	Vitamin K (μg/d)	Thiamin (mg/d)
Infants						
0–6 mo	400*	40*	10*	4*	2.0*	0.2*
7–12 mo	500*	50*	10*	5*	2.5*	0.3*
Children						
1–3 y	**300**	**15**	**15**	**6**	30*	**0.5**
4–8 y	**400**	**25**	**15**	**7**	55*	**0.6**
Males						
9–13 y	**600**	**45**	**15**	**11**	60*	**0.9**
14–18 y	**900**	**75**	**15**	**15**	75*	**1.2**
19–30 y	**900**	**90**	**15**	**15**	120*	**1.2**
31–50 y	**900**	**90**	**15**	**15**	120*	**1.2**
51–70 y	**900**	**90**	**15**	**15**	120*	**1.2**
>70 y	**900**	**90**	**20**	**15**	120*	**1.2**
Females						
9–13 y	**600**	**45**	**15**	**11**	60*	**0.9**
14–18 y	**700**	**65**	**15**	**15**	75*	**1.0**
19–30 y	**700**	**75**	**15**	**15**	90*	**1.1**
31–50 y	**700**	**75**	**15**	**15**	90*	**1.1**
51–70 y	**700**	**75**	**15**	**15**	90*	**1.1**
>70 y	**700**	**75**	**20**	**15**	90*	**1.1**
Pregnancy						
14–18 y	**750**	**80**	**15**	**15**	75*	**1.4**
19–30 y	**770**	**85**	**15**	**15**	90*	**1.4**
31–50 y	**770**	**85**	**15**	**15**	90*	**1.4**
Lactation						
14–18 y	**1200**	**115**	**15**	**19**	75*	**1.4**
19–30 y	**1300**	**120**	**15**	**19**	90*	**1.4**
31–50 y	**1300**	**120**	**15**	**19**	90*	**1.4**

Note: This table (taken from the DRI reports, see www.nap.edu) presents Recommended Dietary Allowances (RDA) in **bold type** or Adequate Intakes (AI) in ordinary type followed by an asterisk (*). An RDA is the average daily dietary intake level sufficient to meet the nutrient requirements of nearly all (97–98 percent) healthy individuals in a group. It is calculated from an Estimated Average Requirement (EAR). If sufficient scientific evidence is not available to establish an EAR, and thus calculate an RDA, an AI is usually developed. For healthy breastfed infants, the AI is the mean intake. The AI for other life stage and gender groups is believed to cover the needs of all healthy individuals in the group, but lack of data or uncertainty in the data prevent being able to specify with confidence the percentage of individuals covered by this intake.

[a] As retinol activity equivalents (RAEs). 1 RAE = 1 μg retinol, 12 μg β-carotene, 24 μg α-carotene, or 24 μg β-cryptoxanthin. The RAE for dietary provitamin A carotenoids is two-fold greater than retinol equivalents (REs), whereas the RAE for preformed vitamin A is the same as RE.

[b] As cholecalciferol. 1 μg cholecalciferol = 40 IU vitamin D.

[c] In the absence of adequate exposure to sunlight.

[d] As α-tocopherol. α-Tocopherol includes *RRR*-α-tocopherol, the only form of α-tocopherol that occurs naturally in foods, and the *2R*-stereoisomeric forms of α-tocopherol (*RRR*-, *RSR*-, *RRS*-, and *RSS*-α-tocopherol) that occur in fortified foods and supplements. It does not include the *2S*-stereoisomeric forms of α-tocopherol (*SRR*-, *SSR*-, *SRS*-, and *SSS*-α-tocopherol), also found in fortified foods and supplements.

[e] As niacin equivalents (NE). 1 mg of niacin = 60 mg of tryptophan; 0–6 months = preformed niacin (not NE).

[f] As dietary folate equivalents (DFE). 1 DFE = 1 μg food folate = 0.6 μg of folic acid from fortified food or as a supplement consumed with food = 0.5 μg of a supplement taken on an empty stomach.

Riboflavin (mg/d)	Niacin (mg/d)[e]	Vitamin B$_6$ (mg/d)	Folate (µg/d)[f]	Vitamin B$_{12}$ (µg/d)	Pantothenic Acid (mg/d)	Biotin (µg/d)	Choline (mg/d)[g]
0.3*	2*	0.1*	65*	0.4*	1.7*	5*	125*
0.4*	4*	0.3*	80*	0.5*	1.8*	6*	150*
0.5	6	0.5	150	0.9	2*	8*	200*
0.6	8	0.6	200	1.2	3*	12*	250*
0.9	12	1.0	300	1.8	4*	20*	375*
1.3	16	1.3	400	2.4	5*	25*	550*
1.3	16	1.3	400	2.4	5*	30*	550*
1.3	16	1.3	400	2.4	5*	30*	550*
1.3	16	1.7	400	2.4[h]	5*	30*	550*
1.3	16	1.7	400	2.4[h]	5*	30*	550*
0.9	12	1.0	300	1.8	4*	20*	375*
1.0	14	1.2	400[i]	2.4	5*	25*	400*
1.1	14	1.3	400[i]	2.4	5*	30*	425*
1.1	14	1.3	400[i]	2.4	5*	30*	425*
1.1	14	1.5	400	2.4[h]	5*	30*	425*
1.1	14	1.5	400	2.4[h]	5*	30*	425*
1.4	18	1.9	600[j]	2.6	6*	30*	450*
1.4	18	1.9	600[j]	2.6	6*	30*	450*
1.4	18	1.9	600[j]	2.6	6*	30*	450*
1.6	17	2.0	500	2.8	7*	35*	550*
1.6	17	2.0	500	2.8	7*	35*	550*
1.6	17	2.0	500	2.8	7*	35*	550*

[g]Although AIs have been set for choline, there are few data to assess whether a dietary supply of choline is needed at all stages of the life cycle, and it may be that the choline requirement can be met by endogenous synthesis at some of these stages.

[h]Because 10 to 30 percent of older people may malabsorb food-bound B$_{12}$, it is advisable for those older than 50 years to meet their RDA mainly by consuming foods fortified with B$_{12}$ or a supplement containing B$_{12}$.

[i]In view of evidence linking folate intake with neural tube defects in the fetus, it is recommended that all women capable of becoming pregnant consume 400 µg from supplements or fortified foods in addition to intake of food folate from a varied diet.

[j]It is assumed that women will continue consuming 400 µg from supplements or fortified food until their pregnancy is confirmed and they enter prenatal care, which ordinarily occurs after the end of the periconceptional period—the critical time for formation of the neural tube.

Sources: *Dietary Reference Intakes for Calcium, Phosphorous, Magnesium, Vitamin D, and Fluoride* (1997); *Dietary Reference Intakes for Thiamin, Riboflavin, Niacin, Vitamin B6, Folate, Vitamin B12, Pantothenic Acid, Biotin, and Choline* (1998); *Dietary Reference Intakes for Vitamin C, Vitamin E, Selenium, and Carotenoids* (2000); *Dietary Reference Intakes for Vitamin A, Vitamin K, Arsenic, Boron, Chromium, Copper, Iodine, Iron, Manganese, Molybdenum, Nickel, Silicon, Vanadium, and Zinc* (2001); *Dietary Reference Intakes for Water, Potassium, Sodium, Chloride, and Sulfate* (2005); and *Dietary Reference Intakes for Calcium and Vitamin D* (2011). These reports may be accessed via http://www.nap.edu.

Dietary Reference Intakes (DRIs): Recommended Dietary Allowances and Adequate Intakes, Elements. Food and Nutrition Board, Institute of Medicine, National Academies

Life Stage Group	Calcium (mg/d)	Chromium (µg/d)	Copper (µg/d)	Fluoride (mg/d)	Iodine (µg/d)	Iron (mg/d)	Magnesium (mg/d)	Manganese (mg/d)	Molybdenum (µg/d)	Phosphorus (mg/d)	Selenium (µg/d)	Zinc (mg/d)	Potassium (g/d)	Sodium (g/d)	Chloride (g/d)
Infants															
0–6 mo	200*	0.2*	200*	0.01*	110*	0.27*	30*	0.003*	2*	100*	15*	2*	0.4*	0.12*	0.18*
7–12 mo	260*	5.5*	220*	0.5*	130*	11	75*	0.6*	3*	275*	20*	3	0.7*	0.37*	0.57*
Children															
1–3 y	700	11*	340	0.7*	90	7	80	1.2*	17	460	20	3	3.0*	1.0*	1.5*
4–8 y	1000	15*	440	1*	90	10	130	1.5*	22	500	30	5	3.8*	1.2*	1.9*
Males															
9–13 y	1300	25*	700	2*	120	8	240	1.9*	34	1250	40	8	4.5*	1.5*	2.3*
14–18 y	1300	35*	890	3*	150	11	410	2.2*	43	1250	55	11	4.7*	1.5*	2.3*
19–30 y	1000	35*	900	4*	150	8	400	2.3*	45	700	55	11	4.7*	1.5*	2.3*
31–50 y	1000	35*	900	4*	150	8	420	2.3*	45	700	55	11	4.7*	1.5*	2.3*
51–70 y	1000	30*	900	4*	150	8	420	2.3*	45	700	55	11	4.7*	1.3*	2.0*
>70 y	1200	30*	900	4*	150	8	420	2.3*	45	700	55	11	4.7*	1.2*	1.8*
Females															
9–13 y	1300	21*	700	2*	120	8	240	1.6*	34	1250	40	8	4.5*	1.5*	2.3*
14–18 y	1300	24*	890	3*	150	15	360	1.6*	43	1250	55	9	4.7*	1.5*	2.3*
19–30 y	1000	25*	900	3*	150	18	310	1.8*	45	700	55	8	4.7*	1.5*	2.3*
31–50 y	1000	25*	900	3*	150	18	320	1.8*	45	700	55	8	4.7*	1.5*	2.3*
51–70 y	1200	20*	900	3*	150	8	320	1.8*	45	700	55	8	4.7*	1.3*	2.0*
>70 y	1200	20*	900	3*	150	8	320	1.8*	45	700	55	8	4.7*	1.2*	1.8*
Pregnancy															
14–18 y	1300	29*	1000	3*	220	27	400	2.0*	50	1250	60	12	4.7*	1.5*	2.3*
19–30 y	1000	30*	1000	3*	220	27	350	2.0*	50	700	60	11	4.7*	1.5*	2.3*
31–50 y	1000	30*	1000	3*	220	27	360	2.0*	50	700	60	11	4.7*	1.5*	2.3*
Lactation															
14–18 y	1300	44*	1300	3*	290	10	360	2.6*	50	1250	70	13	5.1*	1.5*	2.3*
19–30 y	1000	45*	1300	3*	290	9	310	2.6*	50	700	70	12	5.1*	1.5*	2.3*
31–50 y	1000	45*	1300	3*	290	9	320	2.6*	50	700	70	12	5.1*	1.5*	2.3*

Note: This table (taken from the DRI reports, see www.nap.edu) presents Recommended Dietary Allowances (RDA) in **bold type** or Adequate Intakes (AI) in ordinary type followed by an asterisk (*). An RDA is the average daily dietary intake level sufficient to meet the nutrient requirements of nearly all (97–98 percent) healthy individuals in a group. It is calculated from an Estimated Average Requirement (EAR). If sufficient scientific evidence is not available to establish an EAR, and thus calculate an RDA, an AI is usually developed. For healthy breastfed infants, the AI is the mean intake. The AI for other life stage and gender groups is believed to cover the needs of all healthy individuals in the group, but lack of data or uncertainty in the data prevent being able to specify with confidence the percentage of individuals covered by this intake.

Sources: *Dietary Reference Intakes for Calcium, Phosphorous, Magnesium, Vitamin D, and Fluoride* (1997); *Dietary Reference Intakes for Thiamin, Riboflavin, Niacin, Vitamin B6, Folate, Vitamin B12, Pantothenic Acid, Biotin, and Choline* (1998); *Dietary Reference Intakes for Vitamin C, Vitamin E, Selenium, and Carotenoids* (2000); *Dietary Reference Intakes for Vitamin A, Vitamin K, Arsenic, Boron, Chromium, Copper, Iodine, Iron, Manganese, Molybdenum, Nickel, Silicon, Vanadium, and Zinc* (2001); *Dietary Reference Intakes for Water, Potassium, Sodium, Chloride, and Sulfate* (2005); and *Dietary Reference Intakes for Calcium and Vitamin D* (2011). These reports may be accessed via http://www.nap.edu. Reprinted with permission from the National Academies Press, Copyright 2011, National Academy of Sciences.

Answers to Study Questions

Chapter 1
1. a
2. b
3. c
4. b
5. a

Chapter 2
1. c
2. a
3. b
4. d
5. c
6. a
7. c
8. d

Chapter 3
1. a
2. b
3. d
4. d
5. c
6. a
7. c
8. a

Chapter 4
1. b
2. d
3. b
4. b
5. a
6. c
7. d
8. a

Chapter 5
1. b
2. c
3. c
4. c
5. d
6. b
7. c
8. a

Chapter 6
1. b
2. a
3. c
4. b
5. c
6. a
7. d
8. c

Chapter 7
1. c
2. b
3. c
4. b
5. c
6. b
7. a
8. b

Chapter 8
1. a
2. c
3. c
4. a
5. c
6. a
7. a
8. b

Chapter 9
1. b
2. c
3. c
4. d
5. a, c, d
6. c
7. a
8. a

Chapter 10
1. b
2. c
3. b
4. a, d, e
5. a, b, d, e
6. d
7. b
8. a

Chapter 11
1. b
2. a
3. d
4. c
5. b
6. a
7. a
8. c

Chapter 12
1. d
2. a
3. b
4. b
5. a, b, c
6. c
7. a
8. d

Chapter 13

1. d
2. c
3. a
4. b
5. b
6. a, b, c, d, e
7. a
8. a, c, d, e

Chapter 14

1. b, c, d
2. d
3. c
4. a
5. b
6. a, b, c, d, e
7. a, b
8. c

Chapter 15

1. b
2. b
3. a
4. b, c, d
5. b
6. a
7. c
8. b

Chapter 16

1. b
2. c
3. d
4. c
5. c
6. c
7. d
8. b

Chapter 17

1. a
2. a
3. c
4. b
5. b
6. b
7. d
8. d

Chapter 18

1. a
2. a
3. b
4. b
5. b
6. a
7. a
8. b

Chapter 19

1. c
2. d
3. d
4. d
5. a
6. b
7. c
8. a, b, c

Chapter 20

1. b
2. c
3. a
4. a
5. d
6. d
7. c
8. c

Chapter 21

1. a
2. d
3. c
4. c
5. a
6. a
7. b
8. c

Chapter 22

1. d
2. d
3. c
4. a
5. a
6. b
7. d
8. a

Note: Page numbers followed by *b* indicate a box; those followed by *f,* an illustration; and those followed by *t,* a table.